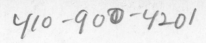

410-900-4201

"The review modules are so helpful because they give me bulleted highlights and concise, nursing information... To top it off, you also get critical thinking exercises! These books are fantastic! They have undoubtedly been the greatest review item I have found."

Kimberly Montgomery
Nursing student

Terim Richards *Nursing student*

"I immediately went to my nurse manager after I failed the NCLEX® and she referred me to ATI. I was able to discover the areas I was weak in, and focused on those areas in the review modules and online assessments. I was much more prepared the second time around!"

Molly Obetz *Nursing student*

"The ATI review books were very helpful in preparing me for the NCLEX®. I really utilized the review summaries and the critical thinking exercises at the end of each chapter. It was nice to review the key points in the areas I was weak in and not have to read the entire book."

Lindsey Koeble *Nursing student*

"I attribute my success totally to ATI. That is the one thing I used between my first and second attempt at the NCLEX®....with ATI I passed!"

Danielle Platt *Nurse Manager • Children's Mercy Hospital • Kansas City, MO*

"The year our hospital did not use the ATI program, we experienced a 15% decrease in the NCLEX® pass rates. We reinstated the ATI program the following year and had a 90% success rate."

"As a manager, I have witnessed graduate nurses fail the NCLEX® and the devastating effects it has on their morale. Once the nurses started using ATI, it was amazing to see the confidence they had in themselves and their ability to go forward and take the NCLEX® exam."

Mary Moss *Associate Dean of Nursing and Health Programs • Mid-State Technical College • Rapids, WI*

"I like that ATI lets students know what to expect from the NCLEX®, helps them plan their study time and tells them what to do in the days and weeks before the exam. It is different from most of the NCLEX® review books on the market."

Contributors

Renee Cantwell, RN, RN, CPHQ, MSN

Education Specialist/Clinical Educator
Cooper Health System
Camden, NJ

Penny S. Cass, RN, PhD

Dean, Division of Nursing
Indiana University
Kokomo, Indiana

Karen DeLeersnyder, RN, BBA

Shawnee Mission Medical Center
Shawnee, Kansas

Bonnie Gantos RN, BSN

Diabetes Educator
Saint Luke's South
Overland Park, Kansas

Susan Simmons Holcomb, PhD, ARNP, BC

Family Nurse Practitioner
Olathe Medical Services, Inc.
Kansas City Kansas Community College
Kansas City, Kansas

Tanya Longaback, RN, BSN

Shawnee Mission Medical Center
Shawnee, Kansas

Gayla H. Love, BSN, RN, CCM

Nurse Educator
Griffin Technical College
Griffin, Georgia

Teresa Y. McPherson, RN, BSN

U.S. Army
Fort Sam Houston, Texas

Kathleen Ohman, RN, CCRN, EdD

Professor of Nursing
College of St. Benedict
St. Joseph, MN

Carol Green Nigro, RN, PhD

Professor of Nursing
Johnson County Community College
Overland Park, Kansas
Textbook Author

Joan Luckmann, RN, MA

Seattle, Washington
Textbook Author

Marcia Reese, RN, BSN

Saint Joseph Medical Center
Kansas City, Missouri

Nancy Schlapman, RN, PhD, MSN, BSN

Coordinator of Baccalaureate and Higher Degree Programs
Indiana University
Kokomo, Indiana

Barbara Kuhn Timby, RNC, MS

Nursing Professor
Glen Oaks Community College
Centerville, Michigan
Textbook Author

Editor-in-Chief

Leslie Schaaf Treas, RN, PhD(c), MSN, CNNP

Director of Research and Development
Assessment Technologies Institute™, LLC
Overland Park, Kansas

Managing Editor

Jim Hauschildt, RN, EdD, MA

Director of Product Development
Assessment Technologies Institute™, LLC
Overland Park, Kansas

Sixth Edition Copyright© 2005 by Assessment Technologies Institute™, LLC. Previous editions copyrighted 1999-2004.

Copyright Notice

Important Notice to the Reader of this Publication

Introduction to Assessment–Driven Review

To prepare candidates for the licensure exam, many different methods have been used. Assessment Technologies Institute™, LLC, (ATI) offers Assessment–Driven Review™ (ADR), a newer approach for customized board review based on candidate performance on a series of content-based assessments.

The ADR method is a four-part process that serves as a type of competency-assessment for preparation for the NCLEX®. The goal is to increase preparedness and subsequent pass rate on the licensure exam. Used as a comprehensive program, the ADR is designed to help learners focus their review and remediation efforts, thereby increasing their confidence and familiarity with the NCLEX® content. This type of program identifies learners at risk for failure in the early stages of nursing education and provides a path for prescriptive learning prior to the licensure examination.

The ADR approach may be preferable to a traditional "crash course" style of review for a variety of reasons. Time restriction is a fundamental barrier to comprehensive review. Because of the difficulty in keeping up with the expansiveness of information available today, a more efficient and directed approach is needed. Individualized review that starts with the areas of deficit helps the learner narrow the focus and begin customized remediation instead of a blanket A-to-Z approach. Additionally, review that occurs sequentially over time may be preferable to after-the-fact efforts after completion of a program when faculty are no longer available to assist with remediation.

Early identification of content weaknesses may prove advantageous to progressive program success. "Smaller bites" for content achievement and a shortened lapse of time between the introduction of course content and remediation efforts is likely to be more effective in catching the struggling learner before it is too late. Regular feedback keeps learners "on track" and reduce attrition rate by identifying the learner who is "slipping." This approach provides the opportunity to tutor or implement intensified instruction before the learner reaches a point of no return and drops out of the program.

Step I: Proctored Assessment

The ADR program is a method using a prescriptive learning strategy that begins with a proctored, diagnostic assessment of the learner's mastery of nursing content. The topics covered within the ADR program are based on the current NCLEX® Test Plan. Proctored assessments are administered in paper-pencil and online formats. Scores are reported instantly with Internet testing or within 24 hours for paper-pencil testing. Individual performance profiles list areas of deficiencies and guide the learner's review and remediation of the missed topics. This road map serves as a starting point for self-directed study for NCLEX® success. Learners receive a cumulative Report Card showing scores from all assessments taken throughout the program—beginning to end. Like reading a transcript, the learner and educator can monitor the sequential progress, step-by-step, an assessment at a time.

Step II: Modular Reviews

A good test is one that supports teaching and learning. The score report identifies areas of content mastery as well as a means for correction and improvement of weak content areas. Eight review modules contain concise summaries of topics with a clinical overview, therapeutic nursing management, and client teaching. Key concepts are provided to streamline the study process. The ATI modules are not intended to serve as a primary teaching source. Instead, they are designed to summarize the material relevant to the licensure exam and entry-level practice.

Learners are taught to integrate holistic care with a critical thinking approach into the review material to promote clinical application of course content. The learner constructs responses to open-ended questions to stimulate higher-order thinking. The learner may provide rationales for actions in various clinical scenarios and generate explanations of why the solution may be effective in similar clinical situations. These exercises serve as the venue to shift from traditional didactic memorization of facts toward the use of analytical and evaluative reason in a client-related situation. The clinical application scenarios involve the learner actively in the problem-solving process and stimulate an attitude of inquiry.

These exercises are designed to provoke creative problem solving for the individual learner as well as collaborative dialogue for groups of learners in the classroom. Through group discussion, learners discover the technique of elaboration. Learners use group dialogue to increase their understanding of nursing content. In study groups, they may pose questions to their peers or explain various topics in their own words, adding personal experiences with clients and examples from previously acquired knowledge of the topic. Together they learn to reframe problems and assemble evidence to support conclusions. Through the integration of multiple perspectives and the synergy involved in the exchange of ideas, this approach may also facilitate the development of effective working relationships and patterns for lifelong learning. Critical thinking exercises for each topic area situate instruction into a problem-solving environment that can capture learners' attention, increase motivation to learn, and frame the content into an application context. Additionally, the group involvement can model the process for effective team interaction.

Step III: Non-Proctored Assessments

The third step is the use of online assessments that allow users to test from any site with an Internet connection. This online battery identifies specific areas of content weakness for further directed study. The interactive style provides the learner with immediate feedback on all response options. Rationales provide additional information about the correctness of an answer to supplement learners' understanding of the concept. Detailed explanations are provided for each incorrect response to clarify topics that learners often confuse, misunderstand, or fail to remember. Readiness to learn is often peaked when errors are uncovered; thus, immediate feedback is provided when learners are most motivated to find the answer. A Performance Profile summarizes learners' mastery of content. Question descriptors for each missed item are used to stimulate inquiry and further exploration of the topic. The online assessment is intended to extend the learners' preparation for NCLEX® in a way that is personally suited to their deficiencies.

Step IV: ATI-PLAN™ DVD Series

This multi-disk set contains more than 28 hours of nursing review material. The DVD content is designed to complement ATI's Content Mastery Series™ review modules and online assessments. Using the ATI-PLAN™ navigational points, learners can easily find the content areas they want to review.

Recognizing that individuals process information in a variety of ways, ATI developed the ATI-PLAN™ DVD series to offer nursing review in a way that simulates the classroom. However, individuals viewing the ATI-PLAN™ DVDs can navigate through more than 28 hours of material to their topics of choice. Nursing review is available at the convenience of the learner and can be replayed as often as necessary to ensure mastery of content.

The regulation of personal learning goals and the ability to plan and pursue academic intentions are the keys to successful learning. The expert teacher is the one who can determine individual learning needs and appropriate strategies to master learning. The ADR program is an efficient method of helping students prepare for the nursing licensure exam using frequent and systematic content review directed by the identified areas of content weakness. The interactive approach for mastery of nursing content focused in the areas of greatest need is likely to increase student success on the licensure exam.

ATI's ADR method parallels the nursing process in concept and in design. Both provide a framework for solving actual and potential problems purposefully and methodically. Assessment ADR-style is accomplished with ATI's battery of proctored assessments. Diagnosis is facilitated by the individual and group score reports the proctored assessments generate. Planning for improving performance in identified areas of weakness incorporates ATI's modular review system. Implementation begins with modular review and culminates in use of ATI's online assessments to validate improvement. Evaluation is reflected in the score reports, and performance can then be strengthened or further improved with the ATI-PLAN™ DVD series. Just like the nursing process, ATI's ADR prescriptive learning method often leads to specific, measurable results and highly desirable outcomes.

Table of Contents

Nursing Management of the Client with Burns

Key Points

- In the United States, 45,000 to 60,000 burned clients are hospitalized annually.
- Up to 7,000 deaths are attributed to burns yearly.
- Very young and elderly clients are most at risk for burn injuries.
- Death rates from burns are much higher among clients from rural and lower-income urban areas.
- Burns are caused by thermal, chemical, electrical and radioactive agents.
- Burns may be superficial-thickness (first-degree burn), partial thickness (second-degree burn), full thickness (third-degree burn) and deep full thickness (fourth-degree burn). Burns are also classified as minor, moderate and major.
- Clients should be transported to the nearest emergency department or to a specialized burn center if the client is pediatric or geriatric. Other conditions whereby specialized burn care is necessary include:
  - Burns that involve the eyes, ears, face, hands, feet or perineum
  - Electrical injuries
  - Inhalation injury
  - Complicated concomitant injuries
  - Cardiac, pulmonary, renal or other chronic metabolic disorders
- Goals of collaborative management:
  - Maintain airway breathing, circulation, and fluid balance.
  - Prevent infection.
  - Support nutrition and healing.
  - Relieve pain.
  - Prevent disability.
  - Prevent complications such as contractures and severe scarring.
  - Prevent anxiety, fear, and depression.
  - Promote feelings of self-worth.
- Important nursing diagnoses (actual or potential):
  - Acute pain
  - Infection
  - Ineffective airway clearance
  - Impaired gas exchange
  - Anxiety and fear
  - Disuse syndrome

- Fluid volume deficit
- Ineffective tissue perfusion
- Decreased cardiac output
- Ineffective breathing pattern
- Altered body image
- Altered self-esteem
- Impaired physical mobility
- Altered nutrition
- Ineffective individual coping
- Dysfunctional grieving
- **Key Terms/Concepts:** Rule of Nines, third spacing fluid shift, Lund-Browder chart, eschar, debridement, escharotomy, fasciotomy, pressure dressings

Overview

Burns are caused by thermal, chemical, electrical, and radioactive agents. Burns result in cellular destruction of the skin layers and subsequent depletion of fluid and electrolytes; loss of temperature regulation; loss of sweat and sebaceous glands; loss of protection to cells, tissues and organs; loss of sensory function; and an altered body image. The extent of the burn is dependent on the type of burning agent, duration of contact, and site of the injury.

Risk Factors

- Exposure to flames, hot liquids, or radiation
- Inhalation or ingestion of acids, alkalosis, or other chemicals
- Contact with electrical current
- Age (children, older adults)
- Sensory deficits
- Smoking
- Lack of smoke detectors in home
- Lack of fire extinguishers in the home
- Poor maintenance of fireplace and wood burning stoves
- Lack of caution when using candles or space heaters

Clinical Manifestations

- **Superficial-thickness:** First-degree burn involving epidermis. Mild to severe erythema, pain, and tenderness eased with cooling; skin blanches with pressure; healing generally occurs within seven days.
- **Partial-thickness:** Second-degree burn involving epidermis and dermis. Large blister formation; edema, pain, and sensitivity to cold air; reddened base with broken, shiny, weeping surface; healing generally occurs within 21 days for superficial partial thickness burns and within 28 days for deep burns; grafting may be required.

- **Full-thickness**: Third-degree burn involving entire dermis and portions of subcutaneous tissue. Dry appearance; deep red, black, brown, or white area with fat exposure; edema; little pain; spontaneous healing will not occur. A dark leather-like covering called eschar will form over the burn area which must be removed. Grafting is required for these burns.
- **Deep full-thickness**: Fourth-degree burn involving injury to muscle and bone. Black, edematous lesion, no pain or blisters, spontaneous healing will not occur, grafting required. If a limb is involved, amputation may be inevitable.
- **Minor burns**: Involves either:
  - Less than 15% of the TBSA (total body surface area) not involving face, hands, feet, or genitalia, or
  - Full-thickness burns that are less than 2% of the TBSA.
- **Moderate burns**: Involves either:
  - Less than or equal to 15% - 25% of the TBSA, or
  - Full-thickness burns that are less than 10% of the TBSA.
- **Major burns**: Involves either:
  - Partial thickness injuries greater than 25% of the TBSA, or
  - Full-thickness injuries involving greater than 10% of the TBSA or face, hands, feet, or genitalia.

Diagnostic and Laboratory Tests

- History and physical exam
- Estimate the extent of burn injury using either the Rule of Nines or the Lund-Browder chart
- Complete blood count (CBC)
- Serum electrolytes
- Blood urea nitrogen (BUN)
- Fasting blood glucose (FBG)—also called: fasting blood sugar (FBS)
- Arterial blood gases (ABGs)
- Pulse oximetry
- Chest x-ray
- Bronchoscopy
- Pulmonary function tests:
  - Air flow (spirometer)
  - Lung volume
  - Diffusion capacity (correlates with body's ability to extract oxygen from the lungs)
  - Electrocardiogram (ECG)
- Urinalysis
- Liver enzyme tests
- Clotting studies

Therapeutic Nursing Management

- Emergency treatment of major burns
  - Shut off electric source.
  - Remove victim from source of burn.
  - Remove items that could continue to burn the client (metal, jewelry, clothing contaminated with chemicals).
  - Assess airway, breathing, and circulation (CPR).
  - Assess for respiratory distress and prepare to intubate if necessary.
  - Maintain body heat and prevent exposure.
  - Cover burned area with sterile or clean cloth.
  - Assess for hypovolemia (decreased BP, increased heart rate and respirations).
  - Monitor ABGs (arterial blood gases) and carboxyhemoglobin levels.
  - Initiate intravenous access.
  - Monitor vital signs.
  - Maintain NPO status.
  - Insert indwelling urinary catheter.
  - Administer pain medication as prescribed.
  - Administer tetanus toxoid as prescribed.
  - Estimate the extent of burn injury using either the Rule of Nines or the Lund-Browder chart.
  - Implement infection control measures/universal precautions.
- Emergency treatment of minor burns
  - Stop burning process (removal from source, application of cool cloth).
  - Administer pain medication as ordered.
  - Administer wound care (cleaning, removing damaging agents, application of antimicrobial medications, sterile dressing).
  - Administer tetanus toxoid as prescribed.
  - Teach client regarding follow-up care.

Hospital Care

- **Prevent:**
  - Prevent shock and it's complications
  - Joint deformity by proper positioning
  - Fluid volume deficit due to third spacing in adjacent tissues
  - Inadequate nutrition due to fluid shifts, tissue damage and hypermetabolic state
  - Wound infection
  - Pain
- **Assess/Monitor:**
  - Laboratory data:
    - Serum electrolytes

- Blood glucose
- Hematocrit
- Hemoglobin
- Blood urea nitrogen (BUN)
- Blood gas
- Protein/albumin
- Fluid balance
- Hypovolemic shock (for 72 hours after the burn)
- Arterial blood gases (ABGs) and carboxyhemoglobin levels
- Signs and symptoms of infection
- Pain control
- Altered self-image, powerlessness, depression, guilt, and anxiety
- **Nursing Activities:**
- Plan course of action based on the severity and extent of client's burns.
- Administer electrolyte replacement as prescribed.
- Implement infection control measures.
- Provide wound care and dressing changes, maintaining sterile technique as prescribed.
- Assess client and immediately report any signs of wound infection.
- Use pressure dressings to prevent edema and scarring.
- Replace fluids as prescribed.
- Provide pain control as prescribed.
- Provide pain medications prior to dressing changes, wound care, and activities that require painful movements.
- Maintain adequate nutrition or hyperalimentation (tube feeding may be necessary with severe burns due to hypermetabolism), airway management and impaired digestion/peristalsis.
- Consult with a dietician to determine client's caloric and protein requirements.
- Encourage the client to order favorite foods that are nutritious.
- Assist the client with eating if injuries impair the client's ability to feed self.
- Assist the client with passive-range-of-motion exercises to prevent contractures and increase mobility.
- Position the client in a neutral body position with minimum flexion to help prevent contractures.
- Use splints if necessary to help client maintain correct positioning. Splints are applied most frequently for the joints of the hands, elbows, knees, neck or ankles.
- Consult with physical therapy and occupational therapy departments to develop an individualized rehabilitation program.
- Assist client for early ambulation to prevent contractures and complications of immobility.
- Obtain assistive devices that will help client to feed and care for self.
- Provide emotional support and encouragement.

- Facilitate consultations with social workers, psychologists, and psychiatrists as necessary
- Arrange for client to meet other clients who have successfully recovered from burn injuries, as in support group.
- Prepare client for escharotomy which is a lengthwise incision made through burn eschar to relieve constriction and improve circulation.
- Prepare client for fasciotomy (incision that extends through the subcutaneous tissue and fascia) if escharotomy has not resulted in adequate tissue perfusion.
- Prepare client for debridement, such as whirlpool for soaking burn injury.

Pharmacology

- Analgesics: morphine sulfate (MSO_4) meperidine: (Demerol)
- Anesthetic agents such as ketamine (Ketalar), pentobarbital sodium (Nembutal), and nitrous oxide for pain reduction.
- Antibiotics (topical and/or systemic)
- Topical antimicrobial agent: silver sulfadiazine (Silvadene), mafenide acetate (Sulfamylon), silver nitrate, triple antibiotic, Bacitracin
- Tetanus prophylaxis: tetanus toxoid
- Enteral or parenteral feedings, that are high in protein to provide a positive nitrogen balance
- Intravenous fluids: Ringer's lactate, normal saline, colloids, and glucose in water
- Electrolytes to correct imbalances
- Topical enzyme debridement: collagenase (Santylo)
- Antiulcerative: ranitidine (Zantac) or other histamine blockers
- Nutritional supplements: multivitamins; zinc, folate, iron

Complications

- Infection, sepsis, disseminated intravascular coagulation (DIC)
- Shock
- Fluid shift called third spacing
- Electrolyte imbalance – sudden shifts in serum potassium levels are especially dangerous due to potential for life threatening cardiac arrhythmias.
- Pneumonia, adult/acute respiratory distress syndrome (ARDS)
- Anemia
- Negative nitrogen balance
- Curling's ulcer (an acute peptic ulcer that sometimes complicates severe burns)
- Disuse syndrome due to burn healing and scarring
- Depression and disturbed body image
- Posttraumatic stress syndrome or disorder (PTSS/PTSD)
- Death
- Renal failure

Age-Related Changes—Gerontological Considerations

- The skin of older clients is thinner and more easily damaged than the skin of younger people, and thus elderly clients are more at risk for extensive burn injuries.
- Elderly clients are at increased risk for development of fluid and electrolyte imbalance and infection is due to the physiological changes that occur with aging.
- Elderly clients may not heal rapidly due to reduced immune function and malnutrition.
- Older clients are at greater risk for complications from burns due to a higher incidence of chronic illnesses, such as cardiovascular diseases and diabetes, which cause decreased circulation, altered tissue perfusion and loss of immune integrity.

Critical Thinking Exercise: Nursing Management of the Client with Burns

Situation: A 42-year-old man is brought into the emergency department following a fire that destroyed the warehouse where he was working. Initial assessment reveals extensive burns covering the majority of his anterior arms, face, and anterior thorax. His burns are a mixture of intact and open blisters with reddened bases and shiny, weeping surfaces. He is awake and alert and complaining of extensive pain and sensitivity to cold air. He has singed nasal hairs, eyebrows, and eyelids; and is hoarse with a brassy cough.

1. Estimate the man's percentage of burns using the Rule of Nines.

2. Which three assessments are of greatest importance during the man's initial care?

_____ Serum electrolytes

_____ Airway

_____ Signs of infection

_____ Body image

_____ Vital signs

_____ Blood glucose

3. Which assessment findings indicate that man may have sustained an inhalation injury?

_____ Frothy urine

_____ Decreased blood pressure

_____ Cough

_____ Open blisters

_____ Facial pain

_____ Hoarseness

4. Match the type of burn with its clinical manifestations:

Deep red, black or brown in color	A. Superficial
<25% TBSA, but >15% TBSA of partial thickness	B. Partial thickness
No pain or blisters	C. Full thickness third-degree burn
Healing occurs within seven days	D. Full thickness fourth-degree burn
Grafting required	E. Moderate
Involves epidermis and dermis	F. Major
Tenderness eased with cooling	
Sensitivity to cold air	
Brown or white fat exposed	
Large blister formation	
Black, edematous lesion	
Skin blanches with pressure	
>10% TBSA of full thickness	
Little pain experienced	
Grafting may be required	

Nursing Management of the Client with Wound Infections

Key Points

- The most important treatment for wound infection is prevention.
- Thorough handwashing is a key factor in the prevention of wound infection.
- In addition to hand washing, application of topical antiseptic agents, universal precautions and wound care using strict surgical asepsis are effective measures for preventing most wound infections.
- Infection results in tissue damage and delays wound healing.
- Goals of collaborative management:
  - Eliminate pathogens and prevent infections.
  - Support nutrition and healing.
  - Prevent complications such as sepsis, septic shock, wound dehiscence and wound evisceration.
- Important nursing diagnoses (actual or potential):
  - Pain
  - Risk for infection
  - Altered nutrition
  - Fatigue and restlessness
  - Activity intolerance
  - Self-care deficit
  - Anxiety and fear
  - Altered body temperature
  - Delayed wound healing
- **Key Terms/Concepts:** Handwashing, standard precautions, asepsis, sterile technique, immune suppression, immune deficiency, dehiscence, evisceration, immunological response, hypertrophic scars, keloid formation, wound contracture, adhesions, antibiotic resistant organisms, negative pressure wound therapy, hyperbaric oxygen therapy

Overview

A wound infection is the presence and growth of microorganisms that results in tissue damage and delays wound healing. When skin integrity is disrupted from trauma or surgery, the risk for infection increases. Wound infections may also develop when there is a break in surgical technique during a surgical procedure or during wound care.

Wounds heal in three phases: the inflammatory phase, the fibroblastic or connective tissue phase and the maturation or remodeling phase. Wounds may also heal by first intention with minimal scarring, second intention with prolonged healing and extensive scar tissue and third intention with delayed wound closure. Wounds are also classified on the basis of color: red wound, yellow wound, black wound or mixed color wound.

Risk Factors

- Age (infants or elderly)
- Chronic stress
- Decreased or compromised circulation
- Trauma, including animal or human bites
- Malnutrition
- Breach in sterile technique
- Contaminated wound prior to surgery or trauma
- Lengthy, complicated surgeries that leave tissues exposed for extended periods of time
- Chronic disease (diabetes mellitus, chronic renal failure, cancer)
- Obesity
- Immune suppression or deficiency (AIDS, corticosteroids, chemotherapy)
- Impaired oxygenation (pulmonary diseases, heart failure, hypovolemia)
- Leukemia
- Anemia
- Poor personal hygiene
- Radiation therapy
- Impaired blood flow (peripheral vascular disease (PVD), peripheral arterial occlusive disease (PAOD)

Signs and Symptoms of Infections

- Redness
- Swelling
- Pain, tenderness
- Warmth
- Malaise
- Purulent drainage
- Elevated body temperature, chills
- Elevated white blood cell (WBC) count
- Elevated I:T ratio (immature neutrophils to total neutrophils)
- Elevated sedimentation rate (the speed of sedimentation rises[ESR])
- Elevated C-relative protein (CRP)

Diagnostic and Laboratory Tests

- History and physical exam
- Wound culture
- Complete blood count (CBC)
- Sedimentation rate (Sed Rate), also called erythrosedimentation rate (ESR): the rate at which red blood cells (RBC) sediment falls to the bottom of a test tube
- C-reactive protein (CRP)
- Serum protein, albumin and protein: albumin ratio in severe cases

Therapeutic Nursing Management

- **Prevent by:**
  - Maintaining asepsis
  - Using good hand washing techniques
  - Universal precautions
- **Assess/Monitor:**
  - Wound appearance
  - Consistency, color, and odor of any drainage
  - For signs of localized infection (pain, erythema, edema, warmth, purulent drainage from wound)
  - For signs of systemic infection (fever, chills, malaise, elevated white blood cell count)
  - Fluid status
  - Nutritional status
  - Vital signs, especially temperature
- **Nursing Activities:**
  - Isolate client from contaminated items provided by roommates or visitors that could infect the wound.
  - Instruct the client to not touch the injured area.
  - Maintain aseptic technique when changing dressings or irrigating wounds.
  - Change the dressing if it becomes wet to avoid "wicking" microbes into the wound.
  - Consider the use of sterile, non-occlusive dressings to promote wound healing.
  - Maintain patency of drains.
  - Maintain adequate hydration and a nutritious diet.
  - Encourage rest.
  - Elevate the injured extremity to reduce edema and promote venous return.
  - Administer antibiotics as prescribed.
  - Administer analgesics and antipyretics as needed.
  - Promote pain relief with nonpharmacologic pain relief measures such as music therapy, guided imagery, relaxation techniques and breathing exercises.

- Administer oxygen if ordered to promote healing in clients with arterial disease, hypovolemia or hypotension.
- Assist with negative pressure wound therapy if ordered. This new type of therapy employs suction to remove drainage and promote wound healing.
- Prepare the client for hyperbaric oxygen therapy if required. Explain that the client will be placed in a chamber with 100% pressurized oxygen to accelerate granulation tissue formation and promote wound healing. A contraindication includes claustrophobia.
- Explain the stages of wound healing to the client, so the client will understand how the appearance of the wound will change as it passes through each stage.
- Encourage early ambulation to enhance circulation and promote healing.
- Teach clients and their families how to reduce the risk of developing antibiotic-resistant infections.

Pharmacology

- Analgesics (opioid or non-opioid)
- Antibiotics (depending on culture/sensitivity results, client allergy, and type or source of wound)
- Nutritional supplements if needed
- Prophylactic antibiotics for clients who are immunosuppressed.

Complications

- Systemic infection
- Septic Shock (life-threatening complication characterized by tachycardia, decreased blood pressure, decreased urine output, fever, and diaphoresis)
- Wound dehiscence (separation of the wound edges at the suture line)
- Evisceration (protrusion of internal organs through a surgical incision)
- Hypertrophic scars
- Keloid formation
- Wound contracture
- Excess granulation tissue ("proud flesh")
- Adhesions
- Loss of limb
- Loss of mobility
- Necrosis of tissues or organ
- Death

Age-Related Changes—Gerontological Considerations

- Elderly clients have an increased risk for wound infection due to alterations in circulation, skin elasticity, healing, and immunologic response.

- With aging, the skin is commonly less sensitive to sensory, tactile, and painful stimuli. For this reason, elderly clients are more prone to secondary complications, including wound infections.
- Older clients are more likely to have chronic medical conditions (cardiovascular, lung, endocrine, or renal) that can compromise wound healing.

Critical Thinking Exercise: Nursing Management of the Client with Wound Infections

Situation: A 39-year-old female underwent a partial bowel resection (removal of the bowel) as treatment for a malignant tumor. Prior to her surgery, she received radiation and chemotherapy in an effort to reduce the size of the tumor. She has lost a significant amount of weight over the past six months and is about twenty pounds under her ideal weight. Currently, her incision is well approximated, free of redness, tenderness or swelling.

1. If noted during wound assessment, which findings must be reported to the surgeon since they indicate the client is developing a wound infection?

   _____ Pallor   _____ Approximation

   _____ Swelling   _____ Erythema

   _____ Tenderness   _____ Serosanguineous drainage

2. Which are the risk factors that predispose this client to development of wound infection?

   _____ Advanced age   _____ Malignant tumor

   _____ Hyperlipidemia _____ Chemotherapy

   _____ Debilitation   _____ Radiation

   _____ Surgery   _____ Septicemia

   _____ Hypertension

3. What is the single most important nursing intervention to protect the woman from developing a postoperative wound infection?

4. List the classical clinical manifestations of system infection in a person who has wound infection.

Nursing Management of the Client with a Wound Dehiscence and Evisceration

Key Points

- Midline abdominal incision is most prone to wound dehiscence.
- Wound dehiscence is the partial or complete separation of the wound edges at the incision line.
- Wound dehiscence typically develops on the 6th to 7th day after surgery because the wound is weakest at this time.
- Wound evisceration is a protrusion of internal organs through the incision.
- Goals of collaborative management:
    - Prevent shock.
    - Prevent anxiety and fear.
    - Prevent evisceration and/or dehiscence.
    - Prevent infection.
    - Surgically close the wound.
    - Promote wound healing.
- Important nursing diagnoses (actual or potential):
    - Impaired skin and/or tissue integrity
    - Impaired wound healing
    - Risk for infection
    - Fear and anxiety
    - Pain
- **Key Terms/Concepts:** Surgical wound, evisceration, wound infection, asepsis

Overview

Wound dehiscence is the separation of the wound edges at the suture line. Wound evisceration is the protrusion of loops of bowel through the suture line. These two surgical complications generally develop with an abdominal incision; complications and delayed healing.

Risk Factors

- Obesity
- Malnutrition
- Abdominal surgery
- Advanced age
- Wound infection

- Diabetes mellitus
- Immunocompromised condition
- Chronic illness
- Excessive postoperative gas or abdominal distention
- Uncontrolled coughing following surgery
- Severe vomiting and retching
- Clogged nasogastric tube, Jackson Pratt, or Hemovac drain
- Excessively tight suturing or other improperly placed sutures
- Not splinting the incision during activity, coughing or vomiting
- Decreased peristalsis
- Invasive abdominal cancer or extensive abdominal surgery

Signs and Symptoms

- Sudden discharge of large amount of serosanguineous fluid from wound associated with wound edge separation with or without organ protrusion.
- Sharp pain in suture line or the feeling of something "giving away."
- A popping sound after turning or coughing.

Diagnostic and Laboratory Tests

- History and physical exam
- Complete blood count (CBC)
- Wound culture (if infection present)

Therapeutic Nursing Management

- **Prevention:**
  - Instruct client to splint the incision when coughing; or with activity or vomiting.
  - Use meticulous aseptic technique when dressing wound, to prevent infection and weakening of wound edge.
  - Have obese clients wear an abdominal binder.
  - Report severe coughing, retching, vomiting, or abdominal distention.
  - Recognize and report signs of infection immediately and obtain a wound culture and complete blood count (CBC).
- **Assess/Monitor:**
  - Vital signs
  - Drainage from wound (color, odor, amount)
  - Wound dressing
  - Approximation of the suture line as well as signs of infection
  - Nausea and vomiting; excessive coughing
  - Abdomen for distention; presence of bowel sounds
  - Nasogastric tube for patency
  - Drainage tubes for patency

- **Nursing Activities:**
  - Instruct another person to notify the surgeon immediately about the client's condition and remain with the client until the surgeon arrives.
  - Provide reassurance
  - If the client eviscerates, treat client for shock. This is a true medical emergency!
    - Place semi-Fowler's supine, or in Trendelenburg position with knees slightly flexed.
    - Start oxygen
    - Secure IV access
    - Place sterile, saline soaked dressings over eviscerated area.
    - Prepare client for surgery
    - Obtain surgical permit

Pharmacology

- Preoperative medications, if needed.
- Antibiotics (if infection present)
- Sedation
- Pain medication

Complications

- Infection
- Shock
- Delayed wound healing

Age-Related Changes—Gerontological Considerations

- Older clients are at greater risk for wound dehiscence than younger clients.
- Older clients may have decreased skin elasticity and decreased circulation, which might retard the healing, placing the client at a greater risk of wound dehiscence or evisceration.

Critical Thinking Exercise: Nursing Management of the Client with a Wound Dehiscence and Evisceration

Situation: A 67-year-old client with long-standing diabetes mellitus underwent surgery to remove an abdominal tumor after being diagnosed with a partial bowel obstruction. The client relates a history of several months of abdominal pain, bloating, nausea, and weight loss. At the time of surgery, he was about 15% below his ideal body weight. The client progressed well during his postoperative period and remained free of incision infection or other complications. On his seventh postoperative day, which was the day he was to be discharged to home, the nurse removed the client's abdominal sutures as ordered by his surgeon. An hour later, the client called the nurse to his room stating when he coughed he felt something "give" at his incision. Inspection revealed a one-inch separation of the client's wound edges.

1. What factors increase the risk for would dehiscence?

2. During what activities is a client most likely to experience wound dehiscence?

3. In what order will the nurse implement the following actions related to the client's wound dehisence?

   ___ Have another nurse notify the surgeon while you remain with the client.

   ___ Cover any protruding coils of intestine with sterile dressings moistened with sterile normal saline; if sterile supplies are not available, use clean towels or dressings.

   ___ Remain calm.

   ___ Document the incident.

   ___ Place the client in bed in semi-Fowler's position with the knees slightly arched. If the wound has not completely opened or has not eviscerated, this position may prevent further tear.

4. How does wound dehiscence differ from wound evisceration?

Nursing Management of the Client with Pressure Ulcers

Key Points

- Prevention is the most important treatment for pressure ulcers.
- Soft tissue damage in the form of a pressure ulcer may develop if a client's skin is exposed to pressure for an extended period of time.
- Pressure ulcers are a significant source of morbidity and mortality among older adults and persons who are immobile.
- Pressure ulcers range from tissue redness to full-thickness skin loss with damage to underlying muscle and bone.
- Goals of collaborative management:
  - Maintain skin integrity.
  - Prevent exposure of tissues to pressure for extended periods of time.
  - Prevent infection.
  - Promote nutrition, hydration, and healing.
  - Promote mobility (when feasible).
  - Prevent recurrence of pressure ulcer.
  - Prevent complications: infection, sepsis, and septic shock.
- Important nursing diagnoses (actual or potential):
  - Pain
  - Impaired mobility
  - Imbalanced nutrition
  - Impaired skin integrity
  - Impaired tissue integrity
  - Ineffective tissue perfusion
  - Risk for infection
  - Anxiety and fear
  - Ineffective individual coping
- **Key Terms/Concepts**: Immobility, staging of pressure ulcers, friction, shearing force, tissue ischemia, tissue necrosis, pressure relieving devices, assistive devices

Overview

A pressure (decubitus) ulcer is an area of soft tissue damage that occurs when pressure is applied to the skin for an extended period of time. Pressure prevents adequate blood supply from reaching tissues, resulting in tissue ischemia and tissue necrosis. The most common sites of pressure ulcer formation are over bony prominences, such as the sacrum, heels, ischial areas, trochanter, and lateral malleoli. The development of pressure ulcers depends on the amount of pressure applied to the client's tissues, the length of time the client's tissues are subjected to pressure, and the ability of the client's tissues to withstand the pressure without breaking down.

Risk Factors

- Immobility
- Older age
- Inadequate nutrition
- Incontinence or excessive moisture
- Anemia
- Skin friction and shearing
- Fever
- Immobility
- Emaciation
- Impaired circulation
- Edema
- Low diastolic blood pressure
- Alteration in cognitive functioning
- Neurological disorders
- Vascular disorders
- Sensory deficits
- Chronic diseases (diabetes mellitus, chronic renal failure, congestive heart failure, chronic lung disease)
- Sedation so that spontaneous repositioning is decreased

Signs and Symptoms

Stage 1: Reddened area on lightly pigmented skin (red, blue, or purple area on darkly pigmented skin) that does not blanch with pressure and returns to normal within 15 to 20 minutes when pressure is relieved, intact skin

Stage 2: Partial-thickness skin loss, shallow crater or abrasion, and clean healing

Stage 3: Full-thickness skin loss involving damage or necrosis of subcutaneous tissue; white, gray, or yellow exudates at base of ulcer; and purulent drainage

Stage 4: Full-thickness skin loss with extensive destruction, tissue necrosis, and damage to muscle and/or bone; black or brown eschar; and purulent drainage

Note: Wounds cannot be staged if they are covered with eschar (a dark, leathery scab or crust made of necrotic tissue) because the wound base is not visible.

Diagnostic and Laboratory Tests

- History and physical
- Complete blood count (CBC) and differential
- Wound culture and sensitivity

- Serum albumin, protein, and protein: albumin ratio

Therapeutic Nursing Management

- **Prevent by**:
  - Using pressure sore preventive measures (pressure relief surfaces and pressure relieving devices)
  - Maintaining adequate fluid and nutritional status
  - Cleansing client's skin immediately if incontinent
  - Encouraging ambulation
  - Repositioning the client every 2 hours
  - Implementing passive or active exercises if the client is immobile
  - Inspecting the integumentary system frequently
- **Assess/Monitor**:
  - For alterations in skin integrity
  - Skin moisture status
  - Incontinence
  - Nutritional status
  - Hydration status
  - Problems with mobility
  - Serum albumen levels
- **Nursing Activities**:
  - Implement pressure sore prevention measures.
  - Maintain clean, dry skin, and wrinkle-free linens.
  - Reposition the client at least every two hours and document position changes.
  - Place pillows strategically, using a bridging technique.
  - Maintain head of bed at or below 30 degree angle (or flat) unless contraindicated to relieve pressure on sacrum, buttocks, and heels.
  - Prevent client from sliding down in bed as this increases shearing forces that pull tissue layers apart and cause damage.
  - Lift rather than pull a client up in bed or in a chair; since pulling creates friction that can damage the client's outer layer of skin (epidermis).
  - Raise client's heels off of the bed to prevent pressure on the heels.
  - Avoid leaving the client in a wheelchair for long periods of time because this position increases shearing forces causing pressure ulcers to develop over the ischial tuberosities. The client may also develop pressure injuries on the feet, especially the heels.
  - Clean and dry skin immediately following urinary or stool incontinence.
  - Apply moisture barrier creams to skin of incontinent clients.
  - Use pressure relief devices such as foam pillows and wheelchair cushions.
  - Cautiously massage reddened areas of skin that are exposed to pressure to enhance circulation.
  - Use assistive devices such as lifts, a trapeze, and turning sheets to help client move without placing excessive pressure on tissues.

- Implement wound care as prescribed.
- Provide 14 mg/kg/day based on energy expenditures to ensure that client receives protein and other nutrients for wound healing.
- Note if serum albumin levels are low because a lack of protein puts the client at greater risk for further skin breakdown, slowed healing and infection at the ulcer site.
- Provide adequate hydration.
- Provide vitamin and mineral supplements as needed.
- Give the client and family emotional support and encouragement.
- Ambulate client as soon as possible and as often as possible.
- Implement active/passive exercises for immobile clients.
- Educate the client and family in measures to prevent recurrence of pressure ulcers.

Pharmacology

- Antimicrobials (topical and /or systemic, as ordered)
- Antiseptics
- Nutritional supplements as needed

Complications

- Advancement to a stage 4 ulcer
- Infection of ulcer
- Tissue necrosis
- Systemic infection
- Septic shock
- Loss of tissue/limb
- Recurrence of pressure ulcers
- Death

Age-Related Changes—Gerontological Considerations

- The aging process is accompanied by decreased skin elasticity, thicker epidermis, thinner dermis, decreased vascularity, and decreased sebaceous gland activity.
- Older clients may have chronic cardiovascular and neurological conditions that limit mobility, weaken tissues subjected to pressure, and retard and prolong wound healing.
- Sensory perceptual alterations and impaired cognitive functioning compromises the older adult's ability to sense or report pressure.
- Inadequate nutrition and fluid intake increases the risk for thin, dry skin, and development of pressure ulcers in elderly clients.

Critical Thinking Exercise: Nursing Management of the Client with Pressure Ulcers

Situation: A 68-year-old female is in a vegetative state after suffering a traumatic brain injury in an automobile accident. She does not respond to verbal commands or pain. She receives nutrition and fluids via a gastrostomy tube. The woman is incontinent of urine and has diarrheal stools. Even though she received very good nursing care and frequent turning, she developed a Stage 3 pressure ulcer on her coccyx.

1. Which of the following statements best describes a Stage 3 pressure ulcer?

   _____ Full-thickness skin loss with extensive destruction, tissue necrosis, and damage to muscle and/or bone.

   _____ A reddened area that does not blanch with pressure and returns to normal within 15-20 minutes when pressure is relieved.

   _____ Full-thickness skin loss and the presence of white, gray, or yellow exudates and purulent drainage at the base of the ulcer.

2. Complete each sentence pertaining to the client's risk factors for skin breakdown.

   The client may be experiencing diarrhea as a result of the _____.

   The nurse should take care to _reposition_ the client at least every _2_ hours to prevent further skin breakdown.

   Adequate amounts of _fluids_ are necessary to support nutrition and aid in wound _healing_.

   Avoid _l_____ the skin over bony prominences; current evidence suggests this may be harmful.

3. Which nursing activities will help promote wound healing?

   _____ Assessing the wound daily   _____ Applying a dressing to the ulcer

   _____ Relieving pressure over the affected site   _____ Maintaining adequate nutrition

   _____ Turning and repositioning q 2-4 hrs   _____ Administering intravenous antibiotics

Nursing Management of the Client with Skin Cancer

Key Points

- Overexposure to the sun (including tanning) is the main cause of skin cancer, especially when it results in sunburn or blistering. Avoidance of sun is the best defense against skin cancer.
- Use of sunscreen, limiting exposure to ultraviolet light, friction, and irritating chemicals can prevent many skin cancers.
- There are three types of skin cancer:
  - Basal cell carcinoma
  - Squamous cell carcinoma
  - Malignant melanoma
- Unlike basal cell and squamous cell carcinoma, malignant melanoma is a dangerous rapidly metastasizing skin cancer.
- The ABCDs of melanoma:
  - Asymmetry: One side does not match the other.
  - Borders: Irregular, ragged, notched or blurred edges.
  - Color: Lack of uniformity in pigmentation. Shades of tan, brown, or black are present.
  - Diameter: The width is greater than 6 mm (about the size of a pencil eraser). Any growth should be a sign for concern.
- Skin cancer can generally be cured if the client is diagnosed and treated early in the course of the disease.
- Goals of collaborative management:
  - Implement early detection and treatment measures.
  - Prevent metastasis.
  - Prevent disfigurement.
- Important nursing diagnoses (actual or potential):
  - Fatigue
  - Impaired skin integrity
  - Impaired tissue integrity
  - Anxiety and fear
  - Body image disturbance
  - Ineffective individual coping
  - Ineffective family coping
  - Anticipatory grieving
  - Hopelessness and lack of control

- Pain
- **Key Terms/Concepts:** Squamous cell carcinoma, basal cell carcinoma, malignant melanoma, ultraviolet radiation, metastasis, cachexia, immunotherapy, chemotherapy, radiation therapy, gene therapy, surgical excision

Overview

Skin cancer is the most common type of cancer in the United States today. It can be a malignant condition that is caused by the uncontrolled growth of cells in specific skin layers. The majority of skin cancers diagnosed are either basal cell carcinoma, benign or squamous cell carcinoma, malignant. These two slower growing types are essentially curable with early detection and treatment. Eighty percent of clients with malignant melanoma, previously considered generally non-curable, may be cured with early diagnosis and treatment.

Risk Factors

- Exposure to ultraviolet light
- Chronic friction to the skin
- Exposure to irritating chemicals, such as coal tar and arsenic
- Fair-skinned persons with freckles who sunburn easily
- Celtic or Scandinavian origin
- Dysplastic or congenital nevi
- Genetic predisposition to malignant melanoma
- Actinic keratosis

Signs and Symptoms

- **Basal cell carcinoma:** Waxy nodule or fleshy bump arising from the basal cells of the epidermis; generally located on the face, neck, or hands. Metastasis is rare in these slow- growing lesions.
- **Squamous cell carcinoma:** Small, red, nodular lesion or scaly patch arising from the epidermal keratinocytes; generally located on upper extremities, lips, and mouth; may infiltrate surrounding structures and metastasize to lymph nodes. This is the second most common type of skin cancer found in fair-skinned persons. When found early and treated properly, the cure rate is very high.
- **Malignant melanoma:** Lesion may be white, gray, black, brown, or blue; changes in characteristics of a mole suggest malignant melanoma. The warning signs include changes in the surface of a mole, scallions, oozing, bleeding, the appearance of a new lesion, spreading of pigment from the border to the surrounding skin, and change in sensation, itching, or tenderness to the site. Extensive metastasis to brain, bone, lungs, liver, or skin can occur and ultimately lead to death.

Diagnostic and Laboratory Tests

- History
- Physical Examination
- Biopsy of skin lesions

Therapeutic Nursing Management

- **Prevent by**:
  - Avoiding excessive sun exposure, using sunscreens, and layering clothing when outside
  - Seeking shade between 10 a.m. and 4 p.m. when the sun's ultraviolet rays are the most intense
  - Wearing light-colored, tightly-woven clothing, and wide-brimmed hats during times of sun exposure
  - Applying sunscreens with sun protection factor (SPF) of at least 15
  - Performing monthly skin self-examination of all parts of the body and immediately reporting skin changes, moles, or suspicious lesions to the primary care provider.
- **Assess/Monitor**:
  - Skin for presence of suspicious lesions
  - Moles that change in size, color, shape, elevation, surface, sensation, and consistency.
- **Nursing Activities**:
  - Teach client to report lesions that do not heal.
  - Teach client to avoid contact with irritating chemicals.
  - Prepare client for surgical excision of the involved tissues if ordered.
  - Provide wound care following surgical excision to promote healing and prevent infection.
  - Report and provide relief for side effects or toxic effects of chemotherapy.
  - Implement postradiation care for clients receiving radiation therapy.
  - Encourage adequate nutrition and fluid intake.
  - Encourage verbalization of fears and concerns.
  - Advise early use of skin protection in childhood because it is estimated that 80% of lifetime sun exposure occurs before age 18 years.
  - Educate clients to keep infants under 6 months of age from prolonged sun exposure. Infants should be protected with sunscreens even if exposure is anticipated to be brief.
  - Teach clients to do periodic self-examinations of the skin. Being familiar with "beauty marks," moles other lesions, and freckles is the key to knowing when a change in appearance occurs. Clients need to report any changes in color, shape, size, or number of moles.
  - Refer client and family to cancer support groups.
  - Schedule the client who is being discharged for a post-surgical checkup and appointments for skin evaluations twice a year.

Pharmacology

- Sunscreen (minimum 15 SPF)
- Chemotherapy: chemotherapeutic agents include dacarbazine (DTIC), temozolomide (Temodal), procarbazine (Matulane), carmustine (BCNU), and lomustine (CCNU)

- Immunotherapy: interferon alfa (Roferon-A)
- Gene therapy which involves repairing or replacing defective genes with normal genes.

Complications

- Metastasis
- Disfigurement
- Infection
- Death

Age-Related Changes—Gerontological Considerations

- Older adults have a significantly increased risk of skin cancer due to cumulative effects of being exposed to the sun over a lifetime.
 - Actinic keratosis is one form of precancerous skin lesion caused by sun exposure. The scaly, whitish lesions on the superficial layer of the epithelium are found in nearly all elderly Caucasians. Topical application of 5-fluorouracil (5-FU, Efudex) is used to remove widespread actinic lesions. Aldara (imiquimod) topical has also been recently approved for treatment of actinic keratosis.

Critical Thinking Exercise: Nursing Management of the Client with Skin Cancer

Situation: A 19-year-old college student visits the student health center because she is concerned about a small, red, nodular epidermal lesion on her arm. The woman relates a history of frequent sunbathing, participation in water sports in the summer, and use of tanning beds in the winter. She is unaware of any close relatives who have a history of skin cancer.

1. Describe the appearance of each skin cancer listed below:

   a. Basal cell

   b. Squamous cell

   c. Malignant melanoma

2. Which factors increase a person's risk for developing skin cancer?

   _____ Using tanning oils when sunbathing

   _____ Applying make-up over sunscreen

   _____ Routinely using a tanning bed

   _____ Wearing clothing that is too tight

3. What is the rationale for teaching a clients to apply SPF 15 sunscreen or higher prior to spending lengthy periods of time in the sun?

Nursing Management of the Client with a Rash

Key Points

- A rash may be localized or generalized to the entire body.
- Rashes have many causes, but are most likely associated with allergic reactions and communicable diseases.
- Clients are at greatest risk for developing a rash when they:
    - Are in contact with an individual who has a communicable disease; direct and/or airborne.
    - Ingest drugs or foods that cause allergic reactions.
    - Are exposed to animals or are stung by insects.
    - Are stressed.
    - Are exposed to a variety of environmental conditions such as extreme or prolonged exposure to heat, cold, or dryness.
- Examples of rashes include diaper rash, drug rash, ecchymotic (hemorrhagic) rash, heat rash, macular rash, maculopapular rash, red rash, rose rash, sunburn-like rash, blistering rash, pustular rash (lesions that are elevated and filled with pus), heat rash (miliaria or prickly heat), and butterfly rash. Rashes are categorized by the type of lesion, primary or secondary, and the rashes characteristics; macular, papular, vesicular, etc.
- Examples of disorders associated with rashes include chickenpox, rubeola, rubella, varicella, roseola, meningitis, toxic shock syndrome, contact dermatitis, eczema, urticaria (hives), scabies, herpes simplex I, herpes simplex II, herpes zoster, impetigo, candidiasis, lupus erythematous, Rocky Mountain spotted fever, and Lyme disease.
- A rash may be difficult to identify in clients with darkly pigmented skin.
- Goals of collaborative management:
    - Obtain a detailed history from the client concerning factors at home, school, or work that may be associated with the development of a rash.
    - Identify causative factors.
    - Discontinue suspected medications.
    - Isolate individuals with a potential communicable disease.
    - Relieve discomfort, itching, and fever.
    - Treat communicable disease if this is the cause.
    - Teach clients to avoid substances and situations that may trigger a rash.
    - Prevent spread of rashes associated with communicable diseases such as meningitis (possible isolation).

- Important nursing diagnoses (actual or potential):
  - Risk for infection
  - Risk for altered body temperature
  - Latex allergy response
  - Impaired tissue and skin integrity
  - Social isolation
  - Risk for loneliness
  - Ineffective management of therapeutic regimen
  - Body image disturbance
  - Anxiety and pain
  - Pain management
- **Key Terms/Concepts**: Communicable disease, allergic reactions, dermatitis, lesions, exanthem, roseola, macular, maculopapular, ecchymotic, pruritus, crusting, scaling, lichenification, topical medications, and antihistamines

Overview

A rash is an eruption of the skin that is associated with a communicable disease or an allergic reaction to drugs, foods, and various allergens in the environment. They are usually temporary. The shade of red and other characteristics of the rash vary with the causative factor. Rashes are sometimes called eruptions, lesions, exanthem, or roseola.

Risk Factors

- Contact with persons with communicable diseases during specific incubation period
- Ingestion of drugs and/or foods that can cause allergic reactions
- Contact with substances that can cause allergic reactions (e.g., soaps, cosmetics, perfumes, plants, poison ivy or oak, lotions, latex gloves, certain foods such as eggs, shellfish, wheat products, milk)
- Allergy to pets
- Exposure to insect bites or ticks
- New or increased stresses
- Hot weather
- Low humidity due to winter weather or air conditioning
- Constrictive clothing
- Use of wool clothing or blankets
- Excessive bathing or showering in hot water
- Sexual relations

Signs and Symptoms associated with Rashes

- Pruritus or severe itching
- Foul odor, possible, if draining
- Petechiae or purpura

- Telangiectasia - dilated small blood vessels
- Angioedema
- Swelling
- Fever
- Tenderness
- Dry skin (xerosis)
- **Specific Lesions:**
  - **Primary:**
    - Macule - small, flat
    - Papule - small (<0.5 cm), raised
    - Nodule - larger than papule
    - Wheal - raised, slightly irregular, hive
    - Vesicle - small (<0.5 cm), clear fluid filled
    - Bulla - larger than vesicle
    - Pustule - pus fluid filled
  - **Secondary:**
    - Erosion - loss of superficial epidermis, does not bleed
    - Ulcer - deeper loss of skin surface, can bleed and scar
    - Scar - replacing damaged tissue by fibrous tissue
    - Lichenification - thickening and roughening of skin with increased furrows
    - Atrophy - thinning of skin with loss of furrows
    - Excoriation - abrasion or scratch

Diagnostic and Laboratory Tests

- History and physical exam
- Medication history including OTC (over-the-counter) drugs
- Dietary history
- Description of home, school, and work environments to identify possible irritants or allergens
- Patch testing - Skin, Radioallergosorbent test (RAST) to identify allergens
- Gram stain and culture to identify rash
- Tzanck smear for vesicular disorders to identify herpes virus
- Wood's (ultraviolet) light to detect fungal infections of the skin and hair
- Potassium hydroxide (KOH) examination if fungal disorder is suspected

Therapeutic Nursing Management

- **Prevention:**
  - Isolate clients with communicable diseases.
  - Instruct clients to avoid individuals with communicable diseases.
  - To prevent eczema (atopic dermatitis), instruct clients to avoid contact

with dyes, cosmetics, skin lotions, permanent press fabrics, deodorant, and other allergens.

- Call primary care provider and discontinue medication that are suspected as allergens.
- Manage stress and avoid unnecessary stress.
- Avoid eating foods such as eggs, milk, peanuts, citrus, corn, seafood, or wheat products if allergic.
- Avoid wearing constrictive clothing and remove wet clothing as soon as possible.
- Avoid wool clothing and blankets.
- Wear clothing made of natural fibers, such as cotton.
- Avoid hot weather and air conditioning.
- Bathe less frequently, but when doing so, add oil to tepid bath water.
- Take quick showers, using tepid water.
- Do not use soap to wash areas of eczema.
- Avoid alcohol-containing lotions, which dry the skin.
- Use rubber gloves dusted on the inside with cornstarch or talcum powder when cleaning house, or use cotton-lined latex gloves.
- Keep skin moisturized.

- **Assess/Monitor:**
  - Location, distribution, and characteristics of rash
  - Color, size, height, and diameter of the lesions
  - Migration pattern of the rash
  - For crusting, scaling, or lichenification
  - For tenderness around area of rash
  - For odor associated with rash
  - For fever if communicable disease present

- **Nursing Activities:**
  - Administer:
    - Therapeutic baths as ordered
    - Systemic medications as ordered
    - Cooling measures to lower fever if necessary
  - Apply:
    - Cool compresses to relieve itching
    - Topical preparations to rash as ordered.
  - Isolate client from other people if he or she has a communicable disease.
  - Instruct client:
    - To keep hands and fingernails clean and nails clipped
    - To avoid touching or scratching the rash
    - To report any sign of infection of the skin
    - Teach client about actions and side effects of all medications and preparations

Pharmacology

- Therapeutic baths (balneotherapy)
  - Water or saline
  - Oatmeal or starch preparations
  - Bicarbonate of soda
  - Emollients (bath oils)
- Burrow's solution compresses
- Potassium permanganate compresses
- Systemic corticosteroids: prednisone, methylprednisolone
- Topical corticosteroids: betamethasone, triamcinolone, fluticasone, hydrocortisone, mometasone, etc.
- Topical antifungals: terbinafine, clotrimazole, ciclopirox, ketoconazole, nystatin and/or systemic antifungals
- Antipsoriatics or eczema medications (immunosuppressants, retinoids, immuno modulators, etc.)
- Scabicides/Pediculicides, if appropriate (permethrin)
- Topical antimicrobials: triple antibiotic ointment, bacitracin, mupirocin
- Systemic antihistamines: First generation - diphenhydramine, hydroxyzine, clemastine, hydroxyzine; Second generation - loratadine, desloratadine, fexofenadine, cetirizine
- Topical antipruritics (calamine lotion, camphor, diphenhydramine, topical corticosteroids)
- Nonsteroidal anti-inflammatory agent (NSAID), if fever present
- Acetaminophen, if fever present
- Systemic antibiotics for secondary infections or if rash related to primary bacterial infection

Complications

- Infection and skin injury due to scratching of lesions
- Secondary bacterial or yeast infections
- Ulceration
- Scarring
- Change in body image due to appearance of rash
- Dehydration due to fever
- Delirium and seizures due to high fever, associated with underlying condition such as meningitis

Age-Related Changes—Gerontological Considerations

- Childhood communicable diseases, especially viral, such as chickenpox, cause many rashes but only chickenpox is known to reappear later in life as shingles (herpes zoster - refer to Chapter 7)

- Eczema is typically more severe during childhood and then gradually improves as the client ages and the client also becomes more aware of allergens that trigger the problem and is able to avoid triggers.
- Elderly clients are at greater risk for medication-triggered dermatitis because they generally take more medications than younger clients.

Critical Thinking Exercise: Nursing Management of the Client with a Rash

Situation: A 25-year-old woman who has recently started employment in a fast-food restaurant is being seen for eczema (atopic dermatitis). The nurse notes patches of dry, red, and scaly skin on the backs of the client's hands and on her arms. The client has a history of eczema, and is allergic to a number of medications and cleaning products. The client states that at her new job she washes her hands frequently with hot water and an antibacterial soap.

1. What measures should the nurse instruct the client to take to avoid exacerbation of her eczema?

2. What nursing diagnoses apply to the care of the client with eczema?

3. What medications will the primary care provider most likely prescribe for this client?

Nursing Management of the Client with Herpes Zoster— Shingles

Key Points

- Herpes zoster is reactivation of latent varicella zoster (chickenpox).
- Acute herpes zoster infection produces painful, and generally, unilateral skin lesions.
- Herpes zoster is potentially transmissible and caution should be exercised around infants, pregnant women who have not had chickenpox, and immunocompromised clients.
- Herpes zoster can be a serious condition that in older adults can produce severe peripheral neuropathy, dissemination, or death.
- Goals of collaborative management:
  - Control pain.
  - Limit viral outbreak.
  - Prevent complications (secondary infections, post-herpetic neuralgia, and blindness).
- Important nursing diagnoses (actual or potential):
  - Pain
  - Impaired skin integrity
  - Risk for infection
  - Altered nutrition possible related to pain and/or medications
  - Anxiety
  - Risk for situational low self-esteem
- **Key Terms/Concepts**: Varicella zoster virus, chickenpox, unilateral skin lesions, immune compromise, antinuclear antibody test titer, wound isolation, secondary infections

Overview

Shingles is a reactivation of dormant varicella zoster virus infection of structures along the dorsal nerve root ganglion. The infection produces painful, usually, unilateral skin eruptions along the affected dermatome associated with the nerve. Following the initial varicella infection, the virus remains dormant in the dorsal nerve root ganglia of the spinal and sensory nerves. If a client becomes immunocompromised for any reason such as stress, trauma, or acute illness; the virus may reactivate and cause an outbreak of shingles. Although more common in the elderly, shingles can occur any age, including children, if the client's immune system becomes compromised.

Risk Factors

- Previous infection with varicella-zoster virus
- Reactivation of varicella-zoster virus
- Immune-compromised state in client who has previously had chickenpox
- Increasing age
- Systemic illness
- Emotional stress
- Trauma
- Poor nutritional state
- Fatigue

Signs and Symptoms

- Unilateral skin lesions along peripheral dermatome (sensory nerve) of spinal cord branching off at face, trunk, thorax, arms
- Pain, burning sensation, or pruritus along dermatome. Classical picture is that burning, pain, or itch precedes breakout of lesions by 24-48 hours.
- Paresthesia
- Fever
- Headache
- Possible visual impairment if trigeminal nerve involvement at ophthalmic branch
- Flu-like symptoms

Diagnostic and Laboratory Tests

- History and physical examination. Lesions are easy to identify by history and clinical picture.
- Skin cultures, if diagnosis unsure
- Antinuclear antibody (ANA) test titer: ANA test results are reported in a titer that indicates how much the test sample can be diluted before the antibodies are no longer detected. Fluorescence techniques are frequently used to actually detect the antibodies in the cells, thus ANA testing is sometimes referred to as fluorescent antinuclear antibody (FANA) testing. Rarely indicated in initial work-up, but maybe helpful if arthritic conditions develop.

Therapeutic Nursing Management

- **Assess/Monitor:**
  - Vital signs
  - Neurovascular status
  - Seventh cranial nerve function
  - Signs of secondary infection
  - Signs/symptoms of peripheral neuropathy

- **Nursing Activities:**
  - Isolate client (exudate contains virus) until vesicles are crusted. Definitely in varicella zoster, controversial in herpes zoster. Only need to potentially isolate from very young, pregnant women who have not had chickenpox, and immunocompromised clients.
  - Maintain strict wound care precautions.
  - Do not rupture blisters if present. Preserving blisters will help to prevent the spread of the virus or the introduction of new infective agents into the blisters.
  - Use air mattress or bed cradle for pain prevention/control.
  - Administer antiviral, analgesic (oral, topical), gabapentin for neuralgia, and antipruritics as prescribed.
  - Control client's pain during acute phase to help prevent posthepatic neuralgia.
  - Administer acetic acid compresses and tepid baths as prescribed.
  - Assist with administration of nerve block for pain control if prescribed.
  - Instruct client to keep nails short.
  - Teach client to avoid scratching lesions.
  - Teach client to wear loose, lightweight clothing and to avoid wool or synthetic clothing.
- **Prevent:**
  - Secondary infection
  - Transmission to other clients/staff

Pharmacology

- Anti-viral agents: acyclovir, famciclovir, valacyclovir
- Antipruritic agents: diphenhydramine, hydroxyzine
- Systemic corticosteroids (controversial)
- Posthepatic neuralgia (gabapentin, lidocaine gel in patch)
- Analgesics (opioid or non-opioid, topical - lidocaine gel in a patch)
- Anti-anxiety agents: diazepam (Valium), chlordiazepoxide (Librium)
- Acetic acid compresses

Complications

- Postherpetic neuralgia, most common
- Keratitis, if ocular involvement
- Skin necrosis of varying depth, rare
- Uveitis, if ocular involvement
- Blindness, if ocular involvement
- Generalized central nervous system (CNS) infection, rare
- Muscle atrophy
- Transient motor paralysis

- Scarring
- Bell's palsy

Age-Related Changes—Gerontological Considerations

- The older adult is at increased risk for post-herpetic neuralgia. Elderly clients may have chronic illnesses (cardiovascular, renal, respiratory, gastrointestinal) or they may have a weakened immune system which leaves them vulnerable to the expression of and complications of herpes zoster.

Critical Thinking Exercise: Nursing Management of the Client with Herpes Zoster—Shingles

Situation: A 59-year-old man is receiving chemotherapy for colon cancer. This morning the man is experiencing pain beneath his right arm and across the right side of his back. The nurse notes the client has several draining lesions that run in a linear pattern across the right side of his back and extending beneath his right arm.

1. What signs are most indicative that the client is experiencing an outbreak of herpes zoster (shingles) rather than an allergic reaction to his chemotherapy?

2. Which nursing activities need to be implemented in response to the client's symptoms?

   _____ Monitor for infection.   _____ Place the client on wound precautions.

   _____ Discontinue the chemotherapy.   _____ Drain the blisters.

   _____ Cover lesions with sterile dressing.   _____ Administer prescribed pain medication.

3. Provide a rationale for each of these nursing activities related to herpes zoster.

   a. Place an air mattress on the client's bed.

   b. Administer an anti-inflammatory agent.

   c. Use acetic acid compound on lesions.

Nursing Management of the Client with Osteoporosis

Key Points

- Osteoporosis is risk factor for fractures among postmenopausal women.
- Early detection and treatment can reduce disability and/or complications associated with osteoporosis.
- Prevention should begin in early adulthood.
- Bone mass density peaks between ages 30-35.
- Goals of collaborative management:
  - Prevent bone demineralization.
  - Prevent deformity.
  - Prevent fractures.
  - Relieve pain.
  - Increase client knowledge.
- Important nursing diagnoses (actual or potential):
  - Potential complications of osteoporosis: fractures
  - Pain management
  - Constipation or other bowel dysfunctions
  - Risk for injury
  - Knowledge deficit
- **Key Terms/Concepts**: Prevention, hormone replacement therapy, anti-inflammatory

Overview

Osteoporosis is a metabolic, age-related disease in which bone demineralization causes loss of bone tissue and decreased bone mass. Bone resorption that exceeds bone formation results in fragile, porous bones that subsequently fracture. There are two categories of osteoporosis: Primary osteoporosis develops in men and women of any age, but usually affects women after menopause and can effect elderly men. Secondary osteoporosis develops in association with other disorders or problems such as hyperparathyroidism, prolonged use of corticosteroids, or prolonged immobility. Although rare, primary osteoporosis has been seen in teenage girls especially those with eating disorders.

Risk Factors

- Menopause
- Aging
- Long-term corticosteroid therapy, thyroid replacement therapy, or administration of anti-seizure medications.

- High caffeine intake
- High alcohol intake
- Possibly high intake of carbonated beverages
- Sedentary lifestyle (lack of physical activity or prolonged immobility, both of which cause rapid bone loss)
- History of falls, fractures, and other injuries
- Smoking
- Insufficient calcium and vitamin D intake or absorption
- Small, thin frame
- Female gender
- Northern European, Caucasian, or Asian heritage
- Hereditary predisposition
- Hyperparathyroidism (PTH triggers release of calcium from bones)
- Acromegaly
- Hyperthyroidism
- History of anorexia nervosa, bulimia, chronic liver disease, or malabsorption syndromes such as celiac disease
- Early or surgically induced menopause

Signs and Symptoms

- Loss of height
- Fractures of the wrist, hip, and vertebral column
- Lower back pain that increases with activity
- Kyphosis, especially of dorsal spine (Dowager's hump)
- Abdominal distention, constipation
- Respiratory impairment
- Pathologic fractures

Diagnostic and Laboratory Tests

- History and physical exam
- Bone density studies, bone mineral density (BMD), dual-energy x-ray absorptiometry (DEXA)
- Magnetic resonance imaging (MRI)
- Computed tomography (CT) scan/computed axial tomography (CAT) scan
- Blood levels of calcium, phosphorus, alkaline phosphatase, and PTH (parathyroid hormone) as well as urinary vitamin D excretion in secondary causes of osteoporosis
- Quantitative ultrasound

Therapeutic Nursing Management

- **Prevention:**
  - Regular weight bearing exercise
  - Intake of high-protein (approximately 0.8 mg/kg/day), high-calcium diet (fish, fowl, dairy products, fortified orange juice, and dark green leafy vegetables)
  - Intake of high vitamin D foods (fortified milk, cold water fatty fish, cereals) to promote calcium absorption.
  - Avoidance of alcohol, caffeine, and tobacco
  - Intake of calcium with vitamin D supplements
  - Hazard free environment that will protect client from falls and fractures
  - Avoidance of high-impact physical activities
  - Spinal support (firm mattress and back brace)
- **Assess/Monitor:**
  - For injury risks
  - For loss of height
  - For extremely stooped posture (Dowager's hump)
  - For lower back pain that increases with activity
  - For pain control effectiveness
  - For abdominal distention and constipation
  - For impaired breathing due to deformities of spine and rib cage
  - For pathologic fractures
- **Nursing Activities:**
  - Administer ERT (estrogen replacement therapy), as prescribed. May no longer be prescribed, risk versus benefit ratio needs to be assessed. Possible use of SERMs (selective estrogen receptor modulators), bisphosphonates, calcitonin, etc.
  - Administer or teach client how to safely take medications for pain relief.
  - Promote a diet that is high in protein, vitamin C, vitamin D, and calcium.
  - Administer dietary supplements as needed.
  - Advise client to stop drinking alcoholic and caffeine beverages and to quit smoking.
  - Encourage the use of assistive devices when gait is unstable.
  - Use protective devices to prevent injury (side rails, walker).
  - Move the client gently when turning.
  - Encourage active/passive ROM (range of motion).
  - Teach client to perform deep breathing exercises to increase pulmonary capacity.
  - Teach client to avoid positions that allow vertebral compression.
  - Encourage the use of a firm mattress.
  - Assist with application of back brace, as prescribed, to provide spinal support.

- Teach client and family to inspect home environment for hazards that can cause falls such as stairs, loose throw rugs, and dangling cords.
- Schedule follow-up physical therapy appointments following discharge
- Refer the client to support groups, community services, and a home health care agency.
- Encourage client to walk, stair climb (if no balance issues), or bicycle daily to increase done mass.
- Encourage client to perform abdominal exercises and practice deep breathing exercises
- Teach client how to lift properly and instruct client to avoid heavy lifting.
- Instruct client to avoid activities such as bowling or horseback riding that may cause vertebral compression and further injury.
- Teach client that swimming, bicycling, low-impact aerobics, and weight training are excellent exercises for preventing osteoporosis.

Pharmacology

- Calcium supplements
- Vitamin D supplements
- Hormone replacement therapy
- Analgesics (opioid or non-opioid)
- Bisphosphonates derivatives: alendronate, risedronate
- Diphosphonate (etidronate)
- Calcitonin
- Selective estrogen receptor modulators: raloxifene
- Parathyroid hormone: teriparatide, injectable only used in severe cases
- Vertebroplasty/kyphoplasty - gluing of osteoporotic fractures

Complications

- Spontaneous fractures
- Pain
- Deformity
- Respiratory compromise

Age-Related Changes—Gerontological Considerations

- Forward thrusting of the head and neck in elderly clients with osteoporosis is due to increased thoracic spine convexity (Dowager's hump).
- Reduction in estrogen production increases the risk of osteoporosis in older women and men, although increase of osteoporosis in men is also due to decrease in testosterone production with age.
- Decreased bone formation and increased bone resorption are factors in the development of osteoporosis in older clients.

- Because older clients tolerate back braces poorly, insure that braces and other assistive devices fit properly and are comfortable.
- Assess elderly clients who are taking NSAIDs for gastrointestinal bleeding and heart failure.
- Loss of height from bone resorption and osteoporotic fractures of the spine.

Critical Thinking Exercise: Nursing Management of the Client with Osteoporosis

Situation: The client is a 50-year-old secretary at a local high school. She has just been diagnosed with osteoporosis based on bone density studies that revealed approximately 30% bone demineralization.

1. List three questions appropriate for the nurse to ask the client regarding her risk factors for osteoporosis.

2. Which of the following activities is most beneficial for the client? Rank in priority with "1" representing the most beneficial.

   _____ Swimming

   _____ Yoga

   _____ Walking

   _____ Tennis

3. The client asks the nurse about taking antacids since they contain calcium. What information is most important for the nurse to give the client in this regard?

Nursing Management of the Client with a Fracture

Key Points

- Fractures occur when bone is subjected to greater stress than it can endure.
- Adjacent structures are affected when bones are fractured.
- Osteoporosis and chronic corticosteroid use are important causes of fracture.
- Goals of collaborative management:
  - Prevent hemorrhage.
  - Prevent deformity and/or loss of function.
  - Prevent complications (fat embolism, neurovascular compromise, deep vein thrombosis).
  - Relieve pain.
  - Support healing process.
  - Maintain urine and bowel elimination.
- Important nursing diagnoses (actual or potential):
  - Pain management
  - Impaired physical mobility
  - Activity intolerance
  - Knowledge deficit
  - Risk for injury
  - Impairment of skin integrity
  - Impaired home maintenance
  - Constipation and other bowel dysfunctions
- **Key Terms/Concepts**: Non-union, acute compartment syndrome (ACS), bone demineralization

Overview

A fracture is a break in bone continuity that occurs when the force exerted on the bone exceeds the strength of the surface to resist the stress. Fractures are accompanied by localized tissue inflammation and muscle spasm. Fractures occur directly from trauma or indirectly from disease. Types of fractures are comminuted, complete, compound (open) compression, greenstick, incomplete and simple (closed).

Risk Factors

- Trauma
- High-risk lifestyle (participation in high-risk sporting activities)
- Malnutrition

- Osteoporosis
- Advanced age
- Decreased circulation
- Immunocompromised status
- Presence of infection (systemic or osteomyelitis)
- Neoplasms
- Corticosteroid therapy
- Cushing's syndrome+
- Falls
- Abuse, physical

Types of Fractures

- **Comminuted**: The bone is splintered or broken into several fragments.
- **Complete**: The bone is completely separated by a break into two parts.
- **Compound (open)**: The skin is broken with or without protrusion of the bone.
- **Compression**: The fractured bone is compressed by another bone.
- **Greenstick**: One side of the bone is fractured and the other side is bent. Commonly occurs in children. (The name for this fracture comes from the analogy of breaking a young, fresh tree branch. The broken branch snaps on one side [the outer side of the bend], while the inner side is bent, and still in continuity.)
- **Incomplete**: The break is partially through the width of the bone.
- **Simple (closed)**: The bone is fractured but the skin is intact.

Signs and Symptoms

- Pain or tenderness over involved area
- Loss of motion
- Crepitus (grating sound when bone is manipulated)
- Obvious deformity
- Edema
- Muscle spasm
- Impaired sensation
- Loss of pulse distal to the fracture
- Protruding bone from the skin
- Damage to underlying structures such as muscles, blood vessels, nerves, tendons, and ligaments.
- Ecchymosis (a subcutaneous collection of blood greater than 1 cm in size outside the vascular tree, and within tissue).
- Shortening of extremity
- Note that with lumbar/sacral fractures there may be loss of bladder or bowel function. With C3 and higher fractures there will likely be an inability to breathe with paraplegia or quadriplegia.

Diagnostic and Laboratory Tests

- History and physical examination
- X-rays
- Bone scans
- Magnetic resonance imaging (MRI)

Therapeutic Nursing Management

- **Prevention:**
  - Avoidance of high-risk activities (e.g., sky diving, high impact sports, rollerblading)
  - Avoidance of safety hazards, especially for older people (e.g., throw rugs, pets under foot, untreated vision problems, side effects of medication)
  - Regular exercise, which strengthens muscles and helps coordination
- **Assess/Monitor client for:**
  - General physical condition
  - Development of respiratory distress, cervical fractures and/or rib fractures
  - Indications of shock
  - Trauma to other body systems
  - Skin color and temperature of injured limb compared with non-injured limb
  - Sensation and movement of injured limb compared with non-injured limb
  - Ecchymosis
  - Swelling of tissues
  - Bleeding
  - Hemorrhage if open fracture
  - Muscle spasms
  - Pain: location, nature, and frequency
  - Pulses distal to injury
  - Elevated temperature
  - Compartment syndrome (worsening pain in extremity, fullness, swelling, tenseness)
  - Anxiety or fear
- **Assess/Monitor casted extremity for:**
  - Foul odor
  - Drainage
  - "Hot spots"
  - Paleness or cyanosis
  - Numbness and tingling
  - Increased pain and burning under cast
  - Change in temperature from warm to cold
  - Pulselessness
  - Excessive edema above or below the cast
  - Decreased movement

- **Assess/Monitor client in a spica body cast for:**
  - Nausea
  - Vomiting
  - Abdominal pain
- **Assess/Monitor client for acute compartment syndrome (ACS)**
  - Increasing pain that is unrelieved by opioid analgesia
  - Increase pain with stretching of the muscle compartment
  - Paresthesias
  - Taut skin over the injured area
- **Nursing Activities:**
  - Provide emergency treatment.
  - Immobilize without altering the position of the deformity.
  - Cover a protruding bone with a sterile dressing or clean cloth.
  - Control bleeding if present.
  - Elevate the limb and apply ice to reduce swelling
  - Administer pain medication as prescribed.
  - Recheck the client's neurovascular status at frequent intervals
  - Prepare client for realignment of bone fragments through casting, splinting, traction, or surgery.
  - Provide care for the client in a cast.
    - Position client so that warm, dry air circulates around and under the cast (support the casted area without pressure under or directly on the cast) for faster drying and to prevent pressure from changing the shape of the cast.
    - Use gloves to touch the cast until cast is completely dry.
    - If any drainage is seen on the cast it should be outlined, dated, and timed so it can be monitored for any additional drainage.
    - Elevate cast above the level of heart during the first 24-48 hours to prevent swelling.
    - "Petal" the cast by placing tape over rough edges to prevent skin irritation.
    - Cut a window in the cast if the client has a wound under the cast so that healthcare providers can assess and care for the wound.
    - If the leg is casted, support foot at a 90-degree flexion angle to prevent foot drop.
    - Observe for and report complications from the cast which include infection, pressure necrosis, circulatory impairment, contracture of joint, muscle atrophy, thrombophlebitis, and thromboembolism.
    - Monitor for neurovascular impairment by assessing for the 5 P's:
  - Progressive pain
  - Pulselessness
  - Paralysis
  - Pallor
  - Paresthesia (numbness and tingling)

- Report these findings immediately to the primary care provider.
- Instruct client with a cast to:
- Exercise joints above and below cast to maintain strength and mobility.
- Inspect skin around cast daily.
- Continue to place adhesive tape over rough edges of cast, as needed.
- Avoid getting the cast wet.
- Avoid dropping articles down into the cast.
- Call primary care provider, or whoever puts cast on, if cast cracks or breaks.
  - Instruct client following cast removal to:
- Remove scaly skin by soaking; avoid scrubbing the area.
- Start a graduated exercise program under supervision of physical therapy department.
- Wear support stockings or elastic bandages on lower extremities to reduce swelling.
  - Provide care for the client in traction.
  - Encourage a diet high in protein and vitamins to promote healing.
  - Encourage isometric exercises to promote muscle tone and strength.
  - Teach appropriate crutch-walking technique as needed.
  - Arrange for follow-up appointments with primary care provider, physical therapist, and social workers if injury has created a job loss or financial problems.

Pharmacology

- Analgesics (use opioids with caution related to respiratory depression)
- Local anesthetics for intercostal nerve block
- Antibiotics (compound fractures, surgical reduction)
- Muscle relaxants: carisoprodol (Soma), cyclobenzaprine (Flexeril), methocarbamol (Robaxin), etc.
- NSAIDs (nonsteroidal anti-inflammatory drugs) for pain and/or swelling
- Acetaminophen for pain, lesser
- Vitamin supplements (especially vitamins C, B, and D) as needed
- Calcium supplements/vitamin D as needed

Complications

- Non-union
- Delayed-union
- Vascular necrosis
- Osteomyelitis
- Paresthesia
- Fat embolism
- Shock
- Infection

- Avascular necrosis
- Deep vein thrombosis
- Acute compartment syndrome (ACS)
- Cast syndrome
- Nerve damage
- Puncture of the lungs, heart or arteries by bone fragments associated with rib fractures

Rib Fracture (most common blunt injury)

- Signs and Symptoms
  - Pain at the site which worsens with inspiration
  - Shallow breathing
  - Splinting of the area of injury with movement, sneezing, laughing, etc.
  - Pain on palpation of the area of injury (may have crepitus on palpation site)
- Diagnostics/Lab Tests
  - History and physical assessment
  - X-ray
- Therapeutic Nursing Management/Client Education
  - No strenuous activity for several days or until rechecked
  - Deep breathing exercises every hour to prevent respiratory complications
  - Use analgesics as ordered, contact the primary care provider if they are not affective when taken as ordered to relieve pain
  - Assist with intercostal nerve blocks performed with local anesthesia for pain relief.
  - Use narcotics for pain relief with caution because narcotics decrease respirations.
  - Assist the client in finding the most comfortable position, generally clients are able to breathe more easily in the Fowler's or semi-Fowlers position
  - Go to the emergency department promptly or notify admitting physician immediately for:
    - Assess/monitor for signs and/or symptoms of pneumothorax/hemothorax:
  - Increased or sudden difficulties in breathing
  - Spitting up or coughing up blood
  - Sudden, sharp, or increased chest pain (without explanation)
- Pharmacology
  - Analgesics
- Complications
  - Hemothorax
  - Pneumothorax
  - Laceration of the liver
  - Atelectasis (from poor lung expansion due to pain)

Hip Fracture

- Hip fractures are the leading cause of hospitalizations for injuries and fractures in older adults.

- Hip fractures are most common in older women with osteoporosis.

- As many as 36% of older clients who have hip fractures die within one year following the fracture. Death may be due to medical complications caused by the fracture or due to the complications of immobility; for example pneumonia. Only 50% of elderly clients are able to resume an independent life after a hip fracture.

- **Types of hip fractures**:
  - Intracapsular fractures that occur within the hip joint.
  - Extracapsular fractures that occur outside the joint capsule. These types of fractures usually result from severe direct trauma of a fall.

- **Signs and Symptoms**:
  - External rotation
  - Shortening of the affected extremity
  - Severe pain and tenderness in the area of the fracture
  - Avascular necrosis caused by disruption of the blood supply to the head of the femur.

- **Basic Therapeutic Nursing Management**
  - Surgical repair is the treatment of choice for hip fractures
  - Prior to surgery, the client's limb may be immobilized by Buck's traction for 24 to 48 hours. Buck's traction helps to relieve painful muscle spasms while the client's condition stabilizes sufficiently to permit surgery.
  - Intracapsular (femur neck) fractures are usually repaired by hemiarthroplasty which involves replacement of the femoral head.
  - Extracapsular fractures are repaired with replacement prostheses, fixed nail plates, sliding nail plates, and intramedullary devices.

- **Preoperative Management and Teaching**:
  - Evaluate and stabilize chronic health problems such as diabetes mellitus, hypertension, pulmonary disease, congestive heart failure, and arthritis.
  - Control painful muscle spasms.
  - Teach clients how to use the overhead trapeze and opposite side rails to turn and move
  - Teach client how to perform out of bed and chair transfers.
  - Begin discharge planning as soon as possible.

- **Postoperative Management and Teaching**:
  - Monitor vital signs, intake and output, pain control, respiratory exercises, and assess the incision for bleeding or infection.
  - Begin ambulating the client on the first or second day with the help of the physical therapist.
  - Encourage the client to use the overhead trapeze when preparing to ambulate.
  - If the fracture was treated with the insertion of a femoral head prosthesis,

take measures to prevent positions that cause hip dislocation. Remind the client not to put on shoes and socks, cross the legs or feet when sitting, sit on low toilet seats, or incorrectly assume a side-lying position.

- If the fracture was treated with pinning, the client will not need to observe dislocation precautions. Weight bearing on the involved leg may be restricted for six to 12 weeks, until x-ray indicates that the fracture has healed adequately.

- **Complications**
  - Nonunion
  - Avascular necrosis
  - Hip dislocation
  - Degenerative arthritis
  - Depression
- **Discharging the Client:**
  - The client must be able to safely use crutches or a walker, transfer into and out of the chair and go up and down stairs to go home.
  - Discharge the client, if necessary, to a subacute unit or rehabilitation center.
  - Arrange for follow-up home care nursing.

Age-Related Changes—Gerontological Considerations

- Increased bone resorption and decreased bone formation lead to the development of osteoporosis and fractures in elderly clients.
- High incidence of osteoporosis occurs in this population, bones become porous and brittle.
- Progressive bone demineralization prolongs healing.
- There is a tendency toward joint stiffness in older clients.
- Muscle mass and strength decrease with age.
- Mobility and range of motion (ROM) is decreased.
- Falling is the most common cause of musculoskeletal injury and fractures in older adults.
- Hip fractures are the leading cause of hospitalizations for injuries in the older adult population.
- Due to a decrease in subcutaneous tissue and fragility of skin, elderly clients are at a higher risk for ulceration/irritation from a cast or splint than younger clients. Instruction in skin assessment should be provided to the client and the family/significant others that may be care providers. The nurse should assess the skin frequently.

Critical Thinking Exercise: Nursing Management of the Client with a Fracture

Situation: A 29-year-old man was admitted to the emergency department for injuries suffered in an automobile accident. Physical examination and radiological studies reveal a fractured left femur just above his knee. The skin is broken, but there is no evidence of bone protrusion. A sterile dressing is covering the open wound.

1. Match the fractures with their correct description:

One part of the bone is compressed by another.	a. Complete
A break is partially through the bone width.	b. Incomplete
One side of the bone is fractured, while the other side is bent.	c. Compound
The bone is broken into two parts and separated.	d. Comminuted
The bone is broken into fragments or splintered.	e. Compression
A bone is fractured beneath intact skin.	f. Simple
A bone is fractured and protrudes through the skin.	g. Greenstick

2. Mark the subjective data with an "S" and the objective data with an "O."

_____ Bone protrusion _____ Impaired sensation

_____ Loss of pulse distal to the fracture _____ Tenderness over affected site

_____ Shortening of the extremity _____ Muscle spasms

3. Prioritize the nursing interventions for this client, with "1" representing the most important intervention.

_____ Immobilize the limb without altering its position.

_____ Control bleeding if present.

_____ Assess pain status.

_____ Assess for other possible problems (internal injuries, head injury, etc.).

_____ Obtain vital signs.

_____ Assist with preparation for cast or surgery as indicated.

Nursing Management of the Client with Total Hip Replacement

Key Points

- Total hip replacement is the most common implant surgery performed.
- Approximately 200,000 total hip replacements are performed in the United States yearly and more than one million are performed internationally.
- Prostheses for hip replacement may be cemented (bone cement holds the prosthesis to the bone), or uncemented (prosthesis is porous, which allows bone to grow into the prosthesis).
- Goals of collaborative management:
  - Provide preoperative preparation and teaching.
  - Prepare the home for client's return following surgery.
  - Prevent postoperative complications.
  - Prevent hip prostheses dislocation.
  - Promote physical rehabilitation and increased mobility following discharge.
- Important nursing diagnoses (actual or potential):
  - Pain management
  - Risk of infection
  - Impaired physical mobility
  - Impaired skin integrity
  - Ineffective management of therapeutic regimen
- **Key Terms/Concepts**: Hip prosthesis, osteoarthritis, joint mobility, arthroscopic examinations, thrombophlebitis, pulmonary embolism, prosthesis dislocation, assistive devices

Overview

Total hip replacement (arthroplasty) is orthopedic surgery that involves removal of the head of the femur followed by the placement of a prosthetic implant. This procedure restores motion to the hip joint and helps to eliminate pain. Prosthetic implants may be "cemented" in place with polymethylmethacrylate which promotes bonding of the prosthesis to the bone. Cemented replacements may loosen in approximately 10 years, requiring the client to undergo more surgery. Younger clients may receive "cementless" replacements to prolong the lifetime of the prosthesis and thus avoid additional surgery.

Risk Factors

- Over 40 years of age
- Chronic joint stress
- Joint abnormalities

- Osteoarthritis
- Obesity
- Lack of physical activity
- Genetic predisposition
- Congenital deformities or dislocations
- Demanding physical occupations such as carpet installation and farming
- History of endocrine, metabolic or inflammatory disease such as rheumatoid arthritis
- Poor posture
- Avascular necrosis (risk factors: alcoholism, corticosteroids, or idiopathic)

Signs and Symptoms Necessitating Surgery

- Severe, chronic pain in the joint
- Loss of joint function and mobility
- Extensive joint destruction
- Infection in the joint
- Contractures
- Sustained fractures

Diagnostic and Laboratory Tests

- History and physical examination
- Complete blood count with differential
- X-rays
- Magnetic resonance imaging (MRI)
- Computed tomography (CT)/computed axial tomography (CAT) scan
- Arthroscopic exam
- Urinalysis

Therapeutic Nursing Management

- **Prevention of osteoarthritis necessitating surgery:**
  - Encourage client to lose weight.
  - Encourage range of motion exercises up to the point of pain.
  - Encourage maintenance of an active exercise program unless inflammation is severe.
  - Encourage good posture and use of appropriate body mechanics.
  - Teach client how to reduce stress on joints.
  - Teach client to avoid or correct hazards in the home such as throw rugs, pets underfoot, and poor lighting.
- **Assess/Monitor:**
  - Vital signs
  - Complete blood count (CBC) with differential

- Drainage from dressing and Hemovac drains
- Use of anticoagulants and antiplatelet medications to prevent thromboemboli
- Affected leg every one-to-two hours for movement, sensation, and circulation (CMS)
- Incision site for signs of infection
- Pain relief (on a scale from 0-10)
- For indications of thrombophlebitis
- For indications of pulmonary embolism
- For indications of hip prosthesis dislocation or loosening

- **Nursing Actions in Addition to Routine Preoperative and Postoperative Care:**
  - Teach client how to walk with crutches or walker prior to surgery.
  - Teach client how to transfer from bed to chair prior to surgery. Instruct client to stand on the unaffected leg and pivot into the chair without bearing weight on the affected leg.
  - Discuss turning and positioning with surgeon prior to surgery.
  - Following surgery, use abduction pillow when available.
  - Elevate the operative leg and apply ice packs as prescribed.
  - Administer an autotransfusion of salvaged perioperative blood within 4 hours of surgery as ordered, with subsequent blood transfusions as needed, typically on the 2nd to 3rd postoperative day.
  - Administer epoetin (Epogen, Procrit) as ordered for anemia.
  - Place affected leg in abducted position and straight alignment following surgery.
  - Prevent hip flexion of more than 90 degrees.
  - Keep client's operative leg extended, supported and elevated when getting client out of bed.
  - Apply support stockings.
  - Administer pain medication prior to activities.
  - Supervise exercises as ordered.
  - If a client has had a total knee replacement, have the client use a continuous passive motion machine for 8 to 12 hours a day post implantation, gradually increasing the client's range of motion from the initial setting. This machine will keep the knee in motion and help to prevent the formation of scar tissue
  - Instruct client to avoid internal/external rotation of the affected leg for 6 months to 1 year following surgery.
  - Instruct client to not cross legs.
  - Instruct client to not twist to reach behind or bend over to pick up objects from the floor.
  - Arrange for home health nurse to assess the client's home for safety prior to discharge.
  - Scatter rubs and dangling electric cords that can cause falls should be removed

- Small pets that can cause falls may need to be boarded.
- Bathroom and bedroom need to be on the first floor.
- Door frames should be wide enough to accommodate a walker.
- Meals on Wheels or a housekeeper and cook may be needed if client lives alone.
- Elevated toilet seats should be installed in client's bathroom.
- Instruct client to avoid sitting in one place for more than 1 hour.
- Remind client to avoid excessive bending, heavy lifting, jogging, and jumping.
- Encourage use of crutches or a walker until full weight bearing is safe.
- Encourage use of adaptive equipment for everyday activities.
- Encourage intake of foods high in vitamin C, and protein, possibly iron if blood loss.
- Arrange for follow-up visits with orthopedic surgeon and primary care provider.
- Remind client to tell technicians about the prosthesis if scheduled for an MRI.
- Have client carry a card verifying presence of the prosthesis, as metal may set off alarms at airports and in security buildings.
- Teach client to assess for and report signs of prosthesis dislocation such as hip pain, shortening of the affected leg and leg rotation.

Pharmacology

- Analgesics: morphine sulfate (MS), meperidine (Demerol)
- Nonsteroidal anti-inflammatory drugs (NSAIDS): Ibuprofen (Advil, Motrin), etc.
- Prophylactic antibiotics: cefazolin (Ancef, Kefzol)
- Anticoagulants: warfarin (Coumadin)
- Low molecular weight heparins: enoxaparin (Lovenox), dalteparin (Fragmin)
- Blood transfusions
- Recombinant human erythropoietin: epoetin (Epogen, Procrit)

Complications

- Wound infection
- Pneumonic
- Hemorrhage
- Thrombophlebitis
- Anemia
- Pulmonary embolism
- Prosthesis dislocation
- Prosthesis loosening

Age-Related Changes—Gerontological Considerations

- Older clients are at greater risk of developing osteoarthritis.
- Older clients have prolonged healing of bones and joints.
- Elderly clients may require rehabilitation in an extended care facility.

Critical Thinking Exercise: Nursing Management of the Client with Total Hip Replacement

Situation: A 72-year-old male client is being discharged home from the hospital following hip replacement surgery. In addition to the prevention of other complications, the staff has made every effort to prevent deep vein thrombosis and pulmonary embolism; the two most common causes of postoperative mortality in older clients. Prior to discharge, the nurse gives the client a list of instructions for positioning, sitting, and ambulating at home. The client is also instructed to use a walker or crutches until weight-bearing is safe, and to employ adaptive devices for everyday activities. Finally, the client is advised to watch for any signs of hip prosthesis loosening or dislocation, and to call the surgeon immediately if such signs occur.

1. Which are the signs and symptoms of deep vein thrombosis?

_____ Pain in the area of thrombus

_____ Fever >101.0° F

_____ Swelling proximal to the site of thrombus

_____ Pallor and cool extremity

_____ Positive Homan's sign

2. Which are the signs and symptoms of pulmonary embolism?

_____ Hemoptysis   _____ Respiratory alkalosis

_____ Bradycardia   _____ Apprehension

_____ Dyspnea   _____ Cough

_____ Subnormal body temperature   _____ Diaphoresis

_____ Respiratory crackles   _____ Pneumothorax

_____ Pleuric pain   _____ Hyperventilation

_____ Cyanosis

3. List several types of adaptive equipment useful for clients who have undergone hip replacement surgery.

4. Which are signs of prosthetic hip dislocation?

_____ Leg shortening

_____ Hypermobility of affected leg

_____ Abnormal rotation

_____ Malalignment

_____ Extremity numbness

5. What measures can be taken to prevent prosthetic hip dislocation?

Nursing Management of the Client Requiring Traction

Key Points

- Properly applied traction is beneficial for maintaining bone alignment.
- Improperly applied traction can harm bones, tissues, and nerves.
- Goals of collaborative management:
    - Promote healing.
    - Prevent injury (tissue necrosis, nerve damage).
    - Restore function.
    - Prevent deformity.
    - Reduce pain.
- Important nursing diagnoses (actual or potential):
    - Impaired physical mobility
    - Pain management
    - Impairment of skin integrity
    - Potential complications of traction (thrombophlebitis, tissue necrosis, nerve damage, infection)
    - Knowledge deficit
- **Key Terms/Concepts**: Counterbalance, anti-inflammatory, alignment

Overview

- **Traction** is a mechanical intervention designed to align bone fragments through the use of weights and pulleys. Traction is also used to keep body parts in anatomical alignment so that healing can occur (e.g., pelvic belt for herniated disk).
- **Skin traction**: Applied directly to the skin by bandages or adhesives.
    - **Buck's traction**: Used to alleviate muscles spasms; immobilizes a lower limb by maintaining a straight pull on the limb with the use of weights (often used with hip fractures prior to surgery).
    - **Cervical skin traction**: Relieves muscle spasms and compression in the upper extremities and neck: uses a head halter and a chin pad to attach the traction.
    - **Bryant's skin traction**: Used to stabilize a fractured femur or correct a congenital hip dislocation in children.
    - **Russell's skin traction**: Used to stabilize a fractured femur before surgery; similar to Buck's traction but provides a double pull with the use of a knee sling.
    - **Pelvic skin traction**: Used to relieve low back, hip, or leg pain and to reduce muscle spasm.

- **Skeletal traction**: Mechanically applied to the bone with pins, wires, or tongs.
- **Balanced suspension traction:**
  - Used with skin or skeletal traction
  - Used with approximate fractures of the femur, tibia, or fibula
- Produced by counterforce other than the client
- Allows for some bodily movement without disrupting the alignment

Risk Factors

- Osteoporosis
- Advanced age
- Immobility
- Hip fracture
- Cervical fracture
- Skull fracture
- Low back pain

Therapeutic Nursing Management

- **Assess/Monitor:**
  - Color, movement, capillary refill, and sensation of affected limb
  - Skin for signs of breakdown
  - Pin insertion sites for signs of infection such as purulent drainage, pain, severe redness and inflammation.
  - For complications of immobilization (renal calculi, constipation, deep vein thrombosis, pneumonia)
  - For pain due to muscle spasms
- **Nursing Activities:**
  - Maintain asepsis when cleaning pin insertion sites.
  - Clean pin sites with sterile normal saline and hydrogen peroxide or povidone iodine per agency protocol.
  - Maintain body alignment and realign if the client seems uncomfortable or reports pain.
  - Countertraction is provided by the client's body weight and must be maintained at all times (the body should be in good alignment without touching the foot of the bed).
  - Avoid lifting or removing weights.
  - Assure that weights hang freely.
  - If the weights are accidentally displaced, replace the weights. If the problem is not corrected, notify the primary care provider or orthopedic technician.
  - Assure that pulley ropes are free of knots and linen.
  - Implement care for client with a fracture.

- Notify primary care provider if client experiences severe pain from muscle spasms unrelieved with medications, repositioning, and/or other medications.
- Perform a neurovascular assessment every eight hours.
- Remove belts, boots, and halters as permitted; at least every 8 hours to inspect the client's skin for signs of irritation, inflammation, or breakdown.
- Consult with primary care provider and physical therapist to institute an exercise program.
- Change client's position every 2 hours.
- Assist client with range of motion (ROM) exercises of unaffected joints several times a day.
- Encourage client to perform deep breathing exercises to prevent respiratory complications.
- Ask the client to use a trapeze bar (if allowed) to raise self off the bed, during linen changes and to use the bedpan.
- Document the length of time the client is in traction, the client's position in bed and the status of the traction setup, including the amount of weights.
- Make certain that the weights are hanging freely.
- Document the client's response to traction.
- Instruct client's family in the care of the client following discharge.
- Arrange for a home health care nurse to assess the client and assist the family with problems and concerns.

Pharmacology

- Analgesics: morphine sulfate (MS), meperidine (Demerol)
- Nonsteroidal anti-inflammatory drugs (NSAIDs): Ibuprofen (Advil, Motrin), ketorolac (Toradol), naproxen (Naprosyn), diclofenac (Cataflam)
- Antibiotics if client develops infection
- Topical antimicrobial agents for clients in skeletal traction for pins
- Muscle relaxants: cyclobenzaprine (Flexeril), carisoprodol (Soma), etc.

Complications

- Compromised skin integrity
- Osteomyelitis
- Infection
- Constipation
- Thrombophlebitis
- Renal calculi
- Pneumonia
- Pulmonary embolism

Age-Related Changes—Gerontological Considerations

- Increased bone resorption and decreased bone formation lead to the development of osteoporosis.
- A high incidence of osteoporosis occurs in this population; bones become porous and brittle.
- Progressive bone demineralization prolongs healing.
- Tendency toward joint stiffness.
- Muscle mass and strength decrease with age.
- Mobility and ROM (range of motion) is decreased.
- Falling is the most common cause of musculoskeletal injury and fractures in older adults.
- Hip fractures are the leading cause of hospitalization for injuries in the older adult population.
- Higher incidence of skin integrity complications with impaired mobility.
- Traction puts elderly clients at risk of pneumonia and pulmonary embolism due to prolonged immobilization.
- Traction may damage the skin and tissues of elderly clients due to decreased circulation to tissues and sensory deficits.

Critical Thinking Exercise: Nursing Management of the Client Requiring Traction

Situation: An 88-year-old man fractured his right hip when he fell on his icy driveway. His right femur is stabilized with balanced suspension skeletal traction. He has a Thomas ring with Pearson attachment and 25 pounds traction on his right leg and 8 pounds of traction on the balanced suspension. The client is receiving oral codeine every 3-4 hours for pain.

1. What assessments does the nurse need to make in regard to each of the following:

    a. Client

    b. Ropes

    c. Pulleys

    d. Weights

2. What signs will alert the nurse the client is developing a wound infection at the pin insertion site?

3. What is the etiology of the nursing diagnoses of the client?

    a. Pain

    b. Risk for constipation

    c. Risk for impaired skin integrity

4. What can the nurse do to prevent skin alterations in any person who is immobilized due to traction?

Nursing Management of the Client with an Amputation

| Key Points |

- Amputation can result from trauma or disease.
- Amputation requires significant physiological and psychosocial adjustments.
- Prosthetic devices allow many clients to regain mobility and function.
- Goals of collaborative management:
  - Reduce pain (actual and phantom).
  - Restore mobility and function.
  - Prevent complications (infection, delayed healing, gangrene, contracture, shock, hemorrhage).
  - Provide early rehabilitation.
- Important nursing diagnoses (actual or potential):
  - Potential complications of amputation (infection, contracture, hemorrhage, shock)
  - Alteration in skin integrity
  - Impaired mobility
  - Pain (actual and phantom)
  - Ineffective individual coping
  - Anxiety and fear
  - Altered family role
  - Altered role at work
  - Depression and psychologic imbalance
  - Dysfunctional grieving
- **Key Terms/Concepts**: Phantom pain

Overview

Amputation is the surgical removal of a limb or part of a limb. Upper extremity amputations are most commonly due to trauma, congenital malformation, or malignancy. Lower extremity amputations are most commonly associated with severe peripheral vascular disease, infection, trauma, congenital deformity, or complicated diabetes mellitus.

Risk Factors

- Diabetes mellitus
- Peripheral vascular disorders
- Arterial insufficiency

- Smoking
- Hypertension
- Hyperlipidemia
- Obesity
- Advanced age
- Malignancy
- Infection (osteomyelitis)
- Trauma (car, motorcycle, or industrial accident)
- Hazardous working conditions

Signs and Symptoms Necessitating Amputation

- Loss of sensation
- Loss of peripheral pulse
- Impaired circulation
- Necrosis
- Gangrene
- Sepsis

Diagnostic and Laboratory Tests

- History and physical exam
- Complete blood count (CBC)
- Ankle/brachial index (determined by dividing ankle systolic pressure by brachial systolic pressure)
- Plethysmography
- Ultrasound
  - 2D (2-dimensional)
  - 3D (3-dimensional)
  - Doppler
- International Normalized Ratio (INR) coagulation studies, as indicated

Therapeutic Nursing Management

- **Assess/Monitor:**
  - Vital signs
  - Distal pulses
  - For insufficient tissue perfusion of affected limb (skin flap color and temperature)
  - For signs of hemorrhage
  - For stump pain
  - For phantom pain
  - For signs of infection such as purulent drainage from wound; fever

- For inflammation (redness and swelling)
- For skin irritation
- **Nursing Activities:**
  - Provide preoperative preparation.
  - Initiate muscle-strengthening exercises.
  - Administer pain medications as prescribed.
  - Teach client about phantom pain and medicate as needed.
  - Perform soft dressing changes until the sutures are removed to keep the incision site clean and dry.
  - Provide residual limb care:
    - Maintain Ace wrap or elastic stump shrinker as prescribed.
    - Wrap the stump distal to proximal to reduce the amount of edema in the stump. Instruct the client and family members/significant others in the proper way to wrap the stump. Stump wrapping or a shrinker bandage is used to minimize edema and shape the stump appropriately.
    - Maintain clean, dry surgical wound until healed.
    - Apply lanolin to dry skin.
    - Progressively apply pressure to end of limb to toughen it.
    - Encourage movement of affected limb.
    - Encourage client to participate in care of limb.
    - Maintain alignment to prevent contractures.
    - Encourage movement of affected limb.
    - Have client perform range of motion exercises on all joints daily as allowed.
    - Do not elevate affected limb on a pillow.
  - Assist with physical mobility and crutch walking.
  - Encourage client to assume a prone position for 30-60 minutes twice a day (if tolerated) to prevent flexion contracture of the hip.
  - Prior to discharge, refer client to a home health care service
  - Offer emotional support during adjustment to limb loss and prosthesis.
  - Allow expression of fears and concerns.
  - Instruct client and the family in the care of the affected limb and prosthesis. Teach client to:
    - Inspect affected limb every day for redness, irritation of skin, and abrasions.
    - Inspect areas that are vulnerable to pressure.
    - Stop use of the prosthesis and call the healthcare provider if affected limb becomes sore or irritated.
    - Wash the affected limb nightly with warm water and use a bacteriostatic soap. Gently rinse and dry the limb and then expose the limb to air for 20 minutes.
    - Wear limb socks that are supplied by the prosthetist and that are not worn or torn.

- Change the sock everyday. Launder socks with a mild soap and dry flat.
- For amputation of lower limbs have client lie prone daily to prevent contractures.
- Refer client to a vocational counselor if client needs to change jobs due to physical limitations.

Pharmacology

- Analgesics: morphine sulfate (MS), meperidine (Demerol)
- Antibiotics
- Bacteriostatic soap

Complications

- Infection
- Contractures
- Hip adduction contracture (rare)
- Skin irritation and breakdown
- Impaired mobility
- Pain
- Phantom pain
- Gangrene
- Delayed healing
- Hemorrhage
- Shock
- Depression

Age-Related Changes—Gerontological Considerations

- Older adults with arthritis may have difficulty applying their prosthesis.
- Some elderly or debilitated clients may not be able to adapt to a prosthesis and will need to use a wheelchair for mobility.
- Injury is more likely related to gait and sensory deficits.
- Older adults are more prone to infection and complications related to immobilization.
- Prolonged healing occurs due to compromised circulation and altered tissue perfusion.

Critical Thinking Exercise: Nursing Management of the Client with an Amputation

Situation: A 24-year-old male is twelve hours post-operation for a below-the-knee amputation of his right leg as treatment for osteogenic sarcoma. His stump is elevated on two pillows and the gauze and elastic dressings are dry and intact. His vital signs are stable and he is controlling his pain with morphine sulfate via a PCA (patient-controlled analgesia) pump.

1. What is the rationale for:

   a. Elevating the client's stump on a pillow for the first 24 hours post op?

   b. Progressively applying pressure to the end of the stump after the incision has healed?

2. Which postoperative assessments does the nurse need to make at least every 2 hours over a period of 12 hours following the client's amputation?

   _____ Client's ability to participate in own care

   _____ Presence and amount of drainage

   _____ The presence of fever

   _____ Signs of situational depression

   _____ Client's response to pain medication

   _____ Presence of stump swelling

   _____ Vital signs

3. The client complains he is experiencing pain in the foot that is no longer there. What is this type of pain called, why does it occur, and what can be done to relieve the pain?

Nursing Management of the Client with Osteoarthritis— Degenerative Joint Disease

Key Points

- Osteoarthritis is a chronic, progressive degenerative disease most commonly involving the hands and weight-bearing joints.
- The bone degeneration is a significant cause of knee, hip, and lower back pain.
- Goals of collaborative management:
    - Prevent disease.
    - Maintain joint mobility.
    - Reduce pain.
    - Prevent joint deformity.
    - Correct joint deformity (total joint replacement).
    - Halt disease progression.
- Important nursing diagnoses (actual or potential):
    - Pain management
    - Impaired mobility
    - Self-care deficit
    - Risk for injury
    - Knowledge deficit
    - Potential complications of drug therapy (gastritis, decreased renal function)
- **Key Terms/Concepts**: Chronic, degenerative, inflammatory, anti-inflammatory

Overview

Osteoarthritis is the progressive degeneration of joints. It is characterized by enzymatic destruction of articular cartilage in peripheral and axial joints. It is a non-inflammatory disease primarily affecting the weight bearing joints. It has no systemic effects. The cause is unknown; but may be secondary to trauma, overuse, infection, or chemicals.

Risk Factors

- Over 40 years of age
- Chronic joint stress
- Obesity
- Trauma
- Hematologic disorders
- Diabetic neuropathy

- Congenital bone or joint abnormalities
- History of endocrine, metabolic, or inflammatory disease
- Genetic predisposition
- Poor posture
- Prolonged corticosteroid use
- Repetitive physical activities

Signs and Symptoms

- Deep, aching joint pain occurring after exercise and relieved by rest
- Joint stiffness, swelling, and limited range of motion
- Joint deformity and instability
- Heberden's Nodes (Hard nodes or nodules or bony swellings which develop around the distal interphangeal joints).
- Bouchard's Nodes (Nodes similar to, but less common than Heberden's nodes, occurring on proximal interphalangeal joints).
- Aching joints related to temperature or humidity changes
- Bony growths at weight-bearing areas
- Early morning stiffness
- Crepitation

Diagnostic and Laboratory Tests

- History and physical exam
- X-rays
- Magnetic resonance imaging (MRI)
- Computed tomography (CT)/computed axial tomography (CAT) scan
- Arthroscopic exam
- Synovial fluid analysis
- Rheumatology profile-rheumatoid factor (RF), anti-nuclear antibody (ANA), Sedimentation rate (ESR), protein (CRP)

Therapeutic Nursing Management

- **Assess/Monitor**:
  - Pain status
  - Functional mobility
  - Dietary intake
  - Depression related to loss of mobility
- **Nursing Activities**:
  - Administer salicylates, NSAIDs (nonsteroidal anti-inflammatory drugs) as prescribed.
  - Teach regarding side effects of salicylates, NSAIDs, and other prescribed medications.

- Maintain functional alignment of joints.
- Immobilize affected joint as needed.
- Allow for adequate rest periods.
- Encourage ROM (range of motion) up to the point of pain.
- Assist with activities that produce pain.
- Encourage use of cane, crutches, or walker.
- Apply cold pack to acutely inflamed joints.
- Apply heat via shower, bath, or warm packs as prescribed.
- Emphasize the need for maintaining good posture and appropriate body mechanics.
- Encourage the use of a firm mattress.
- Encourage clients who are obese to lose weight.
- Encourage well-balanced diet.
- Encourage maintenance of active exercise program as prescribed.
- Discuss complementary and alternative therapies if the client is interested. Examples include movement therapies, herbal drugs, nutritional supplements such as glucosamine and chondroitin, acupuncture, yoga, guided imagery, chiropractics, and massage.
- Teach the need to limit exercise when inflammation is acute and severe.
- Prepare client for surgical procedure (osteotomy, total joint replacement) as needed.
- Provide emotional support and encouragement.

Pharmacology

- Analgesics (opioids and non opioids)
- Nonsteroidal anti-inflammatory drugs: (NSAIDs: diclofenac (Voltaren), ibuprofen (Motrin), naproxen (Aleve), nabumetone (Relafen), etc.
- Salicylates: acetylsalicylic acid (ASA)
- Hyaluronic acid (HA) Synvisc injections to treat osteoarthritis of knee
- Herbal products (alternative therapy), capsaicin cream
- Glucosamine and chondroitin (alternative therapies)
- Muscle relaxants: carisoprodol (Soma), cyclobenzaprine (Flexeril), methocarbamol (Robaxin), etc.
- Epidurals
- Intra-articular corticosteroid injections, no more than 3-4 per year or 12 per joint per lifetime.

Complications

- Partial or total joint dislocations
- Joint fractures
- Chronic pain
- Loss of joint mobility
- Contractures

Age-Related Changes—Gerontological Considerations

- Reduced range of motion during rotation and hyperextension of the hip joint is found in the elderly adult.
- Decreased bone formation and increased bone resorption occur with aging.
- Prolonged healing of bones and joints is related to the aging process.
- Elderly clients with local inflammation and effusion may benefit from injections of corticosteroids into painful joints.

Critical Thinking Exercise: Nursing Management of the Client with Osteoarthritis—Degenerative Joint Disease

Situation: A 57-year-old woman is being evaluated for possible total knee replacement as treatment for her chronic osteoarthritis. The client and two of her four siblings suffer from the same disease with varying degrees of pain and disability. The client is obese and leads a sedentary lifestyle because of her weight.

1. What are the most common risk factors for osteoarthritis?

2. Which pain characteristics are common for osteoarthritis?

_____ Joint stiffness   _____ Deep, aching pain

_____ Pain relieved by rest   _____ Warm, edematous joints

_____ Severe joint deformity   _____ Joint instability

_____ Morning stiffness   _____ Pain following exercise

3. What is the most likely etiology for each of the nursing diagnoses of the client?

   a. Pain

   b. Impaired mobility

   c. Risk for injury

   d. Knowledge deficit

4. Why is it important for clients with osteoarthritis to engage in active stretching exercises?

Nursing Management of the Client with a Head Injury

Key Points

- Skull fractures are often associated with brain injury.
- Head injuries may or may not be associated with hemorrhage.
- Cervical spine injury should always be suspected when head injury occurs.
- Goals of collaborative management:
    - Maintain airway, breathing, and circulation.
    - Maintain cerebral perfusion.
    - Maintain fluid and electrolyte balance.
    - Prevent complications.
    - Maintain cognitive function.
- Important nursing diagnoses (actual or potential):
    - Ineffective airway clearance
    - Potential complication of head injury (seizures, increased intracranial pressure)
    - Altered nutrition
    - Impaired skin integrity
    - Risk for injury
    - Ineffective family coping
- **Key Terms/Concepts**: Glasgow Coma Scale, decorticate, decerebrate, hemiparesis, hemiplegia, quadriplegia

Glasgow Coma Scale			
Eye Opening Response (E)	**Verbal response (V)**	**Motor Response (M)**	
4=Spontaneous	5=Normal Conversation	6=Normal	
3=To Voice	4=Disoriented Conversation	5=Localizes to pain	
2=To Pain	3=Words, but not coherent	4=Withdraws to pain	
1=None	2=No words, only sounds	3=Decorticate posture	
	1=None	2=Decerebrate	
		1=None	
			Total Score
?=E Score	?=V Score	?=M Score	= E+ V+M

Overview

Head injuries (craniocerebral trauma) are among the most frequent and serious of the neurological disorders. Head injuries include: fractures, concussions, contusions, and hematomas. Brain damage can result from secondary changes related to head trauma.

Risk Factors

- Motor vehicle accidents
- Sports injuries
- Assault
- Gunshot wounds
- Falls

Signs and Symptoms

- **Skull fracture**: Cerebrospinal fluid (CSF) leakage from nose or ear, presence of subdural hematoma, indications of increased intracranial pressure (ICP), or positive glucose on test strip.
- **Concussion**: Increased ICP, amnesia, hypotension
- **Contusion**: Increased ICP
- **Hematoma**: Increased ICP, nuchal rigidity, fixed dilated pupil on the affected side, papilledema, hemiparesis, hemiplegia, and leakage of CSF from ears or nose
- Signs of increased ICP include:
  - Decreased level of consciousness
  - Bradycardia
  - Change in respiratory pattern
  - Restlessness
  - Headache
  - Nausea
  - Vomiting
  - Rapid rise in body temperature
  - Widening pulse pressure
  - Increased systolic blood pressure
  - Weakness or paralysis
  - Visual or auditory disturbances
  - Seizures

Diagnostic and Laboratory Tests

- History and physical
- ABGs (arterial blood gases)
- Complete blood count (CBC)
- FBG (fasting blood glucose) (also called: FBS [fasting blood sugar])

- Serum electrolytes
- Magnetic resonance imaging (MRI)
- Computed tomography (CT)/computed axial tomography (CAT) scan
- Electroencephalogram (EEG) – Avoid caffeine and other stimulants prior to the procedure.
- Glasgow Coma Scale
- Cranial nerve testing

Therapeutic Nursing Management

- **Assess/Monitor:**
  - Respiratory status (breathing pattern, CO_2 levels)
  - Neurological status every 15 minutes until client is stable.
    - Vital signs
    - PERLA (Pupils Equal, Round, React to Light and Accommodation)
    - LOC (Loss Of Consciousness)
  - For signs of increased ICP (intracranial pressure)
  - For posturing (decorticate, decerebrate, flaccid)
  - For pain and restlessness
  - For indications of infection
- **Nursing Activities:**
  - Maintain c-spine stability until cleared by x-ray.
  - Maintain patent airway.
  - Elevate head to reduce intracranial pressure.
  - Implement seizure precautions.
  - Instruct client to avoid coughing.
  - Report presence of cerebrospinal fluid (CSF) from nose or ears to client's practitioner.
  - Administer pain medications as ordered in the absence of increased ICP (avoid opioids such as morphine sulfate because it produces respiratory depression, pupillary changes, nausea, and central nervous system clouding).
  - Maintain client safety (side rails up, padded side rails).
  - Provide emotional support.
  - Implement measures to prevent complications of immobility (turn every two hours, footboard and splints).
  - Prepare client for cranial surgery if indicated.

Cranial (Brain) Surgery

- Various procedures can be used for cranial surgery. Options include:
  - Drilling a burr hole
  - Creating a small or large bone flap to permit access to the affected area.
    - Intracranial hemorrhages require surgical evacuation.

- Bleeding that is caused by an aneurysm is treated surgically with clipping or wrapping procedures to excise or support the weakened vessel.
- Preoperative care:
  - Educate the client and family about the procedure.
  - Limit the amount of information you provide the client if the client is very confused.
  - Inform the client that all or part of his/her scalp hair will be shaved.
  - Ensure that consent was obtained either from the client or from a family member who has authority to make decisions for the client, or from both.
- Postoperative care
  - Monitor the client's vital signs, level of consciousness, pupils, motor activity, sensory perception, and verbal responses at frequent intervals.
  - Monitor fluid and electrolyte values and osmolarity to detect changes in sodium regulation, the onset of diabetes insipidus, or severe hypovolemia.
  - Provide adequate fluids to maintain cerebral perfusion. When large amount of IV fluids are ordered, monitor the client carefully for excess fluid volume.
  - Assess for and prevent intracranial pressure; i.e., keep head midline, head of bed elevated, etc.
  - Report any signs of deterioration to the surgeon immediately.
  - Inspect all drainage for bleeding and CSF leakage.
  - Assess the dressing for odor, color and amount of drainage, and check all drains for placement.
  - Clean the scalp with povidone iodine (Betadine) or another antiseptic disinfectant to prevent infections. Then apply an antibiotic ointment.
  - Use an antiseptic soap to wash the scalp once the dressing is removed.
  - Provide the client with wigs, scarves, or turbans to wear once the incision has completely healed.
- Goals following cranial surgery are similar to those for a client who has a head injury and increased intracranial pressure.
  - Nursing diagnoses:
    - Impaired gas exchange
    - Sensory-perceptual alterations
    - Impaired mobility
    - Impaired verbal communication
    - Body image disturbance
    - Self-care deficits
    - Ineffective individual and family coping
    - Ineffective role performance
  - Postoperative complications:
    - ICP

- CSF leakage
- Meningitis
- Seizures
- Prognosis following cranial surgery:
  - If the client survives the acute phase, the extent of recovery depends on the areas of the brain affected and any possible hypoxia and hypoglycemia.
  - Some clients have numerous functional deficits and require extensive rehabilitation.
  - Psychosocial support for the client and significant others is critical.

Pharmacology

- Osmotic diuretics (Mannitol)
- Corticosteroids (Decadron)
- Anti-hypertensives (calcium channel blockers, hydralazine)
- Antipyretics (acetaminophen)
- Anticonvulsants (phenytoin, benzodiazepines), Neurontin, etc.
- Analgesics (use opiates with caution)
- Povidone iodine (Betadine)
- Topical antibiotic
- Systemic antibiotic

Complications

- Brain hypoxia
- Cerebral edema
- Death
- Shock
- Infection
- Motor and/or sensory disability
- Coma
- Cerebrospinal fluid (CSF) flow obstruction
- Intracranial hematoma

Age-Related Changes—Gerontological Considerations

- The presence of dementia or confusion in the older adult may mask signs and symptoms associated with head injury.

Critical Thinking Exercise: Nursing Management of the Client with a Head Injury

Situation: A 31-year-old woman received a closed head injury during an automobile accident approximately six hours ago. Her CT scan indicates she has sustained a contusion of moderate severity to the left side of her brain. She is unresponsive to verbal commands, but does respond to pain. Her blood pressure is 150/68; heart rate 72 bpm; her respirations are 28 per minute and mildly labored.

1. Match the following clinical manifestations with correct head injury:

	a. Nuchal rigidity
Skull fracture	b. Amnesia
Concussion	c. Cerebrospinal fluid (CSF) leakage from the ears
Hematoma	d. Hypotension
	e. Hemiparesis
	f. Fixed, dilated pupil on affected side

2. Which are common signs of increased intracranial pressure (ICP)?

_____ Tachypnea   _____ Decreased body temperature

_____ Restlessness   _____ Headache

_____ Gastric distention   _____ Paralysis

_____ Vomiting   _____ Tachycardia

_____ Seizures   _____ Narrowed pulse pressure

3. List two nursing activities for each of the client's priority nursing diagnosis.

   a. High risk for ineffective airway clearance

   b. High risk for impaired skin integrity

4. List a desired outcome for these nursing diagnoses:

   a. Alterations in nutrition

   b. Risk for complications of head injury

Nursing Management of the Client with an Intracranial Hemorrhage

Key Points

- Intracranial hemorrhage is a significant cause of increased intracranial pressure and resulting disability or death.
- Goals of collaborative management:
  - Maintain airway, breathing, and circulation.
  - Maintain cerebral perfusion.
  - Maintain fluid and electrolyte balance.
  - Prevent complications.
  - Maintain cognitive function.
- Important nursing diagnoses (actual or potential):
  - Ineffective airway clearance
  - Potential complication of head injury (seizures, increased intracranial pressure)
  - Altered nutrition
  - Impaired skin integrity
  - Risk for injury
  - Ineffective family coping
- **Key Terms/Concepts**: Decorticate, decerebrate, hemiparesis, hemiplegia

Overview

Intracranial hemorrhage is bleeding within the cranium most commonly caused by leakage or rupture of an aneurysm, arteriovenous malformation, severe hypertension (cerebrovascular accident), or injury. It is the most common serious complication of blunt craniocerebral trauma. Depending on the site and extent of bleeding, symptoms may appear immediately or within hours to days. Intracranial hemorrhage and subsequent hematoma are classified according to location:

- **Epidural hematoma**: Forms rapidly from an arterial bleed between the dura and the skull from a tear in the meningeal artery
- **Intracerebral hematoma**: Multiple hemorrhages, usually located in the frontal or temporal lobes, from closed head trauma
- **Subdural hematoma**: Forms slowly from a venous bleed beneath the dura from tears in veins crossing the subdural space

Risk Factors

- Arteriosclerosis/atherosclerosis

- Hypertension
- Genetic predisposition
- Trauma
- Obesity
- Diabetes mellitus
- Anticoagulant therapy
- Arteriovenous (AV) malformations aneurysm
- Alcoholism-falls from are a very common cause of subdural hematoma

Signs and Symptoms

- Increased intracranial pressure (ICP)
- Hypertension
- Dilated pupils or unequal pupil size
- Cheyne-Stokes respirations (An abnormal breathing pattern that is first shallow and infrequent [apnea] and then increases gradually to become abnormally deep and rapid [hyperpnea], before fading away [apnea] completely for a brief period. Breathing may stop for about 5 to 30 seconds, before the next cycle of shallow breathing begins).
- Facial drooping
- Nuchal rigidity
- Ataxia
- Change in level of consciousness (LOC)
- Dysphagia
- Changes in speech
- Decreased sensation
- Paralysis
- Hemiplegia
- Unequal strength in extremities
- Decrease in urine specific gravity (related to diabetes insipidus), polyuria

Diagnostic and Laboratory Tests

- History and physical exam
- Magnetic resonance imaging (MRI)
- Computed tomography (CT)/computed axial tomography (CAT) scan
- Glasgow Coma Scale
- Electroencephalogram (EEG)
- Cerebral arteriography
- Electrolytes
- CBC
- Arterial blood gases (ABGs)

- Possible coagulation studies, if was on anticoagulant

Therapeutic Nursing Management

- **Assess/Monitor**:
  - Respiratory status (breathing pattern, CO2 levels)
  - Neurological status every 15 minutes until client is stable
    - Vital signs
    - PERLA (Pupils Equal, Round, React to Light and Accommodation)
    - LOC (Level Of Consciousness)
    - Cincinnati Stroke Scale differentiates LOC into the following categories:
  - 1=Not able to awaken
  - 2=Difficult to arouse
  - 3-Sleeping/arousable
  - 4=Drowsy
  - 5=Wide awake
  - For signs of increased ICP
  - For posturing (decorticate, decerebrate, flaccid)
  - For pain and restlessness
  - For indications of infection
- **Nursing Activities**:
  - Maintain patent airway.
  - Elevate head to reduce intracranial pressure, keep head midline.
  - Implement seizure precautions.
  - Instruct client to avoid coughing.
  - Report presence of cerebrospinal fluid (CSF) from nose or ears to client's practitioner.
  - Administer pain medications as ordered in the absence of ICP (use opiates cautiously because it produces respiratory depression, pupillary changes, nausea, and central nervous system clouding).
  - Maintain client safety (side rails up, padded side rails).
  - Provide emotional support.
  - Implement measures to prevent complications of immobility (turn every two hours, footboard and splints).
  - Prepare client for surgery if indicated.
  - Oxygen

Pharmacology

- Osmotic diuretics (Mannitol)
- Corticosteroids (Decadron)
- Anti-hypertensives
- Antipyretics (acetaminophen)
- Anticonvulsants (phenytoin, benzodiazepines, Neurontin, etc)

- Analgesics (no opioids such as morphine sulfate)
- Nimodipine (for subarachnoid hemorrhage)

Complications

- Hypoxia
- Bowel and/or bladder incontinence
- Hemiplegia
- Aphasia
- Aspiration
- Coma
- Death

Age-Related Changes—Gerontological Considerations

- The increased incidence of cerebral vascular changes and hypertension in older adults predisposes them to intracranial hemorrhage.

Critical Thinking Exercise: Nursing Management of the Client with an Intracranial Hemorrhage

Situation: Three clients are being cared for on the neurosurgery unit. One client has an epidural hematoma, a second has a subdural hematoma, and a third has an intracerebral hematoma. All three are semi-conscious and restless, but stable, and all are demonstrating indications of improvement.

1. Match the type of hematoma with its correct description. There is more than one answer to each type.

Subdural hematoma	a. Multiple hemorrhage
Epidural hematoma	b. From tear in meningeal artery
Intracerebral hematoma	c. Due to closed head trauma
	d. Forms slowly
	e. Between dura and skull
	f. Beneath the dura
	g. In frontal lobe
	h. Forms rapidly
	i. Related to tears in veins

2. Decide if each statement is true or false. Correct false statements.
   a. Shallow, rapid respirations are associated with intracranial hemorrhage.
   b. Diabetes mellitus is a risk factor for intracranial hemorrhage.
   c. Intracranial hemorrhage seldom results in increased intracranial pressure.
   d. Neuro checks should be performed every four hours when intracranial pressure is suspected.

3. All three clients have the nursing diagnosis of "risk for injury related to restlessness." List two nursing actions to protect their safety.

Nursing Management of the Client with Increased Intracranial Pressure (ICP)

Key Points

- Increased intracranial pressure (ICP) is a symptom of disease or injury rather than a disease itself.
- Increased intracranial pressure can rapidly lead to death or permanent disability.
- Goals of collaborative management:
  - Maintain airway, breathing, and circulation.
  - Maintain cerebral perfusion.
  - Reduce intracranial pressure.
  - Maintain fluid and electrolyte balance.
  - Prevent complications.
  - Maintain cognitive function.
- Important nursing diagnoses (actual or potential):
  - Ineffective airway clearance
  - Potential complication of increased intracranial pressure (hyperthermia, herniation, or shock)
  - Altered nutrition
  - Impaired skin integrity
  - Risk for injury
  - Ineffective family coping
- **Key Terms/Concepts:** Papilledema, Babinski reflex, Valsalva maneuver

Overview

Increased intracranial pressure (ICP) can occur from trauma, hemorrhage, tumor growth, edema, inflammation, or hydrocephalus. Increased ICP can impair circulation, interfere with the absorption of cerebral spinal fluid, alter nerve cell function, and lead to brain stem compression and death.

Risk Factors

- Meningitis
- Head injury/trauma
- Brain tumors
- Brain abscesses
- Hemorrhage
- Stroke
- Hydrocephalus

Signs and Symptoms

- Progressive decline in level of consciousness
- Confusion and disorientation
- Drowsiness
- Headache
- Abnormal respirations
- Elevated temperature
- Increased blood pressure and widening pulse pressure
- Bradycardia
- Vomiting
- Papilledema
- Blurred vision
- Pupil changes
- Weakness to hemiplegia
- Positive Babinski reflex (This reflex, initiated by running a blunt, pointed object up the lateral border of the foot, occurs when the great toe flexes toward the dorsum of the foot and the other toes fan out. This is normal in younger children, but abnormal after about 2 years old).
- Seizures
- Restlessness and irritability

Diagnostic Tests

- History and physical exam
- Magnetic resonance imaging (MRI)
- Computed tomography (CT)/computed axial tomography (CAT) scan
- Electroencephalogram (EEG)
- Intracranial pressure (ICP) monitor
- CBC
- Electrolytes
- Arterial blood gases (ABGs)

Therapeutic Nursing Management

- **Assess/Monitor:**
  - Respiratory status for changes (breathing pattern, CO_2 levels)
  - Neurological status every 15 minutes until stable
    - Vital signs
    - PERLA (Pupils Equal, Round, React to Light and Accommodation)
    - LOC (Loss Of Consciousness)
  - For posturing (decorticate, decerebrate, flaccid)
  - Electrolyte and acid-base balance

- **Nursing Activities:**
  - Identify and treat underlying cause.
  - Elevate head of bed 30-45 degrees (avoid Trendelenburg position).
  - Maintain head in neutral position, avoiding flexion and extension.
  - Maintain airway patency.
  - Institute seizure precautions.
  - Caution with use of morphine sulfate.
  - Maintain body temperature.
  - Maintain client safety (side rails up, padded side rails).
  - Provide emotional support.
  - Implement measures to prevent complications of immobility (turn every two hours, footboard and splints).
  - Limit fluid intake.
  - Teach client to avoid sneezing, coughing, and Valsalva maneuver (an attempt to forcibly exhale with the nose and mouth closed).
  - Prepare client for surgery if indicated.
  - Prepare client for mechanical ventilation as indicated.
  - Codeine may decrease cough, which can increase ICP.

Pharmacology

- Osmotic diuretics (Mannitol)
- Corticosteroids (Decadron)
- Anticonvulsants (pentobarbital, Diprivan or other may be used to induce coma for treatment of ICP)
- Stool softeners (docusate sodium)
- Anti-hypertensives (calcium channel blockers, hydralazine, or nitroprusside)
- Antipyretics (acetaminophen)
- Intravenous fluids (avoid hypotonic solutions)
- Electrolyte replacement

Complications

- Seizures
- Cognitive deficits
- Motor deficits
- Sensory deficits
- Coma
- Death

Age-Related Changes—Gerontological Considerations

- Confusion, fatigue, and lethargy due to increased ICP may be difficult to differentiate from other causes in older adults.

Critical Thinking Exercise: Nursing Management of the Client with Increased Intracranial Pressure (ICP)

Situation: A 29-year-old male fell off the roof on which he was working three days ago and received a blunt head injury. He is unconscious, intubated, and receiving mechanical ventilation to support respirations. He has an indwelling urinary catheter and is receiving intravenous fluids and medications, which include Mannitol and Decadron.

1. List four signs of increased intracranial pressure, other than decreased level of consciousness.

2. Match each drug with the reason for its use in treating clients with increased intracranial pressure.

Osmotic diuretics	a. Prevent or control seizures
Corticosteroids	b. Reduce fever
Anticonvulsant	c. Control blood pressure
Stool softeners	d. Reduce inflammation
Anti-hypertensives	e. Prevent fecal impaction
Antipyretics	f. Eliminate excess fluid

3. Which is an achievable outcome for the person with increased intracranial pressure?

    —— Client will be free of intracranial pressure within 24 hours.

    —— Client will be turned every two hours to prevent skin breakdown.

    —— Client will maintain a patent airway throughout hospitalization.

Nursing Management of the Client with a Cerebrovascular Accident (CVA)—Stroke

Key Points

- Mortality from stroke can be significantly decreased by rapid recognition and intervention.
- Clients with history of uncontrolled hypertension are at increased risk for stroke.
- Older adults are at increased risk for stroke.
- Goals of collaborative management:
    - Provide early recognition and treatment.
    - Prevent complications (disability, increased intracranial pressure).
    - Maintain airway, breathing, and circulation.
    - Maintain functional ability.
    - Achieve self-care and communications.
- Important nursing diagnoses (actual and potential):
    - Impaired physical mobility
    - Risk for injury
    - Self-care deficit
    - Altered nutrition
    - Sensory-perceptual alteration
    - Ineffective family coping
    - Ineffective individual coping
- **Key Terms/Concepts**: Hemianopia, dysphagia, dysarthria, aphasia, agnosia, apraxia

Overview

Cerebrovascular accident (CVA), which is also known as acute brain attack, or stroke, is the sudden loss of brain function due to disrupted circulation and oxygenation of brain tissue. Brain cell necrosis varies according to the area of brain involved, the extent of involvement, and the length of time blood flow is interrupted. The primary causes of CVA are:

- **Cerebral hemorrhage**: Rupture of a vessel with bleeding into the brain tissue
- **Embolism**: A blood clot carried from another part of the body to the brain
- **Ischemia**: Impaired circulation and inadequate oxygenation of the brain
- **Thrombus**: Clotting of blood vessels within or supplying the brain

Risk Factors

- Arteriosclerosis
- Hypertension
- Smoking
- Diabetes mellitus
- Sedentary lifestyle
- Use of oral contraceptives
- Cerebral aneurysm
- Obesity
- Coagulation disorders/ anticoagulants
- Hypothyroidism
- Substance abuse
- Sickle cell disease
- Long-term use of corticosteroids
- Arterio-venous malformation (AV)

Signs and Symptoms

- Hypertension
- Headache
- Nausea, vomiting
- Unilateral weakness or paralysis of arm, leg, or face
- Sensoriperceptual deficits
- Hemianopia (blindness of half of visual field)
- Drowsiness
- Urinary incontinence
- Dysphagia (inability or difficulty swallowing)
- Dysarthria (difficulty with speaking)
- Flaccidity, spasticity or rigidity
- Behavioral changes
- Aphasia (receptive or expressive)
- Agnosia (inability to correctly use an object)
- Apraxia (inability to carry out purposeful activities)
- Emotional instability
- Balance problems

Diagnostic Tests

- History and physical exam
- Magnetic resonance imaging (MRI)
- Computed tomography (CT)/computed axial tomography (CAT) scan

- Arteriography and cerebral angiography
- Ultrasound
  - 2D (2-dimensional)
  - 3D (3-dimensional)
  - Doppler
  - CBC
  - PT, PTT, etc, if client has been on anticoagulants or has a coagulopathy

Therapeutic Nursing Management

- **Assess/Monitor**:
  - Neurological status and vital signs every 15 minutes until stable
  - For signs of increased intracranial pressure (ICP)
  - Bowel and bladder function
  - Intake and output
  - Swallowing abilities before feeding (may need to thicken liquids to avoid aspiration)
  - Breath sounds for aspiration pneumonia
  - Reflexes
- **Nursing Activities**:
  - Maintain patent airway.
  - Institute seizure precautions.
  - Position on side with head of bed elevated 15-30 degrees.
  - Maintain non-stimulating environment.
  - Provide assistance with ADLs (activities of daily living) as needed.
  - Assist with communication skills if impaired.
  - Provide safe environment if mobility is impaired.
  - Provide emotional support for client and family.
  - Prevent complications of immobility.
  - Perform range of motion exercises or assist client to physical therapy.

Pharmacology

- Anticoagulants (warfarin, heparin): not for a cerebral hemorrhage
- Antiplatelets (aspirin, ticlopidine, clopidogrel): not for a cerebral hemorrhage
- Antithrombolytic agents (Activase, t-PA): not for a cerebral hemorrhage. Rule out hemorrhagic stroke with magnetic resonance imaging (MRI) before using.
- Hyperosmolar solutions
- Anticonvulsants (phenytoin)
- Stool softeners (docusate sodium)
- Antihypertensives

Complications

- Impaired verbal communication

- Sensory-perceptual deficits
- Constipation and urinary incontinence
- Aspiration pneumonia
- Depression
- Contractures and extremity deformities
- ARDS (acute respiratory distress syndrome) if pneumonia
- Seizures
- Coma
- Death

Age-Related Changes—Gerontological Considerations

- Arteriosclerosis among older adults is related to an increased incidence of stroke.
- Aged adults who have neurologic deficits are at a high risk for falls related to impaired mobility.
- Risk for nutritional deficits related to impaired swallowing occurs in older persons with neurologic deficits.
- Increased risk for behavioral changes, such as emotional instability and depression, are common clinical manifestations.

Assessing Cranial Nerves

Name	Number	Purpose/Findings
Olfactory	1	Identify and detect smell correctly
Optic	2	Vision normal
Oculomotor	3	Pupil reacts to light, eye movement
Trochlear	4	Movement of eye (downward & inward)
Trigeminal	5	Facial sensation
Abducens	6	Lateral movement of eye
Facial	7	Movement of face/symmetry
Acoustic	8	Hearing accuracy and balance
Glossopharyngeal	9	Swallowing, gag reflex, uvula midline
Vagus	10	Voice, talking, swallowing
Spinal Accessory	11	Shoulder movement
Hypoglossal	12	Tongue movement

Critical Thinking Exercise: Nursing Management of the Client with a Cerebrovascular Accident (CVA)—Stroke

Situation: A 50-year-old woman is admitted to the acute care facility after her family finds her in a confused state. Admission assessment reveals a history of hypertension and diabetes mellitus. Her vital signs are BP 190/110, respirations 16, pulse 90, rectal temperature 100.6° F, and Glasgow Coma Scale = 8. She has right-sided weakness with loss of sensory input and facial drooping. Her admitting medical diagnosis is acute brain attack or stroke (cerebrovascular bleed).

1. Which of the following nursing diagnoses are appropriate based on the client's data?

_____ Risk for impaired physical mobility   _____ Risk for injury

_____ Self-care deficit   _____ Altered nutrition

_____ Sensory-perceptual alteration   _____ Ineffective family coping

_____ Ineffective individual coping

2. Prioritize the following nursing interventions, with "1" representing the most important intervention.

_____ Monitor temperature.

_____ Assess neurological status.

_____ Assess respiratory status.

_____ Elevate the client's head to a 45° position (high-Fowler's position).

3. Which signs and symptoms are produced by increased intracranial pressure (ICP)?

_____ Confusion   _____ Restlessness   _____ Constricted pupils

_____ Hiccoughs   _____ Elevated temperature   _____ Narrowed pulse pressure

_____ Bradycardia   _____ Increased respiratory rate   _____ Tetany

4. List three complications that can occur in a client experiencing a stroke.

Nursing Management of the Client with Pain

Key Points

- Pain is a subjective response that can only be rated by the person experiencing the pain.
- Many factors influence a person's perception of pain.
- Acute pain differs from chronic pain.
- Physical and psychological pain produces physiological changes in the body.
- Pain is often under-treated due the nurse's, physician's, client's and family's concerns about addiction.
- Goals of collaborative management:
  - Reduce or eliminate pain.
  - Maximize client's ability to engage in ADLs (activities of daily living).
  - Promote effective respiratory excursions.
  - Maximize range of motion (ROM) and mobility.
  - Optimize individual coping.
  - Enhance rest and sleep.
  - Prevent adverse physiologic effects related to pain.
  - Minimize depression associated with chronic pain.
- Important nursing diagnoses (actual or potential):
  - Pain management
  - Ineffective individual coping
  - Powerlessness and coping mechanisms
  - Self-care deficit
  - Impaired home maintenance management
- **Key Terms/Concepts**: Acute, chronic

Overview

Pain is a subjective response to both physical and psychological stressors. Pain is the most common reason clients seek health care. The expression of pain may be verbal complaints and/or nonverbal actions.

Acute pain: Pain lasting less than six months.

Chronic pain: Constant, intermittent pain that lasts from six months to years.

Risk Factors

- Age
- Sociocultural influences

- Emotional status
- Past experiences with pain
- Overall health

Signs and Symptoms

- Muscle tension
- Tachycardia
- Rapid, shallow respirations
- Increased blood pressure
- Dilated pupils
- Sweating
- Pallor
- Restlessness
- Inability to sleep
- Irritability
- Bracing or guarding of painful area
- Crying
- Moaning
- Social withdrawal
- Decreased mobility
- Sad facial expression
- Denial

Diagnostic and Laboratory Tests

- History and physical
- Psychological testing
- Tests for specific diseases or conditions

Therapeutic Nursing Management

- Assess/Monitor:
  - Pain status
    - Characteristics
    - Location
    - Intensity
    - Quality
    - Patterns
    - Precipitating factors
  - Vital signs for changes indicative of increased pain
  - Utilize pain scales to evaluate intensity of client's pain
    - Simple descriptive pain intensity scales

- Pain rating indexes
- Numerical intensity pain scales
- Faces rating scale: best for children or older adults with cognitive or sensory deficits
- Effectiveness of pain medications
- **Nursing Activities:**
  - Encourage use of relaxation techniques.
  - Provide distraction.
  - Provide massage or therapeutic touch.
  - Encourage verbalization of fears and concerns.
  - Actively listen to complaints and concerns regarding pain management.
  - Provide comfort measures (oral care, bath, linen change).

Pharmacology

- NSAIDs (diclofenac, nabumetone, ibuprofen, naproxen)
- Opiate agonists (codeine, fentanyl, morphine, meperidine, oxycodone, hydrocodone, etc.)
  - Non-opiates (tramadex)
  - Trigger point injections
  - Epidurals
  - Implantable pain medication
  - Lidoderm patches
- Antidepressants (amitriptyline, desipramine, doxepin, venlafaxine)
- Local anesthetics, topical (benzocaine, lidocaine)
- Anticonvulsants (gabapentin [Neurontin])

Complications

- Pain medication addiction/dependency (especially narcotics for chronic pain)
- Sleep deprivation
- Drug tolerance
- Acute pain may become chronic pain
- Lack of pain control
- Immobility
- Depression
- Social isolation
- NSAIDs
  - Renal problems
  - Gastrointestinal bleeding
- Opiates
  - Constipation

Age-Related Changes—Gerontological Considerations

- Failure to alleviate pain in older adults can lead to functional limitations.
- Pain control regimens may be difficult for the older adult to maintain due to increased incidence of memory loss among older adults.
- Age-related changes in the release of neurotransmitters often cause an increase in chronic pain, fatigue, altered sleep and mood.
- Older adults experience lowered pain sensation and decreased response to pain.
- Older adults with altered mentation may have difficulty communicating about pain intensity, quality, and duration.

Critical Thinking Exercise: Nursing Management of the Client with Pain

Situation: A 43-year-old woman is being treated for severe and unrelenting back pain that began about three days ago after she lifted several heavy objects. Upon assessment, the client rates her pain as "8" on a scale of 1-10.

1. What type of pain is the client experiencing? Why?

2. What information needs to be collected from a client experiencing either acute or chronic pain?

3. State the rationale for implementing each of the nursing actions for this client's pain.
    a. Encourage client to report pain before it becomes severe.
    b. Implement pain strategies that have been previously successful.
    c. Instruct the client to call for assistance when getting out of bed to ambulate.

4. Categorize each type of pain as acute or chronic:
    a. Abdominal cramping from gastroenteritis
    b. Bone pain related to cancer
    c. Migraine headache
    d. Toothache

Nursing Management of the Client with a Spinal Cord Injury

Key Points

- The 5th, 6th, 7th cervical, the 12th thoracic, and the 1st lumbar are the vertebrae most frequently involved in spinal cord injury.
- The level of cord involved dictates the consequences of spinal cord injury.
- Spinal cord injuries range from contusions to complete transection of the cord.
- Goals of collaborative management:
    - Provide immediate surgical correction if warranted.
    - Maintain breathing and circulation.
    - Prevent further spinal cord injury by stabilizing head and back.
    - Prevent neurological deficits.
    - Maintain functional abilities.
    - Prevent skin alterations.
    - Maintain bowel and bladder function.
    - Prevent complications (autonomic dysreflexia, neurogenic shock, contractures, and muscle atrophy).
- Important nursing diagnoses (actual or potential):
    - Ineffective airway clearance
    - Ineffective breathing pattern
    - Impaired skin integrity
    - Impaired physical mobility
    - Altered urinary elimination
    - Altered bowel elimination
    - Knowledge deficit
- **Key Terms/Concepts**: Autonomic dysreflexia, neurogenic shock, cord transection, orthostatic hypotension, paraplegia, quadriplegia

Overview

A spinal cord injury is trauma to the spinal cord, which results in complete (transection) or partial disruption of nerve tracts and neurons. Spinal cord injuries are classified according to cause, level of injury, and degree of disruption produced. Injuries may involve contusions, lacerations, or compression of the spinal cord. The majority of spinal cord injuries result from car accidents, falls, or sports injuries.

Risk Factors

- Male
- High-risk lifestyle activities

- Active in sports
- Age (teen to early 20s)
- Alcohol and/or drug abuse

Signs and Symptoms

- Respiratory instability
- Motor and sensory changes below level of injury
- Loss of reflexes below level of injury
- Pain
- Orthostatic hypotension
- Hypercalcemia
- Decreased cough reflex
- Quadriplegia, paraplegia
- Muscle spasms
- Bowel and bladder incontinence
- Urinary retention and bladder distention
- Impotence

Diagnostic Tests and Lab

- History and physical
- X-rays
- Magnetic resonance imaging (MRI)
- Computed tomography (CT)/computed axial tomography (CAT) scan
- Electromyography (EMG)

Therapeutic Nursing Management

- **Assess/Monitor:**
  - Vital signs
  - Neurological status (hand grasp, toe and foot movement)
  - For signs of thrombophlebitis
  - For spinal shock (bradycardia, hypotension, flaccid paralysis, loss of reflex activity below level of injury, and paralytic ileus)
  - For autonomic dysreflexia (hypertension, bradycardia, flushed face and neck, severe headache, nasal stuffiness, dilated pupils, blurred vision, sweating, and nausea)
  - Oxygen saturation levels
  - For bladder distention
  - For indications of altered body image/self concept
- **Nursing Activities:**
  - Maintain patent airway (immobilize neck and spine to prevent further injury).

- Maintain mechanical ventilation as prescribed.
- Encourage deep breathing exercises.
- Perform passive exercises.
- Encourage active exercises.
- Maintain skin integrity.
- Assist with turning as needed.
- Maintain adequate fluid intake.
- Teach self-catheterization.
- Institute bowel retraining as needed.
- Teach regarding sexual function/dysfunction.

Pharmacology

- Glucocorticoids: adrenocortical steroids (dexamethasone [Decadron])
- Vasopressors (norepinephrine, dopamine)
- Muscle relaxants (carisoprodol, methocarbamol, etc.)
- Anti-spasmodics (dantrolene sodium [Dantrium])
- Analgesics (opioid), non opioids and NSAIDs
- Antidepressants (paroxetine, sertraline, bupropion, venlafaxine, duloxetine, etc.)
- Histamine H2-receptor antagonists (ranitidine hydrochloride [Zantac]) to prevent gastric ulcer formation
- Anticoagulants (heparin or low molecular weight heparins for DVT prophylaxis)
- Stool softeners (docusate sodium)
- Vasodilators (hydralazine, nitroglycerin)
- Anti-seizure (gabapentin, etc.)

Complications

- Paralysis
- Autonomic dysreflexia
- Neurogenic shock (spinal shock)
- Contractures
- Muscle atrophy
- Pressure ulcers
- Stool impaction
- Death

Age-Related Changes—Gerontological Considerations

- The skin of the older adult is commonly thin and dry, which may increase the risk for pressure injury.
- Osteoporosis, balance issues, etc
  - More at risk for falls and fractures

Critical Thinking Exercise: Nursing Management of the Client with a Spinal Cord Injury

Situation: While playing football, a 19-year-old college student suffered a 12th thoracic fracture with resulting paraplegia. He has no muscle control of his lower limbs, bowel, bladder, or genital area. He is a week postoperative from spinal stabilization surgery.

1. Which of the following are the primary goals of collaborative management during the acute phase following spinal cord injury?

   _____ Administer morphine sulfate to control pain.

   _____ Maintain physiological stability.

   _____ Teach client about the disease process.

   _____ Prevent alterations in nutrition.

   _____ Prevent further spinal cord injury.

2. The client received high dose glucocorticoid drug therapy when initially admitted to the neuro-surgery unit. Which of the following are risks associated with glucocorticoid therapy?

   _____ UTI (urinary tract infection)   _____ Hypoglycemia

   _____ Fluid retention   _____ Sodium retention

   _____ Decreased appetite   _____ Hypotension

3. What is the etiology for these client problems?

   a. Anxiety

   b. Hopelessness

   c. Powerlessness

4. Define autonomic dysreflexia.

Nursing Management of the Client with Seizures

Key Points

- Seizures are a complex symptom due to brain function disorders, metabolic states, trauma, drugs, and disease.
- Seizure disorders are not associated with intellectual level.
- Goals of collaborative management:
  - Maintain airway and breathing.
  - Prevent seizures.
  - Terminate seizures as rapidly as possible.
  - Restore cerebral oxygenation.
  - Prevent injury.
  - Prevent complications (status epilepticus, aspiration).
- Important nursing diagnoses (actual and potential):
  - Risk for injury
  - Ineffective airway clearance
  - Anxiety and fear
  - Ineffective individual coping
  - Knowledge deficit
- **Key Terms/Concepts:** Status epilepticus, tonic-clonic activity, myoclonic, atonic

Overview

A seizure is a sudden, explosive, disorderly discharge of cerebral neurons, involving motor, sensory, and autonomic responses. The abnormal electrical activity may include all or part of the brain. Tonic-clonic activity is the most common type of seizure in children and adults. The syndrome involving repeated seizure activity is known as epilepsy.

Risk Factors

- Genetic predisposition
- Acute febrile state
- Head injury
- Infection
- Metabolic or endocrine disorders (hypoglycemia)
- Exposure to toxins
- Birth injury
- Trauma

- Brain tumors
- Metabolic disorders
- Hypoxia
- Drug and alcohol withdrawal
- Fluid and electrolyte imbalances

Signs and Symptoms

- Generalized Seizures
    - Tonic-clonic (grand mal): Stiffening or rigidity of muscles lasting 10-20 seconds.
    - Focal seizure: Slow, repetitive jerking of a body part.
    - Absence seizures (petit mal): Sudden brief cessation of all motor activity accompanied by a blank stare.
    - Myoclonic: Brief, generalized jerking of extremities.
    - Atonic: (drop attacks) Sudden, momentary loss of muscle tone
    - Partial Seizures
    - Simple: Conscious, with localized jerking of specific area.
    - Complex: Momentary loss of consciousness with periods of unintentionally altered behavior.
- Memory loss during and immediately following seizure
- Drowsiness or difficulty with arousal for short period of time following seizure
- Incontinence of urine or feces
- Vomiting
- Hypoxia (severe or prolonged seizures)
- Automatism (lip smacking, repeated swallowing)

Diagnostic Tests

- History and physical exam
- Blood and urine tests
- Magnetic resonance imaging (MRI)
- Computed tomography (CT)/computed axial tomography (CAT) scan
- Electroencephalogram (EEG)
- Cerebrospinal fluid (CSF) analysis
- Skull x-rays
- Electrolyte profile
- Drug screen

Therapeutic Nursing Management

- **Prevent:**
    - Seizures by maintaining medication schedules
    - Injury

- Aspiration
- **Assess/Monitor:**
  - Airway and breathing
- **Nursing Activities:**
  - Maintain patent airway.
  - Turn client's head to side and prepare to suction.
  - Loosen restrictive clothing, but do not physically restrain.
  - Protect client from injury (e.g., padded side rails, place standing client on floor and protect head and body).
  - Administer oxygen.
  - Minimize stimuli in environment during a seizure.
  - Administer prescribed medications.
  - Alleviate anxiety.
  - Identify factors that trigger seizures.
  - Document time and duration of seizure.
  - Teach client to avoid alcohol, excessive fatigue, and stress.
  - Refer to appropriate community resources.
  - Encourage verbalization of fears and concerns.
  - Instruct client to wear a medical identification bracelet at all times.
  - Assist with ablation or stereotactic procedures

Pharmacology

- Anticonvulsants (phenytoin, valproic acid, carbamazepine, phenobarbital, oxcarbazepine, clonazepam, topiramate gabapentin, etc.)
- Sedatives (benzodiazepines are also anticonvulsants)

Complications

- Disruption in attention span
- Interference with learning
- Injury
- Aspiration
- Alteration in self-concept
- Status epilepticus

Age-Related Changes—Gerontological Considerations

- Older adults are at higher risk for fractures related to seizure activity.
- Polypharmacy may interfere with effectiveness of anticonvulsants.
- Confusion may prohibit compliance with prescribed medication regimen.

Critical Thinking Exercise: Nursing Management of the Client with Seizures

Situation: A young woman with a history of epilepsy is scheduled to undergo minor outpatient surgery. Before the nurse can obtain data about the woman's seizure history during the admission process, the woman states she is going to have a seizure.

1. What should the nurse do while the client is seizing?

2. What is the rationale for these nursing actions?
   a. Turn the client on her side.
   b. Loosen restrictive clothing.
   c. Minimize external stimuli.

3. Match the type of seizure with its common sign.

Brief, generalized jerking	a. Tonic-Clonic
Localized jerking of a specific area	b. Myoclonic
Rigidity of muscles lasting 10-30 seconds	c. Atonic
Sudden, momentary loss of muscle tone	d. Absence
Slow, repetitive jerking of a body part	e. Simple
Sudden, momentary loss of muscle tone	f. Focal

4. Why is it important to administer seizure medications on time?

Nursing Management of the Client with Alzheimer's Disease

| Key Points |

- Alzheimer's disease is a non-reversible dementia that progresses through three stages.
- Goals of collaborative management:
  - Prevent injury.
  - Maintain nutrition and fluid balance.
  - Maintain communication.
  - Provide socialization.
  - Educate caregivers.
- Important nursing diagnoses (actual and potential):
  - Altered thought processes
  - Risk for injury
  - Altered nutrition
  - Anxiety and fear
  - Self-care deficit
  - Altered family processes
- **Key Terms/Concepts:** Progressive, dementia, degenerative, sundowning

Overview

Alzheimer's disease is a progressive, degenerative neurological disorder commonly causing severe cognitive impairment, behavioral dysfunction, and changes in personality. It is the most common non-reversible form of dementia, beginning insidiously with forgetfulness and progressing to total mental incapacitation.

Dementia, in general, is a condition marked by gradual deterioration of cognitive function, language, personality, and memory. The major types of dementias are associated with Alzheimer's disease, HIV, Parkinson's disease, Huntington's disease, Pick's disease, certain general medical conditions (e.g., cardiopulmonary insufficiency, fluid and electrolyte imbalances), and substance abuse. General interventions for clients with dementia are to provide a safe environment; offer individual, family and group therapy; and administer psychopharmacologic medications.

Risk Factors

- Older age
- Genetic predisposition

Signs and Symptoms

Stage 1: lasts 1-3 years

- Short-term memory loss
- Decreased attention span
- Subtle personality changes
- Mild cognitive deficits
- Difficulty with depth perception

Stage 2: lasts 2-10 years

- Obvious memory loss
- Confusion
- Wandering behavior
- "Sundowning"
- Irritability and agitation
- Decreased spatial orientation
- Impaired motor skills
- Impaired judgment

Stage 3: lasts 8-10 years

- Absent cognitive abilities
- Disoriented to time and place
- Severely altered communication skills
- Impaired or absent motor skills
- Bowel and bladder incontinence

Diagnostic and Laboratory Tests

- History and physical exam
- Magnetic resonance imaging (MRI)
- Computed tomography (CT)/computed axial tomography (CAT) scan
- PET (positron emission tomography) scan
- Electroencephalogram (EEG)
- Psychometric testing

Therapeutic Nursing Management

- **Prevent:**
  - Injuries
- **Assess/Monitor:**
  - Changes in mental status
- **Nursing Activities:**
  - Provide a safe environment.
  - Maintain or improve hygiene, nutrition, and general health.

- Label room contents and belongings.
- Keep routines consistent.
- Schedule frequent rest periods.
- Encourage exercise to maintain mobility.
- Establish communication system with client and family.
- Provide emotional support to the family.
- Keep the client functioning at the highest possible level.
- Prepare for eventual nursing home versus 24 hour in home care

Pharmacology

- Cholinergic agents (tacrine hydrochloride [Cognex], donepezil [Aricept])
- Tricyclic antidepressants (amitriptyline, desipramine, doxepin, nortriptyline)

Complications

- Self-injury
- Exhaustion/sleep deprivation
- Combativeness
- Total loss of independence
- Malnutrition
- Depression

Age-Related Changes—Gerontological Considerations

- Increased risk of severe dementia related to Alzheimer's disease is common among clients over the age of 65.
- Increased risk for falls and injury is related to decreased cognitive function.
- Elderly persons are at increased risk for pneumonia, dehydration, or malnutrition.
- Rule out urinary tract infection (UTI) and possible urosepsis.

Critical Thinking Exercise: Nursing Management of the Client with Alzheimer's Disease

Situation: A 72-year-old man is a resident in a long-term-care Alzheimer's facility. He is in very good physical health, but is unable to care for himself, recognize members of his family, or communicate his needs. An extensive evaluation of the client indicates he is in Stage 2 of the disease process.

1. Match the following characteristics of Alzheimer's disease with the correct stage of the disease process. Use "1," "2" or "3" as your answer.

	"Sundowning"
	Absent motor skills
	Wandering behavior
1 = Stage 1	Difficulty with depth perception
2 = Stage 2	Decreased attention span
3 = Stage 3	Impaired judgment
	Disoriented to time and place
	Irritability and agitation
	Subtle personality changes
	Mild cognitive deficits
	Bladder incontinence

2. If the following statement about Alzheimer's disease is not true, then make the appropriate correction.

   a. Alzheimer's disease is a progressive, inflammatory neurological disorder.

   b. Alzheimer's' disease causes severe behavioral dysfunction and changes in personality.

   c. Alzheimer's disease is an uncommon form of senile dementia.

   d. Alzheimer's disease begins suddenly with forgetfulness and progresses to total mental incapacitation.

3. State the etiology for each of the client's nursing diagnoses:

    a. Risk for injury

    b. Altered nutrition

    c. Self-care deficit

4. Complete the following sentences about clients with Alzheimer's disease:

    a. Older adults with Alzheimer's disease are at increased risk for _____, _____ and _____.

    b. It is important to encourage _____ to maintain _____ as long as frequent _____ _____ are also scheduled.

    c. Family members may feel _____; therefore, it is important for the nurse to provide _____ support.

Nursing Management of the Client with Parkinson's Disease

Key Points

- Parkinson's disease is an important cause of disability and dementia.
- Clients with Parkinson's disease exhibit a characteristic stance and gait.
- Goals of collaborative management:
  - Control symptoms.
  - Maintain functional ability.
  - Prevent complications (aspiration pneumonia, malnutrition).
- Important nursing diagnoses (actual or potential):
  - Self-care deficit
  - Impaired physical mobility
  - Altered nutrition
  - Constipation and other bowel dysfunctions
  - Sleep pattern disturbance
  - Impaired verbal communication
- **Key Terms/Concepts**: Progressive, neurotransmitter, akinesia, anticholinergic

Overview

Parkinson's disease is a common, progressive, disease of the central nervous system that affects males more frequently than females. The cause of the disease is unknown, but involves a deficiency in the production of dopamine, a neurotransmitter. Dopamine is essential in order for brain cells to perform their normal inhibitory functions within the central nervous system. The disease is characterized by tremor at rest, rigidity, and slow motor movements.

Risk Factors

- Older age
- Brain tumor
- Genetic predisposition
- Exposure to environmental toxins including drugs, carbon monoxide and mercury
- Illegal drug use

Signs and Symptoms

- Muscle rigidity
- Akinesia (almost total, or complete, loss of muscle movement)

- Tremor (pill rolling of the fingers) that increases with stress
- Mask-like faces
- Memory loss
- Shuffling gait
- Slow speech
- Difficulty sleeping
- Drooling
- Excessive perspiration

Diagnostic and Laboratory Tests

- History and physical exam
- Magnetic resonance imaging (MRI)
- Computed tomography (CT)/computed axial tomography (CAT) scan
- Electroencephalogram (EEG)
- Therapeutic response to levodopa

Therapeutic Nursing Management

- **Assess/Monitor:**
  - Drug effectiveness
  - Swallowing difficulties
  - Nutrition and hydration status
- **Nursing Activities:**
  - Encourage independence.
  - Encourage use of assistive devices as disease progresses.
  - Provide a safe environment.
  - Establish an effective communication system for client and family.
  - Maintain adequate nutrition and hydration.
  - Promote sleep and rest.
  - Encourage range of motion (ROM) exercises.
  - Assist with activities of daily living (ADLs) as needed.
  - Teach client to stop occasionally when walking to slow down speed and reduce risk of injury.
  - Prepare for possible surgery.
  - Adrenal medullary transplants
  - Thalamotomy
  - Stereotactic pallidotomy
  - Deep brain stimulation

Pharmacology

- Dopamine replacement (levodopa)
- Dopamine agonists (bromocriptine, pergolide, ropinirole [Requip®])

- Monoamine oxidase inhibitor type B (selegiline)
- Anticholinergics (benztropine, trihexyphenidyl, procyclidine)
- Antiviral (amantadine)

Complications

- Injury due to falls
- Malnutrition
- Impaired communication
- Social isolation
- Aspiration pneumonia
- Airway obstruction
- Depression

Age-Related Changes—Gerontological Considerations

- The risk for Parkinson's increases over age 65.
- Signs and symptoms of Parkinson's may be mistaken for normal aging.
- Increased risk for falls occurs with aging normally.

Critical Thinking Exercise: Nursing Management of the Client with Parkinson's Disease

Situation: A 79-year-old male was diagnosed with Parkinson's disease two years ago. In spite of his condition, he is able to live independently with his partner of 59 years. He takes levodopa with carbidopa (dopamine agonist) to control his disease. The couple has two grown children who live nearby to offer assistance when needed. Due to a recent episode of pneumonia, the client is receiving home health visits.

1. Which are considered the classic signs of Parkinson's disease?

_____ Mask-like faces   _____ Akinesia   _____ Memory loss

_____ Shuffling gait   _____ Slow speech   _____ Difficulty sleeping

_____ Muscle rigidity   _____ Drooling   _____ Diaphoresis

_____ Tremor

2. Why is the client at increased risk for the development of pneumonia?

3. Correct any of the following statements which are false regarding Parkinson's disease.

   a. Drug therapy may lose its effectiveness over time.

   b. Clients with Parkinson's disease are at increased risk for malnutrition.

   c. Parkinson's disease is a common, progressive, crippling disease of the peripheral nervous system.

   d. Parkinson's disease affects females more commonly than males.

   e. Levodopa is the drug of choice for treating Parkinson's disease.

Nursing Management of the Client with Myasthenia Gravis

Key Points

- Myasthenia gravis is a progressive autoimmune disease that produces severe muscular weakness.
- Myasthenia gravis is characterized by periods of exacerbation and remission.
- Goals of collaborative management:
    - Control symptoms.
    - Maintain functional ability.
    - Prevent complications (myasthenia crisis, cholinergic crisis, respiratory distress, aspiration pneumonia, malnutrition).
- Important nursing diagnoses (actual or potential):
    - Ineffective airway clearance
    - Ineffective breathing pattern
    - Self-care deficit
    - Impaired physical mobility
    - Altered nutrition
    - Constipation and other bowel dysfunctions
    - Impaired verbal communication
- **Key Terms/Concepts**: Cholinergic, anticholinergic, aspiration, dysphagia, dysarthria, plasmapheresis, autoimmune

Overview

Myasthenia gravis results from the failure of nerve transmission at the neuromuscular junction due to inadequate release of acetylcholine or inadequate response of muscle fibers to acetylcholine. Myasthenia gravis is thought to be an autoimmune disorder and is characterized by periods of remission and exacerbation. It affects women more often than men and occurs generally in the age range of 20-40.

Risk Factors

- Co-existing autoimmune disorder
- Thyroid disorder
- Thymoma

Signs and Symptoms

- Skeletal muscle weakness
- Fatigue

- Weak eye closure
- Drooping eyelids (ptosis)
- Dysphagia
- Dysarthria
- Expressionless face
- Choking, difficulty swallowing
- Neck weakness with head bobbing
- Respiratory distress

Diagnostic and Laboratory Tests

- History and physical exam
- Positive Tensilon (edrophonium chloride) test
- Electromyography (EMG)
- Antinuclear antibody (ANA) test titer: ANA test results are reported in a titer that indicates how much the test sample can be diluted before the antibodies are no longer detected. Fluorescence techniques are frequently used to actually detect the antibodies in the cells; thus ANA testing is sometimes referred to as fluorescent antinuclear antibody [FANA] testing.

Therapeutic Nursing Management

- **Prevent**:
  - Aspiration
- **Assess/Monitor**:
  - For indications of respiratory distress
  - For signs of myasthenia crisis (respiratory distress, increased muscle weakness, difficulty talking or swallowing)
  - For signs of cholinergic crisis (abdominal cramping, diaphoresis, muscle cramps)
  - Lung sounds
  - Ability to swallow
  - Nutritional and fluid status
- **Nursing Activities**:
  - Assist with coughing, turning and deep breathing.
  - Encourage semi-Fowler's position.
  - Maintain hydration.
  - Administer medications 30 minutes before meals to facilitate chewing and swallowing.
  - Thicken liquids to reduce risk of choking.
  - Instruct the client to avoid exposure to infections.
  - Provide the client and family with information about myasthenia gravis and its treatment. Printed brochures for client education are available through the Myasthenia Gravis Foundation.

- Teach the client's family and significant others regarding emergency interventions for respiratory distress, choking.
- Provide emotional support.
- Encourage use of medical identification.
- Prepare client for plasmapheresis if prescribed.
- Prepare client for thymectomy if indicated.

Pharmacology

- Cholinergic agents (edrophonium, neostigmine, pyridostigmine)
- Corticosteroids (prednisone)
- Immunosuppressive drugs (azathioprine)

Complications

- Respiratory distress
- Myasthenia crisis
- Aspiration pneumonia
- Impaired communication
- Corneal ulceration
- Malnutrition
- Cholinergic crisis

Age-Related Changes—Gerontological Considerations

- The weakness associated with myasthenia gravis is greatest after exertion and at the end of the day. Older persons tend to feel most tired at those times; therefore, periods of rest are particularly important for the client to regain strength and recover energy level.
- Arrangement of furniture in the home environment is essential for energy conservation and safety considerations.
- The elderly client may need assistance with taking medications. If the medication is not given on time, the client may become too weak to swallow.
- The elderly client may need assistance with ADLs (activities of daily living); many become immobile and require daily nursing care.
- Myasthenia gravis can also increase the risk of falls related to overexertion and muscle weakness.

Critical Thinking Exercise: Nursing Management of the Client with Myasthenia Gravis

Situation: A 66-year-old male is recovering from myasthenia crisis during which time he suffered respiratory distress requiring mechanical ventilation for several days. The care provider believes an earlier episode of gastroenteritis triggered the crisis.

1. Match the terms associated with myasthenia gravis with the correct definition.

Liberates acetylcholine	a. Cholinergic
Destruction of self	b. Anticholinergic
Difficulty swallowing	c. Aspiration
Filtering of plasma	d. Dysphagia
Blocks acetylcholine	e. Plasmapheresis
Drawing in of fluid	f. Dysarthria
Difficulty speaking	g. Autoimmune

2. What is the rationale for each nursing activity?

   a. Encourage semi-Fowler's position.

   b. Maintain hydration.

   c. Administer medications 30 minutes before meals.

   d. Thicken liquids.

3. Which signs indicate the presence of a myasthenia crisis?

   _____ Respiratory distress   _____ Unusual euphoria

   _____ Difficulty talking   _____ Abdominal cramps

   _____ Muscle spasms   _____ Fever

   _____ Tearing   _____ Increased muscle weakness

   _____ Signs   _____ Difficulty swallowing

Nursing Management of the Client with Multiple Sclerosis (MS)

Key Points

- There are approximately 300,000 cases of multiple sclerosis (MS) in the United States.
- The onset of MS typically occurs between 20 and 40 years of age.
- Twice as many women are diagnosed with MS as men.
- The etiology of MS is unknown.
- There is a family history of MS in 15% of cases.
- The disease follows two major courses: (1) relapsing and remitting, and (2) chronic and progressive.
- There is no cure for the disease.
- Goals of collaborative management:
  - Control symptoms.
  - Prevent complications.
  - Provide adaptive devices to increase mobility and self-care.
- Important nursing diagnoses (actual or potential):
  - Impaired physical mobility
  - Activity intolerance
  - Visual, kinesthetic, tactile, sensory-perceptive alterations
  - Altered thought processes
  - Impaired home maintenance management
  - Ineffective family coping
  - Self-care deficit
  - Altered urinary elimination
  - Self-esteem disturbance
  - High risk for infections
- **Key Terms/Concepts**: Neurologic dysfunction, demyelination, activities of daily living (ADLs)

Overview

Multiple sclerosis (MS) is a chronic, progressive, degenerative, CNS disease that is characterized by intermittent damage of the myelin sheath that covers nerve cell axons. Demyelination impairs the transmission of nerve impulses. The destruction of myelin may be caused by an autoimmune reaction.

Risk Factors

- Infection

- Living in a cold climate
- Physical injury
- Emotional stress
- Pregnancy
- Fatigue
- Familial History

Signs and Symptoms

- Weakness of both lower extremities
- Paresthesias of one or more extremities
- Decreased sensitivity to stimuli to affected extremities
- Loss of vision
- Poor coordination
- Bowel and bladder dysfunction
- Fatigue
- Depression
- Seizures
- Emotional lability
- Sexual dysfunction
- Uhthoff's sign (A temporary worsening of vision and other neurological functions commonly seen in clients with MS, or clients predisposed to MS, just after exertion or in situations where they are exposed to heat.)

Diagnostic and Laboratory Tests

- History and physical exam
- Neurological assessment
- Magnetic resonance imaging (MRI) of brain and spine
- Cerebrospinal fluid (CSF) analysis
- Evoked potentials of optic and auditory pathways

Therapeutic Nursing Management

- **Prevention includes instructing at-risk clients to:**
  - Avoid people with infections.
  - Live in warm climate.
  - Use stress reduction and relaxation techniques.
  - Plan carefully for or avoid pregnancies.
  - Prevent urinary tract infections.
  - Avoid very warm or hot temperatures (Uhthoff's sign) because heat can increase weakness.
- **Assess/Monitor:**
  - Fluid intake and output

- For constipation
- Ability to perform ADLs
- Levels of fatigue as the day progresses
- Evaluate reactions to stress
- **Nursing Activities:**
  - Maintain fluid balance.
  - Provide a high fiber diet.
  - Set up a bowel-training program.
  - Schedule activities early in the day.
  - Provide adequate rest periods.
  - Perform intermittent catheterization if necessary.
  - Collaborate with physical therapy, occupational therapy, and speech therapy departments as needed.
  - Promote use of assistive devices.
  - Remove harmful objects from environment that client may fail to see.
  - Provide adequate lighting.
  - Encourage independence.
  - Suggest community MS support groups for client and family.
  - Stool softeners
  - Pain medications (caution with opiates related to respiratory depression)
  - Possible antidepressants

Pharmacology

- Corticosteroids (prednisone)
- Antispasmodic therapy (dantrolene [Dantrium])
- Interferon (Betaseron)
- Anticonvulsants (carbamazepine [Tegretol])
- Stool softeners (docusate sodium)
- Urinary problems (propantheline)
- Tremors (beta blockers, primidone, clonazepam)
- Hemifacial and dysesthesias (carbamazepine)
- Immunosuppressive agents (azathioprine, adrenocorticotropic hormone, methylprednisolone, cyclophosphamide, cyclosporine)

Complications

- Bacterial infection of lungs and bladder
- Pressure ulcers
- Contractures
- Seizures
- Immobility
- Blindness

Age-Related Changes—Gerontological Considerations

- MS is primarily a disease occurring in young adults.
- MS can interfere with the establishment of families and careers.

Critical Thinking Exercise: Nursing Management of the Client with Multiple Sclerosis (MS)

Situation: A home health care nurse is interviewing a 24-year-old client with newly diagnosed MS. The client is upset over her increasing loss of mobility, decreased visual acuity, and the severe fatigue that worsens as the day progresses. In addition, the client states she is experiencing mood swings she cannot control. As the client has a decreased libido, she is also worried about her relationship with her husband. The client tells the nurse she and her husband had planned a pregnancy, but now they have been forced to put their lives on hold.

1. What initial assessments should the home health care nurse make in regard to the client's MS?

2. What actions should the nurse take to help the client increase mobility and lessen fatigue?

3. What instructional materials and recommendations should the nurse leave with the client and her husband?

Nursing Management of the Client with Meningitis

Key Points

- Bacterial meningitis is a contagious infection.
- Prognosis depends on the supportive care given to the client.
- Goals of collaborative management:
  - Provide early diagnosis and treatment.
  - Eliminate the causative agent.
  - Prevent complications (ICP, sepsis, seizures).
  - Prevent fluid and electrolyte imbalance.
- Important nursing diagnoses (actual and potential):
  - Potential complications of meningitis (ICP, sepsis, seizures)
  - Ineffective airway clearance
  - Ineffective breathing pattern
  - Risk for injury
  - Acute confusion
  - Fluid volume deficit
  - Hyperthermia
  - Impaired physical mobility
  - Pain management
  - Knowledge deficit
- **Key Terms/Concepts**: Sepsis, aseptic, nuchal rigidity, Brudzinski's sign, Kernig's sign

Overview

Meningitis is defined as the inflammation of the meninges (membranes surrounding the brain and spinal cord), which may involve the dura mater, arachnoid, or pia mater. Meningeal inflammation can originate in the bloodstream or from direct extension of another infection or trauma.

Bacterial meningitis, the most common form, is transmitted via respiratory droplet from infected persons. The three types of meningitis include:

- **Aseptic** (viral, lymphoma, abscess, or hemorrhage)
- **Septic** (bacterial)
- **Tuberculosis** (tuberculosis bacillus)

Risk Factors

- Bacterial infections (Neisseria meningitidis, Streptococcus pneumoniae, Haemophilus influenzae)

- Surgery
- Invasive procedures
- Skull fracture or penetrating head wound
- Young age and older age
- Overcrowded living conditions

Signs and Symptoms

Bacterial

- Restlessness, agitation, irritability
- Hemorrhagic purpura, maculopapular rash, petechiae
- Headache
- Nuchal rigidity (stiff neck)
- Chills and high fever
- Photophobia *double vision*
- Seizures
- Increased intracranial pressure
- Back and abdominal pain
- Twitching
- Coma

Viral

- Mild, flu-like symptoms
- Intense headache
- Malaise
- Nausea/vomiting
- Drowsiness
- Nuchal rigidity
- Low-grade fever

Diagnostic and Laboratory Tests

- History and physical examination
- Positive Brudzinski's sign
- Positive Kernig's sign
- Gram stain
- CSF analysis
  - Cell count with differential
  - Total protein
  - Glucose
  - CSF culture
- Cultures to determine cause of infection:
  - Blood

- Throat
- Urine

Therapeutic Nursing Management

- **Assess/Monitor:**
    - Neurological status
    - Vital signs, especially temperature
    - Level of consciousness
    - For signs of seizure activity
    - For signs of increased intracranial pressure
    - Intake and output
    - Dehydration
- **Nursing Activities:**
    - Implement fever reduction measures if necessary.
    - Maintain client safety (padded side rails, oral airway at bedside).
    - Administer pain medication as prescribed.
    - Maintain respiratory isolation until antibiotics have been administered for 24 hours.
    - Report seizure activity.
    - Report meningococcal infections to public health department.
    - Educate the client about and assist with diagnostic testing, specifically in meningitis the lumbar puncture:
        - Confirm that a consent form has been signed, only after assessing the client's understanding of the procedure from discussion it with the physician.
        - Gather all necessary equipment; a sterile lumbar puncture pack, extra sterile gloves, masks and necessary lighting.
        - Be certain the client is comfortable by assessing room temperature, has empty bowels and bladder, and is given pain medication if indicated.
        - Instruct the client to be very still, on his/her side, head to chest, knees flexed; this puts the back in flexion, which creates more space between the vertebrae. The nurse may support the knees and neck to assist the client to stay still for the procedure.
        - Once the procedure is complete, be sure to label the specimens appropriately with the completed requisitions and transport to the lab promptly.
        - During the procedure monitor the client for comfort level.
        - After the procedure the client may be required to lie flat for 8 to 24 hours, monitor the site for swelling or bleeding, monitor the client for headache or changes in neurological status to include assessment of the lower extremities.
        - Document the procedure, the client's level of pain, and how the procedure was tolerated. Also document the correct labeling and transportation of the specimen to the lab.

Pharmacology

- Antibiotics (bacterial infections) (ceftriaxone [Rocephin®] or cefotaxime until culture and sensitivity results are available)
- Anticonvulsants (phenytoin)
- Antipyretics (acetaminophen)
- Analgesics (non-opioid)
- Fluids and electrolytes

Complications

- Seizures
- Airway obstruction and respiratory arrest
- Cardiac dysrhythmias
- Acute tubular necrosis
- Disseminated intravascular coagulation (DIC)
- Cranial nerve palsies
- Acute adrenal hemorrhage (Waterhouse-Friderichsen syndrome)
- Deafness
- Shock
- Dehydration
- Death

Age-Related Changes—Gerontological Considerations

- Increased risk for dehydration occurs with elderly persons, commonly due to diminished thirst.
- Increased risk for secondary complications such as pneumonia
- Increase risk for complications, including death

Lumbar Puncture

- Insertion of a spinal needle through L3-4 interspace into the lumbar subarachnoid space to obtain cerebrospinal fluid (CSF) measure CSF fluid or pressure, or instill air, dye or medications.
- Prior to a lumbar puncture a computerized tomography (CT) or magnetic resonance imaging (MRI) must be done to rule out increased intracranial pressure (ICP). A lumbar puncture done on a client with elevated ICP can lead to cerebral herniation.

Critical Thinking Exercise: Nursing Management of the Client with Meningitis

Situation: A 21-year-old college student is being treated for bacterial meningitis. She complains of a stiff neck and severe headache. Initial assessment by the nurse reveals a positive Kernig's sign and positive Brudzinski's sign.

1. Describe a positive Kernig's sign.

2. Describe a positive Brudzinski's sign.

3. Match the meningitis with the symptoms it produces. Use "V," or "B" as your answer.

	Mild, flu-like symptoms
	Irritability
	Headache
V = Viral Meningitis	Nuchal rigidity
B = Bacterial Meningitis	Drowsiness
	Chills and high fever
	Photophobia
	Seizures
	Low-grade fever
	Back and abdominal pain
	Twitching

4. Identify the following nursing activities as appropriate or inappropriate for the client with meningitis. Correct inappropriate nursing activities.

   a. Monitor vital signs every four hours.

   b. Initiate oxygen therapy.

   c. Institute seizure precautions if there is evidence of seizures.

   d. Initiate protective isolation.

   e. Obtain intravenous access for fluids and medications.

Nursing Management of the Client with Eye Trauma

Key Points

- Wearing appropriate eye gear can prevent many eye injuries.
- Eye injuries can result in permanent blindness.
- Goals of collaborative management:
  - Remove foreign objects (without producing further injury).
  - Prevent further injury.
  - Maintain vision.
  - Prevent infection.
- Important nursing diagnoses (actual or potential):
  - Anxiety and fear
  - Risk for infection
  - Altered sensory perception
  - Knowledge deficit
- **Key Terms/Concepts**: Enucleation, retinal detachment, globe puncture

Overview

Eye trauma occurs as a result of a blunt or penetrating injury to the eye due to foreign bodies, abrasions, chemical splashes, or lacerations.

Risk Factors

- Fireworks/explosives
- Hazardous activity without proper eye protection
- Sports injuries
- Risk-taking behaviors by children
- Working with projectiles such as glass or wood chips, air guns/staple guns

Signs and Symptoms

- Localized pain, headache
- Bleeding from the tissue around the eye
- Bleeding into the aqueous or vitreous humor
- Blurred vision
- Vitreous humor leakage with globe puncture

Diagnostic and Laboratory Tests

- History and physical examination

- Vision tests
- Fluorescence/wood's lamp ascertain abrasions
- Funduscopic exam
- Compute visual exam

Therapeutic Nursing Management

- **Assess/Monitor:**
  - Vision
- **Nursing Activities:**
  - Do not attempt to remove foreign object.
  - Instill eye drops or ointment as prescribed.
  - Prepare client for surgery if indicated.
  - Flush the eye with copious amounts of water in the event of irritating chemical splash.
  - If bleeding or leakage provide rest, darkness, keep blood pressure down

Pharmacology

- Topical antibiotics (bacitracin with polymyxin B, gentamicin, sulfacetamide, erythromycin, quinolones)
- Analgesics (opioid or NSAIDs)
- Avoid topical corticosteroids

Complications

- Partial or total blindness
- Secondary infection
- Retinal detachment
- Corneal ulceration/scar
- Cataracts
- Enucleation
- Optic nerve damage

Age-Related Changes—Gerontological Considerations

- Decreased vision increases risk for injuries.
- Decreased blink reflex
- Increased ocular dryness, decreased production of tears

Critical Thinking Exercise: Nursing Management of the Client with Eye Trauma

Situation: A 37-year-old male accidentally caught a fishhook in his eye while casting for fish. His brother, who was with him at the time, rushed him to the emergency department to have the fishhook removed. The man is in pain and frightened he will lose his sight. His initial assessment reveals no bleeding or loss of fluid from the eye.

1. What is the rationale for each of the nurse's actions?

   a. Leaving the fishhook in place

   b. Placing a patch on the client's uninjured eye

   c. Providing emotional support to the client

2. What can the nurse do to reduce the client's fears?

3. Which are desired client outcomes for this injury? Correct any incorrect/inappropriate outcomes.

   a. Absence of infection

   b. Monitoring vital signs

   c. Maintenance of vision

Nursing Management of the Client with Cataracts

Key Points

- Cataracts decrease vision, potentially leading to falls in older clients.
- Goals of collaborative management:
  - Maintain vision.
  - Prevent infection.
- Important nursing diagnoses (actual or potential):
  - Risk for injury
  - Pain management
  - Knowledge deficit
- **Key Trems/Concept**: Lens opacity, intraocular lens implant

Overview

A cataract is a clouding of the lens of the eye beginning around the outside of the lens and progressing until the entire lens is opaque.

Risk Factors

- Aging
- Diabetes mellitus
- Corticosteroid therapy
- Thorazine
- Eye trauma
- Exposure to heat or radiation
- Sun exposure
- Congenital, rare

Signs and Symptoms

- Inability to see objects clearly
- Loss of red reflex
- Grayish, pearly appearance to the lens
- Vision distortion (dimness, glaring, blurring)

Diagnostic and Laboratory Tests

- History and physical examination
- Eye examination, dilated

Therapeutic Nursing Management

- Prevent injures related to decreased vision.
- Prepare client for surgery if indicated.
- Teach regarding postoperative care.
- Avoid coughing, lifting or straining, after surgery.
- Eye patch, after surgery
- Teach client and his/her significant other how to instill eye drops, if prescribed.
- Provide instructions regarding the need for a new eyeglass prescription.
- Caution the client about driving until depth perception returns, after surgery, as ordered.

Complications

- Eye pain
- Infection
- Blindness

Age-Related Changes—Gerontological Considerations

- Cataracts occur as a result of normal aging.
- Older adults may have difficulty driving and climbing stairs due to impaired depth perception.

Critical Thinking Exercise: Nursing Management of the Client with Cataracts

Situation: A 62-year-old woman who has long-standing diabetes mellitus is being discharged to home following right cataract removal and intraocular lens implant. She is in stable condition and will be staying with her daughter until fully recovered.

1. Which are risk factors for the development of cataracts?

   _____ Hypertension   _____ Diabetes mellitus   _____ Hypothyroidism

   _____ Steroid therapy   _____ Eye trauma   _____ Infection

2. Which statements are true about cataracts? Correct false statements.

   a. Cataract formation is a pathological process that can be prevented if diagnosed early.

   b. Older adults with cataracts are at increased risk for injury due to falls.

   c. A cataract is a clouding that begins around the inside of the lens.

   d. Lenses with cataracts have a grayish, pearly appearance.

3. List the rationale for:

   a. Teaching the client to avoid coughing and lifting when she returns home

   b. Cautioning the client about driving an automobile

   c. Encouraging the client to obtain a new prescription for eyeglasses

Nursing Management of the Client with Glaucoma

| **Key Points** |

- Untreated acute or chronic, abnormally high intraocular pressure (IOP) may lead to permanent blindness.
- Blindness from glaucoma is almost always preventable if detected early in the disease's development.
- The level of vision lost before treatment begins has been found to be unrecoverable.
- Glaucoma may be asymptomatic until late in the disease course.
- Goals of collaborative management:
  - Diagnose early.
  - Lower the IOP.
  - Maintain normal IOP after initial treatment.
  - Control progressive disease.
- Important nursing diagnoses (actual or potential):
  - Pain management
  - Anxiety and fear
  - Knowledge deficit
  - Risk for injury
  - Risk for sensory alteration
- **Key Terms/Concepts**: Open angle, angle closure, intraocular pressure

Overview

Glaucoma refers to a group of ophthalmic conditions that generally produce abnormally high intraocular pressure (IOP) resulting in damage to the optic nerve; however, glaucoma does occur in some clients with IOP in a normal range (14-16 mmHg). Untreated glaucoma leads to gradual loss of the peripheral fields of vision, and subsequent blindness. The two most common types of glaucoma are:

Open Angle Glaucoma (sometimes referred to as: Primary Open Angle Glaucoma [POAG]). This is the most common form of glaucoma, occurring in 90% of persons diagnosed with glaucoma. Generally, both eyes are affected, but not necessarily equally. Generally, there are no early symptoms, with the IOP slowly rising and the cornea adapts without swelling. The fluid within the eye does not drain properly. The elevated IOP causes the optic nerve to slowly degenerate, causing slow, deteriorating loss of vision.

> **Angle Closure Glaucoma** (sometimes referred to as: Acute Glaucoma or Narrow Angle Glaucoma). Caused by an acute blockage of the fluid at the base of the interior angle between the iris and the cornea. Unlike open angle glaucoma, the IOP raises dramatically and very quickly. The iris is pushed forward resulting in a reduction or closure of the angle normally found between the iris and the cornea. This is a medical emergency and may result in permanent loss of vision if IOP is untreated for 24 to 48 hours.

Risk Factors

- Over age 60
- Obstructed outflow of aqueous humor
- Infection
- Tumors
- Hemorrhage
- Eye trauma
- Diabetes mellitus
- Genetic predisposition

Signs and Symptoms

Open Angle

- Insidious onset and slow progression
- Elevated IOP (intraocular pressure) > 21 mmHg
- Mild aching in the eye
- Loss of peripheral vision
- Loss of visual acuity not correctable with glasses
- Seeing halos around lights

Angle Closure

- Ophthalmic emergency
- Rapid onset
- Elevated IOP (intraocular pressure) > 21 mmHg
- Severe unilateral pain and feeling of pressure over affected eye
- Moderate pupil dilation
- Nonreactive to light
- Cloudy cornea
- Photophobia
- Decreased or blurred vision
- Seeing halos around lights

Diagnostic and Laboratory Tests

- Tonometry (measures IOP [intraocular pressure])
- Slit-lamp examination (visualize cornea)
- Gonioscopy (determines angle of anterior chamber of eye)
- Visual field test

Therapeutic Nursing Management

- **Assess/Monitor:**
  - Client's ability to provide self-care and feeding
- **Nursing Activities:**
  - Provide a safe environment.
  - Teach the client the need for carefully following prescribed drug therapy.
  - Assist with pre and postoperative care following surgical or laser interventions.
  - Instruct client to avoid activities that raise intraocular pressure such as heavy lifting, emotional stress, straining at defecation.
  - Instruct client to avoid drugs that dilate the pupils.

Pharmacology

- Topical beta-blocker eye drops (betaxolol [Betoptic], timolol [Timoptic])
- Mydriatic eye drops (epinephrine) for open-angle glaucoma only
- Diuretics (acetazolamide [Diamox])
- Miotic eye drops (pilocarpine, carbachol)

Complications

- Blindness

Age-Related Changes—Gerontological Considerations

- Age-related eye changes are evident with thickening of the lens.
- Sensory functions may decrease with age.
- Arthritis and cognitive impairment may inhibit proper administration of eye drops.

Critical Thinking Exercise: Nursing Management of the Client with Glaucoma

Situation: A 51-year-old man suffered bilateral retinal detachments three years apart. As a result of his two retinal surgeries, he now has secondary, chronic, open-angle glaucoma. His only prescribed medication is Timoptic, a topical beta-blocking agent. He is visiting the outpatient eye clinic for his annual eye examination.

1. Which statements are true regarding glaucoma? Correct false statements.

   a. Glaucoma produces abnormally low intraocular pressure.

   b. Glaucoma can temporarily damage the optic nerve.

   c. The two most common types of glaucoma are open angle and angle closure.

   d. Untreated glaucoma results in gradual loss of vision.

2. Match the clinical manifestation with the correct type of glaucoma. Use "OA" or "AC" for your answers.

OA = Open Angle	Rapid onset
AC = Angle Closure	Mild aching in the eye
	Loss of peripheral vision
	Moderate pupil dilation
	Photophobia
	Halos around lights
	Ophthalmic emergency

3. The nurse establishes teaching outcomes to determine the effectiveness of client education. Which expectations of client understanding are appropriate for the client with glaucoma?

   _____ The procedure for instilling antibacterial eye ointments.

   _____ The need to avoid straining at defecation.

   _____ Signs and symptoms of increased IOP (intraocular pressure).

   _____ How and when to use prescribed medications.

   _____ Clinical manifestations of eye infection.

   _____ Probable need for retinal surgery.

Nursing Management of the Client with Sensorineural Hearing Loss

Key Points

- Sensorineural hearing loss is caused by aging, injuries, ototoxic drugs, or other factors that adversely affect the inner ear, neural structures, and the nerve pathways that lead to the brain stem.
- Sensorineural hearing loss can be partial or complete, resulting in total deafness.
- Sensorineural hearing loss can range from loss of low tones to loss of high tones.
- More than 28 million people in the United States have hearing loss, with 90% of these people experiencing sensorineural hearing loss.
- Goals of collaborative management:
  - Promote aural rehabilitation.
  - Help client to use vision and touch more effectively.
  - Provide hearing aids, implantable hearing devices, and assistive listening devices for use with a telephone, radio, television, or computer.
  - Provide hearing education for lip reading and American Sign Language.
- Important nursing diagnoses (actual or potential):
  - Altered auditory sensory perception
  - Anxiety and fear
  - Impaired verbal communication
  - Diversional activity deficit
- **Key Terms/Concepts:** Cochlea, ototoxic, 8th cranial nerve, presbycusis, audiogram, hearing aids, lip reading, American Sign Language

Overview

Hearing loss may be sensorineural or conductive in origin.

Conductive hearing loss occurs in the external and middle ear, and sounds are blocked from conduction into the inner ear.

Sensorineural hearing loss is due to impaired function of the structures of the inner ear, primarily, the cochlea and 8th cranial (acoustic) nerve.

Risk Factors

- Genetics
- Exposure to excessive noise
- Ototoxic drugs (gentamicin, tobramycin, amikacin, vancomycin, cisplatin, and erythromycin)

- Exposure to measles, mumps, labyrinthitis, or meningitis
- Autoimmune reactions
- Neuromas of the 8th cranial nerve
- Ménière's disease
- Injury to the inner ear
- Head injury
- Presbycusis
- Loss of cortical auditory neurons
- Degeneration of cochlear hair cells
- Decreased vascularity of cochlea

Signs and Symptoms

- History of decreased hearing
- Difficulty understanding words
- Difficulty hearing certain sounds
- Hearing distortion
- Failure to respond to verbal communication
- Constant requests for repeating or clarifying verbal information
- Tendency to speak loudly
- Tilting head to understand conversation
- Tinnitus
- Sensorineural hearing loss on audiogram
- Tympanic membrane is normal
- Understanding of words decreased on audiogram

Diagnostic and Laboratory Tests

- History and physical exam
- Pneumatic otoscopy
- Rinne and Weber tuning fork tests
- Audiometry
- Tympanometry
- Auditory brain stem response test
- Imaging studies

Therapeutic Nursing Management

- **Prevention:**
  - Reduce exposure to excessive noise, use ear plugs when cannot avoid.
  - Avoid prolonged intake of ototoxic drugs.
  - Avoid trauma to ear.
  - Avoid cleaning or putting sharp objects in the ear, including the use of ear

swabs.
- Wear a hard hat or take other safety precautions if job involves risk of head injury.
- Routine ear examinations aid in early diagnosis and treatment of diseases causing sensorineural hearing loss.

- **Assess/Monitor:**
  - Client's hearing acuity level
  - Audiogram or tympanogram findings
  - Use of safety equipment
  - Client's current medications
  - Level of anxiety

- **Nursing Activities:**
  - Facilitate communication with client.
  - Before speaking, gently touch the client or make eye contact.
  - Reduce background noise if possible.
  - Directly face the client or the ear with which the client hears best.
  - Shine a light on your face so the clients can clearly see your lip movement.
  - Use short words and sentences to facilitate lip reading, if needed.
  - Encourage use of hearing aids.
  - Encourage use of assistive listening devices for the radio, television, telephone, and the computer.
  - Encourage social activity.
  - Refer client to community services and support groups that assist the hearing impaired.

Pharmacology

- Nicotinic acid (niacin)
- Antibiotics to treat infections (amoxicillin, amoxicillin with clavulanate)
- Steroids for autoimmune reactions (prednisone)

Complications

- Complete hearing loss
- Total loss of balance
- Vertigo
- Falling
- Abnormal gait
- Meningitis
- Septicemia
- Central Nervous System (CNS) abscess

Age-Related Changes—Gerontological Considerations

- Permanent sensorineural hearing loss is the 3rd most common disorder among individuals who are 65 or older.

- Presbycusis is a progressive hearing loss due to the aging process. It involves atrophy of the cochlea in the inner ear.
  - Hearing loss is gradual and bilateral.
  - Client thinks that the speaker is mumbling (especially words beginning with "f," "s," and "sh").
  - Client experiences inability to hear high-pitched sounds.

Critical Thinking Exercise: Nursing Management of the Client with Sensorineural Hearing Loss

Situation: An 80-year-old male client has been diagnosed with sensorineural hearing loss due to presbycusis. The client is taking niacin and is learning to use a hearing aid. The nurse is also providing the client with a list of community resources for people with impaired hearing.

1. What does niacin do that may help the client with sensorineural hearing loss?

2. Prioritize nursing activities for the client with sensorineural hearing loss, with "1" representing the most important activity

   _____ Encourage client to have extra hearing aid batteries on hand.

   _____ Protect client from injury related to dizziness and falls.

   _____ Teach client how to care for his hearing aid.

   _____ Facilitate communication with the client.

3. Which instructions will the nurse give the client about caring for his hearing aid?

   _____ Keep the hearing aid turned on throughout the day.

   _____ Open the battery compartment at night to avoid draining the battery.

   _____ Monthly cleaning is adequate for the ear mold.

   _____ Completely dry the ear mold before reattaching it to the receiver.

   _____ Avoid wearing the hearing aid if ear infection is present.

4. What should the client do if his hearing aid fails to work?

Nursing Management of the Client with Hypothyroidism

Key Points

- Hypothyroidism is a controllable disease that produces a slowing of the metabolic rate.
- Symptoms associated with hypothyroidism in older adults are often discounted as normal aging.
- Hypnotics and sedatives should be administered with caution to clients with severe hypothyroidism.
- Goals of collaborative management:
  - Recognize and treat early.
  - Restore normal metabolic rate (via medication).
  - Prevent complications (myxedema, hyperthyroidism, hypoglycemia).
- Important nursing diagnoses (actual or potential):
  - Activity intolerance
  - Self-care deficit
  - Risk for injury
  - Altered body image
  - Altered bowel elimination: constipation
  - Knowledge deficit
  - Ineffective individual coping
  - Fluid volume excess
- **Key Terms/Concepts**: Cretinism, myxedema, hypoglycemia

Overview

Hypothyroidism (myxedema) is due to a deficiency in thyroid hormone secretion, which results in reduced metabolic rate. Whereas, hyperthyroidism is the excess secretion of thyroid hormone. When thyroid hormone deficiency occurs in the fetus, the infant may be born with cretinism, a condition that produces impaired growth and mental functioning. The incidence of hypothyroidism increases after age 50.

Risk Factors

- Primary thyroid disease (dysfunction of the thyroid gland)
- Pituitary gland failure
- Hypothalamus failure
- Pituitary gland dysfunction
- Older age

- Female gender

Signs and Syzmptoms

- Extreme fatigue
- Dry skin, brittle nails, hair loss
- Cold intolerance
- Husky voice or hoarseness
- Fluid retention
- Weight gain
- Constipation
- Decreased appetite
- Dyspnea
- Elevation of serum cholesterol and triglyceride levels
- Menstrual disturbances
- Dulled mental processes
- Low blood pressure
- Bradycardia

Diagnostic and Laboratory Tests

- History and physical examination
- Serum thyroid function tests
- Elevated TSH (thyroid stimulating hormone)
  - Low T3 (triiodothyronine) contains 3 atoms of iodine
  - Low T4 (thyroxine) contains 4 atoms of iodine
  - Decreased BMR (Basal metabolic rate)
- Radioactive iodine uptake test (low 131I)
- Thyroid scan, radioscan or scintiscan ("cold" areas)
- T3 resin uptake test (also called: T3RU test) indirectly quantitates--it is inversely proportional to--TBG (thyroxin binding globulin), the protein that carries most of the T3 and T4 in the blood.

Therapeutic Nursing Management

- **Assess/Monitor:**
  - Vital signs
  - Nutritional status
  - Fluid status
- **Nursing Activities:**
  - Maintain warm environment.
  - Alternate activity with rest.
  - Increase fluid intake to 2000 mL/day to prevent constipation.
  - Encourage high fiber diet.
  - Provide emotional support regarding changes in body appearance.
  - Teach the importance of life-long medication regimen.

- Teach avoidance of the use of sedatives or narcotics.
- Teach the signs of thyroid over-medication (tachycardia, nervousness, restlessness, insomnia).
- Teach the signs of thyroid under-medication (fatigue, lethargy, weight gain).

Pharmacology

- Thyroid hormone replacement therapy (levothyroxine sodium [Synthroid])

Complications

- Myxedema coma (persistent, low thyroid production)
- Atherosclerosis
- Hyperthyroidism related to excessive medication
- Hypoglycemia

Age-Related Changes—Gerontological Considerations

- The high prevalence of hypothyroidism in older adults is related to the altered immune function occurring with aging.
- Symptoms of hypothyroidism may be confused with signs of normal aging.
- Increased risk for altered skin integrity.
- Increased risk for constipation.
- Increased risk of coronary artery disease.

Critical Thinking Exercise: Nursing Management of the Client with Hypothyroidism

Situation: A 46-year-old client visits the outpatient clinic for symptoms of fatigue, cold intolerance, dry scaly skin, hoarseness, weight gain, and fluid retention. Based on her symptoms, thyroid studies were obtained that revealed an elevated TSH (thyroid stimulating hormone) and decreased T3 and T4 levels. The client was placed on Synthroid 0.1 mg PO daily and instructed to return to the clinic in one month.

1. Which other clinical manifestations are common with hypothyroidism?

   _____ Hypertension   _____ Decreased appetite   _____ Dyspnea

   _____ Hair loss   _____ Diarrhea   _____ Elevated cholesterol

   _____ Menstrual disturbances _____ Euphoria   _____ Dulled mental processes

2. State the rationale for each nursing activity. Teaching the client:

   a. The importance of maintaining lifelong hormone replacement therapy

   b. Increase her intake of fluids

   c. The signs of thyroid over-medication

3. Which findings best indicate that the client is responding effectively to the prescribed drug therapy?

   _____ Reversal of signs and symptoms

   _____ Absence of drug side effects

   _____ Reported improved quality of life

   _____ Absence of complications

Nursing Management of the Client with Hyperthyroidism

Key Points

- Hyperthyroidism is a thyroid condition that causes an increase in the body's overall metabolic rate.
- Causes of Hyperthyroidism:
    - Graves' disease is the most common form and is due to abnormal stimulation of the thyroid by immunoglobulins.
    - Thyroiditis (common)
    - Emotional shock with thyroid
    - Stress
    - Infection
- The most serious consequences of severe untreated hyperthyroidism leading to thyroid storm which may result in myocardial hypertrophy and heart failure, fever, and mania.
- A goiter (enlarged thyroid gland) occurs when thyroid stimulating hormone (TSH) increases production in an attempt to stimulate the thyroid gland to release thyroid hormone.
- The presence of a goiter does not necessarily mean that the client is hyperthyroid.
- A goiter is an enlargement of the thyroid gland and may be due to tumors or iodine deficiency. Goiters may or may not be associated with hyperthyroidism.
- Graves' disease is the most common form of hyperthyroidism and is due to abnormal stimulation of the thyroid by immunoglobulins.
- Clients using iodide treatment must avoid over-the-counter medications that contain iodide, such as cough medicines, bronchodilators, and salt substitutes.
- Thyroidectomy was once the primary treatment for hyperthyroidism. Currently thyroidectomy is performed when the client is pregnant, has a large goiter, has allergies to antithyroid medications, or is unable to take antithyroid medications.
    - Prior to surgery, the client must be as euthyroid (normal functioning thyroid) as possible in order to reduce the risk of thyroid storm following surgery.
    - Blood pressure, heart rate, and cardiac rhythm should also be stabilized before surgery.
    - Thyroid storm, also knows as thyrotoxic crisis or thyrotoxicosis, is an acute, life-threatening, thyroid hormone induced hypermetabolic state. The symptoms of hyperthyroidism are all magnified in this situation.
- Important nursing diagnoses (actual or potential):
    - Imbalanced nutrition: Less than body requirements
    - Low self-esteem related to appearance

- Altered body image
- Altered body temperature
- Potential for arrhythmias related to hypermetabolic state
- **Key Terms/Concepts**: Cretinism, myxedema, hypoglycemia, Graves' Disease, exophthalmos

Overview

Hyperthyroidism produces an increase in circulating thyroid hormones. Treatment is directed at decreasing thyroid hyperactivity to prevent complications, especially those associated with hypermetabolism and those related to the cardiovascular system. These treatments may include antithyroid medications, radiation, and surgery.

Risk Factors

- Female gender: 3 times more
- Too much thyroid replacement hormone
- Autoimmune
- Toxic multinodular goiter
- Toxic uninodular goiter
- Rare:
  - TSH (thyroid stimulating hormone) pituitary tumor
  - Iodine-induced hyperthyroidism, possibly related to amiodarone administration

Signs and Symptoms

- Early
  - Nervousness
  - Hyperexcitable
  - Apprehensive
  - Palpitations
  - Rapid pulse at rest
  - Hand tremors
  - Insomnia
  - Heat intolerance
  - Skin warm, moist, perspires freely
- Late
  - Severe weight loss
  - Increased appetite
  - Fatigue
  - Changes in bowel function
  - Increased pulse rate
  - Amenorrhea
  - Atrial fibrillation

- Heart failure
- Osteoporosis and fractures
- Exophthalmos (bulging eyes)
- Delirious

Diagnostic and Laboratory Tests

- History and physical examination
- Decreased TSH (thyroid stimulating hormone)
  - Increased T3 (triiodothyronine) contains 3 atoms of iodine
  - Increased Free T4 (thyroxine) contains 4 atoms of iodine
  - Decreased BMR (Basal metabolic rate)
- Radioactive iodine uptake test (increased 131I)
- Thyroid scan, radio scan or scintiscan ("hot" areas)
- Ultrasound guided fine-needle aspiration of nodule, if present
- Soft gland that may pulsate
- Bruit heard over thyroid

Therapeutic Nursing Management

- **Assess/Monitor:**
  - Vital signs: temperature, heart rate, rhythm, blood pressure
  - Heart sounds
  - Intake and output
  - Nutrition
  - Maintain comfortable environment: change bed and clothing as often as necessary, provide cool baths, cool fluids, monitor room temperature
  - Client and family education regarding long term use of antithyroid medications and monitoring for complications of therapy; as well as possible use of thyroid replacement medications if the client becomes hypothyroid
  - Thyroid storm
- **Nursing Activities:**
  - Administer antithyroid medications
  - Prepare for possible thyroidectomy
    - Preoperative Care (thyroidectomy)
  - Administer antithyroid medications and iodine medications, if not previously done.
  - Administer beta blockers or other medications to control blood pressure, heart rate, and rhythm, if needed.
  - Instill methylcellulose eyedrops at bedtime.
  - Provide adequate rest.
  - Provide optimal nutrition.
  - Teach deep breathing and leg exercises.

- Teach client how to support head manually when turning to decrease pressure on surgical suture line.
- Teach client ROM (range of motion) exercises for the neck.
  - Postoperative Care (thyroidectomy)
- Decrease stress on suture line by keeping head midline via use of pillows or sandbags and avoid hypo- or hyper-extension of the neck.
- Keep head-of-bed in semi-Fowler's position to decrease inflammation.
- Keep tracheostomy set, endotracheal tube, laryngoscope, and suction equipment at bedside.
- Be sure that there is a client IV (intravenous) line.
- Provide humidified oxygen as ordered.
- Monitor clients voice quality regularly, as ordered; initially every 30-60 minutes.
- Be prepared to administer calcium gluconate (injury to the parathyroid may occur during thyroidectomy due to its proximity, causing a decrease in serum calcium).
- Monitor for complications of surgical or radiologic ablation of the thyroid such as respiratory obstruction, hemorrhage, hypothyroidism, hypocalcemia (damage to the parathyroid glands), tetany, injury to recurrent laryngeal nerve, and thyroid storm.
- Administer pain medications, calcium replacement, and antipyretics as needed.
- Begin levothyroxine therapy as directed and monitor TSH as ordered.
- Give corticosteroids as needed to reduce swelling.
- Provide information about thyroid replacement medication.
- Schedule follow-up clinic and laboratory appointments.
- Nursing management of thyroid storm usually cased by undertreatment of hyperthyroidism, thyroid surgery, infection, or trauma:
  - Vital signs and cardiac output (if pulmonary artery catheter or non-invasive cardiac output monitoring available)
  - ECG monitoring
  - Arterial blood gases
  - Pulse oximetry
  - Oxygen
  - Intravenous fluids
  - Antithyroid medication - propylthiouracil, iodine
  - External cooling
  - Medications to treat cardiac symptoms - beta-adrenergic blockers, unless contraindicated
  - Hydrocortisone
  - Prepare to treat shock
  - Treat precipitating factors

Pharmacology

- Methimazole
- Potassium iodide SSKI
- Lugol's solution
- Propylthiouracil
- Radioactive iodine 123 I or 131 I
- Beta-adrenergic blockers
- Hydrocortisone

Complications

- Thyroid storm
- Heart failure
- Anxiety, mania

Age-Related Changes—Gerontological Considerations

- Characteristic signs and symptoms of hyperthyroidism may not be demonstrated by the elderly.
- The elderly are more susceptible to the cardiovascular complications of hyperthyroidism.
- Because typical signs and symptoms may be absent in the elderly, hyperthyroidism may be more difficult to diagnose in the elderly.
- Antithyroid agents are more likely to cause granulocytopenia in the elderly.
- Beta-adrenergic agents may increase the likelihood of heart failure in the elderly.

Critical Thinking Exercise: Nursing Management of the Client with Hyperthyroidism

Situation: A 46-year-old male client visits the outpatient clinic for new-onset symptoms of feeling as though his heart is racing, insomnia, and anxiety. Upon further questioning there has been a 10 pound weight loss over the past two weeks without the client dieting. Based on his symptoms, the nurse practitioner obtained thyroid studies, which revealed a decreased TSH (thyroid stimulating hormone) and increased T3 and T4 levels. The client is diagnosed with hyperthyroidism and is scheduled to see an endocrinologist for further evaluation and treatment. In the meantime, the client is placed on Lopressor 50 mg a day.

1. What is the usual treatment for hyperthyroidism?

2. Why did the nurse practitioner place the client of Lopressor?

3. A potential complication of hyperthyroidism is thyroid storm. What signs and symptoms might the client with thyroid storm exhibit and what would the nursing management include?

4. Match the symptoms. Put an arrow next to the sign or symptom.

   (up arrow) = hyperthyroidism

   (down arrow) = hypothyroidism

   a. dry skin _____

   b. heat intolerance _____

   c. constipation _____

exophthalmos _____

e. palpitations _____

f. weight loss _____

g. weight gain _____

h. cold intolerance _____

i. excess perspiration _____

j. amenorrhea _____

k. low blood pressure _____

l. insomnia _____

m. bradycardia _____

n. increased blood pressure _____

Nursing Management of the Client with a Thyroidectomy

Key Points

- Thyroidectomies have been performed since the early 1880s.
- Ideal candidates are young and free from heart disease, diabetes, and renal disease.
- Prior to surgery, the client must be euthyroid (thyroid gland functioning normally) if possible, to reduce the risk of thyroid storm following surgery.
  - Thyroid storm is an acute, life-threatening, thyroid-hormone-induced hypermetabolic state.
  - Thyroid storm is the most extreme case of thyrotoxicosis.
  - Thyrotoxicosis is a syndrome caused by too much free thyroid hormone in the bloodstream.
- Preoperative preparation may take as long as 2 to 3 months.
- Goals of collaborative management:
  - Provide meticulous preoperative assessment and preparation.
  - Prevent postoperative complications such as thyroid storm, hypocalcemia, or hemorrhage.
  - Instruct the client in lifelong hormone replacement therapy.
- Important nursing diagnoses (actual or potential):
  - Pain management
  - Ineffective airway clearance
  - Impaired verbal communication
  - Risk for injury related to tetany
  - Risk for trauma related to head/neck surgery
  - Ineffective management of therapeutic regimen
  - High risk for postoperative complications related to knowledge deficit
- **Key Terms/Concepts:** Euthyroid, hyperthyroidism, thyrotoxicosis, thyroid storm, thyroid replacement therapy

Overview

Hyperthyroidism produces an increase in circulating thyroid hormones. Treatment is directed at decreasing thyroid hyperactivity to prevent complications, especially those associated with hypermetabolism and those related to the cardiovascular system. These treatments may include antithyroid medications, radiation, and surgery.

Risk Factors/Indications for Surgery

- Hyperthyroidism that has not been relieved by pharmaceutical interventions

- Thyroid cancer

Signs and Symptoms Necessitating Thyroidectomy

- Hyperthyroidism
    - Increased appetite
    - Weight loss
    - Fatigue
    - Insomnia
    - Heat intolerance
    - Goiter
    - Arrhythmias
    - Exophthalmos
- Thyroid cancer
    - Hard painless nodule
    - Enlarged thyroid gland
    - Hoarseness or dysphagia
    - Signs of hyper- or hypothyroidism
    - Displaced trachea

Diagnostic and Laboratory Tests

- History and physical exam
- Complete blood count (CBC)
- Radioactive iodine uptake test (low 131I)
- Thyroid scan
- Magnetic resonance imaging (MRI)
- Computed tomography (CT)/computed axial tomography (CAT) scan
- Ultrasound
    - 2D (2-dimensional)
    - 3D (3-dimensional)
- Fine-needle aspiration

Therapeutic Nursing Management

- Preoperative preparation to establish euthyroid status and decrease postoperative complications:
    - Administer antithyroid drugs.
    - Administer iodine preparations.
    - Provide adequate rest.
    - Ensure optimal nutrition.
    - Teach deep breathing and leg exercises.
    - Teach client how to support head manually when turning to decrease pressure on surgical suture line.
    - Teach client ROM exercises for the neck.

- **Assess/Monitor (Postoperative Period):**
    - For complications
    - Vital signs
    - Intake and output
    - Rectal temperature
    - Client's voice for hoarseness or voice weakness
- **Nursing Activities (Postoperative Period):**
    - Decrease stress on suture line.
    - Place client in semi-Fowler's position.
    - Use pillows and sandbags to support head and neck.
    - Advise client to avoid hypo-or hyper-extending the neck.
    - Set up a tracheostomy set, endotracheal tube, laryngoscope, and suction equipment at the bedside.
    - Have ampules of calcium gluconate on hand.
    - Insure that the client has a patent intravenous line.
    - Provide analgesia.
    - Provide humidified supplemental oxygen.
    - Ask client to speak every 30-60 minutes and note voice quality.
    - Provide information about thyroid replacement medication.
    - Schedule follow-up clinic and laboratory appointments.

Pharmacology

- Preoperative:
    - Antithyroid medications (methimazole [Tapazole], potassium iodide [SSKI], propylthiouracil [PTU])
    - Iodine preparations (radioactive)
    - Propranolol (to reduce resting heart rate)
- Postoperative:
    - Thyroid hormone replacement therapy (Synthroid)

Complications

- Respiratory obstruction
- Hemorrhage
- Hypocalcemia
- Tetany
- Injury to recurrent laryngeal nerve
- Thyroid storm (thyrotoxic crisis)

Age–Related Changes—Gerontological Considerations

- Signs of hyperthyroidism may be incorrectly attributed to aging.
- A pre-existing cardiac disorder may be aggravated by hyperthyroidism.
- The elderly are more susceptible to postoperative complications.

...cal Thinking Exercise: Nursing Management of the Client with a Thyroidectomy

Situation: A 25-year-old female client is being admitted to the postanesthesia care unit (PACU) following a thyroidectomy for hyperthyroidism. The nurse places the client in a semi-Fowler's position and is supporting her head and neck with pillows and sandbags. The nurse frequently checks the client's vital signs, and assesses her suture line for strain or bleeding. Once the immediate postoperative period has passed, the client will be transferred to the surgical floor where she will recuperate and learn about lifelong thyroid replacement therapy.

1. Which equipment should the nurse have available at the client's bedside?

_____ Tracheostomy set _____ Sodium bicarbonate

_____ Endotracheal tub _____ Thoracentesis tray

_____ Suction equipment _____ Calcium gluconate

_____ Thyroxine _____ Laryngoscope

_____ Defibrillator

2. Which complications is the client most at risk for immediately following thyroidectomy?

_____ Infection _____ Airway obstruction

_____ Edema of glottis _____ Tetany

_____ Seizures _____ Laryngeal nerve damage

_____ Hemothorax _____ Tracheal compression

_____ Thyroid storm

3. What is the rationale for supporting the client's head and neck with sandbags and pillows?

4. Which are clinical manifestations of thyroid storm?

_____ Fever   _____ Hypertension

_____ Tachycardia   _____ Respiratory distress

_____ Lethargy   _____ Confusion

_____ Coma   _____ Abdominal cramping

_____ Thirst

Nursing Management of the Client with Adrenal Disorders: Cushing's Syndrome and Addison's Disease

| Key Points |

- The adrenal glands, which rest on top of each kidney, are composed of the cortex or outer part of the gland and the medulla or inner part of the gland.
- The adrenal gland secretes glucocorticoids (cortisol), androgens (male sex hormones: testosterone and DHEA) and mineralocorticoids (mainly aldosterone).
  - The secretion of these hormones is regulated by a negative feedback mechanism.
  - The hypothalamus secretes corticotrophin releasing factor (CRF), which then stimulates the pituitary to secrete ACTH (adrenocorticotropic hormone). ACTH then stimulates the adrenal gland (specifically the adrenal cortex) to secrete cortisol.
  - The negative feedback mechanism inhibits CRF and ACTH when the level of adrenal hormones is high and stimulates CRF and ACTH when the level of adrenal hormones is low.
  - Long term use of exogenous steroids interferes with the negative-feedback mechanism.
  - Cushing's syndrome related to pituitary tumor is treated with transsphenoidal hypophysectomy or radiation.
  - Primary adrenal hypertrophy is treated by adrenalectomy.
  - Clients taking exogenous steroids for three or more days require gradual tapering of the medication. Abrupt withdrawal of long term steroids may cause Addisonian crisis, or adrenal crisis.
- Clients who require long term steroid therapy may prevent adrenal shutdown with alternate day therapy.
- The medulla secretes the catecholamines epinephrine and norepinephrine.
- Causes of Addison's Disease, also known as adrenal insufficiency, can be divided into two categories:
  - Primary adrenal insufficiency
  - Secondary adrenal insufficiency
- Causes of Cushing's Syndrome, also known as hypercortisolism, can be divided into two categories:
  - ACTH (adrenocorticotropic hormone)-dependent
    - Pituitary tumor (most common)
    - Non-pituitary or ectopic tumor
    - Hypothalamic or ectopic CRH (corticotropin-releasing hormone) tumor

- ACTH-independent
    - Iatrogenic (cause may be unknown, but most common is overzealous use of exogenous steroid administration; is most common cause of ACTH-independent)
    - Adrenal tumor
    - Nodular adrenal hyperplasia (enlargement)
    - Factitious
- "Pseudo-Cushing's Syndrome" may cause changes in laboratory findings similar to Cushing's Syndrome
    - Depression
    - Alcoholism
    - Estrogen therapy
    - Eating disorders
- Goals of collaborative management:
    - Recognize and treat the underlying cause early.
    - Maintain normal adrenal function.
    - Prevent complications.
- Important nursing diagnoses (actual or potential):
    - Risk for infection
    - Risk for injury
    - Fluid volume excess (Cushing's syndrome)
    - Fluid volume deficit (Addison's disease)
    - Risk for electrolyte imbalance related to fluid losses of diarrhea and/or vomiting (Addison's disease) or volume excess (Cushing's syndrome)
    - Risk of pulmonary edema (Cushing's syndrome)
    - Risk of blood glucose imbalance, hyperglycemia (Cushing's syndrome) and hypoglycemia (Addison's disease)
    - Risk of infections and poor wound healing (Cushing's syndrome)
    - Risk of fracture (Cushing's syndrome)
    - Abnormal changes in blood pressure, hypertension (Cushing's syndrome) and hypotension (Addison's disease)
    - Decreased cardiac output (Addison's disease)
    - Altered nutrition, less than body requirements
    - Fatigue
    - Impaired skin integrity
    - Body image disturbance
    - Activity intolerance
    - Self-care deficit
    - Altered thought processes related to mood swings, irritability, and depression
    - Ineffective individual coping
    - Sexual dysfunction (Cushing's syndrome)
    - Risk for hyperglycemia related to excess glucocorticoid production
    - Self-care deficit related to weakness, fatigue, sleep disturbances, and muscle wasting

- Altered self image related to physical appearance
- Knowledge deficit
- **Key Terms/Concepts:** Cortisol, hyperglycemia, syndrome, buffalo hump, glucocorticoid hormones, adrenocorticoid, ACTH, CRF, negative feedback, hypothalamus, exogenous, Addisonian crisis, tapering of steroids, mineralocorticoid hormones, adrenal insufficiency, glucocorticoid, androgens

Overview

Cushing's syndrome is the term used to describe a constellation of signs and symptoms that results from excessive adrenocortical activity which produces an increase in circulating adrenal hormones. **The treatment of choice is generally and adrenalectomy (or removal of other tumor, if appropriate), however, some cases may respond to radiation or medications. If the etiology is overzealous use of exogenous steroid, then decreasing the dose, cutting back to every-other-day dosing, or a combination may help.**

Addison's disease develops when the immune system makes antibodies that attack the body's own tissues or organs and slowly destroy them. Adrenal insufficiency occurs when at least 90% of the adrenal cortex has been destroyed. Damage to the adrenal glands result in glucocorticoid and mineralocorticoid hormone deficiencies, leading to the signs and symptoms of Addison's disease. **Approximately 80% of Addison's disease is autoimmune related, followed by TB (tuberculosis), HIV (human immunodeficiency virus), a pituitary problem, or abrupt withdrawal of exogenous steroid therapy.**

Treatment of Addison's disease includes administration of medications that will replace or substitute for the hormones not being produced naturally. Aldosterone is replaced with oral doses of a mineralocorticoid. Cortisol is replaced orally with a glucocorticoid, such as hydrocortisone.

Risk Factors

Cushing's syndrome

- Exogenous corticosteroid medications, especially if prolonged usage or excessive dose
- Female gender 8 times more likely
- Female 20 to 40 years of age
- Tumor of the adrenal cortex

Addison's disease

- 80% autoimmune
- Infections such as tuberculosis that destroy or damage the adrenal gland
- Metastatic cancer that spreads to the adrenal glands, usually from the lungs or breasts
- Corticosteroid medications in large enough doses to suppress the hypothalamic-pituitary-adrenal axis, resulting in atrophy of the adrenal gland
- Acquired immunodeficiency syndrome (AIDS)
- Stressful events such as a severe illness, accident, surgery, or other traumatic event can precipitate the development of Addison's disease.

- Pituitary disorder that lead to decreased secretion and/or decreased production of ACTH

Signs and Symptoms

Cushing's syndrome

- Weakness
- Ruddy complexion
- Emotional changes/depression
- Risk for infection, immune suppression
- "Buffalo Hump" due to increased fat deposits in the neck and supraclavicular area
- Muscle wasting of extremities and weakness due to protein catabolism
- "Moon face" appearance related to fluid retention and electrolyte disturbances
- Hyperglycemia and/or diabetes related to excess circulating glucocorticoids
- Hypokalemia, hypernatremia related to excess circulating mineralocorticoids
- Cataracts and glaucoma
- Hypertension and heart failure
- Truncal obesity
- Menstrual irregularities
- Impotence
- Adrenal suppression
- Impaired wound healing
- Skin: thin and fragile with ecchymoses and abdominal striae
- Sleep disturbances due to altered circadian rhythm
- Bone demineralization, osteoporosis, kyphosis, back pain
- Masculine traits in women, increased hair growth, breast atrophy, amenorrhea, related to increase in circulating androgens
- Impotence

Addison's disease

- Chronic, worsening fatigue and muscle weakness
- Loss of appetite and weight loss
- Nausea, vomiting, and diarrhea
- Abdominal pain
- Dehydration
- Low blood pressure causing dizziness or fainting when standing; orthostatic hypotension
- Skin changes including a darkening of the skin (hyperpigmentation), most visible on scars; skin folds; pressure points such as the elbows, knees, knuckles and toes; lips; and mucous membranes
- Alopecia

- Fever
- Irritability, anxiety, and depression
- Salt loss, causing a craving for salty foods
- Hypoglycemia, or low blood sugar, usually more severe in children than in adults
- Irregular or absent menstrual periods

Diagnostic and Laboratory Tests

Cushing's syndrome

- History and physical examination
- 24-hour urinary free cortisol - increased cortisol excretion
- Increased plasma cortisol
- Increased serum sodium and glucose
- Decreased serum potassium
- Elevated cortisol level with Dexamethasone suppression test
- CRH (corticotropin-releasing hormone) stimulation test shows increased ACTH and cortisol if pituitary tumor and no response if ectopic or adrenal tumor
- CT, MRI, and Ultrasound are used to detect adrenal and pituitary tumors

Addison's disease

- History and physical examination
- Decreased plasma cortisol
- Normochromic, normocytic anemia with eosinophilia
- Hyperkalemia, hypochloremia, hypoglycemia
- 24-hour urinary free cortisol - decreased cortisol excretion
- With primary insufficiency; serum levels of cortisol are decreased and ACTH increased and with secondary insufficiency; serum levels of cortisol are increased and ACTH decreased
- Definitive diagnosis is failed response to CRH stimulation test
- Computed tomography (CT)/computed axial tomography (CAT) scan
- Magnetic resonance imaging (MRI of adrenals to detect changes due to tuberculosis, may be noted as calcium deposits on adrenals via MRI or abdominal x-ray)

Therapeutic Nursing Management

- **Assess/Monitor:**
  - For both
    - Vital signs, especially blood pressure and temperature
    - Weight
    - Serum electrolytes
    - Input and output
    - Blood glucose

- **Cushing's syndrome**
  - Signs of infection
  - Skin breakdown related to thinning of skin, fragility, and easy bruising
  - Osteopenia/osteoporosis
  - Response to surgery, radiation, and/or medications
- **Addison's disease**
  - Diarrhea and/or vomiting
  - Skin for changes in pigmentation
  - Mood
  - Stress levels
  - Symptoms of Addisonian crisis:
    - Sudden onset of penetrating-type pain in lower back, abdomen, or legs
    - Severe vomiting and diarrhea
    - Dehydration
    - Hypotension
    - Coma
- **Nursing Activities:**
  - **Cushing's syndrome**
    - Provide emotional support related to body image changes and mood swings.
    - Promote skin integrity.
    - Prevent injury.
    - Encourage intake of a high-protein, high-calcium, low-calorie, low-fat, low-sodium, and high in vitamin D diet.
    - Assist with preparation for surgery if indicated.
    - Prepare for radiation therapy if indicated.
    - Teach client:
      - Importance of not discontinuing corticosteroid medications abruptly
      - Signs and symptoms of excessive or insufficient adrenal hormone
      - Skin care
      - Importance of follow-up with health care provider
      - How to take prescribed medication: dose, side effects, schedule
      - To wear medical alert identification
      - Not to take over-the-counter medications without approval of provider
      - Safety measures related to weakness
  - **Addison's disease**
    - Teach the client to follow the prescribed medications exactly.
    - Provide the client with a high-sodium, low -potassium diet with increased fluids.

- Counsel the client about ways to avoid stressful events and control his or her reactions to stressful events that do occur.
- Instruct client to carry an identification card that states that client has Addison's disease.
    • In case of an emergency, the card should instruct emergency personnel to inject 100 milligrams of cortisol if its bearer is found severely injured or unable to answer questions, and also to give glucose.
    • The card should include the name and telephone number of the physician and the family member or friend to notify in an emergency, after calling 911.
- Advise the client to carry a needle, a syringe, and an injectable form of cortisol for emergencies when traveling and to carry extra glucose if become hypoglycemic.
- Instruct client to increase medication during periods of stress or mild upper respiratory infections; in most cases the dose is doubled.
- Advise client to obtain immediate medical attention for severe infections, vomiting or diarrhea.

Pharmacology

Cushing's syndrome

- Adrenal enzyme inhibitors (aminoglutethimide) used for Cushing's disease caused by a tumor

Addison's disease

- Mineralocorticoids:
    • Fludrocortisone acetate
    • Desoxycorticosterone
- Glucocorticoids:
    • Hydrocortisone
    • Prednisone
- Addisonian crisis
    • Normal saline and dextrose IV (intravenous)
    • Glucocorticoids IV
    • Antipyretics
    • Possible antiemetics

Complications

Cushing's syndrome

- Secondary diabetes mellitus
- Hypertension
- Osteoporosis
- Addisonian crisis
- Shock

- Death

Addison's disease
- Addisonian crisis (acute adrenal insufficiency)
- Osteoporosis due to the excessive use of glucocorticoids
- Hypoglycemia
- Hypotension
- Shock
- Death

Age-Related Changes—Gerontological Considerations

- Older adults have a decreased ability to fight infections.
- Prevalence of chronic disease is greater in the elderly.
- Older adults may have more difficulty managing diabetes mellitus related to Cushing's syndrome.
- Risk for congestive heart failure (CHF) in clients with Cushing's syndrome is increased related to fluid retention.
- Addison's disease occurs in all age groups.
- Weakness may contribute to increased risk of falls.
- Signs of depression, skin changes, and osteoporosis may be incorrectly attributed to aging.
- Elderly clients may need lower doses of adrenal replacement medications with Addison's disease.

Critical Thinking Exercise: Nursing Management of the Client with Adrenal Disorders: Cushing's Syndrome and Addison's Disease

Situation: A 62-year-old woman has been taking 10 mg prednisone PO for over two years to control pulmonary inflammation from COPD (chronic obstructive pulmonary disease). When assessing the client, the nurse notes she has a round-appearing puffy face, a large abdomen, and thin arms and legs. There are multiple bruises on the woman's arms and legs.

1. What is the most common risk factor for Cushing's syndrome?

2. Which are common symptoms of cortisol excess (Cushing's syndrome)?

_____ Weight loss   _____ Weakness

_____ Abdominal striae   _____ Hypoglycemia

_____ Electrolyte imbalance   _____ Excessive hair growth

_____ Bone demineralization   _____ Cataracts

_____ Glaucoma   _____ Hypotension

3. State the rationale for:

   a. Placing the nursing diagnosis "Risk for injury: fractures" on the client's nursing care plan.

   b. Teaching the client to avoid abruptly discontinuing her replacement medication.

Nursing Management of the Client with Diabetes Mellitus

Key Points

- Diabetes mellitus (DM) is a chronic condition, which is characterized by hyperglycemia resulting from defects in insulin secretion, insulin action, or both.
  - Chronic complications include:
    - **Macrovascular**: arteriosclerosis and atherosclerotic changes to moderate and large sized arteries and veins
      Characterized by: coronary artery disease, myocardial infarction, peripheral vascular disease, cerebral vascular disease
    - **Neuropathy**: peripheral nerve dysfunction
      Characterized by: numbness, pain, burning, loss of protective sensation, and possible loss of angle reflexes. May also affect gastric and intestinal motility, erectile function, bladder function, cardiac function, and vascular tone, so may be autonomic as well as peripheral.
    - **Nephropathy**: renal insufficiency
      Characterized by: persistent proteinuria, hypertension, and a progressive decline in renal function; often leads to end stage renal disease (ESRD). Onset occurs before gross proteinuria, so measurements of microalbuminuria are extremely important. Diabetes is the most common cause of ESRD in the United States.
    - **Diabetic retinopathy**: occurs when the microvasculature that nourishes the retina is damaged. May vary from a mild asymptotic form to a severe, rapidly devastating condition.
      Characterized by: visual impairment varying from mild blurring to severe obstruction of vision or even blindness. Retinopathy is the leading cause of new adult blindness in the United States.
  - Four cardinal signs of diabetes mellitus:
    - Polyuria: Water not absorbed from the renal tubules because of osmotic activity of glucose in the tubules
    - Polydipsia: Polyuria causes severe dehydration which causes thirst.
    - Polyphagia: Tissue breakdown and wasting cause a state of starvation which in turn leads to excessive hunger.
    - Weight loss: Primarily in Type 1 diabetes mellitus. Glucose is not available to the cells; thus, the body breaks down fat and protein stores for energy.
  - Consistent control of blood glucose levels within the normal range is correlated with decreased incidence of complications.
  - Goals of collaborative management:
    - Recognize and treat early.

- Normalize blood glucose levels.
- Prevent complications (hyperglycemia, hypoglycemia, diabetic neuropathies, infection, renal failure, hypertension, coronary artery disease, peripheral vascular disease, neuropathy, limb amputation, blindness).
- Prevent skin alterations.
- Important nursing diagnoses (actual or potential):
  - Risk for hyperglycemia, or hypoglycemia
  - Knowledge deficit
  - Impaired skin integrity
  - Risk for infection
  - Risk for fluid volume deficit
  - Altered nutrition
  - Ineffective individual coping
  - Anxiety and fear
  - Potential complications of diabetes mellitus
- **Key Terms/Concepts:** Polyuria, polydipsia, polyphagia, euglycemic, glycosylated hemoglobin, neuropathy, Kussmaul's respirations, orthostatic hypotension

Overview

Diabetes mellitus is a chronic and potentially disabling disorder of carbohydrate metabolism characterized by hyperglycemia and glycosuria due to inadequate production or utilization of insulin. The classifications of diabetes are:

Type I Diabetes Mellitus previously known as Insulin Dependent Diabetes Mellitus (IDDM) or Juvenile-Onset Diabetes. Beta cell destruction occurs. Triggered by an autoimmune response that attacks the islet cells of the pancreas which, in turn, leads to an absolute insulin deficiency. Generally occurs in children and young adults. Onset is usually acute in nature. Accounts for approximately 10% of all cases of DM.

Type II Diabetes Mellitus formerly known as non-insulin dependent Diabetes Mellitus (NIDDM) or adult-onset diabetes. Hyperglycemia develops when the pancreas cannot secrete enough insulin to match the body's needs or when the insulin receptor sites become resistant to insulin. Usually gradual in onset and occurs in people who have several risk factors. Increasing incidence in children with the greatest risk factor being obesity. Women may also have in combination with PCOS (polycystic ovarian syndrome) and adults, in general, may have as part of metabolic syndrome (also known as syndrome X).

Gestational Diabetes occurs as carbohydrate intolerance of varying degrees of severity with onset or first recognition during pregnancy. Gestational diabetes may require insulin or be diet controlled. Usually alleviated with the birth of the child. Women with gestational diabetes are at risk for developing type II diabetes later in life.

Pre-Diabetes Mellitus - previously called Impaired Glucose Tolerance or Impaired Fasting Glucose, blood glucose levels are above the normal range but not into the diabetic range. Often pre-diabetes will become diabetes if not identified and treated early. Approximately 41 million people in the United States fit this definition which is double the current amount of diabetics in the United States!

Risk Factors

- Genetic predisposition
- Obesity, type 2
- Aging, type 2
- Pancreatitis
- Prolonged medication usage such as corticosteroids, methotrexate, etc., type 1
- Pregnancy, gestational
- Viral infections, type 1
- PCOS, type 2
- Metabolic syndrome, type 2

Signs and Symptoms

- Polyuria
- Polydipsia
- Polyphagia
- Weight loss (type 1)
- Blurred vision
- Fatigue
- Headache
- Occasional muscle cramps
- Poor wound healing
- Confusion and changes in mentation

Diagnostic and Laboratory Tests

- Physical examination
- Oral glucose tolerance test (OGTT) 2-hour plasma glucose
- Fasting Plasma Glucose (FBG) - test of choice, minimum of 8 hour fast required
- Random plasma glucose
- Glycated hemoglobin (GHb) testing or Glycosylated hemoglobin (A1C-Glycosylated hemoglobin), measures blood glucose average over 2-3 months.
- Glycated Serum Protein (GSP), measures glucose average for 1-2 weeks. Not currently recommended, needs to be done monthly.
- Lipid Panel, measures total cholesterol, HDL, LDL, and triglycerides
- Urine/Blood ketone, type 1 and/or gestational diabetes
- Serum electrolytes
- Microalbumin, measures renal function, should be done quarterly
- C-peptide, shows how much insulin the body is making, may help determine between type 1 and 2

- Fasting insulin level

Therapeutic Nursing Management

- **Assess/Monitor:**
  - Fasting blood glucose
    - Twice daily if on oral agents
    - Four times daily if on insulin injections
  - Dietary intake (carbohydrate counting or other)
  - Signs and symptoms of hypoglycemia
  - Signs and symptoms of diabetic ketoacidosis (DKA)
  - Signs and symptoms of hyperosmolar hyperglycemia state
  - Skin integrity
  - Risk for falls
  - Mental status/behavior change
  - Diabetes self-care management
  - Visual changes
  - Signs and symptoms of infection
  - Blood pressure
  - Intake and output
  - Literacy/cognitive ability
  - Neuropathy - always assess feet and inside of shoes
- **Nursing Activities:**
  - Encourage self-care.
  - Teach regarding self-administration of insulin and/or oral hypoglycemic agents.
  - Teach regarding specific dietary requirements as prescribed by the primary care provider, the client may be advised to follow the food exchange from the Diabetic Association diet or the dietary guidelines for Americans (Food Guide Pyramid) issued by the U.S. Departments of Agriculture and Health and Human Services.
  - Teach client signs and symptoms of hypoglycemia and insulin shock (headache, jitteriness, diaphoresis, palpitations, weakness, confusion, hunger).
  - Encourage increased intake of dietary fiber.
  - Encourage daily exercise, but be aware that with exercise the client may need to change insulin administration. Exercise promotes the utilization of carbohydrates.
  - Teach regarding alterations in insulin administration if sick, NPO, or physically active. Infection is associated with insulin resistance.
  - Encourage avoidance of smoking to reduce cardiovascular risks.
  - Provide emotional support for family and client related to changes in lifestyle.
  - Encourage regular blood glucose monitoring.
  - Encourage use of a medical alert bracelet or ID card.

- Assist with preparations for islet cell transplant if indicated.
- Administer juice, crackers, milk, or 50% glucose or glucagon IV for hypoglycemic. In general, if blood glucose 50-70 mg/dl give approximately 15 grams of carbohydrate (3-4 glucose tablets, 8 Lifesavers, 4 oz of fruit juice or soda, 8 oz of milk) and if blood glucose < 50 mg/dl give 30 grams of carbohydrate. Be sure client knows to recheck blood glucose every 15 minutes and repeat carbohydrate administration if needed. If client is unable to swallow or is unconscious, family or friends should know how to administer subcutaneous or intramuscular glucagon and call 911 if needed (i.e. the client doesn't respond within 15 minutes and is therefore unable to swallow on his/her own).
- Teach client and family the signs of hyperglycemia, hypoglycemia, and DKA.
- Encourage yearly ophthalmology and podiatry examinations.
- Teach the client to inspect feet and shoes daily.
- Stress the importance of frequent, usually quarterly, visits with the primary care provider or endocrinologist.

Pharmacology and Treatment

- Insulin therapy
  - Very rapid-acting insulin (Humalog/NovoLog) SC: onset within 15 minutes, peak 1 hour, duration 3-4 hours
  - Short-acting insulin (Regular) IV: onset 10-30 minutes, duration 30-60 minutes
  - Short-acting insulin (Regular-Humulin R/Novolin R/Velosulin BR) SC: onset 30-60 minutes, peak 1-5 hours (depending on preparation), duration 6-8 hours
  - Intermediate-acting (Lente & NPH) SC: onset 1-3 hours, peak 4-15 hours (depending on preparation), duration 18-24 hours
  - Long-acting (Ultra-lente/Glargine) SC: onset 4-6 (1 hour for glargine) hours, peak 8-20 hours (none for glargine), duration 24-48 hours (> 24 hours for glargine)
  - Premixed insulin with NPH and regular in doses of 70/30 and 50/50
  - Continuous insulin (Regular or Humalog): pump infusion to meet metabolic needs; bolus dosing, as needed, before meals or snacks based on client's blood sugar
- Oral hypoglycemic agents
  - Sulfonylureas - glyburide, glipizide, glimepiride
  - Non-sulfonylurea secretagogues - repaglinide, nateglinide
  - Biguanides - metformin
  - Alpha-glucosidase inhibitors - acarbose, miglitol
  - Thiazolidinediones - pioglitazone, rosiglitazone
  - Combinations: sulfonylurea & biguanide, thiazolidinedione & biguanide

Complications

Clinical Overview: Chronic hyperglycemia of diabetes is associated with long-term dysfunction, damage, and failure to various organs especially the eyes, kidneys, nerves, and the heart. Individuals with undiagnosed and/or uncontrolled hyperglycemia are also at significantly higher risk for stroke, coronary heart disease, and peripheral vascular disease than the non-diabetic population. They are also at a higher risk for dyslipidemia, hypertension, and obesity.

- Retinopathy
- Nephropathy
- Hypertension
- Diabetic ketoacidosis (DKA)
- Neuropathy
- Myocardial infarction (MI)
- Coronary Artery Disease (CAD)
- Sexual dysfunction
- Peripheral vascular disease (PVD)
- Hypoglycemia
- Slow wound healing/recurrent infections
- Cerebral Vascular Disease
- Gastroparesis
- Gingivitis

Diabetes Mellitus in Older Adults

Overview

Diabetes mellitus often goes undetected in older adults. Many of the physiological changes of aging resemble those of diabetes. Type 2 diabetes in older adults results from impaired insulin release. However, insulin resistance is prominent in obese older adults.

Risk Factors

- People using diuretic, glucocorticoids, or other medications
- People receiving enteral or parenteral nutrition
- Obesity
- Metabolic syndrome
- PCOS

Signs and Symptoms:

- Hyperglycemia (blood glucose usually between 500-800 mg/dl)
- Absence of ketones
- Severe osmotic dehydration

- Mental status changes
- Neurological symptoms such as aphasia, hemiparesis, and seizures
- Gastrointestinal distress such as nausea, vomiting, and/or ileus
- Tachypnea (rapid respirations)
- Serum osmolarity > 28

Treatment

- Rehydration
- Insulin administration (usually slow insulin drip)
- Correction of fluid and electrolyte imbalance
- Treatment of the underlying cause
- Education
- Acid-base correction

Complications:

- Hypoglycemia: Older adults are at a higher risk for medication induced hypoglycemia related to:
  - Inadequate hydration
  - Erratic or inadequate food intake
  - Decreased renal function
  - Decreased intestinal absorption
- Hyperglycemic Hyperosmolar State (HHS): HHS is often overlooked or misdiagnosed related to its similarity to other illnesses. HHS is characterized by hyperglycemia (blood glucose > 500mg/dl), dehydration, and the absence of ketones. Insulin deficiency is not as profound as in diabetic ketoacidosis (DKA). HHS has a 15-20% mortality rate which is 2-3 times higher then DKA

Critical Thinking Exercise: Nursing Management of the Client with Diabetes Mellitus

Situation: A 44-year-old female client has a 25-year history of Type 1 IDDM (insulin-dependent diabetes mellitus). She lives with her husband and two teen-aged daughters. The client has been able to adequately manage her diabetes mellitus, care for her family and work full-time as a cook at the local elementary school cafeteria, where she enjoys cooking and interacting with the children. The client's past medical history includes the usual childhood illnesses, tonsillectomy at age six, and vaginal hysterectomy at age 39 for dysfunctional uterine bleeding secondary to fibroid tumor growth. She is 5'-4" tall and weighs 143 pounds.

1. What are the similarities and differences between Type 1 and 2 diabetes mellitus?

Similarities	Differences
(Examples)	(Examples) Type 1: a. b. c. d. Type 2: a. b. c. d.

2. List the common clinical manifestations that occur from diabetes mellitus, noting those that occur early in the disease process, those that occur late in the disease process.

   a. Early clinical manifestations:

   b. Late clinical manifestations:

3. What are the major consequences of insulin deficiency to each of the following organs/tissues, and what is the overall result of such consequences?

Organ Tissue	Consequence

Additional Information: The client visits her health care practitioner yearly unless she experiences problems. Two years ago she was diagnosed with hypertension secondary to her diabetes mellitus and was placed on the drug metoprolol (Lopressor) 50 mg bid and a low-salt diet to control her blood pressure. Her daily insulin dose was also adjusted because her GHb (glycosylated hemoglobin) was elevated. Other medications include 1 mg estradiol daily and over-the-counter Advil (ibuprofen) for occasional headaches.

4. What does the client's elevated GHb (glycosylated hemoglobin) level imply?

5. What is the relationship between the client's hypertension and her diabetes mellitus?

6. Is there reason for concern about the client's combination of prescribed and over-the-counter medications? Why or why not?

Situation: The client has self-administered 35 units of NPH human insulin and 20 units of Regular human insulin at 7:30 a.m. each morning since her last visit to the clinic, which she feels is controlling her diabetes well. She inconsistently monitors her blood glucose levels because she dislikes pricking her own fingers and believes that she can "feel" when her blood glucose is not within normal limits. The client intakes between 1300 and 1400 calories each day per the American Diabetic Association exchange system, which includes an evening snack.

7. In regard to the client's insulin:

   a. How may she mix her insulin so that she can avoid administering more than one injection?

   b. How does NPH insulin differ from regular insulin?

8. While this client has self-administered her own insulin for years, many clients need to be taught the skill. Cite at least four principles a newly diagnosed diabetic should be taught about insulin and its administration.

9. What is the underlying principle supporting the American Diabetes Association exchange list and how does the client use it to calculate her daily dietary intake?

10. Should the client be counseled regarding monitoring of her blood glucose levels? Why or why not?

11. Clients with Type 1 IDDM occasionally use a sliding scale to determine their insulin needs. What is a sliding scale and what type of insulin is administered when using a sliding scale?

12. Cite at least five signs and symptoms that should be taught to diabetic clients and their significant others because they indicate the presence of hypoglycemia.

13. What are the most common reasons why diabetic clients develop hypoglycemia?

Nursing Management of the Client Requiring Insulin Therapy

Key Points

- People with type 1 diabetes require exogenesis insulin therapy for survival.
- Accuracy of insulin dosages is essential for anyone using insulin.
- Goals of collaborative management:
  - Maintain euglycemia.
  - Prevent complications (hyperglycemia, hypoglycemia).
- Important nursing diagnoses (actual or potential):
  - Knowledge deficit
  - Potential complications of insulin administration (abscess formation, hypoglycemia)
  - Ineffective individual coping
  - Anxiety and fear
  - Ineffective individual management of therapeutic regimen
  - Noncompliance and risk factors
- **Key Terms/Concepts**: Euglycemia, hyperglycemia, hypoglycemia, noncompliance, exogenous, glycosylated hemoglobin, rotation of sites, hypersensitivity

Overview

Insulin is a hormone produced by the beta cells of the Islets of Langerhans in the pancreas. In type 1 diabetes, there is absolute insulin deficiency. Type 2 diabetes, however, ranges from resistance with relative insulin deficiency to a secretory defect with insulin resistance. Insulin is derived from animal or human sources or it is manufactured in a biosynthetic form of human insulin. Various types of insulin are available to provide blood glucose control and meet the needs of people with diabetes. The types available are: rapid, short, intermediate, and long acting. Mixtures are also offered to meet the individual needs of people with diabetes.

Indications for Insulin Therapy

- All individuals with type 1 diabetes
- Individuals with type 2 diabetes not controlled with oral agents
- Women with gestational diabetes not controlled with medical nutrition therapy (MNT)
- Individuals receiving parenteral nutrition
- Treatment of diabetic ketoacidosis (DKA), hyperglycemia hyperosmolar state (HHS)

- Individuals with diabetes secondary to pancreatitis or other illnesses that diminish beta cell function

Diagnostic Tests

- Oral Glucose tolerance test (OGGT) 2-hour plasma glucose
- Fasting plasma glucose (FPG)
- Glycated hemoglobin (GHb) testing or Glycosylated hemoglobin (A1C): measures glucose average over 2 to 3 months.
- Glycated serum protein (GSP): measures glucose average over 1 to 2 weeks
- Lipid panel: measures total cholesterol, HDL, LDL, and triglycerides
- Urine/blood ketone, type 1 and/or gestational diabetes
- Serum electrolytes
- Microalbumin: measures renal function
- C-peptide: shows how much insulin the body is making
- Fasting insulin

Therapeutic Nursing Management

- **Assess/Monitor:**
  - Assess diabetes self-management knowledge and skill level.
    - Medical nutrition therapy (MNT)
    - Self-monitoring of blood glucose (SMBG)
    - Administration of oral agents and/or insulin therapy
    - Urine ketone testing
  - Assess for signs and symptoms of hypoglycemia.
  - Fasting blood glucose (FBG)
  - Assess for signs and symptoms of diabetic ketoacidosis (DKA).
  - Assess for signs and symptoms of hyperglycemia hyperosmolar state (HHS).
  - Assess skin integrity.
- **Nursing Activities:**
  - Provide diabetes self-management training.
  - Teach clients that it is not necessary to aspirate for blood before injecting insulin, to use the abdomen for best absorption, and to rotate sites but do not come within a two-inch radius around the umbilicus. Use of the upper arm, anterior and lateral aspects of the thigh, and the buttocks may still be considered appropriate sites.
  - Teach client and family regarding use of regular insulin for emergencies.
  - Provide information about the use of drugs that potentiate insulin (aspirin, alcohol, oral anticoagulants, oral hypoglycemics, monoamine oxidase inhibitors (MAOI), tricyclic antidepressants, beta blockers).
  - Inform the client to delay insulin administration if breakfast is delayed.
  - Administer juice, crackers, milk or 50% glucose or glucagon IV for hypoglycemia. If blood glucose between 50-70 mg/dl take in 15 grams of carbohydrate (3-4 glucose tablets, 8 Lifesavers, 4 oz of juice or soda, 8 oz

of milk) and if blood glucose < 50 mg/dl take in 30 grams of carbohydrate. Be sure client knows to recheck blood glucose every 15 minutes and repeat carbohydrate administration, if needed. If client is unable to swallow or unconscious, family or friends should know how to administer subcutaneous or intramuscular glucagon and call 911 if needed; i.e. the client doesn't respond within 15 minutes and is therefore unable to swallow on his/her own.

- Teach client and family the signs of hyperglycemia, hypoglycemia, and diabetic ketoacidosis.
- Educate the client about the importance of maintaining prescribed dietary intake.
- Emphasize the importance of maintaining the prescribed activity level.
- Instruct clients that insulin needs may change during periods of stress, pregnancy, illness, or exercise.
- Provide client with opportunities for demonstration and practice of injection techniques.

Pharmacology

- Insulin therapy
  - Very rapid-acting insulin (Humalog/Novolin) SC: onset within 15 minutes, peak 1 hour, duration 3-4 hours
  - Short-acting insulin (Regular) IV: onset 10-30 minutes, duration 30-60 minutes
  - Short-acting insulin (Regular-Humulin R/Novolin R/Velosulin BR) SC: onset 30-60 minutes, peak 1-5 hours (depending on preparation), duration 6-8 hours
  - Intermediate-acting (Lente & NPH) SC: onset 1-3 hours, peak 4-15 hours (depending on preparation), duration 18-24 hours
  - Long-acting (Ultra-lente/Glargine) SC: onset 4-6 (1 hour for glargine) hours, peak 8-20 hours (none for glargine), duration 24-48 hours (> 24 hours for glargine)
  - Premixed insulin with NPH and regular in doses of 70/30 and 50/50
  - Continuous insulin (Regular or Humalog): pump infusion to meet metabolic needs; bolus dosing, as needed, before meals or snacks based on client's blood sugar
  - Insulin should be kept at room temperature, but only for one month - date each bottle when opened. Injecting room temperature insulin is less irritating. Unopened bottles should be refrigerated.
  - When mixing insulin in the same syringe, always draw up the clear (short and rapid acting) insulin first before the cloudy (intermediate acting) insulin.
  - Long acting insulin (ultralente and glargine) should not be mixed with any other insulin.
  - Do not use clear insulin that has become cloudy.

Complications

- Rebound hyperglycemia
- Hypoglycemia
- Diabetic ketoacidosis (DKA)
- Atrophy at injection site (pitting of subcutaneous tissue)
- Hypertrophy (fatty thickening of the lipid tissue)
- Hypersensitivity to insulin (allergies to insulin are rare but may occur as local reactions)
- Infection at injection site

Age-Related Changes—Gerontological Considerations

- Visual and auditory changes or impaired physical mobility may affect the client's ability to perform self-care and insulin administration.
- Older adults with limited financial resources may have difficulty meeting dietary restrictions and providing necessary equipment (syringes, glucose monitoring machine) to remain compliant with treatment regimen.
- There is an increased risk for drug interactions related to polypharmacy among older adults.

Critical Thinking Exercise: Nursing Management of the Client Requiring Insulin Therapy

Situation: A 44-year-old female client has a 25-year history of Type 1 IDDM (insulin-dependent diabetes mellitus). She lives with her husband and two teen-aged daughters. The client has been able to adequately manage her diabetes mellitus, care for her family and work full-time as a cook at the local elementary school cafeteria, where she enjoys cooking and interacting with the children. The client's past medical history includes the usual childhood illnesses, tonsillectomy at age six, and vaginal hysterectomy at age 39 for dysfunctional uterine bleeding secondary to fibroid tumor growth. She is 5' 4" tall and weighs 143 pounds.

1. What are the "classical" early manifestations commonly associated with diabetes mellitus and what other signs and symptoms does the disease produce?

Classical Early Manifestations	Other Signs and Symptoms

2. Cite at least three major consequences that may occur from undiagnosed diabetes mellitus that is not well controlled for long periods of time?

Additional Information: The client visits her health care practitioner quarterly unless she experiences problems. Two years ago she was diagnosed with hypertension secondary to her diabetes mellitus and was placed on the drug metoprolol (Lopressor) 50 mg bid and a low-salt diet to control her blood pressure. Her daily insulin dose was also adjusted because her GHb (glycosylated hemoglobin) was elevated. Other medications include over-the-counter acetaminophen for occasional headaches.

3. Why is it important for the client and nurse to understand the differences between NPH and regular insulin?

4. The client took her insulin at 0730 this morning and it is now 1600. At what time did her insulin take effect, when did it peak and is it still being effective?

| Type of Effect | Insulin Type | | | |
| | Regular | | NPH | |
	Duration (in hours)	Time Frame as Measured on the Clock (Start & Stop)	Duration (in hours)	Time Frame as Measured on the Clock (Start & Stop)
Initial				
Peak				
Duration				
Current (at 1600 hours)				

5. Is this client monitoring her blood glucose often enough? If not, how often should she be monitoring it?

Situation: Four weeks ago the client's mother died following a massive stroke. She is currently responsible for handling her mother's estate and disposing of personal property. This has placed an emotional and physical burden on the client, whose husband is frequently out of town on business. The client isn't sleeping well, and doesn't feel hungry most of the time; consequently, she sometimes forgets to eat when alone.

This evening, when the client's husband returned home, he found his wife lying on the sofa. When he attempted to talk to her he noticed she was pale and sweating profusely. She mumbled something about being tired and having a headache, but her verbalizations were difficult to understand. Upon further questioning, her answers were incoherent. Uncertain about his wife's condition, the husband decided to take her to the emergency department at their local acute care facility.

6. Based on the client's clinical manifestations, what is most likely occurring and why?

7. How can the ED nurse best validate the presence of hyper- or hypoglycemia in this client?

Situation: On arrival at the emergency department, the client remained lethargic and disoriented, mumbling incoherently. Vital signs were assessed, oxygen initiated at 6 L/min per nasal cannula, intravenous access obtained with an infusion of normal saline. Physical assessment revealed:

Client Data		
Vital Signs		
Blood Pressure	128/88	mmHg
Heart Rate	100	bpm
Respirations	28	bpm
Temperature	99.6°	F oral
Electrolyte Panel		
Na	142	mEq/L
K	5.1	mEq/L
Cl	103	mEq/L
Glucose	54	mg/dL
Creatinine	1.0	mg/dL
BUN	15	mg/dL
CBC		
Hgb	12.0	g/dL
Hct	36	%

8. If noted, what signs would alert the nurse that the client's intravenous infusion had infiltrated and what action would be necessary?

   a. Signs of infiltration:

   b. Nursing Activities:

Situation: Hypoglycemia was diagnosed based on the client's assessment and laboratory findings. 1 ampule of 50% dextrose was administered as ordered by the ED physician.

9. Mark an "x" in the box to indicate which priority nursing actions should be implemented immediately following the administration of IV dextrose and why or why not?

Priority	Nursing Action	Why or Why Not
	Insert an indwelling urinary.	
	Monitor for changes in the client's sensorium.	
	Place the client in a supine, flat position.	
	Monitor blood glucose levels every 15 minutes.	
	Reassess vital signs.	
	Monitor for irregular pulse rate.	

10. Why was intravenous dextrose administered to this client rather than a fast-acting carbohydrate such as juice or candy?

11. What signs or symptoms help the nurse differentiate between insulin excess and diabetic coma (insulin deficiency)? What signs and symptoms are similar for both conditions and cannot, therefore, be used to differentiate between the conditions?

Insulin Excess	Insulin Deficiency	Signs and Symptoms that Occur in Both Insulin Excess and Deficiency
Diaphoresis	Polyuria	
Headache	Polydipsia	
Pallor	Polyphagia	
Irritability	Lethargy	
Nervousness	Warm, flushed skin	
Tachycardia	Dry mucus membranes	
Palpitations	Poor skin turgor	
Trembling	Dehydration	
Weakness		
Seizures		

12. While this client is being treated for insulin excess, clients with diabetes mellitus are at increased risk for the development of insulin deficiency. What serious complication is associated with insulin deficiency that must be immediately treated?

Nursing Management of the Client in Hyperglycemic Crises: Diabetic Ketoacidosis (DKA) and Hyperosmolar Hyperglycemic State (HHS)

Key Points

- Hyperglycemia may cause two types of acute, life threatening metabolic crises:
  - Diabetic Ketoacidosis (DKA)
  - Hyperosmolar Hyperglycemic State (HHS)
- A rapid decrease in blood glucose levels can precipitate serious complications:
  - Cerebral edema
  - Electrolytes changes
  - Coma
  - Death
- Goals of collaborative management:
  - Provide early detection.
  - Achieve euglycemia.
  - Prevent fluid and electrolyte imbalances.
  - Restore fluid volume and electrolyte balance.
  - Maintain acid balance.
  - Prevent serious and life threatening complications.
- Important nursing diagnoses (actual or potential):
  - Fluid volume deficit
  - Altered perfusion
  - Respiratory distress
  - Knowledge deficit
  - Altered mental status
  - Anxiety and fear
  - Acid-base imbalance
  - Electrolyte imbalance
- **Key Terms/Concepts:** Euglycemia, ketoacidosis, hyperosmolar hyperglycemic state, Kussmaul's respirations

Overview

DKA and HHS are the most serious metabolic complications related to Diabetes Mellitus. People with Type 1 and Type 2 are at risk. Both DKA and HHS may result in altered mental status, respiratory distress, loss of consciousness, and death. Immediate medical attention is necessary to avoid adverse outcomes.

The mortality rate in DKA is less than 5%, whereas the mortality rate of HHS remains as high as 15%. The most common precipitating factor in development is infection. DKA and HHS can be prevented by access to medical care, proper education, and effective communication with a health care provider during illness.

Diabetic ketoacidosis: Acute condition characterized by hyperglycemia (>250) resulting in breakdown of body fat for energy and an accumulation of ketones in the blood and urine.

Hyperosmolar hyperglycemic state: Acute condition with hyperglycemia (>600), ketones are not present in the blood or urine.

Precipitating Factors

- New onset diabetes mellitus (type 1 or elderly type 2)
- Interruption of insulin regimen
- Infection (most common cause)
- Pancreatitis
- ETOH abuse
- Myocardial infarction (MI)
- Trauma
- Undiagnosed diabetes mellitus
- Non-compliance to diabetes self care
- Cerebrovascular accident (CVA)

Comparison of Signs and Symptoms

Comparison Table of Signs and Symptoms

Signs and Symptoms	DKA	HHS
Age	<40 years	> 40 years
Duration of S/S	< 2 days	Usually > 5 days
Plasma Glucose (mg/dl)	Usually 250-600mg/dl	>600mg/dl
Serum Sodium (mEq/1)	Normal/low	Normal/high
Potassium	High, normal or low	Normal/high
Bicarbonate	Low	High
Ketones	Present 4+ or >	Absence < 2+
Fruity breathe odor	Present	Absence
PH	Low	Normal
Serum Osmolality (mOsm/kg)	<320 mOsm/kg	>320 mOsm/kg
Mental status	Mental status change noted	Mental status change noted
Dehydration	Mild-moderate	Severe
Prognosis	<10% mortality	15% Mortality

Diagnostic and Laboratory Tests

- History and physical examination
- Fasting blood glucose (FBG), also called fasting blood sugar (FBS)
- Serum electrolytes
- Acetone odor on the breath
- Arterial blood gases (ABGs)
- Random plasma glucose

Therapeutic Nursing Management

- **Assess/Monitor**:
  - Blood gases
  - Electrolytes (especially serum potassium)
  - Blood glucose levels
  - Vital signs
  - Urinary output
  - Signs of fluid overload or fluid volume depletion
  - Bowel sounds for ileus
- **Nursing Activities**:
  - Restore and maintain circulatory volume.
  - Administer regular insulin as prescribed. IV insulin is often given with DKA to rapidly lower blood glucose.
  - Correct acidosis if pH is less than 7.1.
  - Correct underlying cause of DKA.

Treatment requirements of DKA & HHS

- Correction of:
  - Dehydration
  - Hyperglycemia
  - Electrolyte imbalances
  - Acid-base imbalance
- Identification of comorbidity precipitating factors:
  - Kussmaul respirations
  - Acetone breathe
  - Intravascular volume depletion
  - Acute abdomen (rebound tenderness, absent bowel sounds)
  - Mentation changes
  - Hyporeflexia
  - Hypotonia
- Frequent client monitoring:
  - Blood glucose
  - Intake and output

- Weight changes
- Electrolytes
- Lactic acid
- Respiratory status, including arterial blood gases (ABG)
- Electrocardiogram monitoring
- Assess and maintain respiratory status.
- Assess circulation.
- Assess presence of ketones bodies.
- Vital signs (orthostatic blood pressure, weight, temperature)
- Identify precipitating factors.
- Evaluate response to therapy.
- Provide education to client and family.

Critical Thinking Exercise: Nursing Management of the Client in Hyperglycemic Crises: Diabetic Ketoacidosis and Hyperosmolar Hyperglycemic State

Situation: A 43-year-old female client has a 24-year history of Type 1 IDDM (insulin-dependent diabetes mellitus). Four weeks ago, the client's mother died, following a massive stroke. The client is currently responsible for handling her mother's estate and disposing of personal property. This has placed a serious emotional and physical burden on the client, whose husband is frequently out of town on business. Since her mother's death, the client has lost ten pounds even though she has been snacking more than usual, is not sleeping well, and is drinking more caffeinated beverages in order to combat her chronic fatigue. Her teenage daughters are supportive of their mother but are involved in numerous school and extra-curricular activities.

1. What is the relationship between stress and blood glucose levels in the diabetic client?

Situation: When the client's husband returned home from work last evening, he found the client sleeping on the sofa. One of the daughters stated that her Mom had complained of a headache and nausea and thought she would feel better if she rested for a while. About an hour later, the client's husband decided to awaken her, only to find that he could not arouse her without shaking her vigorously. The husband called 911 and the client was immediately taken to the emergency department of the local acute care facility.

2. What does the data suggest about the client's physical state?

3. Describe the process of DKA (diabetic ketoacidosis) and list factors that precipitate it.

   a. Process:

   a. Precipitating Factors:

Situation: Upon initial assessment the client was very lethargic, but awoke with shaking. She was disoriented to time and place, but she did know her name. She had rapid, deep respirations, fruity breath odor, and warm, dry, flushed skin with poor skin turgor.

CLIENT DATA		
Vital Signs		
Blood Pressure	86/50	mmHg
Heart Rate	122	bpm
Respirations	28	bpm
Temperature	99.6°	oral
Electrolyte Panel		
Na	128	mEq/L
K	5.9	mEq/L
CL	94	mEq/L
CO2	8	mEq/L
Glucose	593	mg/dL
Creatinine	1.9	mg/dL
Blood urea nitrogen (BUN)	28	mg/dL
ABGs (on room air)		
pH	7.2	
PaCO2	45	mmHg
PaO2	82	mmHg
SaO2	92	%
HCO3	12	mEq/L
Base Excess	-6.2	mEq/L
CBC		
Hgb	14.2	g/dL
Hct	45	%
Other		
Serum osmolarity	330	mOsm/L
Urine osmolarity	970	mOsm/L
Urine ketones		Positive
Serum ketones		Positive

The diagnosis of DKA (diabetic ketoacidosis) is confirmed via the client's assessment and laboratory findings. The client is ordered to receive an infusion of normal saline (NS) at 1 L over the first hour, an insulin drip to run at 5 units per hour, oxygen at 100% FIO_2 per non-rebreather face-mask, placement of an indwelling urinary catheter, hourly blood glucose levels, electrolyte levels, urinary output, blood gas analysis every four hours and vital signs every 15 minutes until stable.

4. The nurse will immediately initiate several essential actions. Cite at least two priority actions and explain why each action is essential at this time.

Nursing Action	Reason for Action (Rationale)

5. Which of the client's clinical manifestations support the presence of fluid volume deficit and why did she develop this complication?

   a. Signs and symptoms of fluid volume deficit:

   b. Factors involved in the development of fluid volume deficit:

6. What acid-base imbalance is the client experiencing based on analysis of her arterial blood gases (ABGs) and how does this imbalance develop?

   a. Type of imbalance:

   b. Compensation:

7. Why is normal saline (NS) the initial fluid of choice for treatment of DKA, and at what point will dextrose be added to the infusion?

8. Calculate the infusion rate of insulin in order to achieve the ordered 5 units per hour if the fluid bag contains 500 mL 0.9% NS and 100 units of regular insulin.

9. Why is it essential the nurse carefully monitor the client's serum potassium levels?

10. Why wasn't the client's acid-base imbalance immediately treated with sodium bicarbonate?

11. Given the client's current physical status, which three nursing diagnoses take precedence at this time?

    Risk for self-care deficit related to fatigue, illness

    Altered nutrition: Less than body requirements

    Fluid volume deficit related to osmotic diuresis secondary to hyperglycemia

    Anxiety related to fear, loss of control

    Knowledge deficit regarding causes of diabetic acidosis

    Risk for injury related to altered mental status

12. After the client's condition has stabilized:

    a. Which three nursing diagnoses will take precedence?

    _____ Risk for self-care deficit related to fatigue, illness

    _____ Altered nutrition: Less than body requirements

    _____ Fluid volume deficit related to osmotic diuresis secondary to hyperglycemia

    _____ Anxiety related to fear, loss of control

    _____ Knowledge deficit regarding causes of diabetic acidosis

    _____ Risk for injury related to altered mental status

    b. Why will priorities change?

13. Why didn't the client's practitioner suspect HHNS (hyperglycemic hyperosmolar nonketotic syndrome) rather than DKA?

14. Which expected outcomes are most realistic for the client during the immediate recovery period following diabetic ketoacidosis and why?

_____ Restoration of fluid balance

_____ Knowledge of pathophysiology of diabetic ketoacidosis

_____ Restoration of acid-base balance

_____ Restoration of normal weight

_____ Decreased anxiety

_____ Absence of complications

_____ Restoration of electrolyte balance

_____ Ability to care for self independently

Nursing Management of the Client with Cardiac Dysrhythmias (Arrhythmias)

Key Points

- Cardiac dysrhythmias are a serious cause of death in clients suffering acute myocardial infarction (MI) and other sudden death disorders.
- Some dysrhythmias are more serious than others:
  - Ventricular tachycardia
  - Ventricular fibrillation
  - Asystole
  - Second-degree II heart block
  - Third-degree AV (atrioventricular) block
- Some dysrhythmias are generally considered benign:
  - Premature atrial contraction (PAC)
  - Premature ventricular contraction (PVC) can result in more serious dysrhythmias in clients with heart disease or history of ventricular tachycardia.
  - Atrial fibrillation with controlled rate
  - First-degree AV block
- Rapid recognition and treatment of serious dysrhythmias is essential to preserve life.
- **Defibrillation** is the delivery of an unsynchronized, direct countershock to the heart during ventricular fibrillation, pulseless ventricular tachycardia, or when PVCs occur in pairs (bigeminy).
- Defibrillation propels the heart's pacemaker to take over and reestablish a perfusing rhythm.
- **Cardioversion** is the delivery of synchronized direct countershock to the heart for the elective treatment of atrial dysrhythmias or ventricular tachycardias with pulse.
- A **cardiac pacemaker** is a battery-powered appliance that electrically stimulates the heart when the natural pacemaker of the heart fails to render a rhythm.
- Pacemakers may be temporary or permanent.
  - The batteries used to power pacemakers usually last 4-12 years.
- Goals of collaborative management:
  - Rapidly recognize and treat dysrhythmias.
  - Restore normal sinus rhythm.
  - Maintain perfusion.

- • Prevent sudden death.
- • Important nursing diagnoses (actual and potential):
  - • Anxiety and fear
  - • Decreased cardiac output
  - • Impaired gas exchange
  - • Impaired management of therapeutic regimen
  - • Risk for infection
  - • Risk for altered body temperature
  - • Altered tissue perfusion, including myocardial infarction
  - • Impaired skin integrity
  - • Fatigue
  - • Death
- • **Key Terms/Concepts**: Dysrhythmia, arrhythmia, antiarrhythmic, isoenzyme, ectopic beat, hypoxia, ischemia, defibrillation, cardioversion, pacemaker

Overview

Dysrhythmias are disturbances in the electrical conduction system of the heart. The dysrhythmia is named according to the site of origin and rate of conduction.

- • Where in the heart's electrical system they occur (site of origin):
  - • SA (sinoatrial) node
  - • Atria
  - • AV (atrioventricular) node
  - • Ventricular
- • By what happens to the heart's rhythm when they occur:
  - • Bradycardia (the heart is beating too slowly: < 60 bpm)
  - • Tachycardia (the heart is beating too rapidly: > 100 bpm, when client is at rest)
  - • Nodal (heart) block
  - • Premature beat
  - • Flutter
  - • Atrial or ventricular fibrillation (heart muscle is quivering and cannot contract normally)
  - • Asystole

Dysrhythmia/Arrhythmia Types		
Originating in:		
Atria	**Junctional**	**Ventricular**
Premature atrial contraction or complexes (PAC)	Atrioventricular (AV) nodal block, 1st degree	Premature ventricular contraction or complexes (PVC)
Atrial flutter	Atrioventricular (AV) nodal block, 2nd degree	Ventricular flutter

Atrial tachycardia (also A-tach)	Type 1	Ventricular tachycardia (also V-tach or VT)
Atrial fibrillation (also A-fib)	Type 2	Ventricular fibrillation (also V-fib)
Sinus tachycardia	High Grade	Premature ventricular complexes (PVC)
Sinus arrhythmia	Atrioventricular (AV) nodal block, 3rd degree HB	
Sinus brachycardia		
Sick sinus syndrome (SSS)		

The rate and rhythm of the heart may be altered by hypoxia, ischemia, autonomic nervous system imbalances, electrolyte imbalances, drug toxicity, or shock. Dysrhythmias may be benign or life threatening.

Risk Factors

- Cardiovascular disease, inherited or acquired
- Chronic renal, hepatic, or lung disease
- Pericarditis
- Drug use or abuse
- Shock
- Electrolyte disturbances
- Fear
- Fever
- Pain
- Anxiety
- Hypoxia
- Infection

Signs and Symptoms

- Dependent upon underlying rhythm and rate; ability to perfuse
  - Decreased perfusion:
    - Chest pain
    - Decreased level of consciousness (LOC)
    - Shortness of breath
    - Hypotension
  - No perfusion:
    - Cardiac arrest

Diagnostic and Laboratory Tests

- History and physical exam

- Electrocardiogram (ECG)
- Holter cardiac monitoring
- Serum electrolytes
- Arterial blood gases (ABGs)
- Myoglobin
- Cardiac enzymes:
    - Troponin
    - CPK: creatine phosphokinase
        - CPK composed of 3 isoenzymes:
            - CPK-1 (also called CPK-BB) concentrated in the brain
            - CPK-2 (also called CPK-MB) found mostly in the heart
            - CPK-3 (also called CPK-MM) found mostly in skeletal muscle
    - LDH: lactic dehydrogenase
    - SGOT: serum glutamic oxaloacetic transaminase (also called AST: aspartate aminotransferase)
- Serum cholesterol
- Lipid profile - The levels of:
    - TC (total cholesterol)
    - Triglycerides
    - VLDL (very low density lipoprotein)
    - LDL (low density lipoprotein)
    - HDL (high density lipoprotein)
    - Ratio:
        - TC/HDL
        - LDL/HDL
- Cardiac stress testing
- Cardiac nuclear scanning
- Cardiac catheterization
- Digital subtraction angiography
- Echocardiogram
- Electro physiological study (EPS)

Therapeutic Nursing Management

- **Prevention**:
    - Reduce risk factors for coronary artery disease.
    - Correct electrolyte imbalances.
    - Treat substance abuse.
    - Manage stress.
    - Manage fever.
- **Assess/Monitor**:
    - Continuous cardiac monitoring

- For indications of decreased cardiac output (fatigue, dyspnea, fainting)
- Serum electrolytes
- Clinical condition, cardiac rhythm, and vital signs before, during, and after defibrillation and cardioversion
- For signs of oversedation during cardioversion
- For pulmonary or systemic emboli following cardioversion
- For signs and symptoms of pacemaker malfunction; dizziness, fatigue, ankle swelling, chest pain, and dyspnea
- **Nursing Activities:**
  - Administer oxygen.
  - Administer prescribed antiarrhythmic or other prescribed drugs.
  - Perform CPR for cardiac asystole or cessation of consciousness and pulse.
    - Determine unresponsiveness in the victim by tapping or gently shaking and shouting, "Are you OK?"
    - If the victim is unresponsive, call out for help and activate the EMS.
    - Position the victim for CPR.
    - Open the victim's airway using the head-tilt-chin method. Look, listen, and feel for breathing.
    - If the victim is not breathing, position your mouth over the victim's mouth; occlude nostrils, forming an airtight seal. Use resuscitation mask if available.
    - Give two slow, full breaths. Uncover the victim's mouth after each breath. Watch the chest rise and fall with each breath.
    - Palpate the carotid artery in the victim's neck for at least 5 seconds to determine whether a pulse is present. If a pulse is present, continue to give breaths at a rate of 10 to 12 per minute.
    - If no pulse is present, begin chest compressions by placing one hand over the lower half of the sternum (avoiding the xiphoid process) and placing the second hand directly on top of the first. Lock elbows and compress the sternum 11/2 to 2 inches before releasing. Repeat the compression and release sequence 15 times at a rate of 80 to 100 compressions per minute.
    - After 15 chest compressions, return to the victim's head and open the airway. Deliver two slow, full breaths. Repeat the sequence of 15 compressions to two breaths until help arrives or pulse and breathing are restored.
    - Reassess for the return of breathing and pulse every few minutes; then resume CPR.
  - **Defibrillate immediately for ventricular fibrillation.**
    - Make certain client is pulseless and apneic before initiating procedure.
    - Position defibrillator machine so that paddles reach client's chest. Properly position defibrillator pads or gel on client's chest.
    - Turn on the defibrillator machine, automated external defibrillator (AED), choose the energy level, charge the machine, direct all personnel to stand clear, and administer the electrical shock.
    - Following defibrillation, document:

- Client's condition prior to intervention
- Pre-procedure rhythm
- Number of defibrillation attempts, energy settings, time, and response
- Post-defibrillation rhythm
- Client's vital signs
- Emergency medications administered, including times and dosages
- Client's condition and state of consciousness following procedure

- **Prepare client for cardioversion if prescribed.**
  - Remove client's dentures or dental bridges if necessary.
  - Administer sedation and oxygen as ordered - patent IV.
  - Prepare cardioverter by plugging into an outlet, turning on power, selecting energy level, and connecting limb leads.
  - Activate the synchronizer and charge button.
  - Apply paddles to chest, direct all personnel to stand clear, and press the discharge button.
  - Obtain postcardioversion ECG, check vital signs, and assess airway patency.
  - Provide reassurance to client and report cardioversion results.

- **Provide preoperative and postoperative care to client receiving a pacemaker.**
  - Arm sling
  - ECG monitor
  - Vital signs

- **Instruct client with a pacemaker to follow these precautions:**
  - Carry a pacemaker ID card at all times.
  - Schedule follow-up visits with primary care provider to check pacemaker function.
  - Avoid being close to high-output electric generators and magnetic equipment such as an MRI machine.
  - Avoid injury or blows to the pacemaker site.

- Offer emotional support to client and family.
- Teach client regarding need for compliance with prescribed drug regimen.
- Teach client and family how to take a pulse and monitor heart rate.
- For the client with a pacemaker, teach client to:
  - Check the heart rate daily by palpating the radial or carotid pulse, as demonstrated by the nurse. If the pulse is lower than the set rate, the client must inform the health care provider immediately.
  - Avoid strenuous movement, especially of the arm in which the pacemaker is inserted.
  - Keep the arm on the side of the pacemaker lower than the head except for brief moments when dressing or performing hygiene.
  - Delay activities such as swimming, bowling, tennis, vacuum cleaning,

carrying heavy objects, chopping wood, mowing or raking the lawn, and shoveling snow for at least eight weeks.

- Avoid sources of electrical interference, which are similar to those that are problematic for people with an automatic internal cardiac defibrillator (AICD).

Pharmacology

- Oxygen
  - Calcium channel blockers (diltiazem, verapamil)
  - Beta-Blockers (propranolol, labetalol)
  - Other anti-dysrhythmic (digoxin, procainamide, amiodarone, adenosine, lidocaine)
- Sedatives (benzodiazepines, thiopental)
- Anticoagulants (heparin, low-molecular weight heparins, warfarin)
- Cardiotonics (epinephrine, isoproterenol)

Complications

- Pulmonary embolism
- Stroke, cerebral vascular embolism (CVA)
- Myocardial infarction (MI)
- Decreased cardiac output
- Heart failure
- Infection at pacemaker site
- Pacemaker malfunction
- Death

Age–Related Changes—Gerontological Considerations

- Risk for heart disease, hypertension, dysrhythmias, and atherosclerosis is increased with aging.
- Increased risk for ectopic beats, tachycardia, and atrial fibrillation occur in older adults.
- Increased risk for CHF (congestive heart failure) is related to long-standing atrial fibrillation often associated with chronic obstructive pulmonary disease (COPD), status postoperative coronary artery bypass grafting (CABG), etc.
- Heart rate variability decreases with age.

Critical Thinking Exercise: Nursing Management of the Client with Cardiac Dysrhythmias (Arrhythmias)

Situation: The nurse is monitoring several clients in the cardiac care unit who are at risk for the development of cardiac dysrhythmias.

1. One of the clients loses consciousness and has no palpable pulse. The cardiac monitor indicates the client is experiencing ventricular fibrillation. Which action will the nurse perform first?

    _____ Document the dysrhythmia.

    _____ Notify the physician.

    _____ Begin CPR.

2. Explain why these nursing diagnoses are appropriate for clients at risk for cardiac dysrhythmias.

    a. Risk for decreased cardiac output

    b. Risk for altered tissue perfusion

    c. Anxiety

3. What are some of the common risk factors, other than cardiac disease, for development of cardiac dysrhythmias?

Nursing Management of the Client Requiring an Electrocardiogram (ECG)

Key Points

- An electrocardiogram (ECG) is obtained by placing electrodes on the client's chest wall and on certain peripheral pulse sites.
- An ECG records the electrical activity of the heart from various angles or positions called leads.
- A 12-lead ECG is a combination of 6 limb leads and 6 chest leads.
- An ECG tracing displays waves called P, Q, R, S, and T-waves, and sometimes a U-wave.
- The first wave, or P wave, indicates atrial muscle depolarization.
- The PR interval is the time it takes for an impulse to travel from the atria to the ventricles, through the atrioventricular (AV) node.
- The Q, R, and S waves (QRS complex) indicate ventricular depolarization.
- The ST segment is the time between the end of ventricular depolarization and the start of ventricular repolarization.
- The T-wave indicates ventricular repolarization or recovery.
- The U-wave indicates late ventricular repolarization and does not normally appear in all leads.
- Normal PR interval measures 0.12-0.20 sec., longer in older clients.
- Normal QRS complex equals 0.08-0.12 sec., but is dependent upon variables such as heart rate and gender.
- OT interval is the total time for ventricular depolarization and repolarization; a normal QT interval equals 0.32-0.44 sec.
- Steps to rhythm analysis:
  - Determine rate
  - Determine regularity
  - P to QRS ratios (is there one P wave for every corresponding QRS, and is the PR the same?)
  - PR interval
  - QRS interval
  - QT interval
- Goals of collaborative management:
  - Obtain an accurate ECG reading.
  - Minimize artifact, which are irrelevant notations produced by muscle twitching.

- Analyze and interpret ECG readings correctly.
- Identify any existing cardiac or lung pathology, medications, or electrolyte imbalances.
- Evaluate client's response to increased activity such as rhythm changes, rate changes, or ST segment changes.
- Important nursing diagnoses (actual or potential):
  - Altered cardiac tissue perfusion due to decreased cardiac output related to ischemia, infarction, or dysrhythmia
  - Knowledge deficit
- **Key Terms/Concepts**: Leads, electrical activity, graphic record, P waves, QRS complex, T-waves, U-wave, PR interval, ST segment, artifact, cardiac pathology

Overview

An electrocardiogram (ECG) is a graphic record of the electrical activity of the heart. The ECG provides important data about the transmission of electrical impulses to the different parts of the heart. In addition, the ECG is a valuable tool for diagnosing abnormal cardiac rhythms and myocardial damage. **Continuous cardiac monitoring is used to evaluate possible dysrhythmias throughout the day. ECG stress testing** measures the heart's reaction to an increased workload imposed by exercise or medication.

Risk Factors Indicating Need for an ECG

- Myocardial infarction (MI)
- Rheumatic heart disease
- Intraventricular conduction defects
- Exercise intolerance
- History of cardiac dysrhythmias

Signs and Symptoms Indicating Need for an ECG

- Abnormal heart rate
- Abnormal heart rhythm
- Chest pain
- Shortness of breath
- Fatigue upon exertion
- Tamponade or pericarditis

Diagnostic Uses of ECG

- Possible cardiomyopathy or enlargement
- Included in routine physical examination for clients at risk for cardiac disease
- ECG provides valuable baseline information prior to surgery.
- May show prior or evolving myocardial infarction or ischemia. Many people may not retain Q waves, an indication of a prior MI.
- Determines presence of dysrhythmias
- Presence of intraventricular conduction defects

- Used with ECG stress testing, whereby the client performs increasing physical activity on a treadmill to evaluate the cardiac response to workload
- Medication (adenosine) can be used for stress testing to simulate physical stress for bedridden clients or those with knee problems, lung disease, etc.

Therapeutic Nursing Management

- **Prevention of ECG Artifacts**:
  - Place leads on a flat, non-bony site on the extremity and chest.
  - Make sure that the lead pads adhere to skin, by correctly preparing skin and shaving hair.
- **Assess/Monitor**:
  - ECG tracing
  - For chest pain or dyspnea during stress test
  - Vital signs, physical status, and ECG during stress testing
  - Heart rhythm continually for critically ill clients, with alarms set to alert nurse to rhythm changes
- **Nursing Activities**:
  - Explain procedure to client.
  - Place client in supine position.
  - Expose client's arms, chest, and limbs.
  - Attach limb lead wires to appropriate limb pad or plate.
  - Use electrode gel or ink, or a prepared conductive pad to identify placement of chest leads.
  - Verify that lead placement is correct.
  - Start electrocardiography machine and record ECG tracing.
  - Turn off machine when tracing is finished, and remove ECG tracing from machine.
  - Disconnect limb leads and chest electrodes.
  - Remove gel from client's skin.
  - Label ECG recording with client's name, date, time of recording, and medical record number.
  - Document procedure and any reactions to procedure in client's record.

Pharmacology

- Electrode gel or ink
- Prepared conductive pads

Age-Related Changes—Gerontological Considerations

- The risk of cardiac pathology increases with age.
- ECG stress testing may cause more cardiovascular symptoms in older clients.
- Older clients have a prolonged PR interval.
- Dysrhythmias are often asymptomatic or present atypically.
- Ischemia and infarction may present asymptomatically or atypically.

Critical Thinking Exercise: Nursing Management of the Client Requiring an Electrocardiogram (ECG)

Situation: As part of his yearly physical examination, a 55-year-old male client is undergoing an ECG (electrocardiogram) exercise stress test. The client is instructed to walk on a treadmill for 30 minutes while the nurse performs an ECG. Prior to the procedure, the nurse obtains the client's baseline blood pressure, pulse rate, and rhythm strip. The nurse carefully monitors the client and ECG tracings throughout the procedure. Once the procedure is over, the nurse helps the client to a resting position, and continues to monitor his ECG and vital signs until they are stable.

1. What is the purpose of ECG stress testing?

2. Which conditions contraindicate the use of ECG stress testing?

_____ Angina pectoris	_____ Heart failure
_____ Myocarditis	_____ Mild hypertension
_____ Bradycardia	_____ Recent acute MI
_____ First-degree heart block	_____ Endocarditis
_____ Severe aortic stenosis	_____ Sinus dysrhythmia

3. Which instructions should the nurse give the client prior to ECG stress testing?

_____ Do not eat or drink for at least 12 hours prior to the test.

_____ Avoid nicotine, alcohol, coffee, and tea on the test day.

_____ Wear loose comfortable clothes and sturdy shoes.

_____ Hold all prescribed medications until after the test.

_____ Report any chest pain or dyspnea during and following the test.

_____ Take a hot shower after completing the test.

4. List the clinical manifestations for which ECG testing must be stopped.

Nursing Management of the Client with Angina Pectoris

Key Points

- Angina pectoris is a warning sign for acute myocardial infarction.
- Women may experience chest pain differently from men; their symptoms may be more subtle.
- Goals of collaborative management:
  - Recognize and treat early.
  - Prevent and reduce pain.
  - Reduce myocardial oxygen demands.
  - Restore cardiac oxygenation.
  - Reduce possibility of MI and premature death.
- Important nursing diagnoses (actual or potential):
  - Pain
  - Altered tissue perfusion due to decreased cardiac output
  - Ineffective breathing pattern
  - Decreased cardiac output
  - Anxiety
  - Fear
  - Knowledge deficit
  - Ineffective management of therapeutic regimen
  - Potential for cardiac dysrhythmias
- **Key Terms/Concepts**: Angina, stable angina, unstable angina, intractable angina, variant angina, cardiomyopathy, anti-platelet therapy

Overview

Chest pain caused by myocardial ischemia due to inadequate myocardial oxygen and blood supply is referred to as angina pectoris. Decreased myocardial blood flow can occur from atherosclerosis or a blood clot. When blood flow to the heart is compromised, the heart muscle is deprived of oxygen, which leads to changes in cellular metabolism and subsequent chest pain. Anginal pain is often described as a tight squeezing, heavy pressure, or constricting feeling in the chest. The pain may radiate to the jaw, neck, or arm. The focus of care is the reduction of coronary oxygen demands and improvement of blood supply. The four types of angina are:

- **Intractable angina** is a persistent, incapacitating pain that is not relieved by conventional treatment methods.
- **Stable angina** (exertional angina) occurs with exercise or emotional stress and is relieved by rest or nitroglycerin.

- **Unstable angina** (preinfarction angina) also occurs with exercise or emotional stress, but it increases in occurrence, severity, and duration over time.
- **Variant angina** (Prinzmetal's angina) is due to coronary artery spasm. It is similar to stable angina, but lasts for a longer period of time.

Risk Factors

- Atherosclerosis
- Coronary artery spasm
- Anemia
- Exercise/sexual activity
- Abuse of stimulants
- Hyperthyroidism
- CHF (congestive heart failure)
- Congenital heart defects
- Pulmonary hypertension
- Left ventricular hypertrophy
- Cardiomyopathy
- Eating a heavy meal
- Emotional stress

Signs and Symptoms

- Chest pain (substernal or precordial, may radiate to the neck, arms, shoulders or jaw, tight squeezing or heaviness in the chest, burning, aching, dull, constant)
- Dyspnea
- Pallor
- Tachycardia and/or palpitations
- Anxiety/fear
- Sweating (diaphoresis)
- Hypertension

Diagnostic and Laboratory Tests

- Rick factor assessment
- History and physical examination
- Stress exercise test or stress echocardiogram
- Lipid profile - The levels of:
  - TC (total cholesterol)
  - Triglycerides
  - VLDL (very low density lipoprotein)
  - LDL (low density lipoprotein)

- HDL (high density lipoprotein)
- Ratio:
  - TC/HDL
  - LDL/HDL
- FBG/ FBS (fasting blood glucose)(fasting blood sugar)
- ECG (electrocardiogram)
- Cardiac enzymes
  - CPK: creatine phosphokinase
    - CPK composed of 3 isoenzymes:
      - CPK-1 (also called CPK-BB) concentrated in the brain
      - CPK-2 (also called CPK-MB) found mostly in the heart
      - CPK-3 (also called CPK-MM) found mostly in skeletal muscle
  - LDH: lactic dehydrogenase
  - Serum glutamic oxaloacetic transaminase (SGOT), also called aspartate aminotransferase (AST)
- Ultrasound (also called cardiac ultrasound or echocardiogram)
  - 2D (2-dimensional)
  - 3D (3-dimensional)
  - Doppler
  - TEE (transesophageal echocardiogram)
- Angiography
- Cardiac catheterization
- Troponin
- Myoglobin

Therapeutic Nursing Management

- **Assess/Monitor:**
  - EKG
  - Location, severity, quality, and duration of pain
- **Nursing Activities:**
  - Teach regarding the use of nitroglycerin (keep in possession at all times, may take every 5 minutes during a 15-minute interval, take prior to vigorous activity).
  - Administer oxygen (4 to 6 L), as prescribed.
  - Encourage rest periods between activities.
  - Assist client with identification of precipitating events.
  - Teach client to seek immediate medical attention if pain does not subside with rest and/or nitroglycerin.
  - Teach client about the disease process and the differences between angina and acute MI.
  - Assist client to identify modifiable cardiac risk factors.
  - Encourage weight loss, smoking cessation, and blood pressure control, if appropriate.

- Teach clients who are taking beta blockers such as atenolol (Tenormin) to check blood pressure on a regular basis.
- Teach client to avoid strenuous exercise or emotional stress when possible.
- Prepare client for diagnostic examinations as prescribed, (i.e. cardiac catheterization [angiogram]).
- Prepare client for revascularization procedures (PTCA/stents).

Pharmacology

- Oxygen
- Vasodilators (sublingual nitroglycerin is the medication of choice)
- Anti-platelet therapy (aspirin, clopidogrel [Plavix], ticlopidine [Ticlid])
- Beta blockers (acebutolol [Sectral], atenolol [Tenormin], metoprolol [Lopressor])
- Calcium channel blockers (amlodipine [Norvasc], nifedipine [Procardia])
- Anticoagulants (heparin, low molecular weight heparins)

Complications

- Myocardial infarction (MI)

Age–Related Changes—Gerontological Considerations

- The incidence of cardiac disease increases with age, especially in the presence of hypertension, diabetes mellitus, hypercholesterolemia, elevated homocystine, HS-CRP (highly sensitive C - reactive protein).
- Older adults may not present with typical signs of angina. Often their symptoms are vague and may be misleading.

Critical Thinking Exercise: Nursing Management of the Client with Angina Pectoris

Situation: A 42-year-old male visits the emergency department stating he developed severe chest pain radiating to his jaw while mowing his lawn. His blood pressure is 140/90, pulse 88 bpm and respirations 26 beats per minute. The nurse administers a prescribed sublingual nitroglycerin tablet and starts oxygen by nasal cannula at 5 L per minute. Within 30 minutes, the client states his pain is relieved.

1. Which instructions should be given to the client before he goes home?

   _____ How to use nitroglycerine at home should his chest pain return

   _____ To take rest periods between activities to prevent chest pain

   _____ To self-administer an antiarrhythmic drug if his chest pain persists

   _____ How to take his own blood pressure and pulse

   _____ The need to make immediate changes in his lifestyle

2. Match the type of angina with the clinical manifestations it produces. Use "V", "S", "U" or "I" as your answers.

V = Variant angina (Prinzmetal's)	Not relieved by conventional methods
S =Stable angina (Exertional)	Lasts for a long period of time
U = Unstable angina	Relieved by rest
I = Intractable angin	Increases in severity over time
	Persistent, incapacitating pain
	Occurs with exercise or stress

3. Which statements are true about angina? Correct any false statements.

   a. Angina may produce pain that radiates to the neck or arms.

   b. Angina is often described as a sharp, unrelenting pain.

   c. Clients with angina are taught to take nitroglycerin every fifteen minutes for severe pain.

   d. Eating a heavy meal can precipitate angina pectoris.

Nursing Management of the Client with Myocardial Infarction (MI)

Key Points

- Acute myocardial infarction (MI) is a major cause of death from coronary artery disease.
- The majority of deaths occur within one hour of symptom onset.
- The intake of one daily aspirin may prevent death from acute myocardial infarction.
- Men and women do not experience the same symptoms associated with myocardial infarction.
- The elderly and diabetics do not always experience symptoms typically associated with myocardial infarction
- Early recognition and treatment of acute myocardial infarction is essential to prevent death.
- Goals of collaborative management:
    - Recognize and treat early.
    - Minimize myocardial damage.
    - Preserve myocardial function.
    - Prevent complications (dysrhythmias, cardiogenic shock).
    - Relieve pain.
    - Reduce myocardial oxygen demand.
- Important nursing diagnoses (actual and potential):
    - Pain
    - Altered myocardial tissue perfusion due to decreased cardiac output
    - Impaired gas exchange
    - Anxiety and fear
    - Knowledge deficit
    - Ineffective individual coping
- **Key Terms/Concepts**: Sudden death, ischemia, infarction (necrosis), cardiogenic shock, cardiac enzymes, cardiac isoenzymes

Overview

A myocardial infarction (MI) is the process by which an abrupt interruption of oxygen to the heart muscle produces myocardial ischemia. Ischemia, persistent or complete, may lead to tissue necrosis (infarction) if blood supply and oxygen are not restored. When cardiac muscle suffers ischemic injury, cardiac enzymes are released into the bloodstream, providing specific markers of myocardial infarction. Ischemia is reversible, whereas infarction is permanent. MIs are classified based on the affected area of the heart (e.g. anterior vs anterolateral); the depth of involvement (transmural vs. nontransmural); the EKG changes they produce (Q wave vs. non-Q wave). Non-Q-wave MIs are more common in older adults and women; they produce smaller changes in cardiac enzymes and less immediate myocardial dysfunction, but have higher incidence of late complications of reinfarction and post-infarction angina.

Risk Factors

- Advanced age
- Under age 60, men are at greater risk
- Hereditary predisposition
- Atherosclerosis
- CAD (Coronary artery disease)
- Hypertension
- Obesity
- Diabetes mellitus
- High serum cholesterol and triglycerides
- Sedentary lifestyle
- Cigarette smoking
- Alcohol abuse
- High-fat diet
- Persistent emotional stress
- History of coronary artery disease
- Race: African American, Native American, Hispanic

Signs and Symptoms

- Acute, crushing or squeezing substernal chest pain unrelieved by rest or nitroglycerin and lasting for more than 15 minutes
- Pain radiating down left arm or up to jaw
- Pallor
- Nausea and vomiting
- Cool, clammy skin
- Diaphoresis
- Dyspnea
- Confusion
- Dizziness
- Fainting
- Anxiety
- Decreased level of consciousness

Diagnostic and Laboratory Tests

- ECG (ischemia-ST segment depression, T wave inversion; injury - ST elevation, possible Q wave formation).
- CK-MB: normal values - 0-3%; >5% - positive for MI.
- Enzymes elevate only after 3-4 hours from onset of symptoms and peak at 18-24 hours.
- History and physical examination
- Electrocardiogram (ECG)
- Cardiac enzymes:
  - Myoglobin
  - Troponins I and T— proteins found in the myocardium that have a high specificity for myocardial injury and rise earlier than CK-MB.
  - CPK (creatine phosphokinase) – an enzyme found in muscle and brain tissue reflects tissue catabolism resulting from cell trauma. The lab test is performed to detect muscle damage. Normal CK is 26-174 U/L.
    - CPK composed of 3 isoenzymes
      - CPK-1 (also called CPK-BB) concentrated in the brain
      - CPK-2 (also called CPK-MB) found mostly in the heart
      - CPK-3 (also called CPK-MM) found mostly in skeletal muscle
  - LDH (lactic dehydrogenase)
  - Serum glutamic oxaloacetic transaminase (SGOT), also called aspartate aminotransferase (AST)
- Cardiac catheterization; angiography
- White blood cell (WBC) count
- ABG analysis
- Lipid profile
  - TC (total cholesterol)
  - Triglycerides
  - VLDL (very low density lipoprotein)
  - LDL (low density lipoprotein)
  - HDL (high density lipoprotein)
  - Ratio
    - TC/HDL
    - LDL/HDL
- Electrolyte profile
- Ultrasound (also called: cardiac sonogram or echocardiogram)
  - 2D (2-dimensional)
  - 3D (3-dimensional)
  - Doppler
  - Transesophageal echocardiogram (TEE)
- Thallium scan (Thallium [a radiopharmaceutical—sometimes referred to as a radioisotope or tracer] is injected into the arterial system. Images are taken

when exercising and at rest using SPECT [single photon emission computed tomography].)

Therapeutic Nursing Management

- **Assess/Monitor:**
  - Vital signs
  - Pain status
  - Cardiac rhythm
  - Laboratory data:
    - Cardiac enzymes
    - Electrolytes
    - ABGs
      - Oxygen saturation levels
  - For complications of acute myocardial infarction (MI), congestive heart failure (CHF), cardiac dysrhythmias
  - For modifiable coronary risk factors
- **Nursing Activities:**
  - Perform admission procedures to a critical or cardiac care unit.
  - Initiate continuous cardiac monitoring.
  - Encourage semi-Fowler's position.
  - Administer nitroglycerin and pain medications as prescribed.
  - Maintain client IV access for emergency medications.
  - Provide rest with gradual return to activities of daily living.
  - Encourage compliance with cardiac rehabilitation plan.
  - Teach client stress reduction measures if appropriate.
  - Educate older clients to notify a health care provider if they experience jaw pain, shoulder pain, or fainting.
  - Offer emotional support to client and family.
  - Prepare for revascularization procedures (PTCA, CABG, TPA, etc.).
  - Prepare for diagnostic procedure such as cardiac catheterization

Pharmacology

- Oxygen
- Nitroglycerin by intravenous infusion
- Analgesics (morphine sulfate [Duramorph, Roxanol])
- Anticoagulants (heparin)
- Anti-platelet medications (aspirin, clopidogrel [Plavix], ticlopidine [Ticlid])
- Thrombolytic agents (streptokinase [Streptase], t-PA)
- Other Anti-dysrhythmic medications to treat specific dysrhythmias
- Sedatives (benzodiazepines)
- Stool softeners
- Beta-blockers or ACE inhibitors-found to be cardioprotective

Complications

- Dysrhythmias
- Congestive heart failure
- Cardiogenic shock
- Death

Age-Related Changes—Gerontological Considerations

- The elderly person often does not feel the intense crushing pain because of altered release of neurotransmitters that occur in the aging process; therefore, many have atypical symptoms.
- Atherosclerotic changes related to aging predispose the heart to poor blood perfusion and oxygen delivery.
- Elderly persons with atherosclerosis typically have well-established collateral circulation in the blood vessels of the heart. For this reason they are often saved the lethal complications associated with myocardial infarction.

Critical Thinking Exercise: Nursing Management of the Client with Myocardial Infarction (MI)

Situation: A 46-year-old man is brought to the emergency department after experiencing sudden, crushing substernal chest pain, which was unrelieved by rest or nitroglycerin. He is pale, cool, clammy, and diaphoretic. He complains of nausea and of the inability to take a deep breath. His blood pressure is 105/80, heart rate 92 bpm, and respirations 28 per minute.

1. What is the rationale for implementing these collaborative interventions for a client who is suffering an acute MI (myocardial infarction)?

   a. Initiate oxygen.

   b. Obtain intravenous access.

   c. Initiate continuous cardiac monitoring.

   d. Administer morphine sulfate.

2. What are the most reliable tests to determine if the client is experiencing a MI (myocardial infarction) or angina?

   _____ Serial electrocardiograms

   _____ Serum electrolytes

   _____ Chest x-ray

   _____ Serum enzyme studies

3. For which three complications is the client most at risk during this early stage of MI (myocardial infarction)?

   _____ Electrolyte imbalance   _____ Sudden death

   _____ Cardiac dysrhythmias   _____ Metabolic acidosis

   _____ Cardiogenic shock   _____ CHF (congestive heart failure)

Nursing Management of the Client with Cardiac Arrest

Key Points

- Ventricular fibrillation is the cause of sudden, non-traumatic cardiac arrest in 80%-90% of victims.
- Other causes of cardiac arrest may include:
  - Lethal arrhythmias (ventricular tachycardias, ventricular fibrillation, asystole)
  - Acute MI/ischemia
  - Electrolyte imbalance
  - Fear, extreme emotional shock
  - Advanced age
  - Choking
  - Electric shock
- Early defibrillation greatly improves the likelihood of a successful resuscitation effort.
- Immediate CPR significantly increases the chances of survival following cardiac arrest.
- Approximately 40% of people who have experienced an out-of-hospital cardiac arrest and who receive emergency care survive the event.
- CPR must be initiated within 4 to 6 minutes of cardiac arrest to prevent brain death due to anoxia.
- Citizens need to be trained to recognize the signs of cardiac arrest, call 911, and initiate CPR.
- Effective basic life support (BLS) combines rescue breathing and chest compressions.
- Advanced cardiac life support (ACLS) assists the client through the stabilization process following the cardiac arrest.
- Automatic implantable cardioverter defibrillators can be surgically implanted in clients who are at high risk for cardiac arrest and sudden cardiac death.
- Goals of collaborative management:
  - Quickly provide oxygen to the vital organs.
  - Restore cardiac output and perfusion.
  - Stabilize the client during the post-arrest period.
  - Diagnose and treat the underlying cause of the cardiac arrest.
- Important nursing diagnoses (actual or potential):
  - Altered cardiopulmonary tissue perfusion due to decreased cardiac output
  - Impaired gas exchange

- Ineffective breathing pattern
- Inability to sustain spontaneous ventilation
- **Key Terms/Concepts**: Ventricular fibrillation, apnea, cardiopulmonary resuscitation (CPR), defibrillation, defibrillator, automated external defibrillator (AED), basic life support (BLS), airway management, ventilation, emergency medical system (EMS), advanced cardiac life support (ACLS)

Overview

Cardiac arrest is the complete cessation of the heart's pumping activity. It usually results from VT and causes sudden cardiac death (occurring within one hour of the onset of cardiovascular symptoms). Whereas the majority of cases are precipitated by VT, some are immediately caused by asystole (cardiac standstill) or pulseless electrical activity (absence of muscle contraction).

Risk Factors

- CAD
- Frequent PVCs, bigeminal PVCs, multifocal PVCs
- Bursts of VT
- Left ventricular hypertrophy
- Ischemia
- Acute MI
- Electrolyte imbalance
- Extreme fear or severe emotional shock
- Drug abuse
- Chocking/electric shock
- Advanced age
- Hypertension
- Diabetes
- Idiopathic hypertropic subaortic stenosis (IHSS)
  - Pneumothorax
  - Aortic dissection/rupture
  - Crushing/blunt chest trauma

Signs and Symptoms

- No pulse or thready pulse
- Apnea or dyspnea
- Unresponsiveness
- Dilation of pupils
- Seizures (sometimes)
- Pain: not always limited to the chest, may be radiating to arm or back
- Diaphoresis
- Pallor

Diagnostic and Laboratory Tests

- Brief, targeted history and physical exam (in clinical setting)
- 12-lead electrocardiogram (ECG)
- Vital signs
- Cardiac enzymes:
  - CPK (creatine phosphokinase)
    - CPK composed of three isoenzymes:
      - CPK-1 (also called CPK-BB) concentrated in the brain
      - CPK-2 (also called CPK-MB) found mostly in the heart
      - CPK-3 (also called CPK-MM) found mostly in skeletal muscle
  - Lactic dehydrogenase (LDH)
  - Serum glutamic oxaloacetic transaminase (SGOT); also called aspartate aminotransferase (AST)
- Arterial blood gases (ABGs)
- Electrolyte panel
- Chest x-ray (later)
- Troponin
- Myoglobin

Therapeutic Nursing Management

- Citizens should be able to recognize a person in cardiac arrest.
- Citizens should be prepared in CPR techniques.
- Nurses should be prepared to respond to a "code" or cardiopulmonary arrest situation.
- Nurses should understand code protocols.
- Nurses should be able to work with emergency equipment on the crash cart.
- Nurses should maintain certification in BLS (ACLS if appropriate).
- Recognize signs of cardiac compromise early.
- Assess effectiveness of interventions continuously.
- Monitor ECG.
- Treat the causes of cardiac arrest:
  - Identify and treat lethal arrhythmias (CPR, defibrillate, administer antiarrhythmic drugs, cardiovert).
  - Identify and correct electrolyte imbalances; administer IV electrolytes.
  - Administer O_2, pain medication, thrombolytics to treat MI.
  - Prepare for angioplasty, CABG, thrombolytics.
- If needed, provide postmortem care.
- Check or clarify do not resuscitate (DNR), advance directives
- **Assess/Monitor:**
  - ABCs (airway, breathing, circulation) before beginning CPR
  - For absence of pulse, apnea, and responsiveness before beginning CPR

- For chest rise with breaths during CPR
- For carotid pulse with compressions during CPR
- ECG continually in clinical setting
- For dysrhythmias in clinical setting
  - **Nursing Actions (In Clinical Settings):**
    - Notify staff of cardiac emergency using code protocol for institution.
    - Respond to emergency code if not at client's bedside.
    - Rush crash cart to bedside.
    - Verify client is in arrested state and identify precipitating factors, as able.
    - Start CPR.
    - Defibrillate client using direct electrical charge if indicated (ventricular fibrillation or pulseless ventricular tachycardia).
    - Assess for return of spontaneous respirations, electrical activity (sinus rhythm) pulse.
    - Monitor ABGs and other lab work as ordered during resuscitative measures.
    - Note response to defibrillation/cardioversion efforts.
    - Note response to medications.
    - Give emergency medications via intravenous route.
    - Give emergency medications via endotracheal tube if tube is in place and no IV access.
    - Give emergency medications via intraosseous route and/or endotracheal tube if intravenous route not available.
    - Orient client to situation when conscious.
    - Document defibrillation procedure and administration of medications.
    - Notify family of client's condition.
    - Notify attending primary care provider.
    - Transfer client to critical care unit for further evaluation and treatment.
    - Initiate postmortem procedures if client does not survive resuscitative efforts.

Pharmacology

- Epinephrine
- Lidocaine
- Atropine
- Supplemental oxygen
- Phenobarbital, phenytoin, or diazepam to prevent or treat seizures
- Antidysrhythmics for dysrhythmias
- Thrombolytics for myocardial infarction (t-PA, streptokinase)
- Vasopressors for hypotension (dopamine, norepinephrine)
- Intravenous fluids (NS, LR)

Complications

- Hypoxemia, anoxia
- Severe neurologic damage
- Dysrhythmias
- Cardiogenic shock
- Rib fractures with or without pneumothorax from cardiac compressions
- Burns from countershocks
- Dental damage or esophageal damage from endotracheal intubation
- Seizures
- Death

Age-Related Changes—Gerontological Considerations

- Older clients are at increased risk for heart conditions that can precipitate cardiac arrest.
- Older clients may not respond as quickly to resuscitation efforts as younger clients and carry a higher post arrest mortality and morbidity.

Critical Thinking Exercise: Nursing Management of the Client with Cardiac Arrest

Situation: A 60-year-old hospitalized male client who had experienced an acute MI three days earlier was in stable condition when he suddenly developed ventricular fibrillation swiftly followed by cardiac arrest. Following verification that the client had arrested, CPR was started immediately. The staff quickly responded to the emergency code, and arrived at the client's bedside with the crash cart. The attending physician defibrillated the client, while the nurse prepared and administered emergency medications via the client's intravenous line. The client responded satisfactorily to the emergency interventions. The nurses documented the event and notified the family of the client's condition.

1. For which purpose is cardiac defibrillation used?

   _____ Cardiac standstill   _____ Premature ventricular contractions

   _____ Ventricular fibrillation   _____ Atrial fibrillation

2. What is an AED (automated external defibrillator), and what is its primary advantage?

3. What are the purposes of ACLS (advanced cardiac life support)?

4. What should the nurse document, following the defibrillation process?

   _____ The presence of family members   _____ The client's condition prior to intervention

   _____ Any known allergies   _____ The pre-procedure rhythm

   _____ The number of defibrillation attempts   _____ The post-defibrillation rhythm

   _____ Vital signs   _____ Intake and output

   _____ Emergency drugs administered

Nursing Management of the Client with Central Venous Pressure (CVP) Monitoring

Key Points

- Normal central venous pressure (CVP) is 2 to 12 mmHg.
- Normal CVP readings are 4 to 10 cm H_2O measured with a water manometer.
- CVP pressure can be estimated by examining for jugular venous distension.
- Goals of collaborative management:
  - Establish a baseline for the transducer position, with 0-point at the level of the right atrium.
  - Obtain an accurate CVP reading.
  - Use CVP measurements to help determine diagnosis and treatment decisions.
  - Prevent complications from procedure.
- Important nursing diagnoses (actual or potential):
  - Altered tissue perfusion
  - Risk for volume imbalance
  - Fluid volume excess
  - Fluid volume deficit
  - Decreased cardiac output
  - Risk for infection
  - Anxiety and fear
- **Key Terms/Concepts:** Estimation of CVP, right atrium, vena cava, CVP catheter, phlebostatic axis, 0-point, workload of heart, fluid overload, right heart failure, vasoconstriction, vasodilation, fluid losses, estimation of CVP

Overview

Central venous pressure (CVP) monitoring measures the pressure in the right atrium of the heart, and is an indirect measure of the workload on the heart's right side. A CVP catheter is passed through a vein into the superior or inferior vena cava. CVP increases with fluid overload from rapid infusion of intravenous fluid, right-sided heart failure or peripheral vasoconstriction. CVP decreases with hemorrhage, fluid loss, or vasodilation.

Risk Factors Necessitating CVP Measurement

- Right ventricular failure
- Constrictive pericarditis
- Cardiac tamponade

- Pulmonary hypertension
- Fluid overload due to very rapid administration of intravenous fluids
- Sodium and water retention
- Fluid losses
- Hemorrhage
- Septic shock
- Severe vasodilation with pooling of blood in extremities
- Vasoconstriction
- Hypertension
- Renal failure

Signs and Symptoms Necessitating CVP Measurement

- Jugular vein distension
- Flat jugular veins
- Manifestations of:
  - Right heart disease
  - Fluid overload
  - Fluid loss
  - Sodium and water retention
  - Hemorrhage

Diagnostic and Laboratory Tests

- History and physical examination
- Estimation of CVP by examining jugular veins

Therapeutic Nursing Management

- **Assess/Monitor**:
  - Baseline vital signs
  - CVP catheter for kinking that could reduce patency
  - CVP reading for accuracy
  - For complications from procedure
- **Nursing Activities**:
  - Place client in supine position and elevate head of bed 15 to 30 degrees when estimating with jugular veins; flat when using manometer transducer.
  - Instruct client to avoid coughing or moving around, as these activities may interfere with obtaining an accurate reading.
  - Help client to relax.
  - Check the connections between the CVP catheter and attachments to make certain they are secure.
  - Mark the phlebostatic axis with an ink mark on the client's chest (4th intercostal space, mid-axillary line).

- When measuring CVP, ensure the zero mark on the manometer is placed at the phlebostatic axis.
- Maintain aseptic technique throughout procedure.
- Document findings.
- Question and troubleshoot any reading that varies significantly from earlier readings.
- Following procedure, change dressing at incision site, maintaining aseptic technique.
- Change intravenous solution, manometer, and tubing according to hospital policy.
- Obtain a chest x-ray (CXR) if client is dyspneic and reports chest pain at insertion site.
- Obtain CXR immediately following placement of CVP catheter if placed at bedside.

Pharmacology

- Antiseptic solution for cleaning skin
- Local anesthetic (lidocaine)
- Antiseptic ointment for dressing

Complications

- Pneumothorax
- Fluid overload
- Hydrothorax
- Pulmonary embolus
- Air embolus
- Sepsis
- Infection at point of insertion
- Dysrhythmias

Age-Related Changes—Gerontological Considerations

- The intravascular volume in elderly clients is often reduced; therefore, the nurse may anticipate a lower CVP reading, particularly if dehydration is a complication.

Critical Thinking Exercise: Nursing Management of the Client with Central Venous Pressure (CVP) Monitoring

Situation: A 55-year-old male client with right ventricular failure is being assessed for increased CVP. During admission, a nurse estimated the client's CVP and determined it was high. The client's CVP was then measured several times over the next 24 hours. The client's CVP ranged from 12 cm H_2O to 15 cm H_2O. However, the next reading was 8 cm H_2O.

1. What does "CVP" stand for, and what does it measure?

2. Clients with which of the following problems are candidates for CVP monitoring?

_____ Acute appendicitis   _____ Hypertension

_____ CHF (congestive heart failure   _____ Acute MI (myocardial infarction)

_____ ARF (acute renal failure)   _____ Tuberculosis

_____ Septic shock   _____ Cardiac tamponade

_____ Hemorrhage

3. What actions does the nurse perform prior to assessing a client's CVP?

4. List at least three factors that can cause a CVP measurement to differ significantly from previous readings.

Nursing Management of the Client with Congestive Heart Failure (CHF)

| Key Points |

- Heart failure occurs when the heart muscle is unable to pump effectively and is divided into systolic and diastolic failure.
- Systolic dysfunction can be divided into right and left causes:
  - Left (more common) - inability of heart to pump effectively
    - Cardiomyopathy
    - Valvular diseases
  - Right
    - Lung diseases
- The most common causes of diastolic dysfunction are coronary artery disease and hypertension.
  - Other causes of diastolic dysfunction include ventricular stiffness, decreased ability of the ventricle to relax, and tachycardia (rapid heart rates).
- Blood cannot circulate to the lungs or body when the cardiac pump is compromised.
- Pump failure can occur on either the left or right side of the heart or on both sides.
- Symptoms differ based on the side of the heart that is dysfunctional.
- Severe disability and morbidity can result from pump failure.
- Goals of collaborative management:
  - Reduce the cardiac workload.
  - Increase the force and efficiency of cardiac contractions or improve cardiac filling.
  - Maintain normal cardiac output.
  - Correct the underlying cause of heart failure.
  - Prevent complications (cardiogenic shock, dysrhythmia, and thromboembolism).
- Important nursing diagnoses (actual or potential):
  - Fluid volume excess
  - Altered tissue perfusion due to decreased cardiac output
  - Activity intolerance
  - Anxiety and fear
  - Ineffective breathing pattern
  - Fatigue and sleeplessness
  - Knowledge deficit

- Powerlessness and hopelessness
- Ineffective individual coping
- **Key Terms/Concepts:** Left-sided failure, right-sided failure, cardiomyopathy, atherosclerosis, dyspnea, orthopnea, hemodynamic, cardiotonic, diastolic dysfunction, systolic dysfunction, inotropic, afterload reduction

Overview

In the absence of valvular disease, pericardial disease, or dysrhythmias; heart failure should be classified by which part of the cardiac cycle is affected, systolic or diastolic. Heart failure is the inability of the heart to maintain adequate circulation to meet the tissue's need for oxygen and nutrients. Systolic dysfunction leading to heart failure, often referred to as congestive heart failure, results from pump failure that is characterized by **impaired contractility.** Diastolic disfunction results from impaired ventricular filling.

Severity of heart failure is graded on the New York Heart Association's functional classification scale indicating how little, or how much, activity it takes to make the client symptomatic (e.g., chest pain, shortness-of-breath):

Class I: Client exhibits no more symptoms with activity than a healthy client would.

Class II: Clients have symptoms with ordinary exertion.

Class III: Clients display symptoms with minimal exertion.

Class IV: Clients have symptoms at rest.

Risk Factors

- Myocardial infarction (MI)
- Coronary atherosclerosis, angina
- Idiopathic dilated cardiomyopathy
- Other cardiomyopathies, may be caused by long-term alcohol abuse, chemotherapy, infection, inflammatory or degenerative muscle disorders
- Valvular heart disease
- Arterial hypertension
- Hypoxia
- Dysrhythmias, long-standing
- Thyroid diseases
- Fluid overload, chronic
- Anemia
- COPD (chronic obstructive pulmonary disease)
- Pulmonary hypertension
- Cor pulmonale

Signs and Symptoms

Left-sided failure

- Dyspnea, orthopnea, nocturnal dyspnea

- Fatigue
- Pulmonary congestion (dyspnea, cough, bibasilar crackles)
- Dry or moist cough
- S3 heart sound (gallop) *first breathing*
- Palpitations, tachycardia, dysrhythmias
- Frothy sputum (may be blood-tinged)
- Mental confusion
- Anorexia

Right-sided failure

- Elevated CVP (central venous pressure)
- Jugular vein distention
- Peripheral edema
- Abdominal distention
- Fatigue, weakness
- Liver enlargement and tenderness
- Weight gain
- Ascites, increased abdominal girth
- Nocturia

Diagnostic and Laboratory Tests

- History and physical examination
- Hemodynamic monitoring (CVP [central venous pressure], right arterial pressure, PCWP [pulmonary capillary wedge pressure], pulmonary artery pressure, cardiac output)
- Pulmonary function tests (PFTs):
  - Air flow (spirometer)
  - Lung volume
  - Diffusion capacity (correlates with body's ability to extract oxygen from the lungs)
- Electrocardiogram (ECG)
- Cardiac enzymes - to rule out MI (myocardial infarction) as a cause of heart failure:
  - CPK: Creatine phosphokinase
    - CPK composed of three isoenzymes:
      - CPK-1 (also called CPK-BB) concentrated in the brain
      - CPK-2 (also called CPK-MB) found mostly in the heart
      - CPK-3 (also called CPK-MM) found mostly in skeletal muscle
- Arterial blood gases (ABGs)
- Serum electrolytes
- CBC (complete blood count) - look for anemia or infection as cause of failure

- TSH (thyroid stimulating hormone) - look at thyroid problems as a cause of heart failure
- Liver function tests:
  - Alkaline phosphatase (ALP), also called: ALK Phos: an enzyme found in the liver, bones and placenta
  - Alanine aminotransferase (ALT), also called serum glutamic pyruvic transaminase (SGPT): an enzyme found primarily in liver cells
  - Aspartate aminotransferase (AST), also called serum glutamic oxaloacetic transaminase (SGOT): an enzyme found in the liver and elsewhere in the body
  - Gamma glutamyl transpeptidase (GGTP), also called GGT or Gamma GT: an enzyme present in the liver, pancreas and kidneys
  - Bilirubin: a waste product formed by the breakdown of red blood cells
  - Albumin: a protein synthesized by the liver
  - Total cholesterol: a substance stored in the liver
  - Total protein: a nutrient normally broken down by the liver and its enzymes
  - Lactic acid dehydrogenase: an enzyme found in the liver
  - Prothrombin time (PT): tests the blood's ability to clot
- Chest x-ray
- Ultrasound (also called: cardiac ultrasound or echocardiogram)
  - 2-D (2-dimensional)
  - 3-D (3-dimensional), to measure both systolic (pumping ability) and diastolic (filling ability) function of the heart
    - LVEF (left ventricular ejection fraction): The proportion, or fraction, of the volume of blood in the left ventricle that is pumped out into the arteries upon each beat. A normal LVEF is 55%-70%.
    - RVEF (right ventricular ejection fraction): The proportion, or fraction, of the volume of blood in the right ventricle that is pumped out to the lungs upon each beat. A normal RVEF is 5%-10% less than the LVEF.
  - Doppler
- Cardiac catheterization, angiography

Therapeutic Nursing Management

- **Assess/Monitor:**
  - For signs of pulmonary and systemic fluid overload
  - SaO_2 (saturation of oxygen)
  - For hemodynamic changes
  - Vital signs
  - Lung sounds for crackles, wheezes
  - Serum electrolytes (especially potassium if receiving diuretics)
  - Daily weight
  - Mental alterations

- Intake and output
- For signs of drug toxicity if receiving cardiotonic drugs
- **Nursing Activities**:
  - Place in high-Fowler's position.
  - Administer oxygen as prescribed.
  - Encourage bedrest until stable.
  - Assist with care and activities of daily living as required.
  - Maintain dietary restrictions as prescribed (fluid intake, sodium intake).
  - Teach clients to ingest foods and drinks that are high in potassium, such as bananas, orange juice, fresh vegetables, strawberries, almonds, and potatoes; unless on ACE (angiotensin converting enzyme) inhibitors or potassium-sparing diuretics.
  - Teach clients who are self-administering digoxin to:
    - Count their pulse for one full minute before taking the medication.
    - Contact the primary care provider if the pulse rate is irregular, or the pulse rate is outside of the limitations set by the provider which is usually less than 60 or greater than 100.
    - Take digoxin dose at 9 p.m. unless otherwise instructed.
  - Provide emotional support to client and family.
  - Encourage vaccinations with pneumococcal vaccine and yearly influenza vaccine.

Pharmacology

- Oxygen; CPAP/BiPAP
- Acute pulmonary edema, use morphine IV
- Loop diuretics (furosemide, bumetanide, torsemide, and ethacrynic acid) if fluid overload present. May need to add metolazone if additional unloading needed.
- Management of systolic dysfunction:
  - ACE (angiotensin converting enzyme) inhibitors (captopril, enalapril, lisinopril, fosinopril, quinapril, ramipril) - decrease afterload making easier for the heart to pump
  - Beta-blockers (carvedilol, metoprolol XL, bisoprolol)
  - Possible addition of digoxin and spironolactone
  - Angiotensin receptor II blockers if client not tolerant of ACE inhibitors
- Management of diastolic dysfunction:
  - Diuretics
  - Nitrates
  - Calcium-channel blockers
  - Beta-blockers
  - ACE inhibitors
- Positive inotropic agents, used to enhance contractility:
  - Cardiac glycosides (digoxin)
  - Sympathomimetic agents (dopamine, dobutamine)

- Phosphodiesterase inhibitors (amrinone, milrinone)
- Anticoagulants (warfarin, heparin, clopidogrel, etc.)
- Vasodilators (hydralazine)

Complications

- Acute pulmonary edema
- Cardiogenic shock
- Systemic and pulmonary emboli
- Pericardial effusion and pericardial tamponade
- Dysrhythmias
- Fluid and electrolyte imbalances due to administration of diuretics
- Sudden death
- Liver failure
- Renal failure
- Coagulopathies

Age-Related Changes—Gerontological Considerations

- Systolic blood pressure is elevated in older adults, putting them at risk for coronary artery disease (CAD) and heart failure.
- The risk for valvular complications is increased in elderly persons with heart failure.
- There is an increased risk for exercise intolerance in older adults with heart failure.
- The presence of other chronic illnesses may mask the presence of heart failure.
- The risk of electrolyte disturbances is related to diuretic use.

Critical Thinking Exercise: Nursing Management of the Client with Congestive Heart Failure (CHF)

Situation: A 72-year-old woman is admitted to the acute care facility for dyspnea, fatigue, and dizziness. She has a history of hypertension and coronary artery disease. She lives independently and reports that her diet consists primarily of canned soups and other pre-packaged foods. Assessment reveals bilateral crackles, irregular heart rate with a bounding pulse at 92 bpm, blood pressure of 190/96, and 4+ pitting edema of both ankles.

1. What risk factors does the client have for congestive heart failure?

2. What is the etiology for each of the client's nursing diagnoses?
   a. Fluid volume excess
   b. Impaired gas exchange
   c. Activity intolerance
   d. Risk for altered skin integrity

3. Prioritize the following nursing interventions, with "1" representing the most important intervention.
   _____ Assess breath sounds and breathing patterns.
   _____ Report laboratory results.
   _____ Assess capillary refill.
   _____ Monitor urine output.
   _____ Place client in high-Fowler's position.

4. How does the drug digitalis help to alleviate the signs and symptoms associated with congestive heart failure?

5. What should the client be taught about her intake of canned soup and pre-packaged food?

Nursing Management of the Client with Hypertension

| Key Points |

- Hypertension is known as the silent killer because many people are unaware that they have hypertension and are asymptomatic.

- The prevalence of hypertension is the same in men and women; but the incidence of coronary artery disease (CAD), a complication of hypertension, is lower in premenopausal women.

- Hypertensive crisis is a severe and abrupt elevation in blood pressure, characterized by a diastolic blood pressure above 120 to 130 mmHg. Some causes of hypertensive crisis include exacerbation of chronic hypertension, preeclampsia, eclampsia, pheochromocytoma, drugs such as cocaine and amphetamines, head injury and the administration of monoamine oxidase (MAO) inhibitors with tyramine-containing foods. Hypertensive crisis is usually treated with the intravenous administration of nitroprusside (Nitropress).

- Hypertensive emergency may develop very quickly, over hours to days. Manifestations include a severely elevated blood pressure accompanied by symptoms that indicate acute target organ damage as well as damage to the central nervous system.

- Hypertensive encephalopathy is associated with a sudden rise in blood pressure as well as severe headache, nausea, vomiting, seizures, confusion, stupor, and coma.

- Goals of collaborative management:
  - Lower blood pressure below 140/90 mmHg or 130/80 mmHg in clients with diabetes, renal disease, heart failure, or CAD.
  - Prevent associated complications.
  - Help the client adhere to plan of care.

- Important nursing diagnoses (actual or potential):
  - Altered health maintenance
  - Knowledge deficit
  - Ineffective individual management of therapeutic regimen
  - Anxiety
  - Sexual dysfunction related to side effects from antihypertensive medications
  - Disturbed body image if stroke occurs

- **Key Terms/Concepts**: Systolic pressure, diastolic pressure, atherosclerosis, brain attack, asymptomatic, transient ischemic attack (TIA), hypertensive crisis, hypertensive emergency, hypertensive encephalopathy, home blood pressure monitoring

Overview

Stage I hypertension is defined as elevation of the systolic blood pressure above 140 mmHg and the diastolic pressure above 90 mmHg on two or more blood pressure measurements. Pre-hypertension is a systolic blood pressure of 120-139 mmHg or a diastolic blood pressure of 80-89 mmHg. Hypertension is a major risk factor for atherosclerotic cardiovascular disease, cerebral vascular accident, renal failure, and heart failure related to blood vessel damage. Hypertension may be a primary disease or secondary to other conditions, such as cardiovascular, renal, or endocrine disease.

Risk Factors

- Modifiable:
  - Cigarette smoking
  - Obesity
  - Stress
  - Greater than moderate alcohol consumption
  - Increased dietary salt intake
  - Diabetes mellitus
  - Medications
- Non-modifiable:
  - Hereditary predisposition
  - Advancing age
  - African-American race
  - Arteriosclerosis
  - Pregnancy

Signs and Symptoms

- Asymptomatic during early stages
- Headache
- Visual disturbances
- Chest pain
- Flushed face
- Epistaxis
- Dizziness

Diagnostic and Laboratory Tests

- History and physical examination
- Blood pressure pattern
- CBC
- Urinalysis
- Lipid profile
- ECG

- Renal arteriograms, ultrasound
- Complete metabolic profile (CMP)
- 24-hour urine protein or spot microalbumin
- Creatinine clearance (A measure of the volume of plasma that is cleared of creatinine in a fixed time period [mL/min]. Because of the unique properties of creatinine [stable plasma concentrations, freely-filtered, not reabsorbed, and minimally secreted by the kidneys], creatinine clearance is used to estimate the glomerular filtration rate [GFR]. The GFR in turn is the standard by which kidney function is assessed.)

Therapeutic Nursing Management

- **Assess/Monitor:**
  - Blood pressure at frequent intervals
  - For visual disturbances and retinal changes
  - Intake and output
  - Renal studies
  - Daily weights
  - Chemistries as ordered: BUN, creatinine, electrolytes
  - Effects of antihypertensives and other medications
- **Nursing Activities:**
  - Assist with identification of modifiable risk factors (diet, salt intake, alcohol, smoking, and sedentary lifestyle).
  - Encourage client to change modifiable risk factors (weight reduction, restrict salt intake, moderate alcohol intake, smoking cessation, and exercise program).
  - Obtain daily weights.
  - Stress importance of compliance with prescribed medication regimen.
  - Watch for signs and symptoms of hypotension in clients on antihypertensive drug therapy, such as dizziness, syncope, tachycardia, fatigue, and weakness.
  - Client education regarding: hypertension (HTW) "silent killer", importance of medication(s), blood pressure monitoring, salt intake, etc.

Pharmacology

- Diuretics (hydrochlorothiazide, etc.)
- ACE inhibitors (captopril, enalapril, lisinopril, quinapril)
- Angiotensin II receptor antagonist (irbesartan, losartan)
- Vasodilators (hydralazine, nitroglycerin)
- Calcium channel blockers (amlodipine, diltiazem, nicardipine, nifedipine, verapamil)
- Beta-blocking agents (atenolol, labetalol, metoprolol, propranolol)
- Alpha-adrenergic blocking agents (doxazosin, prazosin, terazosin)
- Nitroprusside (Nitropress) administered for hypertensive crisis

Complications

- Heart failure (HF)
- Angina
- Peripheral arterial occlusive disease (PAOD)
- Myocardial infarction (MI)
- Renal insufficiency/failure
- Cerebrovascular accident (CVA)
- Transient ischemic attack (TIA)
- Retinal hemorrhage
- Hypertensive crisis
- Hypertensive encephalopathy

Age-Related Changes—Gerontological Considerations

- The risk of developing hypertension increases with aging due to loss of vessel elasticity decreased cardiac output, and heart valve thickening.
- Older clients are more at risk of dehydration and electrolyte imbalances, especially when receiving diuretic therapy. Offering water throughout the day may help to prevent dehydration.
- Pseudohypertension is common in the elderly due to a decrease in vascular compliance.
- Older clients may exhibit "white coat" hypertension due to apprehension.
- Since the elderly are more prone to orthostatic hypertension (decreased baroreceptor sensitivity in the carotid arteries); measurements should be taken in the standing and sitting position, preferable with a 10-15 minute rest period.
- Older clients may not tolerate medications as well due to comorbid conditions.
- Older clients may be less responsive to vasodilators due to vessel rigidity.

Critical Thinking Exercise: Nursing Management of the Client with Hypertension

Situation: During a routine physical examination, a 55-year-old moderately obese male with a 13-year history of Type 2 NIDDM (non-insulin dependent diabetes mellitus) learns he has hypertension. The client is divorced, does not exercise on a regular basis, and has a stressful job. He controls his diabetes mellitus with a daily oral hypoglycemic agent and diet, although he admits he doesn't control his diet as well as he should.

1. Which statements are true about hypertension? Correct any false statements.

    a. Hypertension is a major risk factor for other diseases, such as renal failure.

    b. Maintaining a diastolic pressure below 80 mmHg is a goal of treatment for hypertension.

    c. Moderate smoking has little effect on blood pressure.

    d. Arterial plaque increases peripheral vascular resistance, producing secondary hypertension.

2. What is the difference between primary and secondary hypertension?

3. Which risk factors for hypertension are modifiable?

    _____ Hereditary predisposition   _____ Sedentary lifestyle

    _____ Diabetes mellitus   _____ Gender

    _____ Diet   _____ Race

    _____ Tobacco use   _____ Obesity

    _____ Stress   _____ Advancing age

    _____ Arteriosclerosis   _____ Chronic illness

Nursing Management of the Client with Thrombophlebitis

Key Points

- Thrombophlebitis can occur in either upper of lower extremities; when it occurs in the deep veins it is referred to as deep venous thrombosis (DVT); when it occurs in the superficial veins it is referred to as superficial venous thrombosis or phlebitis.
- DVT is generally more associated with embolization.
- There is growing incidence of DVT in the upper extremities, which carries a higher mortality, due to increased use of subclavian venous access devices.
- The calf is primary place of clot formation (80% of cases) in DVT.
- Venous clots can dislodge, enter the circulation, and cause pulmonary vessel embolic occlusion.
- Goals of collaborative management:
  - Identify and treat disease early.
  - Prevent thrombus fragmentation and embolization of pulmonary vessels.
  - Prevent recurrence.
  - Treat inflammation.
  - Prevent further clotting.
  - Restore venous blood flow.
  - Dissolve existing clots.
- Important nursing diagnoses (actual or potential):
  - Pain
  - Activity intolerance due to pain
  - Altered peripheral tissue perfusion
  - Knowledge deficit
  - Anxiety and fear
  - Self-care deficit
- **Key Terms/Concepts**: Embolization, thrombus, inflammation, venous stasis, altered coagulability, Homan's sign

Overview

Thrombophlebitis is a condition in which a blood clot (thrombus) forms on a vessel wall secondary to inflammation of the vessel. The clot may partially or completely occlude venous blood flow. Thrombophlebitis is a result of three factors:

- Venous stasis
- Increased blood coagulability
- Injury to the vessel wall

Risk Factors

- Bedrest, immobilization
- Intravenous catheters, especially central venous catheters
- Obesity
- Congestive heart failure (CHF)
- Acute myocardial infarction (MI)
- Cerebrovascular accident (CVA)
- Oral contraceptives
- Pregnancy
- Childbirth
- Surgery over age 40
- Surgery, especially involving the abdominal cavity, thoracic cavity, pelvic cavity (especially gynecological), and knee and hip replacement
- Inflammatory bowel diseases
- Dehydration
- Peripheral vascular disease
- Altered coagulability states
- Fractures
- Cancer (breast, pancreas, prostate, or ovary)
- Advanced age
- Prolonged sitting (flying, driving)
- Constrictive clothing
- Superficial venous thrombosis:
  - IV catheter use
  - Repeated venous punctures
  - Acidic/basic IV solutions

Signs and Symptoms

It should be noted that 90% of cases are silent and that the classic signs of pain, edema, erythema, warmth, dilated superficial veins, palpable cord with tenderness, and Homan's sign are not sensitive nor generally positive findings. Be aware of the triad to recognize client's who are at risk: venous stasis, increase in blood coagulation (includes dehydration), and venous vessel wall damage.

- Tenderness and/or dull aching pain in affected extremity, increased by exercise
- Warmth, rubor color over area
- Palpable, hard lump over thrombus
- General malaise, fever, chills
- Marked redness along the course of the vein, usually only with superficial
- Positive Homan's sign
- Enlargement of diameter of affected calf

- Mild tachycardia
- Superficial venous thrombosis:
  - Pain
  - Redness along the course of vein
  - Increased warmth of extremity
  - Palpable cordlike structure along the vein

Diagnostic and Laboratory Tests

- Venous venography, more sensitive in proximal than distal leg veins. Is the most reliable test in asymptomatic clients but requires use of a dye.
- Magnetic resonance direct thrombus imaging (MRDTI) can help detect both proximal and distal thrombus.
- Duplex scanning - rapid, inexpensive, initial procedure of choice to diagnose DVT, may miss small calf thrombi
- Impedance plethysmography (measures changes in the volume of blood in veins, low accuracy)
- D-dimer, laboratory test may be useful when other testing is not available

Therapeutic Nursing Management

- **Assess/Monitor:**
  - Affected extremity for warmth, color, edema, tenderness, and varices.
  - Signs of respiratory distress which may indicate possible embolization to lungs; pulmonary embolism
  - Chest pain which may indicate embolization to the heart and resultant myocardial infarction (MI)
  - Changes in mentation which may indicate embolization to the brain, cerebrovascular accident (CVA)
- **Nursing Activities:**
  - Maintain bedrest.
  - Elevate affected limb.
  - Never massage the affected limb.
  - Apply warm, moist packs to the affected area as prescribed.
  - Administer anticoagulants and anti-inflammatory medications as prescribed.
  - Apply anti-embolic hose.
  - Teach clients to avoid standing or sitting for prolonged periods, massaging affected leg, wearing tight garments, pressure behind the knees, and crossing the legs.
  - Assist clients with performing leg exercises while in bed.
  - Teach client to monitor signs for signs of bleeding if anticoagulant therapy is initiated.
  - Emphasize the importance of compliance with medical treatment plan.
  - Prepare client for surgery if indicated (venous thrombectomy).

Pharmacology

- Analgesics (opioid and/or NSAIDs)
- Anticoagulants (heparin, warfarin, low-molecular weight heparins)
- Thrombolytics (t-PA, urokinase)
- Antibiotics
- Anti-inflammatory (NSAIDs)

Complications

- Pulmonary embolism
- Acute myocardial infarction (MI)
- Cerebral vascular accident (CVA)
- Recurrent DVT
- Post thrombi syndrome
- Death

Age–Related Changes—Gerontological Considerations

- Older adults are at greater risk for thrombophlebitis because of altered mobility, decreased circulation in lower extremities, and increased incidence of cardiac and pulmonary disorders.
- Older adults may develop chronic venous insufficiency as a result of previous episodes of deep vein thrombosis (DVT). Symptoms of chronic venous insufficiency include dependent edema, leathery skin of lower limbs, venous ulcers, eczema ("stasis dermatitis"), pruritus, and loss of leg hair.

Critical Thinking Exercise: Nursing Management of the Client with Thrombophlebitis

Situation: A 43-year-old obese female underwent abdominal surgery two days ago and is now experiencing acute pain in her right calf. The pain is exacerbated by activity and not relieved by rest. The limb is obviously swollen and warm to the touch. Her peripheral pulses are palpable bilaterally. Her routine medications are birth control pills and vitamins.

1. What risk factors does the client have for thrombophlebitis?

2. Prioritize the client's nursing diagnoses, with "1" representing the most important diagnosis.

   _____ Altered tissue perfusion (right lower extremity)

   _____ Risk for impaired skin integrity

   _____ Impaired mobility

   _____ Risk for activity intolerance

   _____ Pain

3. What teaching needs to be done before the client is discharged to home following her recovery?

   _____ Take aspirin daily with anticoagulant therapy.

   _____ Avoid long periods of standing or sitting.

   _____ Massage the limb gently if pain occurs.

   _____ Report blood in the urine or bleeding gums.

Nursing Management of the Client with a Coronary Artery Bypass Graft (CABG)

Key Points

- Coronary artery bypass graft (CABG) is the most frequently performed type of cardiac surgery.
- More than 300,000 CABG surgeries are performed in the United States yearly.
- CABG helps to relieve symptoms, but does not halt the process of atherosclerosis.
- Approximately 80% to 90% of clients are free of pain within one year following CABG.
- 50% of clients are able to return to work following CABG.
- Goals of collaborative management:
    - Preoperative:
        - Restore blood flow to the damaged area of the myocardium.
        - Prepare client for the procedure.
        - Relieve angina pectoris.
        - Preserve the function of the myocardium.
    - Intraoperative:
        - Prevent complications resulting from the use of cardiopulmonary bypass equipment.
    - Postoperative:
        - Prevent postoperative bleeding, infection, pneumonia, and dysrhythmia.
        - Prevent complications related to thoracotomy.
        - Teach client about risk factor education following discharge.
        - Help client return to desirable social and occupational life.
- Important nursing diagnoses (actual or potential):
    - Altered cardiac tissue perfusion due to decreased cardiac output
    - Risk for infection
    - Risk of bleeding
    - Risk of pneumonia
    - Risk of dysrhythmia
    - Risk of thrombophlebitis
    - Risk of hypoxia
    - Ineffective breathing pattern
    - Anxiety/fear
    - Altered thought processes

- Decreased ability to recall information due to anxiety and fear
- Knowledge deficit
- Ineffective management of therapeutic regimen
- **Key Terms/Concepts**: Coronary artery disease (CAD), atherosclerosis, replacement vessels, saphenous vein, mammary artery, revascularize, cardiopulmonary bypass equipment, thoracotomy, minimally invasive surgery

Overview

Coronary artery bypass graft is an invasive surgical procedure that involves revascularization of myocardium using an extracardiac vein (usually saphenous vein) or artery (usually mammary artery) to bypass an obstruction in one or more of the coronary arteries. A median sternotomy is used to gain access to the heart; the heart is stopped, and the cardiopulmonary bypass pump is used to maintain perfusion to the rest of the body. If saphenous vein is used, it is reversed so the valves do not interfere with blood flow, and anastomosed, or grafted, to the aorta and the coronary artery distal to the occlusion. If internal mammary artery is used, its proximal end remains attached to the subclavian artery, and its distal end is excised and anastomosed to a coronary artery distal to the obstruction. After the procedure, the incision is closed, and the client is rewarmed, which stimulates the heart to start beating. The client is then transported to the ICU on a ventilator, has temporary pacing wires sutured in, chest tubes, a Foley catheter, NG tube, IV access, and arterial line.

Risk Factors

- Necessitating CABG
  - Unstable angina
  - Severe left main coronary artery obstruction
  - Triple vessel disease
  - Two vessel disease that does not respond to intervention
- Contraindications for CABG
  - Bleeding disorders
  - Recent myocardial infarction
  - Cardiomegaly
  - Severe heart failure

Signs and Symptoms Necessitating Surgery

- Chronic angina refractory to medical treatment
- Anginal pain that causes severe restrictions affecting quality of life
- Symptoms of left ventricular dysfunction (often due to acute MI): weak pulses, decreased cardiac output, tachycardia, crackles in lungs, decreased urine output, cool pale skin, decreased blood pressure, decreased level of consciousness
- Severe dyspnea

Diagnostic and Laboratory Tests

- History and physical examination

- ECG (electrocardiogram)
- CBC (complete blood count)
- Cardiac enzymes
  - CPK: creatine phosphokinase
    - CPK composed of three isoenzymes:
      - CPK-1 (also called CPK-BB) concentrated in the brain
      - CPK-2 (also called CPK-MB) found mostly in the heart
      - CPK-3 (also called CPK-MM) found mostly in skeletal muscle
  - Lactic dehydrogenase (LDH)
  - Serum glutamic oxaloacetic transaminase (SGOT); also called aspartate aminotransferase (AST)
- Bleeding studies
- Urinalysis
- Chest x-ray
- Pulmonary function tests
  - Air flow (spirometer)
  - Lung volume
  - Diffusion capacity (correlates with body's ability to extract oxygen from the lungs)
- Blood type and cross-match
- Blood urea nitrogen (BUN)
- Arterial blood gases (ABG)
- Complete metabolic profile (CMP)

Therapeutic Nursing Management

- **Prevention of CAD Necessitating CABG:**
  - Stop smoking.
  - Eat a high-fiber, low-fat, low-cholesterol, and low-sodium diet.
  - Exercise daily.
  - Lose weight.
  - Take medications as ordered.
  - Utilize community resources.
- **Assess/Monitor:**
  - Hemodynamic parameters
  - Arterial line pressure readings
  - ECG readings for dysrhythmias
  - ST segment to detect ischemia
  - Chest tubes and chest drainage
  - Drainage from incision
  - Lung sounds and respiratory rate
  - Ventilator settings, respiratory status
  - Urinary drainage from Foley catheter

- Postoperative laboratory studies
- Pacemaker, leads
- IV fluids, medications
- **Nursing Activities:**
  - Preoperative
    - Prepare the client for the surgery, both physically and emotionally.
    - Explain the operative procedure.
    - If possible, arrange for the client and family to tour the intensive care unit.
  - Postoperative
    - Administer intravenous fluids, medications, and blood as ordered.
    - Administer pain medications.
    - Administer oxygen via ventilator and implement ventilator weaning protocols.
    - Suction client if required.
    - Help the client turn, cough, and deep breathe every two hours when extubated.
    - Report any significant changes in client status to the primary care provider.
    - Have emergency equipment ready should it be needed.
    - Gradually wean client from ventilator when ordered.
    - Instruct the client on the care of anti-emboli stockings if they are ordered at discharge.
    - Encourage the client to gradually begin a program of exercise when allowed.
    - Remind the client to avoid lifting anything more than 10 pounds for at least 2 to 3 months following CABG. No driving for six weeks or as ordered.
    - Remind client to not cross legs.
    - Schedule follow-up checkups.
    - Advise the client to avoid risk factors for CAD.

Pharmacology

- Analgesics (morphine sulfate)
- Antibiotics (cefazolin for surgical prophylaxis)
- Oxygen
- Intravenous fluids
- Electrolytes
- Blood pressure medications, inotropic agents, possible antiarrhythmics

Complications

- Bleeding
- Infection

- Respiratory distress
- Gastric distention, ileus
- Transient hyperglycemia
- Delirium
- Sensory disturbances
- Loss of mental ability (memory, attention, concentration)
- Blood dyscrasias (due to heart-lung equipment)
- Pulmonary edema
- Microemboli to the brain
- Mediastinitis
- Hemothorax
- Pneumothorax
- Pericarditis
- Graft closure
- Myocardial infarction
- Dysrhythmias
- Renal failure
- Cardiac tamponade
- Depression

Age-Related Changes—Gerontological Considerations

- Approximately half of CABG surgeries are performed on clients over age 65.
- Elderly clients usually have a 2 to 4 day longer hospital stay than younger clients.
- Clients who are over age 80 are hospitalized for a mean length of 15 days following CABG.
- Older clients have a higher mortality rate.
- The two most common postoperative problems that affect the elderly are multiple drug-drug interactions and decreased stamina.

Critical Thinking Exercise: Nursing Management of the Client with a Coronary Artery Bypass Graft (CABG)

Situation: A 75-year-old client is home after being discharged from the surgical unit following CABG (coronary artery bypass graft) surgery for severe left main coronary artery obstruction. The client is in the process of starting his cardiac rehabilitation program. The home health nurse is giving the client general instructions for self-care following CABG. The client is learning about his medications, how to care for his support stockings, and when to call his physician should problems arise. The nurse is also scheduling the client for a home exercise rehabilitation program.

1. For which problems should the client be instructed to call his physician?

    _____ Elevated temperature for over 24 hours

    _____ Mild fatigue following performance of daily hygiene

    _____ Separation of suture line

    _____ Increased heart rate with exercise

    _____ Foul-smelling drainage from the suture line

    _____ Red, swollen suture line

    _____ Flaking skin around suture line

2. What are support stockings, how often are they worn, and how are they cared for?

3. The client is beginning an at-home exercise rehabilitation program. When and how often will the client exercise? What records will the client need to keep about his exercise and its results?

Nursing Management of the Client with Atherosclerosis— Coronary Artery Disease (CAD)

Key Points

- Atherosclerosis, also known as coronary artery disease (CAD), is the most common arterial disease.
- Atherosclerosis is associated with diabetes mellitus (DM), renal failure, congestive heart failure (CHF), hypertension, and acute myocardial infarction (MI). *heart failure*
- Lack of early clinical manifestations delays identification and treatment of CAD.
- Until a client experiences symptoms, diagnosis is based on history, physical exam, and risk factor assessment.
- Women with CAD are generally about 10 years older than men at the time of presentation; are more likely to have history of diabetes, hypertension, hyperlipidemia, heart failure, unstable anginal patterns; have a greater likelihood of angina being induced by rest or mental stress; are more likely to experience other symptoms in addition to chest pain, such as neck, jaw, back pain and nausea; are more likely to have a delay in seeking and receiving treatment.
- Goals of collaborative management:
  - Manage modifiable risk factors.
  - Control disease progress via medications, exercise, and diet.
  - Prevent complications (DM, renal failure, CHF, hypertension, acute MI).
- Important nursing diagnoses (actual or potential):
  - Altered tissue perfusion
  - Knowledge deficit
  - Anxiety
  - Fear
  - Ineffective individual management of therapeutic regimen
  - Health-seeking behaviors
  - Decisional conflict related to risk factor modification
  - Noncompliance and risk potential
- **Key Terms/Concepts**: Progressive, modifiable risk factors, non-modifiable risk factors

Overview

Atherosclerosis is a progressive narrowing or complete obstruction of major arteries (coronary, peripheral, and cerebral) from deposition of fatty plaques along the inner arterial walls, which leads to decreased tissue perfusion. Atherosclerosis is the major contributing factor to the development of hypertension, angina, myocardial infarction, congestive heart failure, stroke, and death.

Risk Factors

- Non-modifiable:
  - Genetic predisposition
  - Advancing age (65 years of age and older)
  - Gender (males affected earlier than women)
  - Race (African-Americans at increased risk)
  - Menopause
- Modifiable:
  - Hyperlipidemia
  - Obesity
  - Sedentary lifestyle
  - Stress
  - Tobacco use
  - Hypertension
  - Diabetes mellitus

Signs and Symptoms

- May be asymptomatic
- Angina
- Palpitations
- Dyspnea
- Excessive fatigue
- Electrocardiogram (ECG) changes

Diagnostic and Laboratory Tests

- Angiogram, cardiac catheterization
- ECG
- History and physical examination
- Lipid profile - The levels of:
  - TC (total cholesterol)
  - Triglycerides
  - VLDL (very low-density lipoprotein)
  - LDL (low-density lipoprotein)
  - HDL (high-density lipoprotein)
  - Ratio
    - TC/HDL
    - LDL/HDL
- Electrocardiogram (ECG)
- Blood urea nitrogen (BUN)
- Creatinine
- Stress test

- Highly sensitive C-reactive protein (hs-CRP)
- Homocysteine

Therapeutic Nursing Management

- **Assess/Monitor**:
    - Blood pressure
    - Blood glucose levels
    - Peripheral pulses
    - Edema
    - Heart tones
    - Heart rate, rhythm
    - Breath sounds
    - Presence of chest pain
- **Nursing Activities**:
    - Assist client with identification of modifiable risk factors.
    - Encourage client to address modifiable risk factors (smoking cessation; low-fat, low cholesterol, low sodium diet; increase intake of high-fiber foods; participation in aerobic exercise program; weight loss).
    - Teach client about prescribed medications.
    - Provide emotional support and encouragement.
    - Refer to available community resources.

Pharmacology

- Statins (atorvastatin [Lipitor], simvastatin [Zocor]) or other lipid lowering agents
- ACE inhibitors (ramipril [Altace], quinapril [Accupril])
- Antiplatelet agents (aspirin, clopidogrel [Plavix], abciximab [ReoPro])
- Calcium channel blockers (amlodipine [Norvasc])
- Omega-3 polyunsaturated fatty acids
- Antioxidants
- Folates
- Hormone replacement therapy proved more harmful than beneficial; do not initiate for treatment or prevention of CAD in women
- Beta-blockers
- B vitamins, especially B6 and B12

Complications

- Acute myocardial infarction (MI)
- Cerebral vascular accident (CVA), also known as stroke, transient ischemic attack (TIA)
- Renal insufficiency/failure
- Angina pectoris

- Carotid stenosis
- Peripheral arterial occlusive disease (PAOD)
- Death

Age-Related Changes—Gerontological Considerations

- Increased risk of CAD exists for older adults who are physically inactive, have one or more chronic diseases (hypertension, CHF, and diabetes), and/or have lifestyle (smoking and diet) habits that contribute to atherosclerosis.

Critical Thinking Exercise: Nursing Management of the Client with Atherosclerosis—Coronary Artery Disease (CAD)

Situation: A 41-year-old African-American male who smokes two packs of cigarettes a day visits his health care provider because of unusual fatigue and shortness of breath when climbing stairs or exerting himself. He drives a truck for a living and works six or seven days a week. The client's health care provider suspects that the client is experiencing these symptoms due to his smoking and the presence of coronary artery disease.

1. Which statements are true about atherosclerosis? Correct false statements.

   a. Atherosclerosis ultimately leads to decreased tissue perfusion.
   b. Hypertension is a major contributing factor to the development of atherosclerosis.
   c. Atherosclerosis is more common among older adults with chronic illnesses.
   d. It is desirable to have higher LDL levels than HDL levels.

2. Which of the client's risk factors for atherosclerosis are not modifiable?

   _____ Tobacco use   _✓_ Age
   _____ Obesity   _____ Sedentary lifestyle
   _____ Stress producing job   _✓_ Race
   _✓_ Gender

3. Provide rationale for implementing these nursing interventions.

   a. Monitor blood pressure.   *hypertension.*
   b. Monitor blood glucose levels.   *Diabetes*
   c. Help the client to identify risk factors for CAD.

Nursing Management of the Client with Iron-Deficiency Anemia

Key Points

- Iron-deficiency anemia is the most common cause of all the anemias.
- Anemia results in diminished oxygen-carrying capacity and delivery to tissues and organs.
- Goals of collaborative management:
  - Identify and correct the underlying cause.
  - Restore normal hemoglobin and hematocrit levels.
  - Prevent future recurrences.
- Important nursing diagnoses (actual or potential):
  - Activity intolerance
  - Fatigue and restlessness
  - Self-care deficit
  - Risk for injury
  - Knowledge deficit
  - Anxiety and fear
- **Key Terms/Concepts**: Genetic syndrome, nutritional deficiency, malabsorption, cheilosis, pica

Overview

Iron-deficiency anemia is a condition in which iron stores are depleted, resulting in the reduction of hemoglobin and size of red blood cells. Iron deficiency anemia is the most common type of anemia in the world and is a reflection of a disease state, nutritional deficiency, or genetic syndrome.

Risk Factors

- Extensive or prolonged blood loss
- Increased metabolic demands (disease states)
- Gastrointestinal malabsorption
- Pregnancy
- Dietary inadequacy
- Bleeding ulcers
- Intestinal hookworms
- Gastrointestinal tumors
- Menorrhagia

- Chronic alcoholism

Signs and Symptoms

- May be asymptomatic in mild cases
- Fatigue
- Irritability
- Numbness and tingling of extremities
- Dyspnea
- Pallor
- Impaired skin healing
- Low-grade fever
- Brittle, spoon-shaped nails
- Cheilosis
- Smooth, sore, bright red tongue
- Sensitivity to cold
- Brittle and ridged nails
- Pica (persistent eating of substances not normally considered as food [non-nutritive substances] lasting at least one month)

Diagnostic and Laboratory Tests

- History and physical examination
- Complete blood count (CBC) determines:
  - Red blood cells (RBCs): total number
  - White blood cells (WBCs): total number
  - Hemoglobin (Hgb) in the blood: total amount
  - Hematocrit (HCT): percentage of the blood composed of RBCs
  - Mean corpuscular volume (MCV): size of red blood cells
  - Platelet count
  - Differential: test measures the relative numbers of each of the five types of white blood cells (WBCs) in the blood
    - Neutrophils
  - Segmented (mature neutrophils) (also called: polys)
  - Bands (immature neutrophils) (also called: young polys)
    - Basophils
    - Eosinophils
    - Lymphocytes
  - B-lymphocytes
  - T-lymphocytes
    - Monocytes
  - ANC (absolute neutrophil count)
  - Indices calculated from the other measurements:

- MCH (mean corpuscular hemoglobin)—amount of hemoglobin per RBC
- MCHC (mean corpuscular hemoglobin concentration)—hemoglobin amount relative to the size of the cell
- TIBC (Total iron-binding capacity)—reflects an indirect measurement of serum transferring in
- Serum ferritin—measures the amount of ferritin in the blood—indicator of total body iron stores
- Serum iron—measures the amount of iron in the blood

Therapeutic Nursing Management

- **Assess/Monitor:**
  - For activity intolerance
- **Nursing Activities:**
  - Encourage increased intake of dietary iron.
  - Administer iron supplements as prescribed.
  - Provide a restful environment.
  - Provide frequent oral hygiene.
  - Encourage the intake of foods high in fiber.
  - Encourage increased fluid intake.
  - Teach client that supplemental iron is eliminated in stool, so stools will be black in color.
  - Teach client that constipation may occur in response to increased iron intake.
  - Teach client that iron preparations should not be taken with milk or antacids.
  - Teach client that iron preparations should be taken between meals for maximum absorption; may take with food if gastrointestinal upset occurs.
  - Teach client that absorption of iron is enhanced by vitamin C.
  - Teach client that milk and tea decrease iron absorption.
  - Administer parenteral iron as prescribed.

Pharmacology

- Oral iron supplements (ferrous sulfate, ferrous fumarate, ferrous gluconate)
- Parenteral iron supplements (iron dextran [INFeD])
- Oxygen
- Blood transfusions
- Vitamin C supplements (to enhance iron absorption)

Complications

- Cardiovascular decompensation (use of parenteral iron therapy)
- Constipation
- Gastrointestinal distress (gas formation)

- Staining of teeth if taking liquid iron preparations

Age-Related Changes—Gerontological Considerations

- Increased risk for iron-deficiency anemia is related to dietary inadequacy and increased incidence of chronic illnesses, such as gastrointestinal bleeding.

Critical Thinking Exercise: Nursing Management of the Client with Iron-Deficiency Anemia

Situation: A 22-year-old woman volunteers to donate blood at her nearby community blood bank. After the nurse checks the woman's hemoglobin, the woman is informed she cannot donate blood because her hemoglobin level is too low. The client is advised to follow-up with her health care provider, who determines the client has iron-deficiency anemia most likely related to insufficient dietary intake of iron.

1. What are the most common causes of iron-deficiency anemia?

2. State rationale for each of the nursing interventions for iron-deficiency anemia.

   a. Provide frequent oral hygiene.

   b. Encourage the intake of foods high in fiber.

   c. Encourage increased fluid intake.

   d. Teach client that supplemental iron is eliminated in stool.

   e. Teach client that liquid iron preparations should be taken through a straw.

3. When the nurse advises the client to eat organ meats the client replies that she is a vegetarian and does not eat meat or poultry. What other foods can the nurse suggest to the client?

   _____ Signs of infection   _____ Body image

   _____ Carrots   _____ Beans

   _____ Leafy green vegetables _____ Raisins

   _____ Bananas   _____ Molasses

Nursing Management of the Client with Abdominal Aortic Aneurysm (AAA)

Key Points

- Poorly controlled hypertension is an important factor in dissection (rupture) of an aortic aneurysm.
- Early diagnosis is difficult due to absent or subtle clinical manifestations.
- A dissecting aneurysm is a true emergency.
- Goals of collaborative management:
  - Identify and treat early.
  - Prevent dissection.
  - Reduce and control hypertension.
- Important nursing diagnoses (actual or potential):
  - Fear and anxiety
  - Risk for ineffective tissue perfusion (emboli, hemorrhage, shock)
  - Knowledge deficit
- **Key Terms/Concepts**: Dissection, atherosclerosis, embolism

Overview

An abdominal aortic aneurysm (AAA) is localized dilatation of the aortic artery formed at a weak point in the vessel wall. The majority of abdominal aortic aneurysms occur below the renal arteries. Saccular aneurysms project from one side of the artery. Fusiform aneurysms involve dilation of an entire segment of the artery. A dissecting aneurysm develops when a tear in the tunica intima leads to dissection of all layers of the vessel wall. Rupture of an abdominal aortic aneurysm can lead to hemorrhage and death.

Risk Factors

- Atherosclerosis - most common cause
- Hypertension, especially uncontrolled
- Congenital defects
- Genetic predisposition
- Infections (syphilitic or pyogenic)
- Male gender
- Tobacco use
- Increasing age
- Trauma

Signs and Symptoms

- Most clients are asymptomatic
- Low back or middle to low abdominal pain (severe pain is sign of impending rupture)
- Hypovolemic shock (following rupture)
- Pulsating middle to upper abdominal mass (bruit usually auscultated over the mass)
- Decreased or absent pedal pulses

Diagnostic and Laboratory Tests

- History and physical examination
- Angiogram
- Magnetic resonance imaging (MRI)
- Computed tomography (CT)/computed axial tomography (CAT) scan
- Duplex ultrasonography

Therapeutic Nursing Management

- **Assess/Monitor:**
  - Vital signs
  - Pain
  - Pulmonary, cardiovascular, renal, and neurological systems
  - For postoperative complications (arterial occlusion, hemorrhage, infection, ileus, and renal failure)
  - For severe abdominal or back pain which is a sign of impending rupture
  - Peripheral pulses
- **Nursing Activities:**
  - Prepare client for surgery.
  - Provide postoperative care.
  - Provide pain medication as prescribed.
  - Administer antihypertensive medications as prescribed.
  - IV access
  - Oxygen

Pharmacology

- Analgesics (morphine, meperidine)
- Antihypertensives (calcium channel blockers, hydralazine- should not be used with dissecting aorta, ACE inhibitors, beta blockers, sodium nitroprusside)
- Blood transfusions (if rupture occurs)
- Anticoagulants (postoperative)

Complications

- Hemorrhage due to rupture (life-threatening emergency)
- Arterial emboli
- Shock
- Renal failure
- Adult respiratory distress syndrome (ARDS)
- Disseminated intravascular coagulation (DIC), especially if ruptured
- Pneumonia
- Death

Age–Related Changes—Gerontological Considerations

- Increased risk for abdominal aortic aneurysms occurs most often after age 70.
- Increased risk for surgical complications is due to age-related changes.
- Increased risk for hypertension is due to loss of vessel elasticity, decreased cardiac output, and heart valve thickening. Decreased elasticity also increased risk for aneurysm.

Critical Thinking Exercise: Nursing Management of the Client with Abdominal Aortic Aneurysm (AAA)

Situation: A 49-year-old man is being prepared for surgery following his admission to the emergency department for severe abdominal and back pain. He has smoked cigarettes for 34 years and has a history of hypertension controlled by medication. Assessment and radiographic studies reveal the presence of a leaking AAA (abdominal aortic aneurysm).

1. What are the client's risk factors for development of an AAA (abdominal aortic aneurysm)?

2. While all of these interventions are important, which four need to be implemented first, and in what order?

_____ Administering oxygen

_____ Obtaining intravenous access

_____ Inserting an indwelling urinary catheter

_____ Administering pain medication

_____ Initiating a preoperative care plan

_____ Teaching the client about the surgery

_____ Monitoring vital signs

_____ Providing emotional support to the family

3. The client is at increased risk for shock if his aneurysm ruptures. The nurse will, therefore, carefully monitor the client for which serious complications?

_____ Nausea   _____ Hemorrhage

_____ Seizures   _____ Acute renal failure

_____ Hypertensive crisis   _____ Arterial occlusion

Nursing Management of the Client with a Femoral-Popliteal Bypass Graft

Key Points

- The femoral-popliteal area is the site most commonly affected by chronic peripheral arterial occlusive disease (PAOD) in clients who are not diabetics.
- PAOD is caused by atherosclerosis and causes a gradual thickening of the intima and media of arteries, ultimately resulting in the progressive narrowing of the vessel lumen. Progressive stiffening of arteries and narrowing of the lumen decreases the blood supply to affected tissues, and increases resistance to blood flow.
- The exact cause or causes atherosclerosis and PAOD remain unknown.
- Bypass graft surgery helps to slow the arteriosclerotic process, but it is not a cure.
- If bypass surgery fails to restore circulation, the client may need to undergo amputation of the limb.
- Goals of collaborative management:
  - Retard progression of atherosclerosis.
  - Safeguard the lower limbs from injury.
  - Decrease vasospasm.
  - Prevent infection.
  - Improve collateral circulation.
  - Prevent complications from surgery.
  - Assist client in lowering risk factors following surgery.
- Important nursing diagnoses (actual or potential):
  - Pain management
  - Risk for infection
  - Altered peripheral tissue perfusion
  - Impaired skin integrity
  - Activity intolerance
  - Impaired walking
  - Anxiety and fear
  - Ineffective management of therapeutic regimen
- **Key Terms/Concepts:** Peripheral artery occlusive disease (PAD), atherosclerosis, arteriosclerosis, arterial blood supply, intermittent claudication, femoral artery, popliteal artery, collateral circulation

Overview

Managing PAOD encompasses educating client about lifestyle changes, initiating measures to protect the affected extremities, administering drug therapy, performing invasive non-surgical procedures, and surgical procedures. Surgical procedures are reserved for clients who experience severe pain at rest. Claudication interferes with normal circulation, which causes circulatory compromise so severe that there is a danger of loss of the limb.

A femoral-popliteal bypass graft involves suturing graft material around an occluded femoral artery. This procedure improves arterial blood supply to the area normally served by the blocked artery. Graft material may be synthetic or an autogenous vein.

Risk Factors

- Atherosclerosis in lower extremities
- Arteriosclerosis obliterans
- Disease of the femoral or popliteal arteries
- Cigarette smoking
- Hyperlipidemia
- Hypertension
- Diabetes mellitus

Signs and Symptoms Necessitating Surgery

- Intermittent claudication
- Ischemic muscle ache
- Leg pain precipitated by exercise and relieved by rest
- Pain at rest (severe disease)
- Burning pain in extremity
- Paresthesia of toes or feet
- Pallor or blanching of limb upon elevation
- Taut, shiny skin
- Loss of hair on lower leg
- Ulceration and gangrene of lower limb tissues (without revascularization)
- Diminished or absent pedal, popliteal, or femoral pulses

Diagnostic and Laboratory Tests

- History and physical examination
- Complete blood count (CBC)
- Serum electrolytes
- Ultrasound
  - 2-D (2-dimensional)
  - 3-D (3-dimensional)
  - Doppler

- Duplex imaging
- Angiography
- Femoral arteriography
- MRA (magnetic resonance angiography)
- ABI (ankle-brachial index)

Therapeutic Nursing Management

- **Prevention of Risk Factors Associated with PAOD:**
    - Do not smoke.
    - Lose weight, if indicated.
    - Lower cholesterol intake.
    - Reduce intake of saturated dietary fat.
    - Inspect and lubricate feet daily.
    - Wear proper, well-fitted footwear.
    - Avoid extremes of heat and cold to lower limbs.
    - Perform walking exercises 15-30 minutes daily as tolerated.
    - Avoid trauma to lower limbs.
    - Use reverse Trendelenburg's position 10 degrees when in bed.
- **Assess/Monitor:**
    - Vital signs
    - Operative limb every 15 minutes and then hourly
    - Incision site for bleeding or signs of infection
    - ABI (ankle-brachial index) measurements
    - For signs of bypass graft occlusion
- **Nursing Activities:**
    - Administer intravenous fluids as ordered.
    - Administer pain medications.
    - Help the client turn, cough, and breathe deep.
    - Use pillows to cushion the incision.
    - Report any significant changes in client status to the primary care provider.
    - Assist the client to gradually get out of bed and ambulate.
    - Discourage sitting for long periods of time.
    - Wrap legs with ace bandages or use support stockings.
    - Encourage use of a walker initially.
    - Advise the client to completely abstain from smoking.
    - Suggest community services that help smokers abstain.
    - Set up a progressive exercise program that includes walking.
    - Teach techniques of foot inspection and care.
    - Advise client to wear clean, white, cotton socks.
    - Encourage client to avoid risk factors for atherosclerosis.

Pharmacology

- Analgesics (morphine, meperidine)
- Anticoagulants (heparin, warfarin)
- Antiplatelet agents (aspirin, clopidogrel, ticlopidine)
- Antibiotics for surgical prophylaxis (cefazolin)

Complications

- Infection
- Bleeding
- Hematoma
- Deep vein thrombosis
- Embolization
- Compartment syndrome
- Occlusion of bypass graft
- Failure of revascularization
- Lower limb necrosis necessitating amputation

Age-Related Changes—Gerontological Considerations

- Arteriosclerosis obliterans usually affects clients who are 60 to 80 years old.
- Arteriosclerosis obliterans may occur in younger clients with diabetes mellitus.
- The two most common postoperative problems that affect the elderly are multiple drug-drug interactions and decreased stamina.

Critical Thinking Exercise: Nursing Management of the Client with a Femoral-Popliteal Bypass Graft

Situation: A 68-year-old male client with atherosclerosis in his lower limbs has just undergone a femoral-popliteal bypass graft. Upon admission to the PACU (postanesthesia care unit), the nurse monitors the client's vital signs, assesses the operative limb, takes ABI (ankle-brachial index) measurements, and monitors for signs and symptoms of bypass graft occlusion.

1. Which assessments are made hourly following popliteal bypass graft surgery?

   _____ Blood pressure   _____ Limb color

   _____ Limb capillary refill   _____ Oral temperature

   _____ Apical heart rate   _____ Femoral pulse

   _____ Limb peripheral pulses   _____ Limb temperature

   _____ Limb movement

2. How did the nurse calculate the client's ABI (ankle-brachial index) measurement?

3. What is the purpose of obtaining postoperative ABI (ankle-brachial index) measurements on clients who have undergone popliteal bypass graft surgery?

4. What signs and symptoms indicate occlusion of the bypass graft?

   _____ Decreasing blood pressure   _____ Cool, operative limb

   _____ Pallor of limb   _____ Nonpalpable peripheral pulses

   _____ Extremity numbness   _____ Increasing ankle-brachial index measurements

   _____ Extremity twitching   _____ Severe limb pain

Nursing Management of the Client with a Blood Transfusion

Key Points

- Whole blood or components of whole blood can be administered.
- Incompatibility is a major concern when administering blood or blood products.
- Goals of collaborative management:
  - Administer a compatible blood product.
  - Correct the underlying problem for which the blood is being administered.
  - Prevent reactions to the blood or blood product.
- Important nursing diagnoses (actual or potential):
  - Risk for injury
  - Anxiety and fear
  - Potential complications of blood transfusion (febrile reaction, hemolytic reaction, hypersensitivity)
  - Knowledge deficit
- **Key Terms/Concepts**: Incompatibility, febrile reaction, hemolytic reaction, hypersensitivity, thrombocytopenia, ABO typing, Rh typing, autologous transfusion, circulatory overload, urticaria

Overview

A blood transfusion is accomplished using whole blood or blood components. Blood components include packed red blood cells, plasma, albumin, clotting factors, prothrombin complex, cryoprecipitate, and platelets. Clients with Type O blood are referred to as "universal donors", meaning they can give blood to anyone and those with Type AB are known as" universal recipients", meaning they can receive blood from anyone.

Type A+ (read "A positive"): Contains A antigen, contains D antigen, making the Rh factor positive (+). The serum of the blood (plasma) contains antibodies against Type B blood.

Type A- (read "A negative"): Contains A antigen. Does not contain D antigen, making the Rh factor negative (-). The serum of the blood (plasma) contains antibodies against Type B blood.

Type B+ (read "B positive"): Contains B antigen, Contains D antigen, making the Rh factor positive (+). The serum of the blood (plasma) contains antibodies against Type A blood.

Type B- (read "B negative"): Contains B antigen, Does not contain D antigen, making the Rh factor negative (-). The serum of the blood (plasma) contains antibodies against Type A blood.

Type AB+ (read "AB positive"): Contains both A and B antigens, Contains

D antigen, making the Rh factor positive (+). The serum of the blood (plasma) does not contain antibodies.

Type AB- (read "AB negative"): Contains both A and B antigens, does not contain D antigen, making the Rh factor negative (-). The serum of the blood (plasma) does not contain antibodies.

Type O+ (read "O positive"): Does not contain either A or B antigens, Contains D antigen, Making the Rh factor positive (+). The serum of the blood (plasma) contains antibodies against both Type A and Type B blood.

Type O- (read "O negative"): Does not contain either A or B antigens, Does not contain D antigen, making the Rh factor negative (-). The serum of the blood (plasma) contains antibodies against both Type A and Type B blood.

Indications for Transfusions

- Hemorrhagic shock
  - Signs and symptoms include tachycardia and decreased blood pressure.
- Thrombocytopenia/platelet dysfunction
- Anemia
- Surgeries
- Coagulation factor deficiencies (e.g., hemophilia)
- Renal failure, chronic

Diagnostic and Laboratory Tests

- History and physical examination
- Complete blood count (CBC) or hemoglobin and hematocrit
- Arterial blood gases (ABGs)
- ABO and Rh typing, and cross match
- Antibody screen for other than anti-A, anti-B
- Possible cold agglutinins
- Prothrombin time (PT)
- Partial thromboplastin time (PTT)

Transfusion Types

- Transfusion from blood donors
- Autologous transfusion: Client's own blood collected in anticipation of future transfusions (e.g., elective surgery). Can only be used by client.
- Intraoperative blood salvage: Blood loss during certain surgeries can be recycled through a cell saver machine and transfused. Has to be used immediately.

Therapeutic Nursing Management

- **Assess/Monitor:**
    - For previous reactions
    - For first 15 minutes after starting infusion
    - Vital signs
    - Rate of infusion
    - Respiratory status
    - Sudden increase in anxiety
    - Breath sounds
    - Neck vein distention
- **Nursing Activities:**
    - Client teaching: The procedure, symptoms to report during and after the transfusion.
    - Insert at least a 20-gauge intravenous needle in a large vein.
    - Follow blood identification protocol. Two nurses (or nurse and physician) check the order; the client's name and arm band, and compare it to the blood bag; the client's blood type and cross-match, and compare it to the blood bag; compare the number on the requisition to the one on the blood bag; check the expiration date on the blood bag; and examine the unit of blood for gas bubbles, discoloration or cloudiness.
    - Use only normal saline to prime IV tubing.
    - Obtain baseline vital signs prior to infusion.
    - Administer donated blood or self-donated blood (autologous transfusion) as prescribed.
    - Never add medications to blood.
    - Stop transfusion immediately if reaction is suspected: initiate saline infusion, maintain airway patency, and report symptoms (fever, chills, itching, weakness, dyspnea, rash, or cough). Saline infusion should be initiated with a separate line so as not to give more blood from the suspected reaction blood tubing. Save the blood bag with remaining blood and the blood tubing for testing.
    - Change IV tubing after every two units of blood.
    - Infuse blood within four hours to prevent bacterial growth in room temperature blood.
    - A blood warmer may be indicated to decrease potential for hypothermia.

Pharmacology

- Antihistamines (diphenhydramine, hydroxyzine)
- Oxygen
- Emergency drugs (for transfusion reaction)
- Diuretics
- Antibiotics, may be possible if suspected contaminated blood bag

Complications

- Acute hemolytic reaction, most dangerous, most common cause is human error in blood bag labelling or client identification. ABO incompatibility more severe than Rh incompatibility (chills, fever, low back pain, tachycardia, flushing, hypotension, nausea, chest tightening or pain, anxiety, tachypnea, hemoglobinuria. May lead to cardiovascular collapse, acute renal failure, disseminated intravascular coagulation [DIC], shock, death)

- Febrile (non-hemolytic) reaction, most common, (rapid onset of chills and fever, flushing, headache, anxiety)

- Mild allergic reaction (itching, urticaria, flushing)

- Anaphylactic reaction (wheezing, dyspnea, chest tightness, cyanosis, hypotension, shock, death)

- Circulatory overload (dyspnea, chest tightness, tachycardia, tachypnea, headache, hypertension, jugular vein distention, peripheral edema, orthopnea, sudden anxiety, crackles in base of lungs)

- Sepsis (fever, nausea, vomiting, abdominal pain, shock, chills, hypotension, shock if not treated immediately)

- Delayed hemolytic reaction (fever, chills, anemia, jaundice, hemoglobinuria [rare], increased bilirubin, decreased or absent haptoglobin)

- Disease transmission (Hepatitis B and C, HIV, CMV [cytomegalovirus])

- Transfusion-related acute lung injury, rare (fever, chills, severe respiratory distress, bilateral pulmonary infiltrates, can lead to death)

- Iron overload, from chronic transfusions, can lead to organ failure

- Sensitization, from chronic transfusions

Age-Related Changes—Gerontological Considerations

- Increased risk for congestive heart failure and fluid volume excess exists when the elderly person with cardiac dysfunction is receiving a blood transfusion.

- Venous access for blood transfusions may be limited due to age-related vascular and skin changes.

Critical Thinking Exercise: Nursing Management of the Client with a Blood Transfusion

Situation: A 44-year-old man has hemoglobin of 7.8 g/dL due to blood loss secondary to a slowly bleeding gastric ulcer. The bleeding has been controlled and the client is stable. Two successive whole blood transfusions have been prescribed to replace his lost blood volume.

1. Prior to initiating the blood transfusion, it is important for the nurse to assess the client's _____, _____, _____ and _____ _____.

2. The client states he is afraid to receive a transfusion because of AIDS. How should the nurse respond to the client's concern?

3. Match the type of blood reaction with its associated signs and symptoms.

a. Febrile	Chills
b. Anaphylactic	Headache
c. Mild Allergic	Hypotension
d. Acute hemolytic	Rapid onset fever
e. Sepsis	Itching
f. Circulatory overload	Dyspnea
	Cyanosis
	Tachycardia
	Hypertension
	Abdominal pain
	Low back pain

	Shock
	Vomiting
	Tachypnea
	Flushing

4. Prioritize nursing actions for the client who experiences a reaction to a blood transfusion, with "1" representing the first action needed.

_____ Assess vital signs

_____ Open the infusion of normal saline

_____ Notify the client's practitioner

_____ Stop the transfusion

Nursing Management of the Client with Digitalis Toxicity

| Key Points |

- Digitalis is an effective drug that is also potentially dangerous.
- The margin between therapeutic and toxic digoxin levels is very small.
- Goals of collaborative management:
  - Maintain drug levels within the therapeutic range.
  - Minimize side and toxic effects.
- Important nursing diagnoses (actual or potential):
  - Potential complications of digitalis therapy (toxicity)
  - Risk for injury
  - Knowledge deficit
  - Ineffective individual management of therapeutic regimen
- **Key Terms/Concepts**: Toxicity, therapeutic range, polypharmacy, hypokalemia

Overview

Digitalis (digoxin) is a cardiotonic glycoside that promotes increased cardiac output by increasing the force of myocardial contraction and the refractory period of the atrioventricular node. Digitalis toxicity is due to the cumulative effect of digitalis. The onset may be acute or chronic.

Indications for Use of Digoxin

- CHF (congestive heart failure) with atrial fibrillation
- Atrial fibrillation or flutter
- Paroxysmal atrial tachycardia

Signs and Symptoms

- Nausea, vomiting, anorexia, malaise
- Cardiac irregularities (bradycardia, tachycardias, ventricular extrasystoles, partial heart block)
- Diarrhea
- Yellow, green or white halos around lights, diplopia, blurred vision
- ST segment depression and prolonged PR interval on ECG

Contraindications

- Ventricular fibrillation
- Ventricular tachycardia

- Second-degree (intermittent conduction failure) or third-degree (complete conduction failure) AV (atrioventricular) Block
- Electrolyte imbalances (especially hypokalemia, which increases toxicity)
- Impaired renal function
- Drug interactions

Diagnostic Tests to Monitor Drug Action/Toxicity

- Serum digoxin level
- Electrocardiogram (ECG)
- Serum electrolytes
- Blood urea nitrogen (BUN)
- Creatinine

Therapeutic Nursing Management

- **Assess/Monitor:**
  - Rate, rhythm, and character of apical heart beat
  - Blood pressure
  - Lung sounds
  - Edema
  - Daily weights
  - Signs of digitalis toxicity
  - Factors increasing the risk of toxicity (medications, electrolytes, and renal function)
  - Serum digoxin level (drawn just prior to next scheduled dose or at least 6-8 hours after previous dose)
  - Cardiac monitor (if applicable)
- **Nursing Activities:**
  - Withhold drug if apical rate is below 60 bpm or digitalis toxicity is suspected and notify the physician.
  - Teach client how to assess own pulse for rate and regularity.
  - Teach client signs and symptoms of digitalis toxicity.
  - Teach client when to hold medication and notify physician.
  - Encourage use of medication identification bracelet.
  - Encourage the intake of foods high in potassium.
  - Administer Digoxin immune fab (Digibind) if digitalis toxicity is severe (life- threatening).

Pharmacology

- Digoxin Immune Fab (Digibind) an antidote used in clients with life-threatening digoxin toxicity

Complications/Side Effects

- Premature ventricular contractions
- Potassium depletion
- Heart block
- Irregular pulse
- Bradycardia

Age-Related Changes—Gerontological Considerations

- There is an increased risk for toxicity in older clients.
- An increased risk for drug interactions exists for elderly persons due to polypharmacy.

Critical Thinking Exercise: Nursing Management of the Client with Digitalis Toxicity

Situation: A 67-year-old female with a history of congestive heart failure is admitted to the acute care facility due to increased shortness of breath and peripheral edema. Her usual dose of 0.125 mg of oral digitalis has been increased to 0.25 mg PO each morning and evening.

1. Prior to administering the fifth dose of digitalis, the nurse assesses the client's apical heartbeat, which is 54 and irregular. What should the nurse do?

2. Which signs should alert the nurse to the presence of digitalis toxicity?

_____ Constipation	_____ Bradycardia
_____ Yellow vision	_____ Nausea
_____ Hypertension	_____ Leg cramps
_____ Vomiting	_____ Diarrhea
_____ Heart block	

3. Which tests most accurately demonstrate the presence of digitalis toxicity?

_____ ECG (electrocardiogram)	_____ Serum electrolytes
_____ BUN (blood urea nitrogen)	_____ Serum digitalis level

Nursing Management of the Client with HIV/AIDS

Key Points

- Human immunodeficiency virus (HIV) is a generally preventable disease.
- Acquired immunodeficiency syndrome (AIDS) is the disease produced by HIV infection.
- Not all persons who are infected know they are infected.
- There is no cure for HIV infection or AIDS.
- Death from HIV infection is due to relentless opportunistic infections.
- Goals of collaborative management:
  - Identify persons at risk and those who are infected.
  - Prevent opportunistic infections.
  - Prevent transmission of the disease.
  - Restore adequate number of CD4 helper cells.
  - Maintain immune function.
  - Support dying client and family.
- Important nursing diagnoses (actual or potential):
  - Potential complications of HIV infection (opportunistic infections)
  - Fear and anxiety
  - Risk for injury
  - Activity intolerance
  - Ineffective airway clearance
  - Caregiver role strain
  - Ineffective individual and family coping
  - Fatigue and restlessness
  - Diarrhea and other bowel dysfunctions
  - Fluid volume deficit
  - Hopelessness and powerlessness
  - Risk for infection
  - Ineffective management of therapeutic regimen
  - Self-care deficit
  - Altered nutrition, less than body requirements
  - Impaired skin integrity
  - Social isolation
- **Key Terms/Concepts**: Immune, immune deficiency, opportunistic infection, wasting syndrome, modulator, seroconversion

Overview

Acquired immune deficiency syndrome (AIDS) is the most severe form of a continuum of illnesses associated with human immunodeficiency virus (HIV) infection. HIV targets and destroys CD4 helper lymphocytes (cell medicated immunity) and leaves the client at risk for the development of numerous opportunistic infections. HIV is transmitted by direct contact with infected blood or body fluids, especially blood, semen, and breast milk. Persons who are infected with HIV in the absence of opportunistic infections are said to be HIV-infected. Persons with HIV infection coupled with one or more opportunistic infections are said to have AIDS. There is no known cure for HIV infection or AIDS.

Risk Factors

- Unprotected vaginal, anal, or oral intercourse
- Intravenous drug use with contaminated needle
- HIV infected mother to child in utero
- Contaminated needle stick
- Blood and blood product recipients (rare)
- Semen used for artificial insemination (rare)

Signs and Symptoms of HIV Infection/AIDS

- Weight loss
- Generalized, chronic lymphadenopathy
- Fatigue
- Weakness
- Myalgia
- Headache
- Nausea, anorexia
- Dyspnea, cough
- Opportunistic infections
- Wasting syndrome (cachexia)
- Depression
- Dementia/confusion
- Sore throat
- Rash
- Night sweats
- Electrolyte imbalance
- Seizures
- Frequent infections, including fungal or yeast

Diagnostic and Laboratory Tests

- History and physical examination

- ELISA (enzyme linked immunosorbent assay)
- Western Blot test if ELISA is positive. (Since the Western blot test is an antibody detection test, its results will not be accurate until an HIV-infected person seroconverts. Seroconversion describes the process by which the body "reacts" to the viral infection by trying to defend itself through production of antibodies. This process occurs anywhere from 2-12 months after infection with HIV. However, most clients will seroconvert within 6 months. After an infected person has seroconverted, a positive western blot indicates an HIV infection is present.)
- IFA (indirect immunofluorescence assay)
- CD4 count (CD4 count less than 200 indicates need of further testing for HIV)
- CD4/CD8 ratio
- HIV/RNA cell count
- PCR (polymerase chain reaction)
- Complete blood count (CBC)
- Chest x-ray
- Sputum cultures
- Bronchoscopy
- Possible brain, lung, MRI, CT scan

Therapeutic Nursing Management

- **Assess/Monitor**:
  - For risk factors (sexual practices, IV drug use)
  - Client's knowledge of HIV/AIDS
  - Skin integrity
  - For signs and symptoms of opportunistic infections (oral lesions, dyspnea, cough, seizures, skin lesions, fever)
  - Nutritional status
  - Neurological status (dementia, seizures)
  - Respiratory status (cough, dyspnea, breath sounds)
  - Laboratory data to determine drug effectiveness
  - Intake and output
  - Fluid and electrolyte status
  - Pain status
  - Daily weight
  - Response to daily activity
- **Nursing Activities**:
  - Educate the client regarding the need for repeat testing at 3, 6, and 12 months if risk factors are present, even if the first diagnostic test is negative.
  - Teach client regarding transmission of HIV and methods for safer sex with uninfected partners.
  - Identify factors that may interfere with nutrition (anorexia, nausea,

vomiting, oral lesions, and dysphagia).

- Teach regarding self-administration of prescribed drugs, side effects of drugs that must be reported, and compliance with drug therapy.
- Instruct clients who are using highly active anti-retroviral therapy to carefully comply with the drug program and adhere to the dosing schedule to prevent developing resistance to the drugs.
- Encourage activity and rest periods.
- Administer supplemental oxygen as needed.
- Provide analgesia as prescribed.
- Teach client the importance of reporting signs/symptoms of infection immediately.
- Encourage use of constructive coping mechanisms.
- Assist client with identification of support systems.
- Refer client to local or national AIDS support groups or hotlines.

Pharmacology

- Protease inhibitors (indinavir, ritonavir, saquinavir)
- Nucleoside reverse transcriptase inhibitors (zidovudine, didanosine, zalcitabine)
- Nonnucleoside reverse transcriptase inhibitors (nevirapine, delavirdine)
- Antineoplastics for Kaposi's sarcoma (interferon alpha-sa [Roferon-A], interferon alpha 2-b [Intron-A])
- Antibiotics (co-trimoxazole, isoniazid, azithromycin, rifampin)
- Antifungals (amphotericin B, fluconazole, itraconazole)
- Antidiarrheals (opium tincture, diphenoxylate, atropine)
- Antidepressants (sertraline, paroxetine), others
- Analgesics (opioid and nonopioid)
- Appetite stimulants (megestrol, dronabinol)
- Ganciclovir (antiviral for CMV retinitis)

Complications

- HIV encephalopathy
- Wasting syndrome
- Lymphoma of the brain
- Kaposi's sarcoma
- Opportunistic infections:
  - *Pneumocystis carinii pneumonia* (cough, dyspnea, chest pain)
  - *Mycobacterium avium* complex (cough, dyspnea, chest pain)
  - Candidiasis (white patches; painful swallowing; bleeding affecting mouth, esophagus, vagina, and anal region)
  - *Toxoplasma gondii* (seizures, dementia)
  - Viremia, such as Epstein Barr (fatigue, lymphadenopathy)
  - Cytomegalovirus (blindness)

- • Cryptococcus neoformans (fever, stiff neck, nausea, vomiting, seizures)
- • Mycobacterium tuberculosis (cough, fever, dyspnea)
- Social isolation
- B-cell lymphoma
- Death

Age-Related Changes—Gerontological Considerations

- The presence of chronic illnesses complicates the treatment of AIDS and opportunistic infections in older adults.
- Older adults are more susceptible to fluid and electrolyte imbalance, malnutrition, skin alterations, and wasting syndrome than younger adults.

Four Stages of HIV Infection

- Transmission of HIV
- Early or Acute Phase (Caused by primary HIV infection. Lasting from a few days to a few weeks during which time the client may have symptoms resembling acute mononucleosis with fever, sweats, sore throat, and fatigue.)
- Latent or Asymptomatic Phase (possibly lasting years)
- Final or Crisis Phase (With overt AIDS, lasting months or even years, the client is immunocompromised and is susceptible to various infections usually leading to death.)

Critical Thinking Exercise: Nursing Management of the Client with HIV/AIDS

Situation: A 30-year-old client reported to an outpatient clinic for complaints of fatigue and sore throat lasting more than three weeks in spite of frequent rest periods and use of OTC (over-the-counter) cold medications. Physical examination was essentially normal except for the presence of painful white patches in the client's mouth and throat and enlarged cervical lymph nodes. The client's vital signs were a temperature of 100.2° F, heart rate 90 bpm and regular, respirations 16, BP 118/74. Blood samples were obtained for a mononucleosis test and ELISA (enzyme linked immunosorbent assay). It is now one week later and the client must be informed their ELISA test was positive and they have oral candidiasis.

1. What is the significance of the client's positive ELISA test?

2. What further testing is essential at this time?

3. What is the best response to each of the client's questions?

   a. "What is an HIV infection?"

   b. "What is AIDS?"

   c. "Are there medications I can take? If so, what are they?"

   d. "What is oral candidiasis?"

   e. "Am I at risk for other infections? If so, what?"

   f. "Am I going to die?"

4. Cite the two nursing diagnoses that are of highest priority at this time.

   a. Nursing diagnosis # 1

   b. Nursing diagnosis # 2

5. After additional testing, the client is found to have a CD4 T-cell count of 150/mm3 (per cubic millimeter) and an HIV/RNA count of 110,000. What does this mean?

6. What should the client be taught about follow up care?

Nursing Management of the Client with Candidiasis

Key Points

- Candidiasis is an opportunistic infection that can occur in persons with an immature, deficient, or suppressed immune response.
- Candida can affect all age groups.
- Goals of collaborative management:
  - Prevent spread of the infection.
  - Control or eliminate the infection.
  - Correct the underlying immune problem.
  - Prevent recurrence.
- Important nursing diagnoses (actual or potential):
  - Pain management
  - Impaired skin integrity (or mucous membranes)
  - Knowledge deficit
- **Key Terms/Concepts**: Opportunistic, immune suppression, re-infection

Overview

Candidiasis is a secondary fungal infection caused by a strain of candida, most commonly albicans. The organism thrives in a warm, moist environment, such as the mucous membranes of the mouth, vagina, and intestinal tract. When the growth of candida exceeds normal flora, clinical infection may result.

Risk Factors

- Immune suppression (AIDS, cancer, chemotherapy, corticosteroids)
- Diabetes mellitus type 1 (DM1)
- Pregnancy
- Poor hygiene
- Prolonged or frequent use of antibiotics
- Cushing's disease
- Debilitated states
- Infants under six months of age
- Oral contraceptives
- HRT (hormone replacement therapy, Estrogen
- Prolonged periods of tube feeding

Signs and Symptoms

- Affects the outer layers of mucous membranes and skin
- May occur in the mouth, vagina, uncircumcised penis, and between large skin folds
- White patches adhering to tissues that are difficult to remove
- Pruritus, burning, painful sexual intercourse (dyspareunia)
- White, milk-curd, or cheesy appearing discharge

Diagnostic and Laboratory Tests

- History and physical exam
- Culture of discharge or scraping from lesion
- Vaginal smear for microscopic spores and hyphae

Therapeutic Nursing Management

- **Assess/Monitor**:
  - Mucous membranes
  - Skin (especially skin folds)
- **Nursing Activities**:
  - Encourage good personal hygiene.
  - Teach clients regarding potential transmission of fungal infections via sharing of linens or personal care items.
  - Teach clients to thoroughly dry skin folds.
  - Teach clients undergoing treatment for vaginal candidiasis to avoid sexual intercourse or have partner wear a condom until the infection is resolved.
  - Sexual partners may require treatment with an anti-fungal agent simultaneously to prevent reinfection.
  - Teach clients to wear cotton underwear and avoid tight fitting jeans and pants.
  - Encourage the client receiving antibiotics or experiencing recurring vaginal infections to include yogurt or foods containing Lactobacillus acidophilus in their diet to maintain normal vaginal flora but not to take within a few hours of antibiotic or may negate antibiotic. If prone to candidiasis when on antibiotic, can begin anti-candidal treatment at onset of antibiotic.

Pharmacology

- Miconazole (cream, lotion, powder, spray, vaginal suppositories or cream)
- Clotrimazole (cream, lotion, solution, vaginal tablet or cream, oral troche)
- Nystatin (oral suspension, cream, ointment, powder, oral tablet, vaginal tablet)
- Terconazole (vaginal cream or suppository)
- Fluconazole (Diflucan)
- Suspect those with frequent candidiasis infection of possible DM or HIV; assess risk factors and obtain diagnostic work-up as appropriate

Complications

- Secondary infections
- Chronic recurring infections

Age-Related Changes—Gerontological Considerations

- Increased risk for vaginal atrophy is due to decreased mucous-secreting cells following menopause related to changes in estrogen and progesterone.

Critical Thinking Exercise: Nursing Management of the Client with Candidiasis

Situation: A 35-year-old client is undergoing chemotherapy following a modified radical mastectomy for breast cancer. Her mouth is fiery red with white patches on her tongue and oral mucous membranes. She complains of pain when eating and attempting to brush her teeth. Oral candidiasis is suspected.

1. Why is candidiasis considered an opportunistic infection?

2. Which nursing actions will be most effective in addressing the client's oral pain?

_____ Encourage the use of a soft-bristled toothbrush.

_____ Add orange juice or grapefruit juice to the client's diet.

_____ Encourage use of an alcohol-based mouth rinse.

_____ Administer antifungal medications as prescribed.

3. Which statements are true about candidiasis? Correct false statements.

a. Candidiasis is a disease of infants and older adults.

b. Candidiasis is a primary fungal infection caused by candida albicans.

c. Candidiasis commonly occurs in persons with a deficient or immature immune system.

d. Treatment of candidiasis often involves treatment of an underlying immune problem.

Nursing Management of the Client with Systemic Lupus Erythematosus (SLE)

Key Points

- Systemic lupus erythematosus (SLE) is an autoimmune disease with no known cause or cure.
- SLE is characterized by periods of remission and exacerbation.
- Exacerbated disease cannot always be prevented.
- Goals of collaborative management:
  - Identify and initiate treatment early in the disease process.
  - Prevent exacerbations.
  - Control symptoms.
  - Prevent complications of CVA (cerebrovascular accident), renal failure, pulmonary fibrosis.
  - Prevent disease progression.
- Important nursing diagnoses (actual or potential):
  - Risk for infection
  - Potential complications of SLE
  - Activity intolerance
  - Pain management
  - Anxiety and fear
  - Fatigue and restlessness
  - Risk for injury
  - Body image disturbance
  - Self-care deficit
  - Impaired skin integrity
  - Knowledge deficit
- **Key Terms/Concepts:** Autoimmune, progressive, inflammatory, remission, exacerbation

Overview

Systemic lupus erythematosus (SLE) is a chronic, progressive, inflammatory, autoimmune disease that affects the connective tissues of multiple body organs and systems. Affecting females and African Americans most frequently, the disease varies in severity and is characterized by periods of remission and exacerbation.

Risk Factors

- Genetic predisposition
- Pregnancy
- Stress
- Drugs (hydralazine and procainamide produce transient SLE symptoms)
- Female

Signs and Symptoms

- Dry, scaly, reddened "butterfly" rash on face
- Low-grade fever
- Weakness, fatigue, malaise
- Anorexia, weight loss
- Joint tenderness, swelling, and pain
- Photosensitivity
- Proteinuria
- Anemia
- Lymphadenopathy
- Depression

Diagnostic and Laboratory Tests

- History and physical examination
- ANA (antinuclear antibody) test titer (ANA test results are reported in a titer that indicates how much the test sample can be diluted before the antibodies are no longer detected. Fluorescence techniques are frequently used to actually detect the antibodies in the cells, thus ANA testing is sometimes referred to as FANA [fluorescent antinuclear antibody] testing.)
- ESR (Erythrosedimentation rate)
- Serum complement
- CBC
- Urinalysis
- LE (lupus erythematosus) cell prep test

Therapeutic Nursing Management

- Assess/Monitor:
  - Skin for evidence of breakdown
  - For signs of infection
  - Lung sounds
  - Laboratory data
  - Nutritional status
  - Mobility
  - Peripheral edema

- For signs of depression or altered body image
- Renal function
- Blood pressure, cardiac function
- Adverse effects of medications
- Visual changes
- **Nursing Activities**:
  - Teach client
    - To keep skin lesions clean and dry.
    - To avoid exposure to direct sunlight or ultraviolet light
    - Use of sunscreens.
    - The importance of maintaining prescribed medication schedules.
    - To avoid abrupt cessation of glucocorticoid medications.
    - Signs and symptoms of infection (fever, cough, lesions).
    - Signs and symptoms of complications (edema, decreased urine output).
  - Encourage close follow-up care.

Pharmacology

- Salicylates (aspirin, choline magnesium trisalicylate [Trilisate])
- Nonsteroidal anti-inflammatory drugs (NSAIDs) (ketoprofen, diclofenac, ibuprofen nabumetone, naproxen)
- Antimalarial drugs (hydroxychloroquine)
- Corticosteroids (prednisone, methylprednisolone)
- Immune suppressants (azathioprine)
- Antidepressants

Complications

- Anemia
- Glomerulonephritis (Renal failure is the major complication of SLE)
- Pericarditis/myocarditis
- Pleuritis
- Neuritis
- Retinal toxicity/blindness
- Depression/psychosis

Age-Related Changes—Gerontological Considerations

- The diagnosis of SLE may be delayed in older clients who often present with nonspecific symptoms such as fever, fatigue, arthralgias, and weight loss.
- Immune suppressant drugs are less frequently prescribed for older adults with SLE.

Critical Thinking Exercise: Nursing Management of the Client with Systemic Lupus Erythematosus (SLE)

Situation: A 26-year-old female has been admitted to the acute care facility for re-evaluation and control of her systemic lupus erythematosus. She is receiving NSAIDs and prednisone (corticosteroid) to control her symptoms.

1. Why is lupus erythematosus considered an autoimmune disease?

2. Which are common clinical manifestations of lupus erythematosus?

_____ Reddened facial rash   _____ Fever >102°

_____ Weight gain   _____ Anemia

_____ Peripheral edema   _____ Photosensitivity

_____ Headache   _____ Proteinuria

_____ Weakness   _____ Cough

3. Which nursing activities are useful in reducing the pain associated with SLE (systemic lupus erythematosus)?

_____ Performing active range of motion exercises.

_____ Placing heat on the affected joints.

_____ Administering anti-inflammatory agents routinely.

_____ Administering narcotic pain relievers.

4. Which symptoms will be relieved by use of NSAIDs or corticosteroids?

_____ Fever   _____ Joint swelling

_____ Fatigue   _____ Weakness

_____ Joint pain   _____ Anemia

Nursing Management of the Client with Hepatitis (A, B, and/or C)

Key Points

- There are major differences between Hepatitis A Virus (HAV), Hepatitis B Virus (HBV) and Hepatitis C (HCV).
- Hepatitis B and C are the more serious of the hepatitis viruses, possibly leading to liver cancer.
- Prevention is an important aspect of collaborative care.
- Health care workers are at significantly increased risk for contracting hepatitis.
- Goals of collaborative management:
  - Prevent transmission.
  - Provide supportive care.
  - Prevent complications.
  - Immunize susceptible individuals and groups.
- Important nursing diagnoses (actual or potential):
  - Potential complications of hepatitis (ascites, esophageal varices, negative nitrogen balance, liver failure, sepsis, DIC (disseminated intravascular coagulation), cancer, and death)
  - Activity intolerance
  - Self-care deficit
  - Fear and anxiety
  - Knowledge deficit
  - Ineffective individual coping
  - Risk for injury
  - Altered nutrition; less than body requirements
  - Pain management
- **Key Terms/Concepts**: Disease transmission, carrier, infectious, acute, chronic

Overview

Hepatitis A Virus (HAV) and Hepatitis B Virus (HBV) are infectious hepatic diseases.

Hepatitis A: An RNA virus of the enterovirus family. Previously known as "infections hepatitis". Transmitted primarily by the fecal-oral route via contaminated foods or fluids. It has an incubation period of 2-7 weeks, may last 4-8 weeks and is self-limiting.

Hepatitis B: A DNA virus. Previously known as "serum hepatitis". Transmitted primarily through blood, but has been found in semen, vaginal secretions, and saliva. It has an incubation period of 1-6 months. Ten percent of clients with Hepatitis B will develop chronic hepatitis, or become chronic carriers of the disease.

Hepatitis C: An RNA virus, with subgroup genotypes; similar to other RNA viruses in the Flaviviridae virus family. Prior to 1989, the strain could not be identified and so was known as "non-A, non-B". Transmitted primarily through blood. HCV has an incubation period that is variable and ranges from 14-180 days. However, within 1-3 weeks of exposure, LFTs begin to rise. Most clients will begin to demonstrate antibodies to HCV infection within 2-6 months postexposure.

Also, **Hepatitis D, E, F and G are not as common and are not commonly seen in the United States.**

Risk Factors

Hepatitis A - Fecal-Oral transmission

- Poor sanitary living conditions
- Contaminated food, water, or fish
- Inadequate hand washing

Hepatitis B - Mainly blood transmission

- Contaminated blood
- Unprotected sex
- Health care workers, commonly through needle sticks
- Hemodialysis recipients
- Intravenous drug use

Hepatitis C - Mainly blood transmission

- Health care workers
- Contaminated blood products for transfusion, especially before 1992
- IV drug users (most common, 60-70%, cause of new cases)
- Sexually active male homosexuals (although Hepatitis B more common in this population), multiple sexual partners (even in heterosexual, but rare)
- Recipients of organ transplants
- Intranasal snorting of cocaine and sharing intranasal "snorting" devices, small traces of blood contamination
- Body piercing with non-disposable supplies or questionable sterilization techniques; tattooing may also be a risk
- Higher risk of coinfection with HIV infected clients
- 40% unknown
- Hemodialysis

Signs and Symptoms

Hepatitis A

- Clients may be asymptomatic
- Mild, flu-like symptoms
- Low-grade fever
- Fatigue, malaise
- Nausea, anorexia, vomiting
- Jaundice may or may not be present
- Clay-colored stools when jaundice is present
- Headache
- Abdominal pain
- Dark, brown urine
- Pruritus
- Enlarged, tender liver

Hepatitis B

- Clients may be asymptomatic
- Fever
- Loss of appetite, dyspepsia
- Abdominal pain
- Generalized aching
- Weakness, malaise
- Jaundice may or may not be present
- Clay-colored stools when jaundice is present
- Dark-colored urine
- Enlarged, tender liver
- Enlarged posterior cervical lymph nodes

Hepatitis C

- Vast majority are asymptomatic or mildly symptomatic
- Fever
- Malaise
- Nausea and vomiting
- Anorexia
- Jaundice
- Hepatomegaly
- Dark urine
- Transient, pale stools
- Abdominal pain, usually right upper quadrant
- Fatigue
- Joint pain, myalgias

Diagnostic and Laboratory Tests

- History and physical examination
- LFTs (liver function tests)
    - Alanine aminotransferase (ALT); also called serum glutamic pyruvic transaminase (SGPT)
    - Alkaline phosphatase (ALP); also called (ALK Phos)
    - Aspartate aminotransferase (AST); also called serum glutamic oxaloacetic transaminase (SGOT)
    - Increased bilirubin
- Stool analysis for hepatitis A antigen
- Hepatitis panel
    - Hepatitis A
        - Anti-HAV total - positive in acute, recent, and past infections
        - Anti-HAV IgM - positive in acute and recent, negative in past infections
    - Hepatitis B
        - HBsAg and +/- anti HBc IgM with early, acute, and carrier states
        - Anti-HBe, -HBs, and -HBc IgG - present in recovery states
        - HBsAg, HBeAg, HBeAb, anti-HBe and HBV-DNA - all present with chronic states
        - Anti-HBs and +/- Anti-HBc - present in vaccinated clients
    - Hepatitis C
        - Anti-HCV ELISA III or RIBA and HCV RNA (qualitative and quantitative) for genotypes I-IV - present with both acute and chronic states

Therapeutic Nursing Management

- **Prevent**:
    - Transmission (hepatitis vaccine recommended for high risk groups)
    - Prevention of transmission of HAV is proper handling of foods and wastes, and frequent handwashing
    - Prevention of spread of transmission of HBV includes sexual abstinence, use of condoms, careful handling of blood and blood products, as well as properly screening blood products before use. Avoidance of contact with all bodily fluids.
    - Prevention of transmission of CV includes all blood and blood products precautions listed under B as well as no IV and intranasal illicit drug-use paraphernalia sharing.
    - Vaccination against Hepatitis B will also impart immunity against Hepatitis D
    - Vaccinate against Hepatitis A
    - Currently there is no vaccine for Hepatitis C

- **Assess/Monitor:**
  - Activity intolerance.
  - Fluid and electrolyte status
- **Nursing Activities:**
  - Teach client regarding transmission.
  - Group nursing activities, balancing activity with rest.
  - Restrict activity until serum bilirubin and liver enzymes return to normal (Hepatitis B).
  - Provide diet high in calories and carbohydrates, low in fat.
  - Teach client the importance of avoiding alcohol intake.
  - Teach client to seek medical attention if symptoms persist or worsen.
  - Teach client regarding the need for follow-up care.
  - Hospitalization may be required for clients with hepatitis.

Pharmacology

- Antipyretics (acetaminophen)
- Hepatitis A vaccine Immune globulin (for Hepatitis A)
- Hepatitis B vaccine
- Hepatitis B immune globulin (HBIG)
- Antihistamines (diphenhydramine, hydroxyzine)
- Antacids
- Interferon-alpha (Hepatitis B, C)
- Ribavirin (HCV)
- Pegylated interferon-alpha 2b (HCV)
- Antiemetics (meclizine, prochlorperazine)

Complications

- Secondary infection
- Chronic hepatitis
- Carrier state
- Cirrhosis - most commonly with HBV
- Liver cancer - most commonly with HCV, but also with HBV

Age-Related Changes—Gerontological Considerations

- Increased risk for fluid and electrolyte imbalance related to vomiting and diarrhea may lead to more serious consequences in elderly persons.

Critical Thinking Exercise: Nursing Management of the Client with Hepatitis

Situation: A nurse is caring for two clients. One, an older male, has Hepatitis B. The second client, a young female, has Hepatitis A.

1. Match the type of hepatitis (A or B) with the appropriate description.

   _____ The fecal-oral route is the primary route of transmission

   _____ Ten percent of clients infected will develop chronic hepatitis

   _____ A DNA virus

   _____ Contracted from contaminated foods or fluids

   _____ The virus is found in semen, vaginal secretions and saliva

   _____ Incubation period ranges from 2-7 weeks

   _____ Transmitted primarily through blood

2. Match the type of hepatitis (A or B) with its characteristic sign or symptom. Clients may be asymptomatic.

   _____ Low-grade fever   _____ Abdominal pain

   _____ Fatigue, malaise   _____ Dark, brown urine

   _____ Nausea, vomiting   _____ Pruritus

   _____ Anorexia   _____ Enlarged, tender liver

   _____ Jaundice   _____ Dyspepsia

   _____ Clay-colored stools   _____ Mild, flu-like symptoms

   _____ Headache   _____ Enlarged posterior cervical lymph nodes

3. Cite the etiology for the nursing diagnoses that apply to both clients.

   a. Risk for altered nutrition: less than body requirements

   b. Risk for injury: others

   c. Risk for activity intolerance

   d. Abdominal pain

   e. Anxiety/fear

Nursing Management of the Client with Cancer

Key Points

- Cancer may involve the skin, bone, any organ, or blood.
- Carcinomas arise from epithelial tissues.
- Sarcomas arise from mesenchymal tissues.
- Adenocarcinomas arise from glandular organs.
- Leukemias are malignancies of the blood-forming cells.
- Metastasis is the movement of malignant cells from a primary site to distant sites via the circulatory or lymphatic system.
- Chemotherapy is a systemic or regional intervention for cancer using chemicals (cytotoxic drugs).
- Chemotherapy is administered systemically through oral, subcutaneous, intramuscular, and intravenous routes; regionally through topical, intrathecal, intracavitary, or intra-arterial instillations.
- Radiation therapy is a local cancer intervention placing radioactive materials in or near the tumor.
- Radiation therapy may be:
  - The primary treatment
  - An adjunctive treatment in combination with surgery or chemotherapy
  - Palliative
- Many cancers, if diagnosed early, are curable.
- Screening and early diagnosis is the most important aspect of care.
- Goals of collaborative management:
  - Identify and treat early in the disease process.
  - Eliminate the cancer.
  - Restore and maintain normal function.
  - Prevent complications.
  - Provide supportive end-of-life care when cure is not possible.
- Important nursing diagnoses (actual or potential):
  - Potential complications of cancer (wasting syndrome, fractures, metastasis, thrombophlebitis, sepsis)
  - Potential complications of chemotherapy (anemia, toxicity, electrolyte imbalance, leukopenia)
  - Fear and anxiety
  - Activity intolerance

- Risk for injury
- Ineffective airway clearance
- Caregiver role strain
- Ineffective individual/family coping
- Fatigue and restlessness
- Diarrhea and other bowel dysfunctions
- Fluid volume deficit
- Risk for infection
- Ineffective management of therapeutic regimen
- Self-care deficit
- Powerlessness and hopelessness
- Altered nutrition, less than body requirements
- Impaired skin integrity
- Social isolation
- **Key Terms/Concepts:** Wasting syndrome, metastasis, neoplastic disease, neutropenia, leukopenia, carcinomas, sarcomas, leukemias, adenocarcinomas, chemotherapy, radiation therapy, cytotoxic drugs

Overview

Cancer is a **neoplastic** disease process that involves abnormal cell growth and differentiation. The exact cause is unknown, but viruses, physical and chemical agents, hormones, genetics, and diet are thought to be factors that trigger abnormal cell growth. Cancerous cells may invade surrounding tissues and gain access to lymph and blood vessels, allowing it to spread to other areas of the body (metastasis).

Risk Factors

- Genetic predisposition
- Age
- Exposure to environmental and chemical carcinogens
- Exposure to viruses
- Poverty
- Stress
- Diet
- Occupation
- Infection
- Tobacco and alcohol use
- Use of recreational drugs
- Obesity
- Sun exposure

Signs and Symptoms

- Specific to type and location of cancer

- Acute and/or chronic pain (generally late stages)
- Anorexia, cachexia, weight loss, wasting syndrome
- Anemia, neutropenia
- Bruising, hemorrhage
- Infection
- Skin lesions
- Fractures
- Psychological stress
- Seven warning signs spelling CAUTION:
  - C: changes in bowel or bladder habits
  - A: a sore that doesn't heal
  - U: unusual bleeding or discharge
  - T: thickening or lump in the breast or elsewhere
  - I: indigestion or difficulty swallowing
  - O: obvious changes in warts or moles
  - N: nagging cough or hoarseness

Diagnostic and Laboratory Tests

- History and physical examination
- Magnetic resonance imaging (MRI)
- Computed tomography (CT)/computed axial tomography (CAT) scan
- Platelet count
- Complete blood count (CBC), with differential
- Serum electrolytes
- Blood urea nitrogen (BUN)
- Creatinine. Measures the amount of creatinine in the blood. Creatinine is a muscle enzyme. A measure of renal function.
- Liver enzymes:
  - Alkaline phosphatase (ALP); also called ALK Phos, is an enzyme found in the liver, bones and placenta.
  - Alanine aminotransferase (ALT); also called serum glutamic pyruvic transaminase (SGPT) is an enzyme found primarily in liver cells.
  - Aspartate aminotransferase (AST); also called serum glutamic oxaloacetic transaminase (SGOT), is an enzyme found in the liver, and elsewhere in the body.
  - Gamma-glutamyl transpeptidase (GGTP); also called GGT or Gamma GT, is an enzyme present in the liver, pancreas and kidneys.
  - Lactic acid dehydrogenase (LDH); is an enzyme found in the liver.
- Urinalysis
- Blood and urine cultures
- Chest x-ray

- Electrocardiogram (ECG)
- Biopsy
- Endoscopy
- Fluoroscopy
- Radioisotope Scans
- Ultrasound
- 2D (2-dimensional)
- 3D (3-dimensional)
- Positron emission tomography (PET) scan
- Radio immunoconjugate

Therapeutic Nursing Management

- **Prevention**:
  - Promote cancer screening, especially in presence of risk factors.
  - Educate clients regarding early detection, including CAUTION model.
- **Assess/Monitor**:
  - Nutritional status and promote adequate food and fluid intake
  - Pain status. Pain interferes with the clients' sleeping, eating, and ability to care for themselves, or interact with others. Providing pain control can prevent these problems and prevent complications associated with these problems.
  - For altered body image (e.g., mastectomy, hysterectomy, colostomy)
  - For secondary problems (infection, thrombocytopenia, neutropenia, bleeding, skin breakdown, weight loss)
  - For injury
  - Laboratory data
  - For signs of sepsis related to invasive lines or procedures
  - Intake and output and daily weight
  - Clients undergoing chemotherapy for:
    - Side effects and toxic effects of chemotherapy
    - Blood in stools and urine, ecchymotic areas
    - Fever, which may be the only sign of infection
    - Signs and symptoms of stomatitis, esophagitis, mucositis, nausea and vomiting, diarrhea, constipation, weight loss, and effectiveness of therapeutic measures
    - Skin reactions and photosensitivity
    - Hepatotoxicity, cirrhosis, portal hypertension
    - Pulmonary fibrosis, pneumonitis
    - Neuropathies
    - Dysrhythmias, heart failure
    - Changes in level of consciousness
  - Chemotherapy IV injection site for redness and edema

- Client undergoing radiation therapy for fatigue, nausea, anorexia, and skin reactions
- Client undergoing radiation therapy for site-specific side effects such as radiation caries, esophagitis, dysphagia, cystitis
- Client undergoing surgery for postoperative complications
- Client's progress through the stages of grief
- **Nursing Activities:**
  - Provide basic care and assist client as needed.
  - Assure the terminal client and the family (or significant others) that effective pain management will be provided to the client throughout his/her illness.
  - Teach client to maintain adequate oral and body hygiene.
  - Plan activities to conserve client's energy.
  - Teach regarding diagnostic tests and central lines.
  - Provide information to clients undergoing chemotherapy on effects of cytotoxic drugs on cancer cells and bone marrow functioning.
  - Assist the client undergoing chemotherapy by:
    - Administering chemotherapy as prescribed
    - Administering antiemetics and antibiotics as ordered
    - Providing frequent, small, high calorie meals
    - Providing frequent oral hygiene
    - Administering an analgesic if the client has developed mucositis, a condition that makes it difficult for the client to eat and swallow.
    - Assisting the client with hair loss to obtain a wig, hats, or other head coverings
  - Instruct clients undergoing chemotherapy to:
    - Prevent infection by avoiding crowds and people with infections.
    - Use good personal hygiene and hand washing.
    - Use a soft toothbrush and an electric razor.
    - Avoid activities that could cause injury and bleeding.
    - Avoid aspirin and aspirin-containing products.
    - Maintain a nutritious diet and drink adequate fluids.
    - Take an antiemetic about 30 minutes before eating.
    - Immediately report a temperature of over 100 F, sore throat, cough, and chills.
    - Obtain adequate rest.
  - Instruct clients undergoing radiation therapy concerning the goals of treatment, the procedure, risks, benefits, side effects, and symptom management.
  - Advise clients undergoing radiation therapy to:
    - Not remove skin markings used by radiation therapist.
    - Pace activities and receive adequate rest.
    - Avoid hot water, harsh soaps and rubbing of skin.
    - Report side effects that are specific to site receiving radiation.

- Follow-up with primary care provider every 2 to 3 months during the first posttreatment year.
- Provide preoperative and postoperative care to clients undergoing surgery.
- Offer emotional support regarding grieving, loss, and anxiety.
- Refer client to cancer support groups or hospice as appropriate.
- Provide time for the client to express concerns and fears.
- Nursing care of the client with nausea and vomiting (specifically for the cancer client):
  - Encourage the client to eat breakfast. This is often the time they feel best.
  - Maintain NPO status as long as they are vomiting.
  - Encourage or support frequent oral care.
  - Give/encourage clear, cool fluids taken in small amount (continually assess the client's ability to tolerate the fluids).
  - Premedicate or offer antiemetics as needed (and ordered).

Pharmacology

- Antimetabolites (methotrexate, gemcitabine, fluorouracil)
- Alkylating agents (carboplatin, cisplatin, cyclophosphamide, ifosfamide)
- Antibiotics (meropenem, ceftazidime)
- Plant alkaloids (vinblastine, vincristine)
- Hormone antagonists (letrozole, tamoxifen)
- Protein synthesis inhibitors (asparaginase)
- Radiation therapy
- Immune modulators (interferon)
- Antiemetics (granisetron, ondansetron, dolasetron)
- Colony-stimulating factors (filgrastim, sargramostim)

Complications

- Metastases
- Infection/sepsis
- Hemorrhage/shock
- Depression
- Pericardial effusion, cardiac tamponade
- Superior vena cava syndrome
- Spinal cord compression
- Obstructive uropathy
- Fluid and electrolyte imbalance
- Wasting syndrome
- Hyperkalemia
- Death

- Complications related to chemotherapy
- Drug resistance to chemotherapeutic agents
- Complications related to radiation therapy
- Complications related to surgical intervention

Generic Cancer Staging System

- Stage 1: Localized – Usually confined to the organ of origin
- Stage 2: Regional – Extends beyond organ of origin but remains nearby
- Stage 3: Extensive – Has extended beyond regional site of origin crossing several tissue planes or extending distantly via lymphatics or blood
- Stage 4: Widely Disseminated – Often involves the bone marrow or multiple distant organs

Age-Related Changes—Gerontological Considerations

- The highest incidence of cancer occurs in older adults.
- Older adult women most commonly develop colorectal, breast, lung, pancreatic, and ovarian cancers.
- Older adult men most commonly develop lung, colorectal, prostate, pancreatic, and gastric cancers.
- There is increased risk for the development of secondary infections.
- Increased risk for altered skin integrity secondary to radiation therapy exists in older clients.
- Older adults do not heal as quickly as younger adults.

Critical Thinking Exercise: Nursing Management of the Client with Cancer

Situation: A 49-year-old male has a 32-year history of cigarette smoking. He often eats out with associates and typically eats red meat and potatoes. One of his associates is a 51-year-old female whose mother died of breast cancer. She is 40 pounds over her ideal weight because she likes to snack during the day. She is also a heavy coffee drinker.

1. What risk factors does each of these clients have for development of cancer?

    a. Male:

    b. Female:

2. Which statements are true about cancer? Correct inaccurate statements.

    a. Cancer involves abnormal cell growth and differentiation.

    b. Viral agents cause the majority of cancers.

    c. Diet is thought to be a factor that triggers abnormal cell growth.

    d. Metastasis occurs when cancer directly spreads to distant organs.

    e. Cancer may involve the skin, bone, any organ, or blood.

    f. Few cancers are curable even when diagnosed early.

3. What is the rationale for each nursing intervention?

    a. Monitor for secondary problems.

    b. Promote adequate food and fluid intake.

    c. Educate clients regarding early detection, including CAUTION model.

    d. Plan activities to conserve client's energy.

    a. Offer emotional support regarding grieving, loss, and anxiety.

4. What does CAUTION stand for in relation to cancer?

Nursing Management of the Client with Liver Cancer

Key Points

- Primary hepatocellular carcinoma (malignant hepatoma) is one of the most common malignant tumors occurring in the world.
- Liver cancer has a high incidence in parts of Asia and sub-Saharan Africa, and a lower incidence in Western countries.
- The exact etiology of primary liver cancer is unknown.
- If the cancer is confined to one lobe, liver resection may be performed as a palliative measure, with up to 90% of the liver being removed.
- 30%-40% of clients are candidates for liver lobe resection.
- Following liver resection, clients may survive for five years or longer.
- Liver cancer has a very poor prognosis without surgery, with survival ranging from a few months to one year.
- Goals of collaborative management:
  - Identify the cancer and treat early in disease process.
  - Prevent complications of disease.
  - Prevent complications from chemotherapy and surgery.
  - Provide supportive end-of-life care.
- Important nursing diagnoses (actual or potential):
  - Fear and anxiety
  - Death anxiety
  - Anticipatory grieving
  - Hopelessness and powerlessness
  - Social isolation
  - Risk of infection
  - Activity intolerance
  - Risk for injury
  - Caregiver role strain
  - Ineffective management of therapeutic regimen
  - Self-care deficit
  - Altered nutrition, less than body requirements
  - Pain management
  - Risk for impaired skin integrity
  - Fatigue and sleeplessness
  - Ineffective individual/family coping

- **Key Terms and Concepts**: Primary source, primary hepatocellular carcinoma, cirrhosis, liver biopsy, liver lobe resection, metastases

Overview

Liver cancer is a malignancy of the liver. Liver cancer may be primary in nature; resulting from a tumor of the liver itself, or it may develop secondarily to the spread of cancer from another site. Cancer cells spread to the liver via the portal system or the lymphatic channels.

Risk Factors

- Male gender
- Heredity
- Chronic Hepatitis B (for primary liver cancer)
- Hepatitis C
- Cigarette smoking (especially combined with alcohol ingestion)
- Hemochromatosis
- Use of androgenic steroids
- Exposure to vinyl chloride and similar chemicals
- Ingestion of aflatoxins (peanuts or peanut products contaminated with *Aspergillus* or *Aspergillus* parasiticus)
- Type II glycogen storage disease

Signs and Symptoms

- No symptoms in early stages
- Jaundice
- Pruritus
- Anorexia
- Nausea and vomiting
- Weight loss
- Fatigue
- Abdominal pain
- Abdominal mass in right upper quadrant
- Ascites

Diagnostic and Laboratory Tests

- a-fetoprotein (AFP or alpha-fetoprotein), which acts as a tumor marker to distinguish primary from secondary liver cancer
- Liver function tests:
  - Alkaline phosphatase (ALP), also called ALK Phos, is an enzyme found in the liver, bones and placenta.
  - Alanine aminotransferase (ALT), also called serum glutamic pyruvic

transaminase (SGPT), is an enzyme found primarily in liver cells.

- Aspartate aminotransferase (AST), also called serum glutamic oxaloacetic transaminase (SGOT), is an enzyme found in the liver, and elsewhere in the body.
- Gamma-glutamyl transpeptidase; also called (GGT or Gamma GT) is an enzyme present in the liver, pancreas and kidneys
- Bilirubin: a waste product formed by the breakdown of red blood cells
- Albumin: a protein synthesized by the liver
- Total cholesterol: a substance stored in the liver
- Total protein: a nutrient normally broken down by the liver and its enzymes
- Lactic acid dehydrogenase (LDH): an enzyme found in the liver
- Prothrombin time: tests the blood's ability to clot
- Liver biopsy
- Ultrasound
  - 2D (2-dimensional)
  - 3D (3-dimensional)
  - Doppler
- Magnetic resonance imaging (MRI)
- Computed tomography (CT)/computed axial tomography (CAT) scan
- Hepatic arteriography
- Endoscopic retrograde cholangiopancreatography (ERCP)
- Hepatic scintigraphy

Therapeutic Nursing Management

- **Prevention:**
  - Promote cancer screening, especially in presence of risk factors.
  - Use of condoms
  - Hepatitis B vaccine
  - Avoidance of high risk behaviors such as IV drug abuse, non-use of condoms
  - Encourage prompt diagnosis and treatment of Hepatitis B and Hepatitis C.
  - Advise client to stop smoking and drinking alcohol.
  - Advise client to avoid exposure to vinyl chloride and similar chemicals.
  - Advise client to avoid eating peanuts or peanut products since they might be contaminated with Aspergillus or Aspergillus parasiticus.
  - Advise client to avoid use of androgenic steroids.
- **Assess/Monitor:**
  - Client for signs of fatigue
  - Nutritional status
  - Laboratory data
  - Client for signs of depression or anticipatory grief

- Client for pain
- Vital signs, platelet count, and prothrombin levels prior to liver biopsy
- For complications following liver biopsy
- For postoperative complications following liver resection
- For complications following radiation therapy
- For nausea and vomiting following chemotherapy
- Bleeding

- **Nursing Activities:**
  - Place client on bedrest and promote conservation of energy.
  - Teach client relaxation exercises and guided imagery techniques.
  - Provide a diet high in calories and carbohydrates and low in fat, sodium, and protein.
  - Provide small frequent feedings to help reduce nausea and promote caloric intake.
  - Administer pain medications as necessary with caution.
  - Relieve symptoms of skin irritation and pruritus.
  - Prepare client and family for liver biopsy, liver resection, radiation, or chemotherapy as appropriate.
  - Provide care before, during, and following liver biopsy.
    - Place client in supine or left lateral position with right arm extended above the head.
    - Ask client to inhale fully before biopsy needle is inserted and then hold breath while primary care provider obtains specimen of liver tissue.
    - Apply pressure dressing following removal of needle and turn client to right side.
    - Maintain client on bedrest for 8 to 24 hours.
    - Provide postoperative care if a liver resection is performed. Monitor site for bleeding, infection.
    - Provide antiemetics following chemotherapy as needed.
  - Offer emotional support to client and family as they pass through the stages of grief.
  - Refer the client to support groups or hospice as appropriate.

Pharmacology

- Sedation prior to liver biopsy (benzodiazepines)
- Vitamin K following liver biopsy to reduce risk of bleeding (phytonadione)
- Chemotherapy (doxorubicin, etoposide)
- Continuous chemotherapy infusion to the liver through the hepatic artery via an intravenous pump
- Pain medications (meperidine)
- Antiemetics (granisetron, ondansetron, dolasetron)

Complications

- Hemorrhage, bile peritonitis, or pneumothorax following liver biopsy
- Lung metastases
- Metastases to regional lymph nodes, adrenals, kidneys, heart, pancreas, bone and stomach
- Hepatic encephalopathy
- Severe depression
- Postoperative complications
- Complications following chemotherapy
- Complications following radiation therapy
- Infection/sepsis, disseminated intravascular coagulation (DIC)
- Death

Age-Related Changes—Gerontological Considerations

- Liver cancer is most prevalent among clients over 50 years of age.
- Older clients are at greater risk of complications following surgery for cancer.

Critical Thinking Exercise: Nursing Management of the Client with Liver Cancer

Situation: A 65-year-old male client is being evaluated for possible primary hepatocellular carcinoma. The client is slightly jaundiced, and he has been experiencing nausea, anorexia, and abdominal pain. His health care provider has also discovered a small abdominal mass in the right upper quadrant. The client is scheduled for a liver biopsy.

1. Which are accurate steps for the nurse to take when preparing a client for a liver biopsy?

   _____ Instruct the client to take nothing by mouth for one to two hours prior to the procedure.

   _____ Explain the procedure, its purposes and risks.

   _____ Discuss how important it is for the client to follow instructions during the procedure.

   _____ Administer sedation an hour and a half prior to the procedure.

   _____ Assist the client into a supine or left lateral position.

2. Which are clinical manifestations of pneumothorax during liver biopsy?

   _____ Decreased respiratory rate   _____ Pleuritic chest pain

   _____ Shoulder pain   _____ Inability to inhale

   _____ Shortness of breath   _____ Decreased breath sounds

3. Why are pain medications administered with caution to clients with liver cancer?

4. What is the etiology of the client's nursing diagnoses?

   a. Risk for impaired skin integrity:

   b. Self-care deficit:

   c. Altered nutrition: Less than body requirements:

   d. Pain:

Nursing Management of the Client with a Common Cold or Influenza

- The common cold is a very contagious respiratory infection that is caused by over 100 rhinoviruses.
- Influenza or "the flu" is a highly contagious respiratory infection that is caused by one of only three different influenza virus types.
  - Type A, the most common type, is divided into many subtypes. Different subtypes of type A strike every year, account for about 80% of all cases of flu, and also cause the most severe illness.
  - Type B also strikes every year and causes occasional small outbreaks.
  - Type C causes only mild illness, similar to the common cold.
- Influenza can be a serious illness whereas the common cold is generally benign.
  - There is no known cure for the common cold.
  - Treatment for colds and the flu focus on relieving the symptoms and preventing complications of the flu such as pneumonia.
  - Antibiotics have no effect on the viruses resulting in colds or the flu.
  - Antiviral therapy (oseltamivir, zanamivir, amantadine, rimantadine) can be given to clients who contract influenza A in certain circumstances (within 48 hours of symptom onset) to shorten the course, lessen the severity, and lessen the complications associated with the flu.
- The Centers for Disease Control and Prevention (CDC) recommend a flu shot every year for infants over 6 months of age, adults over age of 50, and for anyone with a chronic disease. In general, the flu shot can be recommended for anyone, but high risk groups are 6-23 months of age, children on long-term aspirin therapy, clients over 50 years of age, and clients with chronic diseases.
- Goals of collaborative management:
  - Prevent complications (bronchitis, pneumonia).
  - Relieve symptoms.
  - Prevent the spread of infection to other people.
  - Promote adequate rest and nutrition.
- Important nursing diagnoses (actual or potential):
  - Activity intolerance
  - Pain management
  - Ineffective airway clearance
  - Fatigue and restlessness
- **Key Terms/Concepts**: Contagious, inflammation, flu shot, bronchitis, pneumonia

Overview

The common cold (acute viral rhinitis) is a highly contagious viral infection that produces inflammation of the upper airway, primarily the nasal mucosa. Colds generally peak in September and January.

Influenza is a highly contagious respiratory viral disease that is much more serious than the common cold. The CDC recommends flu shots yearly for most people. Nasal immunization for influenza can be used in certain populations.

Risk Factors

- Exposure to the virus via coughing, sneezing, use of contaminated equipment
- Inadequate hygiene, especially hand washing
- Lack of rest, sleep, and nutrition
- Physical or emotional stress

Signs and Symptoms

Colds

- Nasal congestion
- Headache
- Cough
- Lethargy, fatigue
- Fever, usually low-grade
- Sore throat

Influenza

Major symptoms of influenza are headache, sore throat, fever, cough, and body aches.

- Nasal congestion
- Fever, usually greater than 101
- Cough
- Chills
- Hoarseness
- Laryngitis
- Sore throat
- Muscle aches, body aches
- Loss of appetite
- Fatigue
- Headache

Diagnostic and Laboratory Tests

- History and physical examination
- Nasal swab for Influenza A

Therapeutic Nursing Management

- **Prevention**
  - Annual flu shot
  - Good hand-washing skills
  - Coughing/sneezing into elbow rather than hand
- **Assess/Monitor:**
  - Hydration
  - Nutrition
  - Fever
  - Breath sounds for pneumonia in influenza clients
- **Nursing Activities:**
  - Encourage increased fluid intake.
  - Teach the need for hand washing and hygiene.
  - Encourage avoidance of crowds during peak seasons.
  - Encourage rest and a nutritious diet.

Pharmacology

- Nasal decongestants (oral pseudoephedrine, nasal phenylephrine for no more than 3 days)
- Analgesics (acetaminophen, ibuprofen, naproxen)
- Antipyretics (acetaminophen, ibuprofen)
- Antitussives
- Antiviral agents for influenza
- Zinc lozenges
- Increase fluid intake

Complications

Common Cold
- Secondary bacterial infections of the sinuses, throat, or lungs

Influenza
- Pneumonia
- Reye's Syndrome if aspirin used, especially with children

Age-Related Changes—Gerontological Considerations

- Older adults experience more severe symptoms related to colds and influenza and secondary complications, such as bronchitis and pneumonia.
- Increased risk for dehydration and electrolyte imbalance due to fever, especially in the elderly population.
- Colds tend to last longer in older adults because of decreased immunity.
- The Centers for Disease Control (CDC) recommends yearly flu shots for all individuals over the age of 50.

Critical Thinking Exercise: Nursing Management of the Client with a Common Cold or Influenza

Situation: A 71-year-old woman who lives with her daughter is exposed to a child who has a cold when they visit nearby relatives. The woman has already had pneumonia this winter and she is concerned about becoming ill again.

1. In general, which interventions may help the client to avoid contracting a cold during cold season?

   _____ Gargling with mouthwash   _____ Obtaining adequate rest

   _____ Increasing her fluid intake   _____ Taking prophylactic aspirin

   _____ Taking zinc after exposure   _____ Washing her hands frequently

2. If the client develops a cold, which activities may speed her recovery?

   _____ Vitamin supplements   _____ Increased rest

   _____ Well-balanced diet   _____ Antibiotics

   _____ Restricted fluid intake   _____ Pallor

Nursing Management of the Client with Rheumatoid Arthritis

| Key Points |

- Chronic, painful, inflammatory disorder of the peripheral joints, ligaments, tendons, muscles, and blood vessels.
- Autoimmune disease with no known cause or cure.
- Characterized by exacerbations and remissions.
- Goals of collaborative management:
  - Reduce pain.
  - Maintain joint mobility.
  - Prevent joint deformity.
  - Control the autoimmune process.
  - Prevent complications (muscle atrophy, vasculitis, and paresthesia).
- Important nursing diagnoses (actual or potential):
  - Pain management
  - Self-care deficit
  - Self-esteem disturbance
  - Altered body image
  - Risk for injury
  - Knowledge deficit
  - Potential complications of drug therapy (infection, gastritis)
  - Ineffective individual coping
- **Key Terms/Concepts**: Autoimmune, chronic, systemic, inflammatory, exacerbation, remission

Overview

Rheumatoid arthritis is a chronic, systemic, inflammatory, autoimmune disorder that primarily involves peripheral joints and their surrounding ligaments, tendons, muscles and blood vessels. Altered immune complexes deposited in the synovial membranes produce inflammation, which results in tissue destruction and subsequent joint deformity and fusion. The disease is characterized by periods of exacerbation and remission.

Risk Factors

- Female gender
- Age 20-50
- Genetic predisposition
- Native American

Signs and Symptoms

- Insidious onset
- Fatigue
- Malaise
- Low-grade fever
- Anorexia
- Particular joint stiffness after inactivity, especially in the morning
- Edema, warmth, and congestion of affected joints
- Tender, painful joints
- Diminished joint function
- Joint deformity
- Vasculitis
- Pulmonary fibrosis
- Pericardial disease
- Depression
- Pain MCP (metacarpophalangeal), DIP (distal interphalangeal) joints in hands
- Neuropathy
- Scleritis
- Splenomegaly

Diagnostic and Laboratory Tests

- History and physical examination
- Rheumatoid factor (RF)
- ESR (Erythrosedimentation rate)
- Complete blood count (CBC)
- Serum complement
- Serum electrophoresis
- ANA (antinuclear antibody) test titer. (ANA test results are reported in a titer that indicates how much the test sample can be diluted before the antibodies are no longer detected. Fluorescence techniques are frequently used to actually detect the antibodies in the cells, thus ANA testing is sometimes referred to as FANA [fluorescent antinuclear antibody] testing.)
- X-rays
- Synovial fluid analysis
- C-reactive protein (CRP)
- HLA-DR4 (human leukocyte antigen) - 70% of Caucasian clients are seropositive

Therapeutic Nursing Management

- **Assess/Monitor:**
  - Joints for pain, mobility, deformities, and contractures

- Vital signs
- Weight
- Response to medications
- **Nursing Activities:**
  - Administer disease modifying antirheumatic drugs (DMARDs), salicylates, NSAIDs, and other medications as prescribed.
  - Encourage frequent rest periods.
  - Splint acutely inflamed joints.
  - Encourage compliance with prescribed exercise program.
  - Encourage active ROM exercises.
  - Encourage use of cane, crutches, or other assistive devices.
  - Encourage the client to perform activities in the order of their priority, thereby accomplishing the most important tasks while still conserving energy.
  - Apply cold compresses to acutely inflamed joints.
  - Apply heat via shower, bath, or moist warm packs as prescribed.
  - Teach regarding side effects of immunosuppressive medications.
  - Apply splints correctly, as prescribed.
  - Prepare client for surgery as needed (synovectomy, joint reconstruction, total joint arthroplasty).
  - Provide emotional support and encouragement.
  - Refer to Arthritis Foundation or support group as appropriate.

Pharmacology

- NSAIDs (diclofenac, ibuprofen, naproxen, nabumetone)
- Anti-malarials (hydroxychloroquine)
- Gold injections
- Glucocorticoid steroids (prednisone)
- Immunosuppressive agents (methotrexate, azathioprine)
- Salicylates (aspirin)
- Analgesics (opioid or nonopioid)
- Cytotoxic (chemotherapy) agents (cyclophosphamide)
- Disease modifying antirheumatic drugs (DMARDs) - include penicillamine, gold salts, immunosuppressants such as those listed above, and hydroxychloroquine. These medications differ from NSAIDs in that they alter the disease process by reducing ESR (erythrocyte sedimentation rate) and rheumatoid factor (RF). However, these drugs work slowly and have a low margin of safety, so careful monitoring must be carried out.
- Other immune system modifiers: tumor necrosis factor (TNF) blocker (etanercept, adalimumab, infliximab) and interleukin-1 receptor antagonist (anakinra)
- Complications
- Joint deformity

- Spontaneous tendon rupture
- Muscle atrophy
- Sjögren's syndrome
- Pericarditis
- Vasculitis
- Fibrotic lung disease
- Paresthesia

Age-Related Changes—Gerontological Considerations

- Reduced range of motion during rotation and hyperextension of the hip joint occurs commonly in older adults.
- Decreased bone formation and increased bone resorption are related to physiologic changes of aging.
- Prolonged healing of bones and joints occurs with aging.
- Elderly clients who contracted RA in their early to middle adult years may be very limited in mobility due to contractures.
- Body systems, especially the cardiovascular and pulmonary, can be affected negatively enough to shorten life-span.
- Side effects of medications to treat RA may also affect the elder client's health and general wellbeing.

Critical Thinking Exercise: Nursing Management of the Client with Rheumatoid Arthritis

Situation: A 47-year-old woman visits the outpatient clinic due to exacerbation of her rheumatoid arthritis. She has joint tenderness, symmetrical joint swelling, and subcutaneous nodules.

1. What symptoms, in addition to those being experienced by the client, are common with rheumatoid arthritis?

2. Which laboratory values are likely to be elevated when a client is experiencing exacerbated rheumatoid arthritis?

_____ Erythrosedimentation rate (ESR)	_____ Red blood cell (RBC) count
_____ White blood cell (WBC) count	_____ Antinuclear antibody (ANA) titer
_____ Serum complement	_____ C-reactive protein (CRP)

3. What is the rationale for applying ice to the client's inflamed joints, rather than heat?

4. What is the desired client outcome for each nursing intervention?

   a. Encouraging active range of motion exercises.

   b. Administering salicylates or NSAIDs as prescribed.

   c. Splinting inflamed joints.

Nursing Management of the Client Requiring Immunizations

Key Points

- The organs of the immune system include the bone marrow, thymus gland, lymph nodes, spleen, tonsils, and mucosal lymphatic tissues.
- Immunity may be natural or acquired, active or passive, humoral or cell-mediated.
- Natural immunity (innate immunity or genetic immunity) is inherited and has been programmed into the person's DNA.
- Acquired immunity (adaptive immunity) can be active or passive and it can develop at any time.
- Active acquired immunity results from the development of antibodies or sensitized T-lymphocytes that neutralize or destroy pathologic organisms. This form of immunity may follow natural exposure to an invading organism, or artificial exposure resulting from the injection of a vaccine.
- Passive acquired immunity is a temporary form of immunity acquired by either the injection of antibodies into an unprotected individual, or by the passage of antibodies from mother to fetus through the placenta. Antibodies are also contained in mother's milk.
- Humoral immunity involves the response of B-lymphocytes followed by the production of antibodies, which combat invading antigens. The primary immune response develops upon an individual's first exposure to a particular antigen. The secondary immune response occurs upon the second and all ensuing exposures to a particular antigen.
- Cell-mediated immunity (CMI) involves the action of T-cells. CMI destroys virus-infected cells and cancer cells, and it can cause delayed hypersensitivity reactions.
- Immunodeficiency disorders are characterized by a failure of the immune system to fight infection and cancer. These disorders may be inherited or they may result from an acquired disease that damages the immune system.
- Autoimmunity is the body's ability to tolerate the antigens that are present on its own cells.
- Autoimmune disease develops when the body's normal tolerance of the antigens present on its own cells disappears, resulting in the production of autoantibodies which attack normal cells (e.g. rheumatoid arthritis).
- Allergic reaction is a reaction that results from hypersensitivity to an antigen.
- Immunization may be passive or active.
- Immunobiologicals include antigenic substances such as vaccines and toxoids or antibody-containing substances such as globulins and antitoxins.
- Passive immunization is temporary, and is promoted by the injection of antibodies, which act to protect the person against specific bacteria, viruses, or

toxins. Passive immunity can come from pooled human immune globulin, specific immune globulin, and antitoxin.

- Human immune globulin is a sterile antibody solution made from human blood. Used for immunization against diseases such as measles and hepatitis A.
- Specific immune globulin is antigen-specific, such as hepatitis B immune globulin, rabies immune globulin, or tetanus immune globulin.
- Antitoxins are antibodies derived from serum of animals immunized with specific antigens, such as with diphtheria.

- Active immunization is long-lasting, and is characterized by the body's ability to make its own antibodies against microorganisms. Active immunity is derived from a vaccine or toxoid.

  - Live attenuated vaccine is a modified disease producing virus or bacteria that usually does not cause an illness, but is still strong enough to replicate and produce immunity. Examples include measles, mumps, rubella, polio, and varicella vaccines.

- Goals of collaborative management:
  - Identify immunocompromised clients who are at risk of infection.
  - Prevent infection and restore the immune response.
  - Prevent and treat hypersensitivity reactions.
  - Relieve multisystem symptoms and prevent joint destruction from autoimmune disorders.
  - Follow the recommendations of the Advisory Committee of Immunization Practices (ACIP), National Coalition for Adult Immunization, and Center for Disease Control (CDC).
  - Educate clients about maintaining vaccinations and to receive vaccinations prior to foreign travel. Identify what vaccinations are needed and what other medications and precautions should be taken. This can be done by visiting http://www.cdc.gov under travel.
  - Identify contraindications for client's use of a vaccine.

- Important nursing diagnoses (actual or potential):
  - Risk for infection at the injection site
  - Risk for injury
  - Altered protection
  - Risk for impaired skin integrity
  - Pain management
  - Impaired physical mobility
  - Activity intolerance
  - Fatigue
  - Ineffective management of therapeutic program
  - Social Isolation

- **Key Terms/Concepts**: Innate immunity (natural immunity), adaptive immunity (acquired immunity), active acquired immunity, passive acquired immunity, humoral immunity, cellular immunity, radioassay tests, immunocompromised, autoimmune disease, adult immunizations, vaccines, allergic reaction, hypersensitivity, Advisory Committee on Immunization Practices (ACIP)

Overview

The **immune system** is composed of cells and proteins that protect the body from harmful bacteria, viruses, and fungi. It also helps to control the growth of cancer cells. Further, an improperly-working immune system promotes the development of allergies and hypersensitivity reactions. A strong immune system helps protect against rejection problems that can complicate organ and graft transplant surgery. The immune system can also see the body as "foreign" and "attack" itself, leading to autoimmune diseases.

- **Immunity** is the state of being protected against infectious diseases due to the development of humoral or cell-mediated immunity.
- **Immunization** is the process of promoting or providing immunity in an individual against certain infectious diseases.

Risk Factors

- Indications for adult vaccinations
    - Health care worker
    - Aging, over 50 years old, 65 and older, all adults
    - Chronic health care conditions
    - Foreign travel
    - Day care worker
    - Food handler
    - Some vaccines were not available when we were children
    - Contact with blood or body fluids and not previously vaccinated against hepatitis B
    - Women wishing to get pregnant and have never had varicella zoster (chickenpox) or measles (MMR-measles, mumps, rubella)
- Contraindications for adult vaccinations
    - Previous anaphylactic reaction
    - Moderate or severe acute illness, especially if fever present, on an antibiotic, or on an oral or injectable steroid
    - Pregnancy (with some vaccines)
    - Breastfeeding (with some vaccines)
    - Immunocompromised state due to:
        - Cancer
        - Leukemia
        - Lymphoma
        - HIV
        - Use of immunosuppressive drugs
- Specific contraindications per adult vaccine
    - Tetanus, diphtheria (Td)
        - Precaution with Guillain-Barré syndrome less than or equal to 6 weeks after last Td
    - MMR
        - Pregnant or may become pregnant in 1 month

- Known severe immunodeficiency
- Caution if less than or equal to 11 months since receiving antibody-containing blood product
- Caution with history of thrombocytopenia or thrombocytopenic purpura
- Hepatitis B
  - As above
- Hepatitis A
  - Pregnancy
- Varicella
  - Substantial suppression of cellular immunity
  - Pregnant or going to become pregnant within 1 month
  - Caution if less than or equal to 11 months since receiving antibody-containing blood product
- Influenza
  - Intranasal, which is live-attenuated, can only be given to clients age 5-49 who are healthy, non-pregnant, non-asthmatic or other chronic condition, and non-health care workers
  - Egg allergy
  - Guillain-Barré syndrome history
- Pneumococcal
  - As above
- Meningococcal
  - As above

Signs and Symptoms

- Immune System and Autoimmune Disorders
  - Fever
  - Symptoms of recurrent infections
  - Symptoms of lymphoma or Kaposi's sarcoma
  - Symptoms of recurrent allergies
  - Lymphadenopathy
  - Splenomegaly
  - Joint pain (rheumatoid arthritis)
- Immunization Reactions
  - Anaphylactic reaction
  - Pain and swelling at injection site
  - Slight fever
  - Irritability
  - Malaise

Diagnostic and Laboratory Tests

- History and physical examination
- White blood cell (WBC) count, and differential
- Immune cell function studies
- T- and B-lymphocyte assays
- Immunoglobulin assays
- ELISA (Enzyme Linked Immunosorbent Assay)
- Radioimmunoassay
- RAST (radioallergosorbent test)
- RIST (radioimmunosorbent test)
- Lymphangiography
- Skin testing for allergies
- Food allergy testing

Therapeutic Nursing Management

- **Prevention**:
  - Prevent opportunistic infections in immunocompromised clients by encouraging clients to take antibiotics as ordered.
  - Prevent hypersensitivity reactions by writing known allergies on the client's health record, and by having client wear a special identification bracelet.
  - Administer immunosuppressive medications as ordered to help prevent graft rejection.
  - Prevent the spread of infectious diseases by having clients maintain vaccinations as recommended by the Advisory Committee on Immunization Practices (ACIP).
  - Prevent vaccination reactions by first taking a history of previous anaphylactic or neurologic reactions to specific vaccines.
- **Assess/Monitor**:
  - Assess need for Td at each client visit.
  - Assess allergies to medications, vaccinations, and eggs at each visit; record.
  - Assess for previous medical history of Guillain-Barré syndrome.
  - Be aware that a cough that persists for greater than 2-3 weeks in an adult, especially in the fall-winter, may be related to pertussis and waning of immunity from childhood immunization. Clients should receive antibiotics accordingly.
  - Clients following a vaccination for any untoward reaction to the vaccine
- **Nursing Activities**:
  - Administer antibiotics to immunocompromised clients as ordered.
  - Instruct immunocompromised clients to avoid people with infectious disorders.
  - Administer drug therapy and arrange for physical therapy to control symptoms associated with autoimmune disorders; e.g., rheumatoid arthritis.

- Teach clients how to desensitize a room in order to control environmental allergens that cause hypersensitivity reactions.
- Encourage clients to receive recommended vaccinations prior to foreign travel.
- Administer hepatitis A vaccine as ordered to clients who have chronic liver disease, are food handlers or health care workers, use illicit drugs, or travel outside of the United States.
- Administer hepatitis B vaccine to adolescents, adults engaging in high-risk sexual activities, workers who come in contact with blood, health care workers, and international travelers.
- Encourage older clients to receive an influenza vaccine yearly, and the pneumococcal vaccine if at risk of developing pneumonia. Because of the vaccine shortage of 2004, the ACIP (Advisory Committee on Immunization Practices) modified the recommendations that all clients should get influenza vaccination to (December 17, 2004) all persons from 50-64 years of age and high-risk, including occupational and household risk or inhabitants.
- Health care workers and those in close contact with the public, and all clients, should be encouraged to obtain influenza vaccine yearly.
- Those at high risk for developing pneumonia, or those who have had multiple bouts of pneumonia should be encouraged to obtain the pneumococcal vaccine.
- Provide all adolescents and adults with a tetanus-diphtheria booster shot every 10 years if they received the primary series of shots earlier.
- Provide all adults born in 1957 or later who are ≥ 18 years of age and all women of childbearing age with at least one measles, mumps, and rubella dose if there is no proof of immunity.
- Advise college-bound students, especially if they will reside in a dormitory, to obtain the meningitis vaccine.
- Provide all susceptible adults and adolescents with 2 doses of the varicella vaccine, one month apart, for chickenpox.
- Advise clients who work in a tick-infested habitat, or perform duties that bring them into contact with ticks to receive the Lyme disease vaccine.

Pharmacology

- Bacterial vaccines
  - Bacillus Calmette-Guérin (BCG) vaccine
  - Pneumococcal polysaccharide vaccine
  - Hemophiles B conjugate vaccine
  - Cholera vaccine
  - Meningococcal vaccine
  - Typhoid vaccine
  - Staphylococcus Phage Lysate vaccine
- Viral vaccines
  - Hepatitis A vaccine

- Hepatitis B vaccine
- Poliovirus vaccine
- Influenza virus vaccine
- MMR (Measles, mumps, rubella)
- Varicella (chickenpox)
- Mixed respiratory vaccine
- Toxoids
  - Tetanus toxoid
  - Diphtheria toxoid
  - DTP (Diphtheria, tetanus toxoids and pertussis vaccine)
    - DTaP, introduced in 1997, is about 10 times less likely to cause certain adverse reactions (such as fever, vomiting, and mild seizures) than DTP. The DTP contains the whole, inactivated pertussis bacteria, while the DTaP uses only the parts of the bacteria that help develop immunity but leaves behind all other components that may have been responsible for many of the DTP's adverse effects. The "a" in DTaP stands for acellular, which means there are no whole pertussis bacteria in the vaccine.
- Investigational vaccines
  - Lyme disease vaccine removed from the market; underused and not highly effective
  - Melanoma vaccine
  - Escherichia coli vaccine
  - Hepatitis C vaccine
  - Pseudomonas vaccine
  - HIV vaccine
  - Vaccines against certain cancers and rheumatoid arthritis

Complications

- Immune and autoimmune disorders
  - Opportunistic infections
  - Cancer (lymphoma)
  - Joint deformity
  - Muscle atrophy
- Hypersensitivity reactions
  - Anaphylactic shock
  - Graft rejection (acute or chronic)
  - Graft-versus-host disease
  - Blood transfusion reactions
- Vaccinations
  - Local anaphylactic reaction (Arthus reaction)
  - Anaphylactic shock

Age-Related Changes—Gerontological Considerations

- The ability to produce antibodies in response to antigens (humoral immunity) decreases with age, making older adults more susceptible to infections. Because of a depressed immune system, older adults are also at higher risk for complications resulting from infections such as the development of the secondary infection of pneumonia following the primary infection of influenza.
- Killer T-cell activity (cell-mediated immunity) decreases with age and is linked to an increased risk of cancer in older adults.

Critical Thinking Exercise: Nursing Management of the Client Requiring Immunizations

Situation: An 18-year-old female who recently graduated from high school is visiting her primary care provider prior to taking a vacation in Mexico. Afterwards, the teenager plans to start a job as a waitress in a fast-food restaurant while attending college. The nurse is preparing to administer appropriate immunizations.

1. Prior to administering immunizations, what questions should the nurse ask the client?

2. What immunizations should this 18-year-old client receive?

3. What immunizations should older clients receive?

4. What are the signs and symptoms of an anaphylactic reaction to a vaccine, and what is the emergency treatment?

Nursing Management of the Client Undergoing Angiography and Angioplasty

Key Points

- Angiogram/angiography is done prior to angioplasty.
- Angioplasty (also known as percutaneous transluminal angioplasty or PTCA) is used as an alternative treatment for cardiac arterial bypass graft (CABG) approximately 50% of the time.
- If one or two arteries are blocked, angioplasty can be performed; if more vessels are blocked or if CAD is diffuse, CABG is usually performed.
- The advantages in comparison with CABG are that an angioplasty is:
  - Less expensive
  - Less invasive
  - Faster to perform
  - Reduced length of hosipitalization
- The main disadvantage of angioplasty is:
  - Restenosis occurs 20-30% of the time within 6 months (unless a stent is placed in the artery).
- In more than 75% of all angioplasties performed, a stent is placed in the artery to prevent restenosis; stents can be covered with medication that prevents scar tissue formation and restenosis (drug-eluting stents).
- The goal of angioplasty is to reduce vessel obstruction to 50% of arterial lumen.
- Angioplasty can be performed on an elective basis to treat CAD or on emergency basis to treat MI.
- Goals of collaborative management:
  - Prevent ischemia/infarction/MI.
  - Increase blood flow to the myocardium.
  - Eliminate anginal pain.
  - Prevent restenosis.
  - Prevent post-procedural complications.
- Important nursing diagnoses (actual or potential):
  - Altered myocardial tissue perfusion due to coronary artery blockage
  - Pain
  - Activity intolerance
  - Knowledge deficit
- **Key Terms/Concepts**: Angioplasty, angiogram, myocardial infarction, coronary artery disease, hematoma, dysrhythmia

Overview

An angiogram, also called a cardiac catheterization, is a diagnostic procedure used to evaluate the presence and degree of coronary artery blockage. During an angiogram, a catheter is inserted in the client's groin (femoral artery) and threaded into the right or left coronary artery and into the left ventricle. A dye is then injected under x-ray revealing coronary artery plaque; additionally, left ventricular function can be checked.

An angioplasty is an invasive procedure performed to open up a blocked coronary artery and restore blood flow to the myocardium. Once the catheter is threaded into the affected artery, a balloon is inflated to stretch the arterial lumen and the adhering plaque, thus widening the arterial lumen. A stent is often placed to prevent the artery from collapsing immediately or restenosis (hardening) later.

Risk Factors

- CAD
- Previous or potential MI
- Advancing age
- Hypertension
- Diabetes
- Hyperlipidemia
- Obesity
- Sedentary lifestyle

Signs and Symptoms Necessitating the Procedure:

- Chest pain
- Palpitations
- Dyspnea
- ECG changes that may be indicative of ischemia/infarction (ST elevation and widened QRS complex)

Diagnostic and Laboratory Tests

- History and physical
- ECG
- Lipid profile
- Total serum cholesterol
- CPK

Therapeutic Nursing Management

- Assess/Monitor:
  - Chest pain during angioplasty
  - Dysrhythmias during angioplasty

- MI or restenosis by means of continuous ECG monitoring during and after the procedure
- Dye reaction/allergy (anaphylaxis)
- Coagulation labs to determine when to pull the sheath
- Insertion site for signs of hematoma
- Bleeding or artery perforation during/after the procedure
- Oxygen levels
- Pulses, color, sensation, capillary refill distal to access site after the procedure
- Intake and output
- Inability to urinate lying down. Be prepared to catheterize the client if they are unable.
- Light-headedness, bradycardia, hypotension, diaphoresis, fainting during sheath removal; keep atropine at bedside in case of fainting
- **Nursing Activities:**
  - Check for allergy to dye, iodine, shellfish
  - Teach what to expect before, during, and after the procedure
  - Perform a head-to-toe assessment
  - Maintain bedrest until advised (usually 6-8 hours)
  - Keep the extremity straight to ensure the sheath remains intact.
  - Encourage fluid intake to promote dye excretion
  - Administer pain medication for discomfort
  - Apply pressure after sheath removal (usually 20 to 30 minutes of direct pressure) or with use of a hemostasis device.

Pharmacology

- Pain medication as prescribed
- Oxygen
- Dye
- Anticoagulants

Complications

- Chest pain
- MI during or after the procedure
- Dysrhythmia
- Thromboembolism
- Shortness of breath
- Hematoma formation or infection at sheath insertion site
- Bleeding or tear in the lining of the artery
- Restenosis
- Fainting with sheath removal
- Allergy to dye

Age-Related Changes—Gerontological Considerations

- Older adults are at higher risk for CAD and MI; therefore are more likely to need angioplasty
- Recovery time may be longer
- An older adult may be at higher risk for intra- and postprocedural complications

Critical Thinking Exercise: Nursing Management of the Client Undergoing Angiography and Angioplasty

Situation: The client arrived to the intensive care unit following a PTCA. He still has a sheath in place is alert and oriented and his only complaint is that he is tired of lying still.

1. The client is asking you if he can sit up or take a couple of steps. What is your answer?

2. You have done your head-to-toe assessment with particular emphasis on the extremity where the sheath is. The client's pulses are already weak due to advanced CAD. Every time you come to check them, you are not sure which spot to look at and if the pulses are present at all. What will you assess in that extremity and what interventions can you provide?

3. In an hour, the client states that he needs to urinate, but cannot do so lying down. What intervention can the nurse provide in this instance?

Nursing Management of the Client with Bronchitis

Key Points

- Acute bronchitis is a relatively common disorder among adults usually as a sequela to an upper respiratory infection.
- Chronic bronchitis is an important component of chronic obstructive pulmonary (lung) disease.
- Cigarette smoking is one of the most significant risk factors for developing chronic bronchitis.
- Goals of collaborative management:
  - Provide early recognition and treatment.
  - Prevent the development of chronic bronchitis.
  - Assist the client with smoking cessation.
  - Prevent complications (bronchiectasis, COPD [chronic obstructive pulmonary disease]).
- Important nursing diagnoses (actual or potential):
  - Ineffective breathing pattern related to dyspnea, hypoxia
  - Ineffective airway clearance related to narrowed bronchioles
  - Risk for infection related to ineffective airway clearance and exposure to infectious irritants
  - Pain related to chest discomfort
  - Anxiety and fear related to difficulty breathing
  - Knowledge deficit related to prescribed medications/regimen
  - Activity intolerance related to fatigue and restlessness
  - Altered nutrition: less than body requirements related to loss of appetite
- **Key Terms/Concepts**: Acute, chronic, exacerbation, inflammation, (COPD) chronic obstructive pulmonary disease

Overview

Bronchitis, classified as acute or chronic, is an inflammation of the bronchi and bronchioles caused by continuous exposure to infectious or noninfectious irritants, especially smoke. People with impaired physiologic defense mechanisms and cigarette smokers are more susceptible to bronchitis. Acute bronchitis is usually related to an upper respiratory infection and is characterized by a nonproductive cough that usually becomes productive. Chronic bronchitis is a major component of COPD (chronic obstructive pulmonary disease) and is defined as a productive cough lasting at least three months and occurring for two consecutive years.

Risk Factors

- Tobacco use
- Exposure to respiratory pollutants
- Exposure to cigarette smoke
- Viral or bacterial upper respiratory infection
- Surgical procedures
- Medications
- Malnutrition

Signs and Symptoms

- Acute Bronchitis
  - Productive cough
  - Diffuse rhonchi/wheezes
  - Dyspnea
  - Chest pain
  - Low-grade temperature
- Chronic Bronchitis
  - Productive cough, most pronounced in the mornings
  - Increased dyspnea and use of accessory muscles
  - Later stages of the disease, cyanosis often accompanied by right ventricular failure
  - Reddish-blue skin color (also associated with right ventricular failure)

Diagnostic and Laboratory Tests

- History and physical examination
- Chest x-ray
- Sputum culture
- Bronchoscopy

Therapeutic Nursing Management

- **Assess/Monitor:**
  - Respiratory status (frequent assessment of respiratory status with vital signs, auscultate breath sounds noting presence of wheezing and basilar crackles)
  - For compromise
  - For changes in sputum (color, appearance, thickness)
  - Body temperature
  - For signs and symptoms of infection
- **Nursing Activities:**
  - Goal is to facilitate recovery and prevent secondary infections
  - Provide rest.

- Provide humidified air.
- Increase fluid intake (avoiding milk).
- Facilitate removal of secretions.
- Encourage smoking cessation.
- Prophylactic vaccination against pneumonia, influenza
- Administer antibiotics for current infections as prescribed.
- Minimize exposure to environmental irritants.
- Instruct/assess understanding of signs/symptoms that may indicate worsening infection.
- Teach importance of following a prescribed medical regimen.

Pharmacology

- Mucolytics/expectorants (guaifenesin)
- Bronchodilators (albuterol inhaler)
- Antibiotics (macrolides, cephalosporins, levofloxacin)
- Antipyretics (acetaminophen, ibuprofen)
- Corticosteroids (prednisone, methylprednisolone)

Complications

- Pneumonia
- Bronchiectasis

Age-Related Changes—Gerontological Considerations

- Increased risk for bronchitis is secondary to colds and influenza.
- Increased risk for infections may occur due to age-related changes in immune response.
- Older adults have decreased numbers of cilia and weakened cough responses.
- Older adults are prone to dehydration, which places them at increased risk for thicker mucous.

Critical Thinking Exercise: Nursing Management of the Client with Bronchitis

Situation: A 32-year-old woman with a 16-year history of cigarette smoking is experiencing her third episode of bronchitis within the past 12 months. She has a productive cough that has persisted between episodes of acute illness, fever, chest discomfort, and fatigue. Her chest x-ray is negative, but her WBC (white blood cell) count is elevated. Based on her data, the medical diagnosis of bronchitis is established. Her health care provider prescribes an albuterol sulfate inhaler and antibiotic therapy.

1. What is the most important information to provide the client about her recurrent episodes of bronchitis?

2. Cite three nursing activities to help reduce the client's risk for future episodes of bronchitis.

3. Differentiate between acute and chronic bronchitis.

4. What type of bronchitis is the client experiencing? Provide rationale for your answer.

Nursing Management of the Client with Pneumonia

Key Points

- Pneumonia is an inflammatory process of the lung parenchyma.
- Pneumonia may be a primary disease or complication of another disease.
- Persons of all ages are susceptible to pneumonia, but it is more common in infants, older adults and in people with debilitating diseases.
- Despite use of antibiotics, pneumonia is still a significant cause of death among older adults.
- There are two major types of pneumonia:
    - Community-acquired pneumonia (CAP). The onset of CAP occurs while the client is still out in the community or within the first 48 hours of hospitalization.
    - Hospital-acquired pneumonia (HAP) which occurs after the first 48 hours of hospitalization.
- Community-acquired pneumonia, although more responsive to antibiotic therapy, is more common than hospital-acquired pneumonia and is the sixth leading cause of death in the United States.
- HAP, also known as nosocomial pneumonia has 20 to 50% mortality.
- Immobility is a significant contributing factor for development of pneumonia.
- Goals of collaborative management:
    - Prevent pneumonia.
    - Provide early recognition and treatment.
    - Restore and maintain respiratory function.
    - Prevent complications (respiratory failure, sepsis).
    - Prevent recurrence.
- Important nursing diagnoses (actual or potential):
    - Ineffective breathing pattern related to respiratory muscle fatigue/hyper-hypoventilation
    - Ineffective airway clearance related to inflammation and presence of secretions
    - Impaired gas exchange related to decreased functional lung tissue
    - Impaired oral mucous membrane related to dry mouth from mouth breathing, decreased fluid intake
    - Pain related to pleurisy (chest pain), coughing, and breathing
    - Anxiety related to illness, difficulty breathing, knowledge deficit
    - Knowledge deficit related to risk factors predisposing person to pneumonia, treatment

- • Activity intolerance related to imbalance between oxygen supply and demand
- • Altered nutrition: less than body requirements related to loss of appetite
- • Risk for deficient fluid volume related to inadequate intake of fluids
- • **Key Terms/Concepts**: Aspiration, community-acquired pneumonia (CAP), hospital acquired pneumonia (HAP), infectious pneumonia, noninfectious pneumonia, respiratory failure, sepsis

Overview

Pneumonia is an acute inflammatory process of the lung parenchyma (the respiratory bronchioles and alveoli) that results in edema of lung tissue and movement of fluid into the alveoli. The source of inflammation can be infectious or noninfectious. Bacteria, viruses, fungi, protozoa, and other microbes can lead to infection. Microbes can enter the lung via a number of routes, including inhalation, the bloodstream, or spread from an adjacent locus of infection. The most common means of entry is aspiration of secretions containing microbes. Noninfectious causes of pneumonia include aspiration of food or fluids, inhalation of toxic or irritating gases, oversedation, and inadequate ventilation.

Risk Factors

- • Chronic underlying disease (e.g., COPD)
- • Severe acute illness (e.g., influenza) or other acute illness such as sinusitis
- • Recent anesthesia
- • Immune deficiency or suppression, such as AIDS, corticosteroid use
- • Exposure to infectious agents
- • Smoking
- • Dysphagia
- • Tracheostomy
- • Aspiration
- • Exposure to pulmonary pollutants
- • Immobility
- • Older age
- • Cold climates

Signs and Symptoms

- • Rapidly rising fever, chills
- • Productive cough with purulent, rust-colored, blood-tinged, or greenish sputum
- • Diaphoresis
- • Tachycardia
- • Tachypnea
- • Fatigue, weakness
- • Night sweats
- • Pleural pain (sudden onset of severe, sharp pain in chest, increases with breathing and coughing)

- Dyspnea
- Crackling breath sounds
- Decreased SAO_2
- Cyanosis, late sign

Diagnostic and Laboratory Tests

- History and physical examination
- CBC (complete blood count), WBC (white blood cell) count, and differential
- Chest x-ray
- Sputum culture/sputum gram stain
- Fiberoptic bronchoscopy may be done to obtain a sputum specimen or to remove secretions
- Blood culture, if bacteremia suspected
- ABGs (arterial blood gases) analysis
- Pulmonary function test
- Pulse oximetry

Therapeutic Nursing Management

- **Prevention/Teaching**:
  - Teach clients to prevent pneumonia by:
    - Avoiding large crowds during flu season and getting flu shots.
    - Receiving pneumococcal vaccine if older and at risk of pneumonia.
    - Instruct/assessing understanding of importance of hand washing and proper disposal of sputum.
    - Eating a nutritious diet.
  - Prevent aspiration of food, fluids or medications in at-risk clients, which can cause aspiration pneumonia.
  - Prevent contamination of aerosol inhalents.
  - Instruct on importance of medical follow-up and adherence to medical regimen
  - Prevent infection and mechanical trauma from oropharyngeal and nasopharyngeal suctioning.
- **Assess/Monitor**:
  - Respiratory status and monitor for compromise (tachypnea, use of accessory muscles)
  - Need for oropharyngeal or nasopharyngeal suctioning (restlessness, labored respirations, diaphoresis, adventitious breath sounds)
  - Monitor vital signs every two hours or as ordered
  - Monitor for fever, chills, night sweats
  - Monitor color, consistency, and amount of sputum
  - Assess nutritional status
  - Monitor/assess older adults for altered mental status, dehydration, and

signs/symptoms of organ failure or compromise related to decreased oxygen availability.

- Therapeutic response to oxygen therapy and aerosol treatments, and antibiotics or other medications

- **Nursing Activities:**
  - Encourage bed rest.
  - Encourage increased fluid intake.
  - Encourage deep breathing.
  - Position in semi-Fowler's position.
  - Administer oxygen therapy as prescribed.
  - Suction client as necessary via oropharyngeal or nasopharyngeal routes.
    - Use a sterile suction catheter, and discard catheter after each insertion.
    - Do not store suction catheters in any type of solution, including antibacterial solutions.
    - Use sterile gloves for the suctioning procedure.
    - Administer oxygen before, during, and after suctioning, as ordered.
  - If using the same catheter, suction the major bronchi first before suctioning the mouth and nose to prevent contamination of the lungs.
  - Vacuum pressures should not exceed 80-120 mmHg.
  - Insert catheter during inhalation and apply intermittent vacuum while withdrawing catheter.
  - Insertion, suctioning, and removal of catheter should not exceed 10 to 15 seconds.
  - Provide periods of rest.
  - Instruct client how to use nebulizers or metered dose inhalers for aerosolization.
  - Teach signs and symptoms of secondary infection.
  - Teach regarding antibiotic therapy (bacterial infections).

Pharmacology

- Immunizations (pneumonia, influenza)
- Antibiotics (organism-dependent - macrolides, cephalosporins, quinolones for CAP, aminoglycosides, quinolones, penicillins, beta-lactams, vancomycin, macrolides generally given IV for HAP)
- Bronchodilators (beta2 agonists)
- Corticosteroids (inhaled, oral, and intramuscular or intravenous)
- Mucolytics/Expectorants (guaifenesin)
- Antipyretics (acetaminophen, ibuprofen)
- Nasal decongestants (pseudoephedrine)
- Oxygen

Complications

- Atelectasis

- Pleural effusion
- Cardiac dysrhythmias
- Suctioning – infection, hypoxia leading to cardiac dysrhythmias, increased intracranial pressure, changes in blood pressure, etc.
- Respiratory failure, renal failure, heart failure
- Embolism – pulmonary embolism, myocardial infarction
- Bacteremia which may lead to meningitis, arthritis, endocarditis, pericarditis, and peritonitis in up to 10%
- ARDS (acute/adult respiratory distress syndrome)
- Shock
- Death

Age-Related Changes—Gerontological Considerations

- Changes of aging affect respiratory function and ability to fight infection.
- Increased risk for ineffective airway clearance is related to decreased cough reflex and muscle strength.
- Increased risk for pneumonia (primary or secondary) is due to age-related changes in lungs, such as decreased lung cilia and muscle strength. Drier mucous membranes decrease cilia function and increase the risk for inflammation and infection. Adequate hydration is important, as it helps liquefy secretions and aids in expectoration.
- Kyphosis and calcification of costal cartilage are common changes that cause restriction of the expansion of the thoracic cavity.
- Intercostal muscles and diaphragm lose elasticity resulting in decreased ability to breathe deeply and cough.
- As the elasticity of airways and alveoli decreases, the alveoli thickens and pulmonary blood decreases, resulting in an increased risk for impaired gas exchange, including a widening of the normal alveolar-arterial gradient (A-a gradient).
- Inactivity and immobility increase the risk of secretions pooling, thereby increasing the risk for pneumonia.
- Older clients often have trouble expectorating, which may lead to difficulty in breathing and make specimen retrieval more difficult.
- Neurologic changes associated with stroke and other conditions increase risk for aspiration pneumonia.
- Signs and symptoms of pneumonia are often atypical:
  - Fever, cough, and purulent sputum are often absent.
  - Generalized symptoms such as lethargy, chills, chest pain, tachypnea, vomiting and exacerbation of pre-existing conditions should be viewed with suspicion as they could indicate pneumonia. Main sign may be a change in LOC or mentation.
  - Obtain a chest x-ray and CBC if pneumonia is suspected.

Critical Thinking Exercise: Nursing Management of the Client with Pneumonia

Situation: An 88-year-old woman underwent a hip pinning four days ago after she fell and fractured her hip. She has a poor appetite and refuses to eat or drink most of the time. While the nurse was attempting to feed the woman two days ago, the woman moved her affected hip and gasped with pain. As she did, she aspirated the milk she was holding in her mouth and began coughing violently. Today the woman is lethargic, has an oral temperature of 101°F, crackling lung sounds on the left, and an elevated heart rate. It is determined the woman has pneumonia.

1. Complete these sentences:

   Pneumonia may be a _____ disease or _____ of another disease.

   _____ is a significant cause of _____ among _____ adults.

   _____ is a significant _____ factor for development of _____.

   Pneumonia related to a _____ substance in the _____ is known as _____ pneumonia.

2. Prioritize the client's nursing diagnoses, with "1" representing the most important diagnosis.

   _____ Altered nutrition: less than body requirements
   _____ Ineffective breathing pattern
   _____ Anxiety/fear
   _____ Pain
   _____ Knowledge deficit

3. How does the woman's pneumonia differ from other types of pneumonia?

4. What assessments does the nurse need to make that directly relate to the client's pneumonia?

_____ Skin integrity	_____ Temperature
_____ Urine output	_____ Peripheral pulses
_____ Heart rate	_____ Lung sounds
_____ Gag reflex	_____ Pain status

Nursing Management of the Client with Asthma

Key Points

- Asthma is a chronic inflammatory disorder of the airways that varies from mild, intermittent episodes to severe life-threatening events.
- It involves episodic increased tracheobronchial, or airway, responsiveness to various stimuli, resulting in widespread inflammation, narrowing of the airways (bronchoconstriction), and increased secretions.
- Asthma is classified as extrinsic or intrinsic.
- Although more common in children than adults, about 5% of the adult population is affected with asthma.
- Asthma may be a significant component of chronic obstructive pulmonary (lung) disease in the adult.
- The diagnosis of asthma is based primarily on the client's history and a high index of suspicion since client's with asthma generally have normal lung function (PFTs – pulmonary function tests) when not having an asthma exacerbation (attack).
- Goals of collaborative management:
  - Provide early recognition and treatment.
  - When an acute episode occurs, direct therapy at restoring airway patency and alveolar ventilation.
  - Prevent complications (respiratory collapse, status asthmaticus).
  - Prevent recurrence.
- Important nursing diagnoses (actual or potential):
  - Ineffective breathing pattern related to inadequate lung ventilation
  - Ineffective airway clearance related to bronchospasm and bronchoconstriction
  - Impaired gas exchange related to airway narrowing, edema and increased secretions
  - Anxiety and fear related to hypoxia and difficulty breathing
  - Knowledge deficit related to possible triggers, self-management
  - Activity intolerance related to ineffective respirations
  - Ineffective individual/family coping related to chronic disease
- **Key Terms/Concepts**: Acute, chronic, inflammatory, airway hyperresponsiveness, extrinsic asthma, and intrinsic asthma, status asthmaticus, bronchoconstriction, metered-dose inhaler

Overview

Asthma is a chronic inflammatory disease of the airways characterized by hyperresponsiveness, mucosal edema, bronchoconstriction, and excessive secretions. It is classified as extrinsic or intrinsic. Extrinsic is caused by external factors, such as environmental allergens (pollens, dust, feathers, etc.); intrinsic is from internal causes, not fully understood but often triggered by respiratory infection. Asthma can result from an altered immune response or increased airway resistance and altered air exchange. An acute asthma exacerbation may last from minutes to hours with symptom-free periods in between acute attacks. Asthma can present at any age, but most commonly begins in childhood. Asthma may be a significant component of chronic obstructive pulmonary disease (COPD) in adults. Asthma may be intermittent or persistent with symptoms ranging from mild to severe. A stepwise approach is used to both classify asthma based on frequency and severity and to guide treatment. If symptoms of asthma worsen, a step up in care is done; if symptoms improve, stepping down in treatment is carried out.

Risk Factors

- Hereditary predisposition
- Allergic rhinitis – approximately 78% of asthma clients complain of allergies and 58% of allergic clients complain of asthma
- Exposure to environmental irritants, dust, smoke
- Hypersensitivity to pollens, bee stings, foods, drugs, mold
- Respiratory infection – especially otitis media, sinusitis
- Sensitivity to aspirin and NSAIDs (non-steroidal anti-inflammatory drugs)
- Cold, dry air
- Exercise
- GERD (gastroesophageal reflux disease)

Signs and Symptoms

- Wheezing
- Cough
- Chest tightness/pain
- Wheezing or cough with exercise, exposure to cold, exposure to possible irritants, etc.
- Frequent bouts of "bronchitis"
- Waking up at night with coughing or wheezing
- Snoring
- GERD complaints

Diagnostic and Laboratory Tests

- History and physical examination
- ABG (arterial blood gas) analysis, rare unless status asthmaticus suspected
- Pulse oximetry

- CBC (complete blood count), to rule out other causes of shortness-of-breath
- Sputum culture, to rule out infectious source of breathing difficulty
- Pulmonary function tests
- Peak flow (peak expiratory flow rate) if unable to obtain PFTs
- Hypersensitivity testing, allergy testing for possible immunotherapy (allergy shots) if allergies are main triggers
- Bronchoprovocation testing, if diagnosis unsure
- Chest x-ray, to rule out other causes of shortness-of-breath such as pneumonia, cardiomyopathy

Therapeutic Nursing Management

- Assess/Monitor:
  - Respiratory status (assess vital signs and lung sounds every two to four hours).
  - Cardiac status
- Nursing Activities:
  - Initiate intravenous access.
  - Administer other prescribed medications/breathing treatments.
  - Administer humidified oxygen.
  - Decrease anxiety.
  - Place in high-Fowler's position.
  - Increase fluid intake.
  - Instruct client to recognize triggering agents.
  - Eliminate causative agents when possible (dust, pets, smoke, pollen, stress).
  - Include teaching about the specific medications prescribed and their expected effects.
  - Instruct clients about procedures (PFTs, nebulizer treatment, and other respiratory treatments such as percussion and postural drainage).
  - If client is a smoker, initiate teaching about the effects of tobacco smoke on asthma.
  - Instruct client on prevention of infections (adequate rest, good nutrition, and stress management to help maintain immune function).
  - Encourage yearly vaccine for influenza, consider pneumococcal pneumonia.
  - Provide referral for local support groups for continued teaching and support as needed.
  - Teach client regarding self-management:
    - Avoidance of triggers
    - Instruction on use of Peak Flow Meter (if ordered)
    - Asthma Action Plan – use of Zone System
      - Green – client at 80 to 100% predicted of PEFR (peak expiratory flow rate) or breathing without difficulty, able to complete daily activities

- • Yellow – client at 50(60) to 80% of predicted PEFR or having some difficulty with breathing such as wheezing, coughing, or shortness-of-breath
  - • Red – client at 50% or below predicted PEFR or having severe difficulty breathing
- - Medications
  - • Controller medications – used for clients with persistent symptoms, inhaled corticosteroids, step 4/sever persistent inhaled corticosteroids, and long acting beta2 agonists. Alternatives include leukotriene receptor antagonist, cromolyn (mast cell inhibitor) by nebulizer, and theophylline (methylxanthines).
  - • Rescue medications – short acting beta2 agonists
  - • Oral corticosteroids – under certain conditions for acute, sever exacerbations
- - Proper inhaler use – dependent upon type of inhaler, with or without spacer device. Very important. Most clients do not properly use their inhaler. Should go over technique at each office visit.
  - • Metered dose inhaler (MDI)
  - • Auto inhaler – combination inhaler/spacer
  - • Dry powder inhalers (DPIs)
  - • In general, inspiration with all inhalers, if no spacer used, should be deep and long (over 3-5 seconds). Type of inhaler dictates if inhalation is fast or slow, generally MDIs utilize slow inhalation and DPIs a quicker inhalation. Techniques include "closed" mouth and "open" mouth. In closed mouth the inhaler is placed in the mouth before actuation. In open mouth the inhaler is placed 1-2" or 2 finger widths away from the mouth before actuation. After inhaling, the breath is then held for 8-10 seconds.

Pharmacology

- • Beta2 agonists
- • Anticholinergics
- • Corticosteroids
- • Leukotriene receptor antagonists
- • Mast cell inhibitors
- • Methylxanthines
- • Antihistamines (especially when allergies trigger asthma)
- • Oxygen

Complications

- • Respiratory failure
- • Respiratory acidosis
- • Hypoxia

- Pneumothorax
- Status asthmaticus
- Death

Age-Related Changes—Gerontological Considerations

- Lung and airway changes as a part of aging make pulmonary problems more serious in the older adult. One problem thought to be related to aging is a change in the sensitivity of beta-adrenergic receptors. When stimulated, these receptors relax bronchial smooth muscle and cause bronchodilation. As these receptors become less sensitive, they no longer respond as quickly or as strongly to naturally occurring agonists and beta-adrenergic medications. Increased risk for respiratory complications is related to decreased muscle strength required for coughing and deep breathing.

- Asthma was thought previously to rarely develop in the elderly. However, it is now estimated to be as prevalent in the elderly as in young adults; yet the risk of hospitalization due to asthma is twice as high in the elderly as in the young adult and death related to asthma is 11 times greater in elderly than in the young adult!

- Elderly clients with asthma may not have complete reversibility of their asthma.

- The elderly have a higher incidence of near-fatal asthma episodes related to delay in diagnosis and treatment, decreased cardiac function from normal aging, decreased respiratory function that normally occurs with aging, blunted chemoreceptors needed for hypoxic ventilatory drive, and possible decreased perception of difficulty with breathing. These changes along with other comorbid factors may make the elderly much more vulnerable to fatality associated with asthma exacerbations.

Critical Thinking Exercise: Nursing Management of the Client with Asthma

Situation: A 59-year-old man lives in a cool, dry part of the country. Upon visiting his daughter who lives in a warm, humid part of the country, the man begins to experience chest tightness, wheezing, and a hacking, non-productive cough. The man has a history of asthma and allergy to molds.

1. Which are the common risk factors for asthma?

    _____ Colds   _____ Dust

    _____ Genetics   _____ Smoking

    _____ Mold   _____ Drugs

    _____ Exercise   _____ Humid air

2. What is the etiology for the client's nursing diagnoses?

    a. Ineffective breathing pattern

    b. Anxiety/fear

    c. Fatigue

3. Prioritize the following nursing interventions for the client experiencing an asthmatic attack, with "1" representing the first intervention to implement.

    _____ Offer emotional support

    _____ Raise the head of the bed

    _____ Establish a patent airway

    _____ Assess vital signs

Nursing Management of the Client with Status Asthmaticus

Key Points

- Status asthmaticus is characterized by an acute episode of bronchospasm that greatly increases the workload of breathing.
- Individuals between 40 and 60 years of age with a history of asthma, and children younger than two years of age are more susceptible to status asthmaticus.
- Approximately 10% of clients admitted to the hospital with status asthmaticus require treatment in an ICU (Intensive Care Unit) and mechanical ventilation.
- Hypersensitivity to aspirin may precipitate an attack.
- Pathophysiology of status asthmaticus involves decreased diameter of the bronchi, and a ventilation-perfusion abnormality.
- Goals of collaborative management:
  - Provide immediate recognition and emergency treatment.
  - Correct hypoxemia.
  - Improve ventilation.
  - Prevent respiratory failure.
- Important nursing diagnoses (actual or potential):
  - Ineffective breathing pattern related to changes in lung ventilation (decreased lung expansion and emptying)
  - Ineffective airway clearance related to bronchospasm, bronchoconstriction, increased mucus secretion and airway edema.
  - Impaired gas exchange related to airway narrowing and edema
  - Risk for infection related to ineffective airway clearance
  - Anxiety related to difficulty breathing (hypoxia) and fear of death
  - Ineffective health maintenance related to therapeutic regimen
- **Key Terms/Concepts:** Bronchospasm, severe dyspnea, hypoxemia, hypoventilation, hypercapnia, acidosis, respiratory failure, arterial blood gases (ABGs), mechanical ventilation

Overview

Status asthmaticus is a severe, persistent, and life-threatening attack of asthma, which is refractory to regular treatment. Without aggressive therapy, status asthmaticus can lead to respiratory failure with hypoxemia, hypercapnia, respiratory acidosis, and inability to ventilate. Subsequently, the client may require intubation and mechanical ventilation along with aggressive pharmacologic therapy to sustain life.

Risk Factors

- Upper and lower respiratory infections
- Exposure to triggers
- Ingestion of aspirin or other NSAIDs (Non-steroidal anti-inflammatory drugs)
- Abrupt cessation of corticosteroid or theophylline therapy
- Abuse of aerosol treatments
- Poor control of asthma over several days or weeks
- Undiagnosed asthma

Signs and Symptoms

- Severe, prolonged dyspnea
- Severe inspiratory and expiratory wheezing
- Non-productive cough
- Hypertension
- Orthopnea
- Diminished breath sounds
- Nasal flaring
- Prolonged expiration
- Tachypnea
- Use of accessory muscles of breathing
- Intercostal retractions
- Inability to speak in complete sentences
- Inability to perform pulmonary assessment such as spirometry or peak expiratory flow
- Sinus tachycardia
- Severe restlessness and apprehension
- Exhaustion
- Inaudible breath sounds with reduced wheezing and an ineffective cough may signify impending respiratory arrest

Diagnostic and Laboratory Tests

- History from family member and physical examination
- Pulmonary function tests:
  - Air flow (spirometer)
  - Lung volume
  - Diffusion capacity (correlates with body's ability to extract oxygen from the lungs)
- ABG (arterial blood gas) analysis
- Examination of sputum (in a client with asthma shows the presence of many eosinophils and other WBCs)

- Chest x-ray
- Pulse oximetry
- ECG (Electrocardiogram)

Therapeutic Nursing Management

- **Prevention**:
    - Teach client:
        - To avoid allergens and environmental triggers.
        - To modify causative household environment agents.
        - To use prophylactic medications correctly.
        - To avoid exposure to respiratory infections.
        - Initiation and adherence to Asthma Action Plan
        - That early treatment of respiratory infections is vital to preventing asthmatic exacerbations.
        - To maintain adequate hydration at home.
        - To monitor PEFR (peak expiratory flow rates) daily using a Peak Flow Meter.
        - To contact primary care provider or go to Emergency Department when asthma symptoms are not controlled by usual measures (e.g., use of an inhaler) or have fallen into the red zone on action plan.
- **Assess/Monitor**:
    - Respiratory status continually until exacerbation resolved (rate, depth, chest movement or excursion and breath sounds; SaO2)
    - Client's cough effort and sputum for color consistency, and amount
    - For changes in level of consciousness
    - Skin color, turgor and temperature
    - Vital signs
    - ABGs (arterial blood gases)
    - Pulmonary function test results, not usually possible during statis
    - Pulse oximetry
    - PEFR (peak expiratory flow rates) (usually not possible during statis)
- **Nursing Activities**:
    - Provide constant reassurance.
    - Position in Fowler's, high-Fowler's, or orthopnea position..
    - Provide a quiet environment as free of allergens as possible.
    - Administer humidified low-flow oxygen via Venturi mask or nasal cannula.
    - Administer intravenous infusions.
    - Administer nebulizer treatments.
    - Administer prescribed medications.
    - Provide endotracheal suctioning as needed.
    - Assist with intubation and mechanical ventilation if indicated by blood gases.

- Develop an action plan with the family in the event of another severe asthma attack.
  - Before discharge, Asthma Action Plan should be developed or revised to prevent recurrence.

Pharmacology

- Intravenous corticosteroids (methylprednisolone)
- Beta2 agonists, hourly or continuously with or without inhaled anticholinergic
- Oxygen
- Intravenous infusions
- Possible use of IV methylxanthines
- In special or severe cases, use of magnesium IV, paralytic agents, or anesthetic agents may be used to reverse severe bronchospasm and inflammation when ventilation is essentially impossible and the client is impending respiratory arrest.

Complications

- Respiratory acidosis
- Respiratory infection
- Atelectasis
- Ventricular arrhythmias
- Pulmonary hypertension and pulsus paradoxica
- Metabolic alkalosis
- Pneumothorax
- Cardiac arrest
- Respiratory failure

Age-Related Changes—Gerontological Considerations

- Older clients may have pre-existing cardiovascular or respiratory problems that can complicate treatment for status asthmaticus.

Critical Thinking Exercise: Nursing Management of the Client with Status Asthmaticus

Situation: A 45-year-old female client with status asthmaticus has just been transferred to the ICU (Intensive Care Unit) from the emergency department. The client's husband states his wife has been experiencing episodes of asthma for several days, which have not been relieved by using her metered-dose inhaler. The client is experiencing severe dyspnea and wheezing. In addition, the client is restless and very fearful.

1. Prioritize nursing activities for the client, with "1" representing the activity to implement first.

_____ Administer prescribed medications.

_____ Use calm, reassuring approach.

_____ Maintain patent airway.

_____ Administer oxygen.

_____ Monitor for drug side effects.

2. How does status asthmaticus differ from the usual asthma attack?

3. What is the purpose of increasing intravenous fluid intake in the client suffering status asthmaticus?

4. Which are goals of mechanical ventilation for the client with status asthmaticus?

5. What is the purpose of administering these drugs to clients with status asthmaticus?

    a.   Corticosteroids

    b.   Theophylline

Nursing Management of the Client with Chronic Obstructive Pulmonary Disease (COPD)

Key Points

- Chronic obstructive pulmonary disease (COPD) is a significant cause of morbidity and mortality in the United States.
- COPD is not an individual disease, but a group of several diseases that result in obstructed airflow.
- COPD is characterized by diminished inspiratory and expiratory lung capacity.
- Symptoms usually develop when a client is in their 40s, and progress to disability by their 50s and 60s.
- Primary cause is cigarette smoking; usually about 30 to 35 years between onset of smoking and development of symptoms
- Prevention is an important component of treatment.
- Goals of collaborative management:
    - Provide early recognition and treatment; to a certain extent, airway obstruction can be reversed and disability minimized early in the disease.
    - Restore maximum respiratory function.
    - Prevent complications (respiratory failure, pneumonia).
    - Prevent recurrence.
- Important nursing diagnoses (actual or potential):
    - Ineffective breathing pattern related to airway obstruction
    - Ineffective airway clearance related to excessive secretions, fatigue, and ineffective cough
    - Impaired gas exchange related to diminished airway size, alveolar membrane changes, respiratory muscle fatigue
    - Anxiety and fear related to loss of control during exacerbation of the disease, breathlessness
    - Ineffective health maintenance related to deficient knowledge regarding the disease
    - Activity intolerance related to fatigue, imbalance between oxygen supply and demand
    - Potential complications of COPD (chronic obstructive pulmonary disease)
    - Imbalanced nutrition: less than body requirements related to decreased intake due to dyspnea
    - Self-care deficit related to fatigue secondary to increased work of breathing
    - Ineffective individual/family coping related to reluctance to accept responsibility

- Noncompliance related to reluctance to accept responsibility for changing detrimental health practices, such as tobacco abuse
- Powerlessness related to progressive nature of the disease
- **Key Terms/Concepts:** Progressive, obstructive respiratory/pulmonary disease, emphysema, chronic bronchitis, asthma, cystic fibrosis, bronchiectasis

Overview

Chronic obstructive pulmonary disease (or chronic obstructive lung disease) is a chronic, progressive, irreversible group of obstructive airflow diseases (asthma, chronic bronchitis, emphysema, cystic fibrosis, and bronchiectasis) that produce increased airway resistance, and permanent lung distention. However, asthma is generally considered reversible and non-progressive, especially if under control. Obstructive lung disease typically affects middle-aged and older adults. Cigarette smoking is clearly implicated as a primary cause. Most commonly COPD refers to emphysema and/or chronic bronchitis. Emphysema is a disease of the distal or terminal airways and involves the lung parenchyma. Chronic bronchitis is a persistent cough with sputum production, on most days, for at least three months during the previous two years.

Risk Factors

- Cigarette smoking
- Chronic exposure to air pollutants (coal, cotton, grain)
- Chronic lung infections
- Nutrition
- Genetic predisposition – alpha 1 antitrypsin deficiency, cystic fibrosis

Signs and Symptoms

- Most common symptom may be gradual, progressive, exertional dyspnea
- Productive cough, dyspnea, and exercise intolerance
- Wheezing
- Rhonchi
- Increased sputum production
- Hemoptysis
- Decreased breath sounds
- Recurrent respiratory infections
- Tachypnea
- Tachycardia
- Barrel chest, increased A-P (anterior-posterior) diameter
- Use of accessory muscles
- Cyanosis
- Orthopnea
- Hypoxia
- Fatigue

- Peripheral edema
- Chronic weight loss with emaciation
- Possible signs and symptoms of right heart failure if long-standing

Diagnostic and Laboratory Tests

- History and physical examination
- Pulmonary function tests:
  - Air flow (spirometer)
  - Lung volume
  - Diffusion capacity (correlates with body's ability to extract oxygen from the lungs)
- ABG (arterial blood gas) analysis
- CBC (complete blood count), WBC (white blood cell) count, and differential
- Serum alpha 1-antitrypsin levels: (COPD clients with a family history of obstructive airway disease, those with an early onset, women, and nonsmokers should be screened)
- Pulse oximetry
- Chest x-rays
- Sputum cultures
- Bronchoscopy
- Thoracic computed tomography (CT) may be ordered to localize emphysematous changes in the lungs and/or to rule out lung cancer.

Therapeutic Nursing Management

- **Assess/Monitor:**
  - Respiratory status and oxygenation needs
  - Vital signs
  - Nutritional status
  - For effectiveness and side effects of prescribed medications
  - For respiratory compromise
- **Nursing Activities:**
  - Teach purse-lip, diaphragmatic, or abdominal breathing techniques.
  - Administer oxygen as prescribed. (Avoid high levels of oxygen. Hypoxemia is the stimulus for respiration via carotid chemoreceptors. If PaO2 levels are elevated, the drive to breathe may be suppressed, causing apnea).
  - Position client for maximum ventilation and to mobilize secretions.
  - Teach respiratory exercises.
  - Assist with postural drainage, percussion, and vibration.
  - Encourage fluid intake up to 2000-3000 mL/day, if not contraindicated.
  - Instruct on proper nutritional needs:
    - Client with emphysema has an increased protein and caloric requirement.

- Adequate protein and calories should be divided into five or six small meals per day. Large meals may increase shortness-of-breath by increasing activity level.
- Assist with activities as needed.
- Avoid respiratory irritants.
- Encourage and/or assist with smoking cessation.
- Teach client signs and symptoms of hypoxia.
- Teach use of medications and inhalers (a spacer used with an inhaler can assist in the delivery of the medication deeper into the airways, using each dose more efficiently).
- Teach client regarding signs and symptoms associated with secondary infection.
- Teach client to avoid extremes in temperature or humidity.
- Instruct client to avoid contact with those with an active respiratory infection.
- Instruct on the importance of receiving immunizations for prevention of influenza and pneumonia.

Pharmacology

- Immunizations (pneumonia, influenza)
- Antibiotics (when bacterial infection present)
- Bronchodilators (ipratropium, albuterol, salmeterol)
- Corticosteroids
  - Oral or intravenous: prednisone, methylprednisolone
  - Inhaled: fluticasone, beclomethasone, triamcinolone
- Oxygen, possible for persistent SaO_2 below 90% or PaO_2 below 60 mmHg

Complications

- Respiratory insufficiency or failure
- Pneumonia
- Atelectasis
- Pulmonary hypertension
- Cor pulmonale
- Pneumothorax
- CHF (congestive heart failure)
- ARDS (acute respiratory distress syndrome)
- Death

Age-Related Changes—Gerontological Considerations

- Increased risk for respiratory failure and inadequate airway clearance is due to decreased ciliary action and muscle strength.
- Classic symptoms of COPD (productive cough, fever, chest pain) may be absent.

- Increased risk for pneumonia secondary to COPD may present with confusion and general deterioration.
- More common in the elderly and more common to progressively worsen. Require frequent monitoring and follow-up

Critical Thinking Exercise: Nursing Management of the Client with Chronic Obstructive Pulmonary Disease (COPD)

Situation: A 60-year-old male is being treated for COPD (chronic obstructive pulmonary disease). Assessment reveals a thin, frail man with a barrel chest who leans forward to breathe. Breath sounds are decreased bilaterally and the client is tachycardic with a respiratory rate of 36. Low dose oxygen therapy, an aminophylline drip, and bed rest have been prescribed.

1. Place an "S" in front of those nursing diagnoses that are **supported** by the client's data and a "P" in front of those that are **possible**, but unsupported by the client's data.

   _____ Ineffective airway clearance   _____ Activity intolerance

   _____ Anxiety/fear   _____ Ineffective individual/family coping

   _____ Fatigue   _____ Powerlessness

   _____ Potential complications of COPD   _____ Knowledge deficit

   _____ Ineffective individual/family management of therapeutic regimen

   _____ Altered nutrition: less than body requirements

   _____ Self-care deficit

2. What is the rationale for administering low-dose oxygen to the client?

3. Which criteria will the nurse use to evaluate the effectiveness of the client's oxygen therapy?

   _____ Reduced dyspnea   _____ Improving respiratory rate

   _____ Normal skin color   _____ Mental alertness

   _____ Increased fluid intake   _____ Quiet sleep

   _____ Pink nail beds   _____ Increased appetite

4. Prioritize the following nursing interventions, with "1" representing the most important intervention.

_____ Initiate infusion of intravenous antibiotic as prescribed.

_____ Check O_2 saturation.

_____ Auscultate breath sounds.

_____ Administer acetaminophen (Tylenol) for fever as prescribed.

_____ Collect and send sputum specimen to laboratory for culture.

5. What is the purpose of the aminophylline drip and what symptoms will it help improve or eliminate?

Nursing Management of the Client with Hemothorax/ Pneumothorax

Key Points

- Air or blood in the pleural space prevents lung expansion and subsequent exchange of oxygen and carbon dioxide.
- Tension pneumothorax is a medical emergency because both respiratory and circulatory systems are affected. Hemothorax is frequently found in association with an open pneumothorax and is then called a hemopneumothorax.
- Goals of collaborative management:
    - Remove air or blood from the pleural space to normalize pulmonary function
        - The most definitive and common form of treatment of pneumothorax and hemothorax is to insert a chest tube and connect it to water-seal drainage until the lung reinflates.
    - Maintain ventilation and perfusion.
    - Maintain fluid balance.
    - Prevent recurrence.
- Important nursing diagnoses (actual or potential):
    - Ineffective breathing pattern
    - Ineffective airway clearance
    - Anxiety and fear
    - Knowledge deficit
    - Fatigue and restlessness
    - Risk for infection
- **Key Terms/Concepts:** Pneumothorax, closed pneumothorax, open pneumothorax, tension pneumothorax, hemothorax, hemopneumothorax, water-seal drainage

Overview

Both conditions result in partial or complete collapse of the lung.

- **Hemothorax** is the accumulation of blood within the chest cavity. Causes of hemothorax include chest trauma, lung malignancy, complications of anticoagulant therapy, pulmonary embolus, and tearing of pleural adhesions.
- **Pneumothorax** is the accumulation of air within the pleural space producing increased intrathoracic pressure and decreased vital capacity. This condition should be suspected after any blunt trauma. There are several types:
    - Closed pneumothorax has no associated external wound. The most

common form is a spontaneous pneumothorax caused by rupture of small blebs on the visceral pleural space (rupture of an apical pleural bleb).

- Open pneumothorax occurs when air enters the pleural space through an opening in the chest wall. Examples include blunt or sharp trauma such as a stab wound or gunshot wound and surgical thoracotomies.
- Tension pneumothorax may result from either an open or a closed pneumothorax. Intrathoracic pressure increases, the lung collapses, and the mediastinum shifts toward the unaffected side. This can occur from mechanical ventilation and resuscitative efforts.

Risk Factors

- Blunt, crushing, or penetrating chest injury
- Interstitial lung disease (COPD, emphysema)
- Liver or kidney disorders that cause hypoproteinemia
- Invasive thoracic procedures (thoracentesis)
- Insertion of central venous catheter or pulmonary artery catheter
- Mechanical ventilation

Signs and Symptoms

- Sudden onset of pleuritic pain
- Tachypnea, dyspnea
- Use of accessory muscles
- Anxiety, apprehension
- Absence of breath sounds on affected side
- Hypotension
- Tachycardia
- Cyanosis
- Subcutaneous emphysema
- Hemothorax: dullness to percussion
- Tension pneumothorax: hyper-resonance to percussion, neck vein distention, tracheal deviation
- Shifting of the mediastinum to the unaffected side with compression of the great vessels

Diagnostic Tests

- History and physical exam
- Chest x-rays
- ABG (arterial blood gas) analysis
- Pulse oximetry

Therapeutic Nursing Management

- **Assess/Monitor:**
  - Chest tube placement and function (water seal drainage)
  - Respiratory status and oxygen saturations
  - For respiratory compromise
  - Chest tube insertion site for redness, pain, infection, and crepitus
  - Chest tube for amount of drainage if hemothorax or hemopneumothorax
- **Nursing Activities:**
  - Assess for early identification of persons at risk.
  - Administer oxygen as prescribed.
  - Position in high-Fowler's position.
  - Prepare client for surgery if necessary.
  - Explain all procedures.
  - Provide emotional support to client and family.

Complications

- Hypoxemia
- Respiratory failure
- Decreased cardiac output
- Death

Age-Related Changes—Gerontological Considerations

- Ventilation-perfusion imbalance results from the presence of blood with hemothorax or trapped air with pneumothorax. Poor oxygenation can lead more quickly to serious consequences in the older adult because many have decreased pulmonary reserves. If untreated, hypoxemia, respiratory acidosis and death can occur rapidly.

- The clinical presentation is similar to the older adult with congestive heart failure. In both conditions, the client exhibits dyspnea, distended neck veins, pallor with poor circulatory perfusion and coughing. However, the distinguishing characteristic of pneumothorax and hemothorax from heart failure is the rapid deterioration in respiratory status; this is a true medical emergency requiring prompt intervention.

Critical Thinking Exercise: Nursing Management of the Client with Hemothorax/Pneumothorax

Situation: A 25-year-old man is admitted to the trauma unit following a motorcycle accident in which he suffered rib fractures and a pneumothorax. He has a chest tube in place on the right that is connected to water seal drainage with 20 cm of suction.

1. Match the description with the type of problem it produces. Use "P", "H" or "B" as a response.

P = Pneumothorax	Air enters the pleural space due to trauma or disease
H = Hemothorax	Produces collapse of the lung or portion of the lung
B = Both	Trauma allows blood to collect in the pleural cavity
	Causes increased intrathoracic pressure
	Results in decreased vital capacity
	May be spontaneous or traumatic

2. Of the following, which four assessments are of highest priority for the client with a chest tube in place?

_____ Respiratory status   _____ Oxygen saturations

_____ Bowel sounds   _____ Urinary output

_____ Pain   _____ Appetite

_____ Fever   _____ Anxiety

3. While getting out of bed, the client pulls his chest tube out of his chest wall. What is the first response on the part of the nurse, to this incident?

4. Which nursing diagnoses need to be placed on the client's care plan?

_____ Risk for ineffective breathing pattern

_____ Risk for ineffective airway clearance

_____ Anxiety/fear

_____ Risk for activity intolerance

_____ Risk for infection

Nursing Management of the Client with Acute Respiratory Distress Syndrome (ARDS)

Key Points

- ARDS is a sudden and progressive form of acute respiratory failure characterized by non-cardiac pulmonary edema and progressive refractory hypoxemia.
- The alveolar capillary membrane becomes damaged and more permeable allowing fluid to leak into the interstitial spaces and alveoli.
- Incidence of acute/adult respiratory distress syndrome (ARDS) in the United States is estimated at more than 150,000 cases yearly.
- Despite supportive therapy, the mortality rate from ARDS is approximately 50%.
- The exact etiology for damage to the alveoli is unknown.
- ARDS is referred to as shock lung, wet lung, and post-traumatic lung.
- The phases of ARDS pathophysiology are:
    - (1) Injury or exudative phase: interstitial and alveolar edema and atelectasis
    - (2) Reparative or proliferative phase: 1 to 2 weeks after the initial lung injury, influx of granulocytes, monocytes, and lymphocytes and fibroblast proliferation as part of the inflammatory response; increased pulmonary vascular resistance and pulmonary hypertension may occur
    - (3) Fibrotic phase: occurs 2 to 3 weeks after the initial lung injury; chronic or late stage, diffuse scarring and fibrosis resulting in decreased lung compliance.
- Goals of collaborative management:
    - Identify and treat the underlying cause of the syndrome.
    - Maintain adequate oxygenation.
    - Treat the cause (drug overdose, infections, or inhaled toxins).
    - Provide aggressive respiratory support.
    - Provide fluid management with intravenous solutions as needed.
    - Provide nutritional support.
    - Prevent complications.
- Important nursing diagnoses (actual or potential):
    - Ineffective breathing pattern
    - Ineffective airway clearance
    - Impaired gas exchange
    - Altered tissue perfusion: cardiopulmonary related to damaged alveolar-capillary membrane
    - Risk for fluid volume excess
    - Altered nutrition: less than body requirements

- Anxiety and fear
- **Key Terms/Concepts:** Alveolar-capillary membrane damage, hypoxemia, pulmonary edema, injury or exudative phase, reparative or proliferative phase, fibrotic phase

Overview

Adult/acute respiratory distress syndrome (ARDS) is a sudden and progressive type of acute respiratory failure. The underlying pathology in ARDS is acute lung injury resulting from an unregulated systemic inflammatory response to acute injury or inflammation. ARDS may also develop as a consequence of multiple organ dysfunction syndromes (MODS). Inflammatory cellular responses and biochemical mediators damage the alveolar-capillary membrane. This damage develops rapidly, often within 90 minutes of the systemic inflammatory response and within 24 hours of the initial insult causing severe dyspnea, hypoxemia, reduced lung compliance, pulmonary edema, and atelectasis. The two risk factors most commonly associated with ARDS are gram-negative septic shock and aspiration of gastric contents. Clients with multiple risk factors are 3 to 4 times more likely to develop ARDS.

Risk Factors

- Direct lung trauma
  - Pneumonia
  - Prolonged inhalation of smoke or other toxic substances
  - Lung contusion
  - Aspiration of gastric contents
  - Fat embolus
  - Near drowning
- Indirect lung trauma
  - Shock
  - Sepsis
  - DIC (disseminated intravascular coagulation)
  - Drug overdose
  - Increased intracranial pressure
  - Multisystem trauma
  - Cardiopulmonary bypass
  - Anaphylaxis

Signs and Symptoms

- Initial presentation is insidious (several hours to 1-2 days)
- Cough
- Restlessness
- Progressive dyspnea
- Tachypnea
- Fine scattered crackles

- As ARDS progresses:
  - Labored breathing and dyspnea
  - Intercostals and suprasternal retractions
  - Altered sensorium due to elevated $PaCO_2$ and decreased PaO_2
  - Adventitious breath sounds (scattered to diffuse crackles)
  - Tachycardia
  - Hypotension
  - Cyanosis
  - Pallor
- Late stage: profound respiratory distress requiring endotracheal intubation

Diagnostic and Laboratory Tests

- History and physical exam
- ABGs (arterial blood gases)
- Chest x-ray
- Serum electrolyte levels
- Insertion of pulmonary artery catheter for monitoring of pulmonary artery, pulmonary artery wedge pressures, and cardiac output
- Hemoglobin
- Hematocrit

Therapeutic Nursing Management

- **Prevention**:
  - Monitor respiratory status in at-risk clients.
  - Begin immediate intervention upon diagnosis of ARDS to prevent complications.
- **Assess/Monitor**:
  - For lung congestion by monitoring depth and rhythm of respirations, adventitious sounds, and jugular vein distention
  - For cyanosis
  - For peripheral edema
  - Mechanical ventilator sounds, alarms, and connections hourly
- **Nursing Activities**:
  - Initiate continuous hemodynamic monitoring (critical care environment).
  - Provide oxygen therapy.
  - Provide oxygen saturation monitoring.
  - Provide continuous mechanical ventilation via ET (endotracheal tube) with PEEP (positive end-expiratory pressure) as ordered.
  - Administer intravenous fluids cautiously.
  - Record intake and output and daily weight.
  - Suction as necessary.
  - Reposition the client every two hours.

- Provide reassurance and emotional support.
- Administer sedation as needed.
- Teaching (focuses on the acute illness period):
  - Teach slow pursed-lip breathing techniques.
  - Explain all procedures, tubes, equipment, and therapeutic interventions to the client and family.
  - Provide reassurance to client and family that mechanical ventilation are temporary measures.
  - Provide factual information about ARDS and its prognosis.
  - Explain the importance of rest.
  - Explain the purpose and side effects of all medications.
  - If client has been a smoker, stress the importance of avoiding cigarette smoking in the future.

Pharmacology

- Oxygen
- Inotropic drugs (dobutamine or dopamine)
- Sedatives (benzodiazepines)
- Antibiotics (if bacterial infection present)
- Diuretics (furosemide)
- Corticosteroids

Complications

- Sepsis
- Pulmonary emboli
- Nosocomial pneumonia
- ARF (acute renal failure)
- Cardiac arrhythmias
- Oxygen toxicity
- Gastrointestinal bleeding secondary to stress ulcers
- Anemia
- Lung fibrosis
- Tracheal ulceration from ET (endotracheal) tube
- Malposition or inadvertent extubation of ET tube
- Pulmonary barotrauma from continuous mechanical ventilation
- MODS (multiple organ dysfunction syndrome)
- Death

Age-Related Changes—Gerontological Considerations

- Older adults are at a higher risk of developing respiratory failure because of the reduction in ventilatory capacity that accompanies aging, especially if other risk factors are present.

- In older adults, the PaO_2 falls further and the $PaCO_2$ rises to a higher level before the respiratory system is stimulated to alter the rate and depth of breathing. This delayed response predisposes to the development of respiratory failure.

Critical Thinking Exercise: Nursing Management of the Client with Acute Respiratory Distress Syndrome (ARDS)

Situation: A 40-year-old male in acute respiratory distress has been admitted to the ICU (Intensive Care Unit) following an automobile accident during which he suffered direct lung trauma. The client has been placed in a prone position and his vital signs and ABG (arterial blood gas) values are being continuously monitored. The client initially received oxygen via a mask with a high flow system, but he is now on a mechanical ventilator using PEEP (positive end-expiratory pressure). The client is extremely anxious and is also frustrated that he cannot speak due to the placement of an endotrachea tube.

1. Which of the client's symptoms indicates his ARDS is progressing?

_____ Hypertension	_____ Intracostal retraction	_____ Bradycardi
_____ Tachypnea	_____ Complaints of nausea	_____ Blurred vision
_____ Tachycardia	_____ Warm, dry skin	_____ Changes in sensorium
_____ Pallor	_____ Cyanosis	_____ Non-productive cough

2. What does PEEP stand for and what does it do?

3. Which is/are the primary purpose(s) for monitoring the client's ABGs (arterial blood gases)?

_____ To determine if the client is being adequately oxygenated

_____ To assess the client's fluid balance

_____ To establish what medications are needed

_____ To identify the clinical findings associates with hypoxemia

4. List at least three nursing interventions to allay the client's anxiety, fear, and frustration.

Nursing Management of the Client with Acute Respiratory Failure

Key Points

- Respiratory failure is not a disease, but rather a consequence of severe respiratory dysfunction.
- In respiratory failure, the lungs are unable to oxygenate the blood and remove carbon dioxide adequately to meet the body's needs, even at rest.
- Respiratory failure can result from inadequate ventilation of the alveoli, impaired gas exchange, or a significant ventilation-perfusion mismatch.
- COPD is the most common cause of respiratory failure.
- Other lung diseases, chest injury, inhalation trauma, neuromuscular disorders, and cardiac conditions can also lead to respiratory failure.
- Prevention is an important aspect of treatment.
- Goals of collaborative management:
  - Correct the underlying cause or disease process.
  - Support ventilation.
  - Correct hypoxemia and hypercapnia.
  - Provide early recognition and treatment.
  - Prevent recurrence.
- Important nursing diagnoses (actual or potential):
  - Ineffective breathing pattern related to excessive secretion, decreased level of consciousness, presence of an artificial airway, neuromuscular dysfunction and pain.
  - Ineffective airway clearance related to neuromuscular impairment of respirations, pain, anxiety, decreased level of consciousness, respiratory muscle fatigue and bronchospasm
  - Impaired gas exchange related alveolar hypoventilation, intrapulmonary shunting, V/Q mismatch and diffusion impairment
  - Anxiety and fear related to artificial airway, feeling of dyspnea
  - Knowledge deficit related to underlying cause or disease process
  - Fatigue related to increased respiratory effort
  - Altered nutrition: less than body requirements related to poor appetite, shortness of breath, presence of artificial airway, and increased caloric requirements
  - Self-care deficit related to critical illness
  - Impaired physical mobility related to the presence of multiple tubes, wires and monitors

- Activity intolerance
- Ineffective individual/family coping
- Decreased cardiac output
- Decreased cerebral perfusion
- **Key Terms/Concepts:** Hypoxemia, hypoxia, hypercarbia, acid-base imbalance, V/Q mismatch, shunt, hypoventilation

Overview

Respiratory failure occurs when the lungs cannot eliminate carbon dioxide from the alveoli, resulting in hypoxemia, hypercapnia and inadequate O_2/CO_2 exchange. The major function of the respiratory system is gas exchange, the transfer of oxygen (O_2) and carbon dioxide (CO_2) between the atmosphere and the blood. Respiratory failure results when one or both of these gas exchanging functions are inadequate. Respiratory failure can be classified as hypoxemic or hypercapnic. Hypoxemic respiratory failure is defined as a PaO_2 of 60mmHg or less when the client is receiving an inspired O_2 concentration of 60% or greater. Hypercapnic respiratory failure is defined as a $PaCO_2$ above 45 mmHg in combination with acidemia (pH less than 7.35). Four physiologic mechanisms may cause hypoxemia and subsequent hypoxemic respiratory failure: V/Q mismatch, shunt, diffusion limitation, and hypoventilation of which V/Q mismatch and shunt are the most common causes. Hypercapnic respiratory failure results from an imbalance between ventilatory supply and ventilatory demand. Many different diseases can cause a limitation in ventilatory supply and can be grouped as abnormalities of the airways and alveoli, abnormalities of the CNS, abnormalities of the chest wall, and neuromuscular conditions.

Risk Factors

- Direct injury to the lungs, airways, or chest wall
- Defect in the brain's respiratory control center
- Neuromuscular disorders (multiple sclerosis, myasthenia gravis, Guillain-Barré syndrome)
- CNS dysfunction (stroke, cerebral edema, head injury, increased intracranial pressure meningitis)
- Chemical depression (opioid analgesics, sedatives, anesthetic agents)
- Kyphoscoliosis
- Massive obesity
- Sleep apnea
- External obstruction/constriction
- Intrapulmonary causes
  - Airway disease
  - Asthma
  - Ventilation-perfusion mismatch
- Cardiac disorders, cardiopulmonary bypass surgery
- Near drowning
- Pneumonia

- Asthma
- Aspiration
- Fat emboli
- Sepsis
- Intravascular coagulation
- Trauma
- Excessive smoke inhalation
- Burns, about the face and/or chest
- Massive blood transfusions

Signs and Symptoms

- Dyspnea
- Orthopnea
- Restlessness
- Headache, confusion
- Rapid, shallow respirations
- Hypoxemia, hypercarbia/hypercapnia, respiratory acidosis
- Cyanosis
- Pale, cool, clammy skin or warm flushed skin
- Tachycardia progressing to bradycardia
- Dysrhythmias
- Decreased level of consciousness; can progress to coma
- Abnormal lung sounds (pulmonary edema)
- Peripheral and conjunctival hyperemia (vasodilation)
- Papilledema
- Neuromuscular irritability

Diagnostic and Laboratory Tests

- History and physical examination
- Pulmonary function tests:
    - Air flow (spirometer)
    - Lung volume
    - Diffusion capacity (correlates with body's ability to extract oxygen from the lungs)
- Chest x-ray
- ABG (arterial blood gas) analysis
- Chemistry panel
- Blood and sputum cultures (if indicated)
- CBC with differential, if indicated

Therapeutic Nursing Management

- **Assess/Monitor:**
  - ABGs (arterial blood gases)
  - Oxygen saturation levels
  - Respiratory status (rate and other vital signs, assess for signs of respiratory distress)
  - Mental status
- **Nursing Activities:**
  - Establish and maintain airway.
  - Support ventilation.
  - Administer oxygen as prescribed.
  - Suction the client as needed.
  - Obtain a specimen for culture if the sputum appears purulent.
  - Identify and treat underlying problem.
  - Place in high-Fowler's position.
  - Avoid medications that depress respirations.
  - Prepare for mechanical ventilation if condition worsens.
  - Encourage deep breathing.
  - Minimize activities and energy expenditures.
  - Provide emotional support to client and family.

Pharmacology

- Oxygen
- Bronchodilators (short-acting beta$_2$ agonists)
- Corticosteroids (methylprednisolone)
- Sodium bicarbonate (if metabolic acidosis present)
- Anti-anxiety agents (benzodiazepines)
- Diuretics (furosemide), if indicated
- Antibiotics (in presence of underlying infection)

Complications

- Hypotension
- Decreased cardiac output
- Infection
- Pneumothorax
- ARDS (acute/adult respiratory distress syndrome)
- Death

Age–Related Changes—Gerontological Considerations

- Older adults are at higher risk of developing respiratory failure because of the reduction in ventilatory capacity that accompanies aging, especially if other risk factors are present. In older adults, the PaO_2 falls further and the $PaCO_2$ rises to a higher level before the respiratory system is stimulated to alter the rate and depth of breathing. This delayed response predisposes to the development of respiratory failure.

- Increased risk for secondary infections and respiratory failure occurs related to respiratory diseases.
- Increased risk for ventilator dependence.

Critical Thinking Exercise: Nursing Management of the Client with Acute Respiratory Failure

Situation: While caring for an older client with COPD (chronic obstructive pulmonary disease), the nurse notes that he is unusually lethargic, diaphoretic, and difficult to rouse.

1. What is the client's primary risk factor for developing respiratory failure?

2. Assuming that all need to be performed, prioritize the order of performance of nursing actions for the client, with "1" representing the most important.

   _____ Place the client in a high-Fowler's position.

   _____ Establish a patent airway.

   _____ Change the damp sheets beneath the client

   _____ Administer prescribed oxygen

   _____ Obtain intravenous access.

3. What are the two highest priority client outcomes for the client experiencing respiratory failure?

   _____ Preventing infection

   _____ Correcting underlying cause

   _____ Restoring ventilation and oxygenation

   _____ Preventing recurrence

4. List four other signs and symptoms commonly associated with respiratory failure.

Nursing Management of the Client with Pulmonary Edema

Key Points

- Pulmonary edema is a life-threatening complication that requires immediate collaborative management.
- Severe left ventricular failure causes backup of blood into the left atrium and the pulmonary circulation.
- Cardiogenic factors are the most common cause of pulmonary edema:
    - Left heart failure
    - Ischemic heart/disease/myocardial infarction
    - Valvular disorders
    - Hypertension
    - Cardiomyopathy
    - Dysrhythmias
    - Fluid overhead
    - Endocarditis, myocarditis
    - Cardiac tamponade
- Pulmonary edema may also be due to non-cardiogenic causes:
    - Shock
    - Trauma
    - Sepsis and disseminated intravascular coagulation
    - Aspiration pneumonia
    - Inhaled toxic substances
    - Drug overdose
    - High-altitude sickness
    - Pancreatitis
    - Embolism
    - Neurogenic
    - Oxygen toxicity
    - ARDS (acute/adult respiratory distress syndrome)
    - Renal failure
- Goals of collaborative management:
    - Provide early recognition and treatment.
    - Correct the underlying disorder.
    - Reduce total circulating fluid volume.
    - Restore and maintain ventilation and perfusion.

- Prevent recurrence.
- Important nursing diagnoses (actual or potential):
  - Ineffective breathing pattern
  - Ineffective airway clearance
  - Anxiety and fear
  - Fatigue and restlessness
  - Altered nutrition: less than body requirements
  - Self-care deficit
  - Activity intolerance
  - Ineffective individual and family coping
  - Decreased cardiac output
  - Decreased cerebral perfusion
  - Fluid volume excess
- **Key Terms/Concepts:** Left-sided heart failure, hypoxemia

Overview

Pulmonary edema is a severe, life-threatening accumulation of fluid in the alveoli and interstitial spaces of the lung. It is a complication of various heart and lung diseases and usually occurs from increased pulmonary vascular pressure secondary to severe cardiac dysfunction. Fluid from the left side of the heart backs up into the pulmonary vasculature and results in extravascular fluid accumulation in the interstitial space and alveoli. Non-cardiac pulmonary edema can occur from barbiturate or opiate overdose, post-pneumonectomy, post-evacuation of pleural effusion, inhalation of irritating gases, and rapid administration of intravenous fluids; or from other entities previously mentioned.

Risk Factors

- Atherosclerosis
- Acute MI (myocardial infarction)
- Hypertension
- Valvular heart disease
- Post-pneumonectomy
- Post-evacuation of pleural effusion
- Toxic inhalants
- Acute respiratory failure
- Left-sided heart failure
- High altitude exposure or deep sea diving
- Trauma
- Sepsis
- Drug overdose
- Fluid volume overload

Signs and Symptoms

- Restlessness, inability to sleep
- Anxiety
- Dyspnea and labored breathing
- Hypoxemia
- Persistent cough with pink, frothy sputum
- Tachypnea
- Cyanosis, later stage
- Crackles, rales (wheezes may be heard in more severe cases)
- Weak, rapid pulse
- Neck vein distention
- Sense of suffocation
- Ashen gray color
- Confusion, stupor

Diagnostic and Laboratory Tests

- History and physical examination
- ABG (arterial blood gas) analysis
- SaO_2
- Chest x-rays
- Hemodynamic testing (pulmonary artery capillary pressure, wedge pressure, cardiac output)
- CBC with differential possible
- Chemistry profile, possible
- Urinalysis, possible

Therapeutic Nursing Management

- **Assess/Monitor:**
  - Respiratory status for respiratory compromise
  - Intake and output
  - Hemodynamic status (pulmonary capillary wedge pressures, cardiac output)
  - Blood work as indicated
- **Nursing Activities:**
  - Maintain patent airway.
  - Administer oxygen as prescribed.
  - Restrict fluid intake.
  - Position client in high-Fowler's position with feet and legs down.
  - Establish intravenous access.
  - Administer morphine sulfate for anxiety and dyspnea.

- Administer diuretics for fluid overload.
- Administer pulmonary vasodilators if indicated.
- Administer cardiac inotropic agents or antihypertensive agents as indicated.
- Prepare to administer emergency medications.
- Provide emotional support for client and family.
- **Client teaching:**
  - Teach/assess understanding of effective breathing techniques.
  - Teach/assess understanding of medications:
    - Include family members if this is a long-term problem (i.e. cardiac disease).
    - Teach importance of continuing to take medications even if client is feeling better.
    - Teach common side effects and reasons to contact physician.
  - Teach/assess understanding of low-sodium diet and fluid restriction.

Pharmacology

- Diuretics (furosemide, bumetanide)
- Vasodilators (Nitroprusside, nitroglycerin)
- Oxygen
- Cardiac glycosides (digoxin)
- Dobutamine
- Antihypertensives, possible ACE (angiotensin converting enzyme) inhibitors
- Morphine sulfate
- Carvedilol (possible beta-blocker used to increase cardiac output and reduce pulmonary congestion – used for left heart failure)

Complications

- Hypotension
- Acute respiratory failure
- ARDS (acute/adult respiratory syndrome)
- Death

Age–Related Changes—Gerontological Considerations

- Increased risk for pulmonary edema occurs related to decreased cardiac output and CHF (congestive heart failure).
- Increased risk for fluid and electrolyte imbalances occurs when the client receives treatment with diuretics.
- Intravenous infusions must be administered at a slower rate to prevent circulatory overload.

Critical Thinking Exercise: Nursing Management of the Client with Pulmonary Edema

Situation: A 51-year-old man with a history of CHF (congestive heart failure) arrives at the emergency department after a two-day illness, during which time he developed severe dyspnea. He has distended neck veins, audible bilateral crackles, is restless and confused to place and date. The nurse immediately recognizes the client is suffering from pulmonary edema.

1. Which priority nursing diagnoses need to be added to the client's care plan based on the data provided?

   _____ Ineffective breathing pattern   _____ Anxiety/fear

   _____ Risk for activity intolerance   _____ Fatigue

   _____ Ineffective individual/family coping   _____ Altered nutrition: less than body requirements

   _____ Decreased cardiac output   _____ Decreased cerebral perfusion

   _____ Fluid volume excess   _____ Self-care deficit

2. What other clinical manifestations is the client likely to experience?

   _____ High fever   _____ Productive cough

   _____ Frothy sputum   _____ Bradycardia

   _____ Cheyne Stokes respirations   _____ Cyanosis

   _____ Wheezing   _____ Hot, dry skin

   _____ Ashen gray color   _____ Stupor

1. What is the rationale for administering each medication/drug to the client experiencing pulmonary edema?

   a. Oxygen

   b. Morphine sulfate

   c. Diuretics

   d. Digitalis

   e. Dobutamine

Nursing Management of the Client with a Pulmonary Embolism

Key Points

- Pulmonary embolism (PE) is a life-threatening complication of thrombophlebitis, which may result from surgery or immobility.
- Pulmonary embolism is the most common pulmonary perfusion abnormality
- Most pulmonary emboli (90-95%) arise from thrombi in the deep veins of the leg, most commonly the femoral or iliac veins.
- Less common causes of pulmonary emboli include fat emboli, air emboli, amniotic fluid, and tumors, and devices such as shearing off of IV catheters.
- Can present as one of three syndromes:
    - Acute cor pulmonale – massive embolism, obstructing 60-75% of pulmonary circulation.
    - Pulmonary infarction – submassive embolism, but complete obstruction of a distal branch of the pulmonary circulation.
    - Acute and unexplained dyspnea – clients who do not present with acute cor pulmonale or pulmonary infarction.
- Early diagnosis and appropriate treatment reduce mortality to 5%.
- Untreated PE carries a 30% mortality rate; however, 10% die within the first hour.
- Goals of collaborative management:
    - Provide early recognition and treatment.
    - Prevent further growth or multiplication of thrombi in the lower extremities.
    - Prevent embolization from the upper or lower extremities to the pulmonary vascular system.
    - Stabilize and maintain oxygenation and cardiac function.
    - Prevent complications (dysrhythmias, hypotension, and cardiac decompensation).
    - Maintain fluid and electrolyte balance.
    - Assist with ventilation if needed.
- Important nursing diagnoses (actual or potential):
    - Impaired gas exchange
    - Decreased cardiac output
    - Fear and anxiety
    - Self-care deficit
    - Activity intolerance
    - Altered nutrition: less than body requirements
    - Ineffective individual/family coping

- **Key Terms/Concepts**: Embolectomy, embolization, thrombus, hypoxemia, cardiac decompensation, ventilation-perfusion mismatch, atelectasis, thrombolytics, low-molecular weight heparin.

Overview

A pulmonary embolism is caused by a thrombus dislodging and traveling through the venous circulation, passing through the right side of the heart, and entering the pulmonary artery, or branch, where it becomes lodged. The embolus obstructs pulmonary blood flow, causing a V/Q mismatch; an area of the lung is ventilated, but not perfused. The subsequent obstruction hinders oxygenation of blood, atelectasis develops, pulmonary vascular resistance increases and arterial hypoxia develops. Pulmonary embolism usually occurs in clients identified to be at risk such as those with prior thrombophlebitis, history of recent surgeries, recent pregnancy/childbirth, women taking contraceptives on a long-term basis, and those with a history of congestive heart failure, obesity, or immobilization.

Risk Factors

- Deep vein thrombosis
- Surgery (orthopedic, pelvic, gynecological, abdominal)
- Hypercoagulability (anemia, estrogen therapy, birth control pills, smoking)
- Prolonged immobility
- Pregnancy
- Women taking contraceptives on a long-term basis
- Obesity
- CHF (congestive heart failure)
- Advanced age

Signs and Symptoms

- Sudden onset of unexplained dyspnea, tachypnea, or tachycardia
- Pleuritic chest pain
- Cough
- Hemoptysis
- Fever
- Apprehension
- Diaphoresis
- Pulmonary crackles
- Hypotension
- Syncope
- Cyanosis
- Accentuation of pulmonic heart sound
- Sudden change in mental status (as a result of hypoxemia)
- Massive emboli may result in
- Sudden collapse of the client

- Shock
- Pallor, severe dyspnea
- Crushing chest pain
- Cardiopulmonary arrest and death

Diagnostic and Laboratory Tests

- First Line:
  - Electrocardiograph (ECG)
  - Chest x-ray
  - ABG (arterial blood gas) analysis
  - Ventilation/perfusion scan/Lung scintigraphy.
  - Pulmonary angiography. Safer than in previous years, but should only be utilized in those clients who cannot be positively diagnosed via scan.
  - Electrocardiography may be beneficial in those clients in whom massive embolism is suspected.
  - Venous ultrasound, to identify thromboembolism
  - Prothrombin Time (PT); partial prothrombin time (PPT), also sometimes referred to as partial thromboplastin time (PTT), as well as Activated partial thromboplastin time (aPTT)
  - Impedance plethysmography, to identify thromboembolism
  - D-dimer serum test (a product of fibrin degradation, when thrombus or embolus is present, plasma D-dimer concentrations are elevated)

Therapeutic Nursing Management

Prevention:
- Identification of clients at risk

Assess/Monitor:
- For positive Homans' sign, unreliable test for thrombophlebitis, see chapter on thromboembolism
- Vital signs
- Respiratory status
- For signs of respiratory compromise
- For signs of shock
- For signs of hypoxia
- For signs of bleeding
- Urinary output of less than 30 mL/hour
- PT and PPT levels, CBC

Nursing Activities:
- Provide bed rest in semi-Fowler's position.
- Administer oxygen via nasal cannula or mask as prescribed.
  - Prepare for possible endotracheal intubation in severe cases.
  - Report abnormal ABG (arterial blood gas) and laboratory data.

- Encourage deep breathing exercises.
- Apply TED (antiembolism) stockings, pneumatic stockings or other.
- Administer pain medications as prescribed.
- Administer anticoagulants as prescribed.
- Administer fluids intravenously until urinary output is 30 mL/hour or more, indicating that fluid resuscitation is adequate.
- Client teaching
  - Teach/assess understanding of techniques to avoid venous stasis.
  - Frequent position changes
  - Wear loose clothing.
  - Regular physical activity
  - Avoid crossing legs.
  - Teach proper application of antiembolism hose.
  - Smoking cessation
- Medications
  - Teach/assess proper technique for administering low-molecular weight heparin SQ, as needed.
  - Teach/assess understanding of Coumadin therapy.
  - Importance of taking medications at same time each day.
  - Importance of monitoring lab values to ensure efficacy.
- Prepare the client for surgical intervention if needed, embolectomy and/or vena cava filter.
- Provide emotional support to client and family.

Pharmacology

- Anticoagulants (heparin, warfarin, low molecular weight heparins - LMWH). Heparin is initial treatment of choice, although LMWH can be used in non-massive cases of PE.
- Thrombolytic therapy (urokinase, streptokinase, t-PA) for use in massive PE with shock and/or hypotension
- Analgesics (opioid or non-opioid)
- Dobutamine and dopamine if low cardiac output and normal blood pressure
- Vasopressors if low blood pressure

Complications

- Hemorrhage
- Pulmonary infarction
- Acute cor pulmonale
- Recurrent thromboembolism with pulmonary embolism
- Treatment failure or recurrence requiring vena cava filter
- Respiratory arrest
- Death

Age-Related Changes—Gerontological Considerations

- Increased risk of complications occurs related to decreased elasticity of the lungs and chest wall.
- Increased risk for pulmonary embolism occurs related to venous stasis, poor circulation, and immobility.
- Increased risk for venous stasis is related to decreased efficiency of lower extremity vein valves.

Critical Thinking Exercise: Nursing Management of the Client with a Pulmonary Embolism

Situation: A 65-year-old woman returned to her room at 2:00 p.m. yesterday following an abdominal hysterectomy. Her vital signs have been stable and her dressings dry and intact. She was up to the side of the bed and ambulated a few feet before returning to bed. A few minutes later, she turned on her call light stating she was having difficulty breathing. The nurse found the client anxious, tachycardic, diaphoretic, gasping for air, and complaining of chest pain.

1. Which diagnostic tests help differentiate between pulmonary embolism and heart attack?

   _____ Oxygen saturation   _____ Ventilation-perfusion scan

   _____ Electrocardiogram (ECG) _____ White blood cell (WBC) count

   _____ Pulmonary angiography   _____ Serum electrolytes

2. What known risk factors does the client have for development of pulmonary embolism?

   _____ Deep vein thrombosis   _____ Surgery

   _____ Hypercoagulability   _____ Prolonged immobility

   _____ Advanced age   _____ Obesity

3. There is sufficient data to support placing which nursing diagnoses on the client's plan of care?

   _____ Decreased cardiac output

   _____ Altered nutrition: less than body requirements

   _____ Fear/anxiety

   _____ Self-care deficit

   _____ Impaired skin integrity

   _____ Impaired gas exchange

   _____ Ineffective individual/family coping

Nursing Management of the Client with Tuberculosis (TB)

Key Points

- Tuberculosis (TB) is an infectious disease caused by Mycobacterium tuberculosis.
- TB is a potentially chronic pulmonary and extrapulmonary infectious disease acquired by inhalation of a dried droplet nucleus containing a tubercle bacillus into the alveolar structure of the lung.
- Despite being curable and preventable, TB is still a major public health problem in the United States.
- Multidrug-resistant strains of M. tuberculosis and epidemic proportions of TB among clients with human immunodeficiency virus (HIV) infections have contributed to the resurgence of TB.
- Tuberculosis may affect any organ in the body, but primarily affects the lungs.
- Initial infection with tuberculosis occurs within 2-10 weeks of exposure.
- The tuberculosis bacillus may lie dormant for many years before producing disease.
- Individuals at risk for TB infection include urban, homeless residents of inner-city neighborhoods, migrant workers, close contact with infected individuals, immigrant within past 5 years, (especially from Asia, Africa and Latin America), those in institutions, older adults, health care workers, the socioeconomically disadvantaged and medically underserved of all races. Approximately 90% of primary infections of TB will remain latent. Clients with latent TB are not infectious. Latent TB may become active disease after periods of stress, where the immune system is altered.
- Those at risk for the development of active TB disease from infection include immunocompromised individuals, especially those with HIV; IV drug abusers; clients with cancers, chronic renal failure, or diabetes mellitus; malnourished, chronic corticosteroid use or use of immunosuppressive medications
- Goals of collaborative management:
    - Provide early detection.
    - Provide accurate diagnosis.
    - Provide effective treatment of the disease.
    - Prevent transmission.
    - Eradicate the infection.
    - Maintain respiratory function.
    - Prevent complications.
    - Restore functional ability.
- Important nursing diagnoses (actual or potential):
    - Noncompliance and potential risk of spread of infection

- Knowledge deficit
- Activity intolerance, if active disease
- Impaired gas exchange, if active disease
- Fatigue and restlessness, if active disease
- Fear and anxiety
- Ineffective individual/family coping
- Altered health maintenance
- Altered nutrition: less than body requirements
- Risk for injury
- **Key Terms/Concepts**: Contagious, droplet infection, immunosuppressed, chemotherapy, latent infection, dormant infection, active disease, host, extrapulmonary

Overview

Tuberculosis (TB) is an infectious disease caused by *mycobacterium tuberculosis* bacillus. While primarily a lung infection, tuberculosis may disseminate throughout the body, including the kidneys, bones, adrenal glands, lymph nodes, and meninges. It is usually spread via airborne droplets, which are produced when the infected individual coughs, sneezes, or speaks. Infection may occur when a susceptible host breathes in air containing droplet nuclei and the contaminated particle eludes the normal defenses of the upper respiratory tract to reach the alveoli. As the bacteria multiply, they spread through the lymphatic system to regional lymph nodes, the bloodstream, and throughout the body, stimulating any immune response. If the initial immune response is not adequate, control of the organisms is not maintained and clinical disease results. Tuberculosis infection is different from tuberculosis disease. Although infection always precedes the development of active disease, only about 10% of infections progress to active disease. Tuberculosis infection is characterized by the presence of mycobacteria in the tissue of a host who is free of clinical signs and symptoms and who demonstrates the presence of antibodies against the mycobacteria. Tuberculosis disease manifests as pathological and functional signs and symptoms indicating destructive activity of mycobacteria in host issue. Certain individuals are at a higher risk for clinical disease, including those who are immunosuppressed, those receiving cancer chemotherapy or long-term corticosteroid therapy or have diabetes mellitus. Tuberculosis may remain dormant for years. Reactivation of TB can occur if the host's defense mechanisms become impaired. The reasons for reactivation of TB are not well understood, but they are related to decreased resistance found in older adults, individuals with concomitant diseases, and those who receive immunosuppressive therapy.

Risk Factors

- Direct exposure to *mycobacterium tuberculosis* bacillus
- Immunocompromised status (HIV/AIDS, cancer, the elderly, corticosteroid drugs)
- Crowded living conditions
- IV drug use
- Alcohol abuse

- Malnourishment
- Low socioeconomic levels/medically underserved
- Advanced age
- Chronic illness
- Institutionalization (long-term care facilities, prisons, mental health facilities)
- Persons with increased risk of developing active TB after infection
- Diabetes
- Chronic renal failure
- Underweight (more than 10% below ideal body weight)
- Prolonged use of corticosteroids
- Alcoholics, IV drug users, cocaine and crack users
- Health care workers

Signs and Symptoms

- Asymptomatic early in the disease process
- Nonproductive cough progressing to purulent sputum and hemoptysis
- Low-grade fever
- Night sweats
- Pleuritic chest pain
- Weight loss
- Anorexia
- Fatigue and malaise

Diagnostic and Laboratory Tests

- History and physical examination
- Chest x-ray
- Sputum smear and culture (acid-fast bacilli)
- Mantoux skin test (read in 48 to 72 hours) (also known as PPD)
- QuantiFeron – TB blood test
- Bronchoscopy

Therapeutic Nursing Management

- **Prevention**:
  - Prevent transmission to self or others
  - Public health teaching
  - Teach clients and their families
    - Means to prevent disease transmission
    - Screening close contacts for infection
    - Enhance their willingness and ability to comply with treatment.

- **Assess/Monitor:**
  - Respiratory status
  - Nutritional status
  - Fluid status
  - Effectiveness of drug therapy
  - Compliance of client with chemotherapy regimen
- **Nursing Activities:**
  - Promote airway clearance.
  - Assist client to cough and take deep breaths.
  - Administer oxygen as prescribed.
  - Administer antituberculosis medications as ordered.
  - Encourage increased fluid intake and a well-balanced diet.
  - Ensure the use of personal protective devices, and respirator mask to reduce the risk of transmission.
  - Implement respiratory isolation (negative pressure room), until client has received medication for 2 to 3 weeks.
  - Make referrals as necessary (i.e., smoking cessation, Alcoholics Anonymous, drug treatment facilities, hospice).
  - Teach client regarding the disease process, medication regimen and drug side effects.
  - Emphasize the need for maintaining medication regimen.
  - Teach client regarding transmission (mouth care, covering mouth when coughing and sneezing, proper disposal of tissues and hand washing).
  - Teach the client the need for close, follow-up care.

Pharmacology

- Isoniazid (INH)
- Rifampin (RIF)
- Pyrazinamide (PZA)
- Ethambutol (EMB)
- Streptomycin – not as widely used due to increased resistance
- Resistance or treatment failure – fluoroquinolone, injectable streptomycin (unless known resistance) amikacin, kanamycin, capreomycin and p-aminosalicylic acid (PAS), cycloserine, or ethionamide
- Vitamin B6 (pyridoxine) to prevent toxicity from isoniazid
- PPD testing and 2-step PPD testing in individuals such as health care workers who will be retested periodically (second PPD done 1-3 weeks after first test, both should be negative, if second test is positive, client is considered infected and should be treated.)
- BCG (Bacille Calmette-Guérin) vaccine, given in foreign countries against TB, is now not considered a contraindication to PPD testing.

Complications

- Extrapulmonary tuberculosis
- Miliary TB (necrotic Ghon complex erodes through a blood vessel, large number of organisms invade the blood stream and spread to all body organs)
- Pleural effusion
- Bronchopleural fistula
- Tuberculosis empyema
- Pneumothorax
- Tuberculous pneumonia (large amounts of tubercle bacilli in lung and lymph nodes)
- Other organ involvement
- Death

Age-Related Changes—Gerontological Considerations

- Atypical presentation often occurs in older clients, such as altered mentation or unusual behavior, fever, anorexia, and weight loss.
- Increased incidence of tuberculosis exists among older adults in long-term care facilities, older immigrants, and immunosuppressed older adults and should be watched closely for drug-resistant strains of tuberculosis.
- Increased risk of reactivation of tuberculosis is related to chronic illnesses and corticosteroid drug use. Recurrence of active tuberculosis, signs and symptoms are often vague and include loss of appetite and weight loss.
- Increased risk for altered health maintenance is related to inability to follow strict medication regimens.

Critical Thinking Exercise: Nursing Management of the Client with Tuberculosis (TB)

Situation: A 74-year-old woman who lives independently developed night sweats, loss of appetite, and chronic nonproductive cough. After losing more than ten pounds and undergoing numerous tests, the client was diagnosed with tuberculosis.

1. Which statements are true about tuberculosis? Correct any false statements.

   a. Tuberculosis is a contagious disease that is highly sensitive to current chemotherapies.

   b. Tuberculosis may affect any organ in the body, but primarily affects the lungs.

   c. Initial infection with tuberculosis occurs within 6-12 weeks of exposure.

   d. Dormant *tuberculosis bacillus* can be killed by prolonged chemotherapy.

   e. Tuberculosis is transmitted via respiratory and gastrointestinal secretions.

2. Provide an etiology for each of the client's nursing diagnoses:

   a. Noncompliance

   b. Activity intolerance

   c. Impaired gas exchange

   d. Fatigue

   e. Fear/anxiety

   f. Altered nutrition: less than body requirements

3. The client is placed on Isoniazid (isonicotinic acid hydrazide ([INH]) and Rifampin (RIF). What parameters will the nurse use to determine the effectiveness of the drugs?

Nursing Management of the Client with Atelectasis

Key Points

- Atelectasis is a preventable complication of immobility.
- Atelectasis is the airless condition of the lungs due to obstruction or hypoventilation.
- Atelectasis may be acute or chronic and is the most common postoperative complication.
- Other causes of atelectasis include pneumothorax, pleural effusion, or tumor; loss of pulmonary surfactant and inability to maintain open alveoli.
- Goals of collaborative management:
  - Provide early recognition and treatment.
  - Restore and maintain oxygenation.
  - Prevent complications (respiratory distress, respiratory failure).
- Important nursing diagnoses (actual or potential):
  - Ineffective breathing pattern
  - Impaired gas exchange
  - Decreased cardiac output
  - Fear/anxiety
  - Self-care deficit
  - Activity intolerance
  - Impaired skin integrity
  - Altered nutrition: less than body requirements
  - Ineffective individual/family coping
  - Knowledge deficit
  - Fatigue and restlessness, if active disease
  - Altered health maintenance
  - Risk for injury
- **Key Terms/Concepts**: Hypoventilation, immobility, bronchus

Overview

Atelectasis is a state of partial or total lung collapse and airlessness that may be acute or chronic. The most common cause of atelectasis is obstruction of the bronchus ventilating the affected lung tissue. Obstruction may affect only a small segment of a lung or the entire lobe.

Risk Factors

- COPD
- Supine positioning/prolonged bed rest
- Mechanical ventilation
- Hypoventilation secondary to pain, mucous plug, excessive or thick secretions
- Inability to breathe deeply
- Respiratory depression from narcotics and relaxants
- Abdominal distension
- May follow abdominal surgeries, lung surgery, open heart surgery
- Compression by tumor, aneurysm, or enlarged lymph nodes
- Smoking
- Obesity
- Older age group
- Respiratory tract infection

Signs and Symptoms

- Dyspnea
- Anxiety
- Cyanosis
- Tachycardia
- Tachypnea
- Hypoxemia
- Hypotension
- Fever
- Pain on the affected side
- Pulmonary crackles
- Decreased breath sounds over the affected area

Diagnostic and Laboratory Tests

- History and physical examination
- Chest x-ray
- CT scan
- Bronchoscopy to remove an obstructive cause

Therapeutic Nursing Management

- **Assess/Monitor:**
  - Respiratory status including rate, breath sounds, spirometry
  - Nutritional status
  - Fluid status

- **Nursing Activities:**
  - Encourage coughing, turning and deep breathing every 2 hours following anesthesia and surgery.
  - Encourage mobility.
  - Position on the unaffected side with the involved side uppermost to promote drainage.
  - Reposition clients every 2 hours if on bed rest; in cases of prolonged immobility, consider specialty bed.
  - If not contraindicated, encourage fluids to help liquefy secretions.
  - Encourage use of incentive spirometry at least every 2 hours.
  - Suction if needed to remove thick secretions.
  - Administer humidified oxygen as ordered.
  - Perform chest percussion and postural drainage.
  - Assist with insertion of the chest tube, or thoracentesis, if necessary.
  - Administer analgesics.
  - Encourage early ambulation (unless contraindicated).
  - Teach client and family (especially for people at high risk for developing atelectasis) pulmonary care measures, fluid intake and avoidance of infections.

Pharmacology

- Antibiotics (if bacterial infection present)
- Bronchodilators
- Mucolytic (acetylcysteine) agents
- Analgesics (opioid or non-opioid), use caution since opioids may decrease respiratory drive and/or depth of respiration

Complications

- Respiratory acidosis
- Pneumonia
- Respiratory failure
- Death

Age-Related Changes—Gerontological Considerations

- Increased risk for development of atelectasis is related to decreased lung tissue elasticity and decreased functional reserve. Loss of abdominal muscle use decreases cough effectiveness. A decreased vital capacity leads to atelectasis. Decreased mobility also contributes to pneumonia and atelectasis. Prognosis is dependent upon age and pre-existing illness of the client.

Critical Thinking Exercise: Nursing Management of the Client with Atelectasis

Situation: A 27-year-old man who underwent abdominal surgery is reluctant to move because of incisional pain. He coughs frequently because he is a cigarette smoker. He complains he cannot take a deep breath because it hurts. The nurse is concerned that he is going to develop atelectasis.

1. Why is it essential that postoperative clients take deep breaths and ambulate as early as possible?

2. What are the client's risk factors for atelectasis?

3. What are the common clinical manifestations of atelectasis?

_____ Diaphoresis   _____ Dyspnea

_____ Anxiety   _____ Bradycardia

_____ Hypertension   _____ Tachypnea

_____ Decreased breath sounds   _____ Fever

4. List at least three nursing actions that can prevent the development of atelectasis?

Nursing Management of the Client with Lung Cancer

Key Points

- Lung cancer is the leading cause of death in both men and women, accounting for 28% of all cancer deaths.
- Lung cancer primarily affects people between the ages 50 and 75.
- Cigarette smoking is related to approximately 80 to 90% of all lung cancers.
- Tumors may result from metastasis anywhere or may appear as primary tumors (metastasis from the colon and kidney is common).
- 80 to 90% of tumors are linked to cigarette smoking.
- Mortality depends on the type of cancer and size of tumor when diagnosed.
- Lung cancer is treated with surgery, radiation therapy, and chemotherapy.
- Treatment is based on type and extent of disease.
- Lung cancer has a poor prognosis, especially for clients with small cell carcinomas.
- The overall 5-year survival rate for lung cancer is only 14%.
- Goals of collaborative management:
  - Prioritize prevention of the disease, as lung cancer typically has reached an advanced state at the time of diagnosis and the prognosis is generally poor.
  - Prevent or decrease environmental and occupational risks.
  - Support treatment decisions based on the tumor location, type of cancer cell, staging of the tumor and the client's ability to tolerate treatment.
  - Surgical intervention provides the only significant chance for a cure in most forms of lung cancer (in small-cell lung cancer).
  - The goal of surgical intervention is to remove all tumorous tissue, including lymph nodes.
  - Ease respiratory symptoms.
  - Reduce pain and discomfort.
  - Maintain quality of life.
  - Provide emotional support.
  - Prevent complications.
  - Assist client and family with anticipatory grieving process.
- Important nursing diagnoses (actual or potential):
  - Ineffective breathing pattern
  - Impaired gas exchange
  - Altered nutrition: less than body requirements
  - Impaired physical mobility

- Pain management
- Risk of infection
- Risk for injury
- Fear and anxiety
- Anticipatory grieving
- Caregiver role strain
- Ineffective individual/family coping
- Fatigue and restlessness
- Ineffective management of therapeutic regimen
- Impaired skin integrity
- **Key Terms/Concepts**: Hypoventilation, immobility, bronchus

Overview

The pathogenesis of primary lung cancer is not well understood. More than 90% of cancers originate from the epithelium of the bronchus (bronchogenic carcinoma). They grow slowly and it takes 8-10 years for a tumor to reach 1 cm in size, which is the smallest detectable lesion on an x-ray. Therefore, the poor long-term survival rate is due to the fact that most lung cancers are diagnosed at a late stage, when metastasis is present. Only 15% of clients have small tumors and localized disease at the time of diagnosis. Lung cancer can eventually metastasize into the pleural space, pleural cavity, and other thoracic organs. Lung cancers are classified according to their histologic cell type:

- Small cell carcinoma (oat cell), which is the most aggressive of all lung cancers, accounting for 20% of all cases
- Squamous cell cancer (epidermoid), accounting for 30% of all cases
- Adenocarcinoma, accounting for 40% of all cases
- Large cell carcinoma, accounting for 10% of all cases

Risk Factors

- Cigarette smoking accounts for 85% of all lung cancer deaths (directly related to the total exposure to cigarette smoke as determined by the number of years of smoking, number of cigarettes smoked per day, depth of inhalation, and the tar and nicotine content of the cigarettes).
- Family history of lung cancer can give rise to lung cancer, even if the client did not smoke.
- Air pollution
- Pre-existing pulmonary diseases:
  - Tuberculosis
  - Bronchiectasis
  - COPD (chronic obstructive pulmonary disease)
- Exposure to:
  - Passive smoke
  - Beryllium
  - Chromium

- Coal distillates
- Cobalt
- Iron oxide
- Mustard gas
- Petroleum distillates
- Radiation
- Tar
- Nickel
- Uranium
- Radioactive isotopes
- Polycyclic hydrocarbons
- Vinyl chloride
- Metallurgical ores
- Asbestos fibers

Prevention:

- Instruct clients at risk to:
    - Stop smoking.
    - Avoid passive smoke.
    - Avoid air pollution.
    - Avoid contact with asbestos and other environmental exposures.
- Educate clients regarding early signs of lung cancer.
- Promote cancer-screening programs.
- Schedule yearly physical examinations.

Signs and Symptoms

- Peripheral lesions
- Few cancers are found by routine chest x-ray.
- If lesions perforate the pleural space, there will be a pleural effusion and severe pain.
- Central lesions:
    - Originate from larger branch of the bronchial tree
    - Cause obstruction or erosion of the bronchus
    - Present with hemoptysis (coughing up blood), dyspnea, fever, chills
    - Wheeze may be auscultated on affected side.
    - Phrenic nerve involvement will cause paralysis of the diaphragm.
- Metastasis
    - Presents with weight loss
    - Usual sites
        - Liver
        - Bone
        - Esophagus
        - Brain

- Other symptoms may include:
  - Chronic cough
  - Rust-colored or purulent sputum
  - Hoarseness
  - Dysphagia (if tumor invades mediastinum)
  - Pleural effusion
  - Pain (type will depend on location of tumor)
  - Fatigue
  - Recurrent pneumonia
  - Recurrent bronchitis
  - Specific symptoms depend on the location and type of lung cancer.

Diagnostic and Laboratory Tests

- History and physical examination
- Detailed history of cigarette smoking
- Chest x-ray
- Sputum cytology
- CBC, liver function studies, and serum electrolytes, including calcium
- MRI (magnetic resonance imaging)
- CT/CAT (computer tomography/computed axial tomography) scan and spiral computed tomography may be able to pick up cancers earlier.
- PET (Positron emission tomography) scan
- Bronchoscopy/mediastinoscopy
- Percutaneous needle biopsy
- Lung biopsy
- Thoracentesis
- Nuclear scan
- Ultrasound
  - 2-D (2-Dimensional)
  - 3-D (3-Dimensional)
- Carcinoembryonic antigen titer
- Tumor staging

Therapeutic Nursing Management

- **Assess/Monitor:**
  - Vital signs
  - Respiratory rate, depth, and rhythm
  - Pulse oximetry
  - Use of ancillary muscles to breathe
  - Breath sounds
  - Client's level of pain (frequently)

- Laboratory reports
- Oxygen saturation
- Arterial blood gases (ABGs)
- For changes in mental status (restlessness, irritability, confusion)
- Nutritional status
- Fluid and electrolyte status
- Body weight

- **Nursing Activities Postoperatively**:
  - Assess for postoperative complications following pulmonary surgery.
  - Assess for adequate pain control.
  - Determine respiratory status, coughing, postural drainage, incentive spirometry, and need for suctioning.
  - Monitor and maintain effective mechanical ventilation.
  - Observe dressing and incision for bleeding and drainage.
  - Maintain patency of chest tubes and the integrity of closed drainage system (assess site for redness, pain, infection, and crepitus).
  - Record type and amount of chest tube drainage.
  - Check wound for excessive drainage or signs of infection following chest tube removal.
  - Build activity tolerance following surgery.
  - Provide frequent monitoring of intake and output.
  - Assess for side effects resulting from chemotherapy.
  - Assess for side effects resulting from radiation therapy.

- **Nursing Activities**:
  - Teach the client and family the warning signals of lung cancer:
    - Persistent cough
    - Any change in respiratory patterns, or dyspnea out of proportion to exertion
    - Blood in the sputum, blood streaked or frank hemoptysis
    - Rust-colored or purulent sputum
    - Chest, shoulder, or arm pain
    - Recurring episodes of pleural effusion, pneumonia, or bronchitis
  - Recommend programs that will help client quit smoking.
  - Prepare client for diagnostic tests.
  - Prepare client for chemotherapy and radiation therapy.
  - Promote adequate food and fluid intake.
  - Instruct the client in diaphragmatic breathing.
  - Provide preoperative teaching and care.
  - Instruct clients regarding chest tubes (except for pneumonectomy), drainage tubes, oxygen therapy, and mechanical ventilation.
  - Provide postoperative care.
  - Immediately report pulmonary or cardiac postoperative complications to surgeon.

- Monitor for signs of wound infection.
- Provide pain control.
- Administer antibiotics as ordered.
- Provide humidification as needed.
- Make certain that connections between chest tubes, drainage tubing, and drainage collection bottles are tight.
- Take precaution that drainage bottles are never elevated to level of client's chest.
- Encourage client to cough and deep breathe, sit up in bed, perform arm/shoulder exercises, and ambulate following surgery.
- Offer emotional support and encouragement.
- Order daily chest x-rays following removal of chest tubes.
- Upon discharge, refer client to a home health care agency.
- Refer to cancer support groups or hospice as appropriate.

Pharmacology

- Radiation therapy
- Chemotherapy (vincristine, cyclophosphamide, etoposide, cisplatin)
- Bronchodilators (albuterol)
- Pain medications (opioid or non-opioid)
- Antibiotics (if infection present)
- Antipyretics
- Antiemetics (for nausea)

Complications

- Airway obstruction
- Atelectasis
- Pulmonary embolism
- Cardiac dysrhythmias
- Hemorrhage
- Hemothorax
- Paraneoplastic syndrome
- Pleural effusion
- Pulmonary abscess
- Pneumonia
- Recurrent bronchitis

Age-Related Changes—Gerontological Considerations

- Lung cancer primarily develops in clients who are 50 to 75 years old.
- Older clients are at greater risk of complications following surgery for cancer.
- For many individuals who have lung cancer, little can be done to significantly prolong their lives.

- Constant pain becomes a major problem; therefore measures used to relieve pain must be initiated and maintained.

Critical Thinking Exercise: Nursing Management of the Client with Lung Cancer

Situation: A 68-year-old male client who has smoked three packs of cigarettes a day since his teen years is seeing his physician for pulmonary symptoms including dyspnea and a chronic productive cough. The client also states he has pain in his chest, shoulder, and back. The physician suspects the client has lung cancer and is ordering diagnostic tests.

1. What are the warning signals of lung cancer that the nurse may teach the client and family?

2. What can the nurse do to help chronic smokers overcome habitual tobacco use for lung cancer prevention?

3. How may the nurse educate the client to perform diaphragmatic breathing?

4. Describe the most common surgical procedures that are used to remove tumors of the lung.

    a. Wedge resection:

    b. Segmental resection:

    c. Lobectomy:

    d. Pneumonectomy:

5. What outcomes should the client with lung cancer experience following interventions?

Nursing Management of the Client with Laryngeal Cancer

Key Points

- Squamous cell carcinoma is the most common malignancy of the larynx.
- Laryngeal cancer comprises 2% of all cancers.
- About 5% of all cancer diagnoses involve the head and neck.
- Untreated cancer of the head and neck is a fatal disease, with untreated clients usually dying within 2 years of diagnosis.
- Laryngeal cancer occurs in people over age 60 with 90% occurring in men. However, the incidence in women has increased markedly over the years due to the number of women who are heavy smokers.
- With early diagnosis and treatment, as many as 80 to 90% of small cord lesions may be cured.
- Precise therapy is determined, once the cancer is staged.
- The type of surgical approach used for laryngeal cancer is based on site, size, and degree of tumor invasion of the larynx.
- The goals of surgical intervention are to remove the tumor, maintain airway patency, and provide for optimal cosmetic appearance.
- Surgical procedures for laryngeal cancer:
    - Laser surgery
    - Partial laryngectomy
    - Total laryngectomy
    - Radical neck dissection
- Goals of collaborative management:
    - Maintain a patent airway.
    - Maintain adequate nutrition.
    - Prevent complications from therapy.
    - Relieve pain.
    - Allay anxiety and fear.
- Important nursing diagnoses (actual or potential):
    - Impaired verbal communication related to removal of the larynx
    - Fear and anxiety related to diagnosis and surgery
    - Ineffective airway clearance related to retained secretions or local edema
    - Potential for impaired gas exchange related to ineffective clearing of secretions and increased work of breathing
    - Impaired swallowing related to odynophagia (painful swallowing) or surgery (swallowing is no longer an automatic function and needs to be relearned)

- Impaired tissue integrity related to altered circulation, nutritional deficit, tumor invasion and radiation
- Body image disturbance related to change in appearance following surgery
- Pain related to pressure of the tumor on surrounding tissues
- Ineffective individual/family coping related to situational crisis
- Sensory-perceptual alterations: gustatory and olfactory related to changed breathing pattern and interrupted innervation
- Knowledge deficit related to laryngeal cancer and laryngectomy
- Altered tissue perfusion
- Altered nutrition: less than body requirements related to dysphagia or odynophagia (painful swallowing)
- Extreme fatigue
- Social isolation
- Risk of infection
- Alteration in body image
- Ineffective management of therapeutic regimen
- Feelings of powerlessness
- Death anxiety
- **Key Terms/Concepts:** Head and neck disease, hoarseness, dysphagia, odynophagia, metastasis, neoplastic disease, laryngectomy squamous cell carcinoma, radical neck dissection

Overview

Laryngeal cancer, limited to the true vocal cords, is slow growing because of decreased lymphatic supply. However, elsewhere in the larynx there is an abundance of lymph tissue. Cancer in these tissues spreads rapidly and metastasizes early to the deep lymph nodes of the neck. When metastasis occurs, it is most commonly to the lungs or liver. Laryngeal cancer may occur in any of the 3 areas of the larynx; the glottis, the supraglottis, and the subglottis. The 2 major risk factors for laryngeal carcinoma are prolonged use of alcohol and tobacco.

Risk Factors

- Age
- History of heavy smoking
- Prolonged use of alcohol
- Use of chewing tobacco, pipe smoking, and/or marijuana
- Exposure to carcinogenic chemicals toxins or radiation
- Frequent and prolonged vocal straining
- Chronic laryngitis
- Complete neglect of oral hygiene
- Genetic predisposition

Prevention:
- Promote cancer screening, especially when risk factors are present.

- Instruct individuals with prolonged hoarseness or lumps in neck area to see a primary care provider for evaluation.
- Advise client to stop smoking and drinking alcohol.

Signs and Symptoms

- Hoarseness that persists for more than 2 weeks (usually earliest symptom)
- Persistent cough
- Change in voice quality
- Feeling of lump in throat
- Difficulty swallowing
- Color changes in the mouth or tongue to red, white, gray, dark brown, or black
- Persistent or unexplained oral bleeding
- Burning sensation when drinking citrus juices or hot liquids
- Neck masses
- Unilateral sore throat
- Persistent unilateral ear pain
- Anorexia and weight loss
- Halitosis
- Dysphagia (late)
- Airway obstruction (late)

Diagnostic and Laboratory Tests

- History and physical exam
- Complete blood count (CBC) with differential, urinalysis, complete metabolic profile
- Indirect and direct laryngoscopy
- Panendoscopy (performed with anesthesia to define the extent of the tumor)
- Bronchoscopy
- MRI (magnetic resonance imaging)
- Computed tomography (CT)/computed axial tomography (CAT) scan
- Chest x-ray
- Barium swallow
- Multiple biopsy specimens

Therapeutic Nursing Management

- **Assess/Monitor:**
  - Respiratory system (rate, breath sounds, pulse oximetry)
  - Blood gas values and results of pulmonary function tests
  - Position for optimal air exchange (Fowler's and semi-Fowler's position)
  - Ability to swallow

- Nutritional status and weight
- Intake and output
- Pain status
- For secondary problems (infection, bleeding, skin breakdown, and weight loss)
- For anxiety, depression, or grief
- Laboratory results
- **Nursing Activities**:
  - Prepare client for diagnostic tests, surgery, radiation, or the chemotherapy process and outcomes.
  - Monitor respiratory status, encourage deep breathing and coughing, elevate HOB, and maintain humidification.
  - Promote adequate nutrition and hydration.
  - Perform tracheal suctioning.
  - Perform tracheostomy care as needed.
  - Promote adequate rest.
  - Provide analgesia as needed to relieve pain.
  - Teach client to protect the stoma.
  - Maintain IV fluids and/or enteral feedings.
  - Teach the client to initiate a swallow; swallowing is no longer an automatic function and needs to be relearned.
  - Encourage the client and family members to express their fears and anxieties.
  - Refer to cancer support groups or hospice as appropriate.

Pharmacology

- Radiation therapy
- Chemotherapy (carboplatin, cisplatin, cyclophosphamide, vincristine)
- Antibiotics (if infection present)
- Analgesics (opioid)
- Sedatives (benzodiazepines)

Complications

- Metastasis
- Infection/sepsis
- Pharyngeal stridor
- Depression
- Death

Age-Related Changes—Gerontological Considerations

- Older adults have the highest incidence of cancer.
- Older adults heal more slowly than younger adults; wound breakdown is a common complication because of poor nutrition and altered circulation.

- Inactivity and immobility increase the risk of stasis pooling of respiratory secretions, thereby placing them at increased risk of secondary infections (i.e., pneumonia).
- This population may be less tolerant to side effects of radiation and chemotherapy.

Critical Thinking Exercise: Nursing Management of the Client with Laryngeal Cancer

Situation: A 50-year-old woman, who has been singing in various church and civic choirs for the past 30 years, developed a raspy voice. Since the problem interferes with her ability to sing, she decided to seek medical attention. Visualization of the woman's throat reveals the presence of a small nodule on the client's vocal cord.

1. What questions should the nurse ask the client in order to gain additional data about her hoarseness?

2. What additional assessments need to be made?

3. The presence of laryngeal cancer is verified via biopsy and a hemi-laryngectomy is scheduled. What is a hemi-laryngectomy and how does it differ from a total laryngectomy?

4. How can the nurse help the client prepare for the needed surgery?

Nursing Management of the Client with a Laryngectomy

Key Points

- Laryngectomy, removal of the larynx, may be necessary to treat the client with laryngeal cancer.
- A partial laryngectomy may be employed for tumors localized to a portion of the larynx with limited metastasis to regional lymph nodes.
- Advanced laryngeal tumors are treated with surgery and radiation or with surgery alone.
- Radical neck dissection is performed when the client is at risk of metastasis to the cervical lymph nodes.
- The goals of surgical intervention are to remove the tumor, maintain airway patency, and provide for optimal cosmetic appearance.
- Goals of collaborative management:
  - Prepare client for vocal changes or loss of normal speech following surgery.
  - Maintain an open airway via a tracheostomy tube.
  - Prevent complications (infection, hemorrhage, and airway obstruction).
- Important nursing diagnoses (actual or potential):
  - Impaired verbal communication
  - Fear and anxiety
  - Anticipatory grieving
  - Pain management
  - Ineffective airway clearance
  - Impaired skin/tissue integrity
  - Altered oral mucous membranes
  - Impaired swallowing, with risk for aspiration
  - Altered nutrition: less than body requirements
  - Fatigue and restlessness
  - Social isolation
  - Risk of infection
  - Body image disturbance
  - Altered sexuality patterns
  - Ineffective management of therapeutic regimen
  - Ineffective individual/family coping
- **Key Terms/Concepts:** Larynx, epiglottis, vocal cords, radical neck dissection, tracheostomy, artificial larynx, esophageal speech, tracheoesophageal puncture

Overview

Laryngectomy is removal of the entire larynx (voice box) and the preepiglottic region and a permanent tracheostomy is performed. Radical neck dissection frequently accompanies total laryngectomy on the same side of the neck as the lesion to decrease the risk of lymphatic spread. Depending on the extent of involvement, extensive dissection and reconstruction may be performed. Surgical procedures for laryngeal cancer include:

- **Cordectomy/cordal stripping**: excision of a vocal cord
- **Total laryngectomy**: the entire larynx is removed along with the epiglottis, thyroid cartilage, several tracheal rings and the hyoid bone; creation of a permanent tracheostomy, which leaves the client unable to use normal speech
- **Radical neck dissection**: tissue is removed from the lower edge of the mandible down to the clavicle, including cervical lymph nodes, the sternocleidomastoid muscle, internal jugular vein, cranial nerve XI and submaxillary salivary gland
- **Laser surgery**: irradiation of small laryngeal tumors
- **Partial laryngectomy**: excision of one-half or more of the larynx
- **Hemilaryngectomy**: a partial laryngectomy performed when the malignancy is less than 1 cm and extends beyond the vocal cords, but within the subglottic area
- **Supraglottic laryngectomy**: a form of partial laryngectomy in which the superior portion of the larynx is excised from the false vocal cords to the epiglottis

Risk Factors/Indications for Laryngectomy

- Cancer of larynx
- Chronic alcoholism and heavy use of tobacco increase the risk of developing laryngeal cancer.
- Airway obstruction

Signs and Symptoms Indicating Need for Laryngectomy

- Hoarseness that persists for more than two weeks (usually earliest symptom)
- Persistent cough
- Change in voice quality
- Feeling of lump in throat
- Difficulty swallowing
- Color changes in the mouth or tongue to red, white gray, dark brown, or black
- Persistent or unexplained oral bleeding
- Burning sensation when drinking citrus juices or hot liquids
- Neck masses
- Unilateral sore throat
- Persistent unilateral ear pain
- Anorexia and weight loss

- Halitosis
- Advanced lesions may cause a sore throat, dyspnea, dysphagia, and cervical adenopathy.
- Airway obstruction (late)

Diagnostic and Laboratory Tests

- History and physical exam
- Complete blood count (CBC) with differential, urinalysis, SMA-20
- Indirect and direct laryngoscopy
- Panendoscopy (performed with anesthesia to define the extent of the tumor)
- Bronchoscopy
- MRI (magnetic resonance imaging)
- Computed tomography (CT)/computed axial tomography (CAT) scan
- Chest x-ray
- Barium swallow
- Multiple biopsy specimens

Therapeutic Nursing Management

- **Assess/Monitor**:
  - Respiratory status and check for compromise every 1-2 hours
  - Arterial blood gases and pulse oximetry
  - Nutritional status including intake and output, and daily weights
  - Ability to swallow
  - Signs of infection at operative site as well as pneumonia
- **Nursing Activities**:
  - Provide analgesia as ordered.
  - Encourage deep breathing and coughing.
  - Elevate HOB, place client in high-Fowler's or Fowler's position to enhance respirations.
  - Maintain humidification of inspired gases.
  - Maintain an adequate fluid intake.
  - Perform tracheal suctioning using sterile technique.
  - Perform tracheostomy care as needed and per protocol noting that clients with laryngectomies normally have uncuffed tracheostomy tubes.
  - Administer prophylactic antibiotics as ordered.
  - Administer oxygen as prescribed. (Avoid high levels of oxygen. Hypoxemia is the stimulus for respiration. If PaO2 levels are elevated, the drive to breathe may be suppressed, causing apnea.)
  - Maintain IV fluids and/or enteral feedings.
  - Teach the client to initiate a swallow by placing a small amount of food on the back of the tongue.
  - Provide privacy during initial attempts at eating.

- Reinforce and clarify information provided by the client's physician about the extent of the cancer, and proposed surgery.
- Emphasize that a total laryngectomy results in a loss of speech and that the client will breathe through a permanent stoma in the neck.
- Point out that surgery will affect the client's sense of taste and smell, and eating in the initial postoperative period.
- Teach pursed-lip breathing techniques.
- Discourage tobacco use, especially cigarettes.
- Encourage participation in a progressive, low-impact exercise program.
- Teach relaxation techniques.
- Provide emotional support to client and family; refer to counseling and/or support group.

Pharmacology

- Antibiotics (cefazolin for surgical prophylaxis)
- Analgesics (morphine, meperidine)
- Anti-depressants

Complications

- Risk of injury to the auditory or facial nerve with possible loss of hearing and facial expression on the affected side
- Damage to the spinal accessory nerve may cause shoulder drop on the affected side.
- Poor wound healing
- Infection
- Excessive coughing or vomiting of blood
- Airway obstruction
- Tracheostomy stenosis
- Pharyngocutaneous fistula
- Pharyngeal stricture
- Disfigurement
- Depression

Age-Related Changes—Gerontological Considerations

- Wound healing proceeds more slowly in the elderly client; wound breakdown is a common complication because of poor nutrition and altered circulation.
- The elderly are more susceptible to postoperative complications.
- Inactivity and immobility increases the risk of stasis pooling of respiratory sections, thereby placing them at increased risk of secondary infections (i.e., pneumonia).
- Older clients may find it more difficult to learn new methods of speech following laryngectomy.

Critical Thinking Exercise: Nursing Management of the Client with a Laryngectomy

Situation: The 62-year-old client who was diagnosed with laryngeal cancer earlier has been transferred to the surgical unit from the PACU (Post Anesthesia Care Unit) following a total laryngectomy. The client has a tracheostomy, and a nasogastric tube is attached to suction. The nurse suctions the client's tracheostomy tube every two hours, deflates the tracheostomy cuff every eight hours during expiration, and changes the tracheostomy tube daily. Although the nurse is trying to communicate with the client using a magic slate, the client is very apprehensive and frustrated because he cannot speak. The nurse assures him he will be meeting with a speech therapist as soon as he feels stronger.

1. What are some likely etiologies for the client's preoperative nursing diagnoses?

   a. Anxiety:

   b. Knowledge deficit:

   c. Risk for ineffective individual coping:

2. Prioritize the client's postoperative nursing diagnoses, with "1" representing the most important diagnosis.

   _____ Knowledge deficit

   _____ Risk for altered nutrition

   _____ Anxiety

   _____ Risk for ineffective airway clearance

3. Why is it necessary to deflate the tracheostomy cuff during exhalation?

4. Describe the three speech methods available to clients following laryngectomy.

   a. Artificial larynx (electrolarynx):

   b. Esophageal speech:

   c. Tracheoesophageal puncture (TEP):

Nursing Management of the Client with Emphysema

Key Points

- Emphysema is a chronic, progressive lung disease characterized by destruction of the alveolar walls and capillaries and permanent enlargement of the air spaces.
- A component of pulmonary connective tissue, lung elastin, is destroyed by an enzyme which then causes decreased pulmonary surface area available for gas exchange.
- Emphysema symptoms usually develop when the client is in their 40s with disability increasing by age 50 to 60.
- Cigarette smoking is the most common cause of emphysema and chronic bronchitis.
- There is a lag of 30 to 35 years, on average, between taking up smoking and the onset of signs and symptoms.
- Emphysema or other obstructive lung diseases can lead to cor pulmonale, an abnormal cardiac condition characterized by hypertrophy of the right ventricle.
- Most clients with emphysema usually have chronic bronchitis; both conditions are significant components of COPD (chronic obstructive pulmonary disease); clients may also have asthma.
- In general, COPD is an irreversible process; however, smoking cessation is the only certain way to prevent COPD and to slow its progression.
- Goals of collaborative management:
  - Provide early recognition and treatment.
  - Restore maximum respiratory function.
  - Prevent complications (respiratory failure, pneumonia).
  - Treatment generally focuses on easing the symptoms and is based on the degree of obstruction and the extent of disability.
- Important nursing diagnoses (actual or potential):
  - Ineffective breathing pattern
  - Ineffective airway clearance
  - Anxiety and fear
  - Knowledge deficit
  - Fatigue and restlessness
  - Potential complications of emphysema
  - Altered nutrition: less than body requirements
  - Self-care deficit
  - Activity intolerance
  - Ineffective individual/family coping

- Ineffective individual/family management of therapeutic regimen
- **Key Terms/Concepts**: Progressive, chronic cor pulmonale, alpha 1-antitrypsin enzyme, chronic obstructive pulmonary disease, chronic bronchitis

Overview

Emphysema is a chronic lung disease that is characterized by abnormal, permanent enlargement of air spaces, destruction of alveolar walls, and reduced capillary perfusion. Enzymes that degrade protein (proteases) alter or destroy the alveoli and the small airways by breaking down elastin. The bronchi, bronchioles, and alveoli become inflamed as a result of chronic irritation. Because of bronchiole lumen narrowing, air becomes trapped in the alveoli during expiration, causing alveolar distention. The alveoli then rupture and scar, losing their elasticity. Oxygen in arterial blood decreases (hypoxia) and CO2 increases (hypercarbia). Deficiency of alpha 1-antritrypsin, an enzyme that normally inhibits the activity of proteolytic enzymes and tissue destruction in the lungs, leads to an early onset of emphysema, often before age 40. Cessation of cigarette smoking in the early stages is probably the most significant factor in slowing the progression of the disease.

Risk Factors/Indications for Laryngectomy

- Cigarette smoking
- Genetic predisposition (alpha-1 antitrypsin deficiency)
- Environmental exposure to air pollutants
- Advanced age
- Chronic respiratory infections

Signs and Symptoms

- Dyspnea (initially dyspnea on exertion)
- Minimal coughing
- Sputum production (initially very little, later in the disease copious amounts)
- Breath sounds diminished, hyperresonant
- Lung crackles, wheezes
- Fatigue, weakness
- Tachypnea with use of accessory muscles
- Assumes a position of sitting or leaning forward
- Expiratory phase of the respiratory cycle is prolonged
- Tachycardia
- Hypoxemia
- Hypercarbia/hypercapnia
- Barrel chest
- Pursed lip breathing
- Anorexia, weight loss
- Finger clubbing (in advanced stages)

Diagnostic and Laboratory tests

- History and physical examination
- Pulmonary function tests:
  - Air flow (spirometer)
  - Lung volume
  - Diffusion capacity (correlates with body's ability to extract oxygen from the lungs)
- Arterial blood gas (ABG) analysis
- Complete blood count (CBC) with differential
- Alpha 1-antitrypsin assay
- Pulse oximetry
- Chest x-rays
- Sputum cultures
- Bronchoscopy

Therapeutic Nursing Management

- **Assess/Monitor**:
  - Respiratory status
  - ABGs (arterial blood gases)
  - Pulse oximetry
  - Nutritional status
  - Fluid status
- **Nursing Activities**:
  - Teach pursed-lip breathing techniques.
  - Administer prophylactic antibiotics as ordered.
  - Place client in high-Fowler's position to enhance respirations.
  - Administer oxygen as prescribed. (Avoid high levels of oxygen. Hypoxemia is the stimulus for respiration. If PaO2 levels are elevated, the drive to breathe may be suppressed, causing apnea.)
  - Chest physiotherapy
  - Encourage oral intake of fluids (to help liquefy secretions) if not contraindicated.
  - Use of humidifier
  - Allow for sufficient rest periods and assist in ADL.
  - Increase intake of high-protein, high-calorie diet divided into five or six small meals per day.
  - Drink fluids between meals rather than with meals to reduce gastric distention.
  - Perform frequent oral hygiene.
  - Assist with pulmonary rehabilitation (physical therapy, bronchial hygiene, nutrition, educational topics such as smoking cessation, counseling, vocational rehab, etc.).
  - Encourage participation in a progressive, low impact exercise program.

- Discourage tobacco use, especially cigarettes, refer for behavior modification.
- Encourage client to get a yearly flu shot.
- Teach relaxation techniques, understanding of disease process, smoking cessation, etc.
- Provide emotional support to client and family (referral to support groups).

Pharmacology

- Immunizations (pneumonia, influenza)
- Bronchodilators (short acting and long acting beta2 agonists and anticholinergics)
- Corticosteroids – PO or IV (prednisone, methylprednisolone), Inhaled (fluticasone, beclomethasone, triamcinolone)
- Oxygen
- Diuretics, if fluid overload
- Anti-anxiety
- Antibiotics (if bacterial infection present)

Complications

- Acute exacerbations of chronic bronchitis
- Cor pulmonale (hypertrophy of the right side of the heart with or without heart failure)
- Right-sided heart failure
- Acute respiratory failure
- Peptic ulcer and gastroesophageal reflux
- Pneumonia
- Oxygen toxicity
- Death

Age-Related Changes—Gerontological Considerations

- In the older adult, alveolar membranes atrophy and may collapse, producing large, air-filled spaces and a decreased total surface area of the pulmonary membranes.
- Respiratory rates generally increase in older adults as respiratory reserves decrease.
- Clients with advanced COPD/emphysema often become fatigued and dyspneic with minimal activity, including eating. At the same time the increased work of breathing raises their metabolic demands and more calories are required to meet their body's needs.
- Poor nutrition status further impairs the immune system and increases the risk of a complicating infection.
- Increased risks for fluid and nutritional deficits are related to fatigue and dyspnea.

Critical Thinking Exercise: Nursing Management of the Client with Emphysema

Situation: A 62-year-old retired coal miner is being treated for advanced COPD (chronic obstructive pulmonary disease). He has dyspnea with minor exertion, obvious barrel chest, wheezing, tachypnea, and tachycardia.

1. Which statements are true of emphysema? Correct any false statements.

   a. Emphysema is an acute, rapidly progressive lung disease.

   b. Emphysema and bronchitis rarely occur in the same client.

   c. Prevention is an important component of treatment.

   d. Restoring maximum respiratory function is a goal of collaborative management.

   e. Emphysema is characterized by permanent shrinkage of air spaces.

2. Based on the client's data, the nurse is correct in placing which nursing diagnoses on the client's care plan?

   _____ Ineffective breathing pattern   _____ Anxiety/fear

   _____ Fatigue   _____ Potential complications of emphysema

   _____ Self-care deficit   _____ Activity intolerance

   _____ Altered nutrition: less than body requirements

   _____ Ineffective individual/family coping

3. "Ineffective airway clearance" is included as a nursing diagnosis on the client's plan of care. Which nursing activities best address this nursing diagnosis?

   _____ Encourage the client to take short, shallow breaths.

   _____ Teach the client to use relaxation techniques.

   _____ Encourage increased fluid intake.

   _____ Position the client flat in bed for maximum ventilation.

   _____ Administer high-dose oxygen therapy.

Nursing Management of the Client Requiring Oxygen Therapy

Key Points

- The goal of oxygen therapy is to achieve an oxygen saturation of 90% or greater without oxygen toxicity.
- A PaO_2 of about 60 mmHg usually allows adequate oxygen to meet the needs of body tissues.
- With continued high levels of oxygen delivery, surfactant synthesis is impaired, and the lungs become less compliant (more stiff) and may lead to hypoventilation in clients with chronic hypercapnia.
- The client who is hypoxemic and also has chronic hypercarbia (increased partial pressure of arterial carbon dioxide) requires lower levels of oxygen to prevent decreased respiratory effort, unless on mechanical ventilatory support.
- Clients with chronic COPD may require as little as 1 to 3 liters of oxygen per nasal cannula or 28% per Venturi mask to correct hypoxemia.
- Goals of collaborative management:
  - Restore and/or maintain cellular oxygenation through ventilation and perfusion.
  - Prevent complications of oxygen therapy (oxygen toxicity).
- Important nursing diagnoses (actual or potential):
  - Risk for injury
  - Impaired gas exchange
  - Fear and anxiety
  - Altered tissue perfusion
- **Key Terms/Concepts:** Hypoxia, hypoxemia, oxygen toxicity, hypercapnia, COPD (chronic obstructive pulmonary disease), partial pressure, FIO_2 (fraction of inspired oxygen), hypercarbia

Overview

Oxygen (O_2) is a colorless, odorless, tasteless gas that constitutes 21% of the atmosphere. Used clinically, it is a potent drug prescribed by providers to augment cellular ventilation and to relieve symptoms of hypoxemia. Therapeutic oxygen is prescribed when the oxygen needs of the body cannot be met by atmospheric or "room air" alone. Oxygen therapy is used for both acute and chronic respiratory conditions associated with decreased blood and tissue oxygen levels as indicated by decreased partial pressure of arterial oxygen (PaO_2) levels or by decreased arterial oxygen saturation (SaO_2). The goal of oxygen therapy is to use the lowest fraction inspired oxygen (FiO_2) to obtain the most acceptable oxygenation without causing the development of harmful side effects. Prolonged exposure to a high level of PaO_2 may result in oxygen toxicity. The amount and route of administration are based on the individual needs of the client. Oxygen is administered by mask, nasal cannula, tent, hood, or mechanical ventilation.

Risk Factors

- Hypoxia
- Hypoxemia
- Severe bleeding
- Trauma
- Respiratory diseases
- Postanesthesia

Signs and Symptoms Indicating Need for Oxygen

- Restlessness
- Respiratory distress (dyspnea/ nasal flaring)
- Pallor
- Cyanosis (dark-skinned clients will have a grayish cast to skin)
- Rapid, shallow breathing
- Confusion, stupor, coma
- Tachycardia
- Cardiac dysrhythmias
- Increased pulse rate; as hypoxia advances, bradycardia results
- Increased rate and depth of respiration; as hypoxia progresses, shallow, slow respirations develop
- Elevated blood pressure; if O_2 deficiency is not corrected, blood pressure will decrease
- Use of accessory muscles
- Wheezing
- Lung crackles
- Clubbing

Diagnostic Tests

- ABG (arterial blood gas) analysis
- Pulse oximetry
- Chest x-ray
- Pulmonary function tests:
  - Air flow (spirometer)
  - Lung volume
  - Diffusion capacity (correlates with body's ability to extract oxygen from the lungs)

Therapeutic Nursing Management

- **Assess/Monitor:**
  - For impediments of oxygenation
  - For signs of oxygen toxicity
  - For correct oxygen liter flow and correct position of device
  - For the effectiveness of oxygen therapy
  - Client's anxiety related to need for oxygen
  - For skin breakdown from oxygen device
  - Skin integrity for breakdown (nares, ears, neck)
- **Nursing Activities:**
  - Teach the client regarding the purpose of oxygen.
  - Promote oxygenation by appropriate positioning (high-Fowler's or semi-Fowler's).
  - Teach techniques to enhance breathing.
  - Encourage deep breathing and use of incentive spirometry following surgery.
  - Arrange for home use of oxygen.
  - Instruct client and family about use of oxygen at home.
  - Be sure that no flammable object, such as a cigarette, is used around oxygen.
  - Petroleum products should not be used on the lips of someone receiving oxygen since they are potentially flammable.

Complications

- Oxygen toxicity (nonproductive cough, substernal pain, nasal stuffiness, nausea and vomiting, fatigue, headache, sore throat and hypoventilation)
- Drying of nasal passages if nasal cannula used
- Absorption atelectasis (nitrogen is washed out of the alveoli and replaced with O_2)
- Infection (use of heated nebulizers or humidifiers support the growth of bacteria)
- Oxygen induced hypoventilation/carbon dioxide narcosis (respiratory center loses its sensitivity to elevated CO_2)
- Necrosis of nares from prolonged use of nasal cannula
- Loss of skin integrity related to prolonged mask usage
- Acute respiratory distress (high concentrations of O_2 inactivate pulmonary surfactant)

Age-Related Changes—Gerontological Considerations

- Increased risk for compromised ventilation and respiration is due to calcification of rib cartilage, skeletal changes, reduced numbers of alveoli, decreased elastic recoil of the lungs, and greater dead space within the lungs.

- Ill-fitting masks, related to decreased subcutaneous facial fat, may interfere with older adults receiving their prescribed amount of oxygen.
- Increased risk for dehydration in the elderly may cause dry mucous membranes.
- Increased risk for skin alterations related to oxygen equipment is due to decreased subcutaneous tissue and elasticity.

Critical Thinking Exercise: Nursing Management of the Client Requiring Oxygen Therapy

Situation: An older man is receiving oxygen therapy via a nasal cannula while being treated for exacerbated COPD (chronic obstructive pulmonary disease). The oxygen is prescribed to run at 2 L per minute.

1. How can the nurse prevent the client's skin from breaking down beneath the oxygen tubing?

2. Why is low-dose oxygen therapy prescribed for a person with COPD (chronic obstructive pulmonary disease) even though they may be experiencing difficulty breathing?

3. Prioritize the nurse's activities for the client receiving oxygen, with "1" representing the first activity to be implemented.

   _____ Assess for skin alterations beneath oxygen tubing.

   _____ Place client in Fowler's position.

   _____ Teach client relaxation to enhance breathing.

   _____ Encourage client to participate in his/her own care.

Nursing Management of the Client with Arterial Blood Gas (ABG) Abnormalities

> ## Key Points

- Arterial blood gases (ABGs) are measured to determine oxygenation status and acid-base balance.
- Acid-base balance is crucial to the effective functioning of the body systems; severe imbalances can be lethal to the client.
- ABG analysis includes the pH which represents the amount of free hydrogen ion (H+) available in the blood (normal value 7.35 to 7.45); the PaO_2 which represents the partial pressure of the oxygen dissolved in arterial blood (normal value 80 to 100 mmHg), the $PaCO_2$, which represents the partial pressure of carbon dioxide in arterial blood (normal value 35 to 45 mmHg), and the HCO_3, which represents the concentration of bicarbonate in the blood, normally 22-26 Eq/L.
- The SaO_2 is also calculated during this analysis and is the percentage of oxygen combined with hemoglobin compared with the total amount it could carry (normal value >95%).
- Chemoreceptors located in the medulla, and peripheral chemoreceptors located in the carotid and aortic bodies, respond to changes in hydrogen ion (H+) concentration (acidosis) and to changes in PaO_2, pH and $PaCO_2$ to increase or decrease the respiratory rate in an attempt to maintain normal acid-base balance.
- Both metabolic and respiratory compromise can result in altered arterial blood gases (ABGs), acid-base balance, and corresponding change in pH.
- Goals of collaborative management:
  - Restore and maintain acid-base balance.
  - Correct the underlying cause.
  - Prevent complications of acid-base imbalance.
  - Maintain oxygenation and ventilation.
- Important nursing diagnoses (actual or potential):
  - Anxiety and fear related to breathlessness
  - Ineffective breathing pattern related to hyperventilation
  - Impaired gas exchange related to alveolar hypoventilation
  - Ineffective airway clearance related to thick pulmonary secretions and fatigue
  - Fluid volume deficit secondary to excessive gastrointestinal fluid loss
  - Altered renal/peripheral tissue perfusion related to hypovolemia
  - Decreased cardiac output secondary to dysrhythmias
  - Knowledge deficit related to appropriate use and potential side effects of medications

- **Key Terms/Concepts**: Oxygenation saturation, base excess, metabolic compromise, respiratory compromise, acidosis, alkalosis, buffering mechanism, respiratory compensation mechanism, metabolic or renal compensation, partial pressure

Overview

Arterial blood gas (ABG) analysis measures the oxygen and carbon dioxide content of arterial blood by various methods to assess the adequacy of ventilation and oxygenation and the acid-base status of the body. The body is not tolerant of wide changes in pH and is working constantly to maintain the pH range between 7.35 and 7.45. A normal pH is maintained if the ratio of bicarbonate (HCO_3) to carbon dioxide (CO_2) remains at approximately 20:1 (HCO_3/CO_2). The body has three mechanisms to maintain acid-base balance: (1) the buffering mechanism, which represents chemical reactions between acids and bases to maintain a neutral environment, (2) the respiratory compensation mechanism, which increases or decreases alveolar ventilation to rid the system of excessive acid or retain carbon dioxide, and (3) the metabolic or renal compensation mechanism which controls the rate of elimination or reabsorption of hydrogen and bicarbonate ions in the kidney. Oxygen saturation is also measured which is important in determining the amount of oxygen available for delivery to the tissues. Oxygen saturation of hemoglobin is normally 95% or higher. The partial pressure of arterial oxygen, normally 80 to 100 mmHg is increased in hyperventilation and decreased in cardiac decompensation, chronic obstructive pulmonary disease, and certain neuromuscular disorders. The partial pressure of carbon dioxide, normally 38 to 45 mmHg, may be higher in emphysema, chronic obstructive pulmonary disease, and reduced respiratory center function; it may be lower in pregnancy and in the presence of pulmonary emboli and anxiety. Blood for ABG analysis can be obtained by arterial puncture or from an arterial catheter typically placed in the radial or femoral artery.

Normal Values of Arterial Blood Gases			
Blood pH	Acidity - Alkalinity	7.35-7.45	pH
$PaCO_2$ or PCO_2	Partial pressure of carbon dioxide	35-45	mmHg
PaO_2 or PO_2	Partial pressure of oxygen	80-100	mmHg
HCO_3	Bicarbonate level	22-26	mEq/L
SaO_2	Oxygen saturation (bound to hemoglobin)	96-98	%

("Pa" or "P" stands for "Partial" and "Sa" stands for "Saturated")

Risk Factors/Indications

- Inadequate oxygenation
- Chronic obstructive pulmonary disease (chronic bronchitis, emphysema)
- Conditions precipitating an increase in hydrogen ion (H+) concentration
    - Diabetic acidosis
    - Uremia
    - Ingestion of acidic drugs

- Lactic acidosis
- Conditions precipitating a decrease in bicarbonate (HCO3) levels
  - Diarrhea
  - Gastrointestinal fistulas
  - Loss of body fluids
  - Drugs causing loss of alkali
  - Hyperaldosteronism
- Conditions that result in a decrease in acid:
  - Ingestion of alkaline drugs
  - Loss of gastric fluids (vomiting or NG suctioning)
  - Treatment with steroids
  - Diuretic therapy
  - Binge-purge syndrome
- Conditions that result in an increase in acid:
  - Severe hydration
  - Severe infection/sepsis
  - Severe trauma
  - Diabetic ketoacidosis
  - Hepatic failure
  - Shock
- Conditions that result in respiratory acidosis
  - Alveolar hypoventilation (respiratory depression: e.g., head injury, overdose, oversedation, decreased ventilation)
  - Altered diffusion/ventilation-perfusion mismatch
- Conditions that result in respiratory alkalosis:
  - Alveolar hyperventilation (anxiety, fear, pain, hypoxia, head injury, fever, mechanical ventilation)
- Acute and chronic illnesses
- Traumatic injuries
- Fever
- Dehydration
- Fluid and electrolyte imbalance
- CPR
- Sepsis
- Shock

Signs and Symptoms of Acid-Base Imbalance

- Metabolic acidosis: Kussmaul's respirations, headache, hyperkalemia
- Metabolic alkalosis: dizziness, confusion, tetany, convulsions
- Respiratory acidosis: hyperpnea, headache, confusion, drowsiness, coma
- Respiratory alkalosis: Lightheadedness, tetany, convulsions

- Inadequate oxygenation:
    - Respiratory: tachypnea, dyspnea, use of accessory muscles, and retraction of interspaces on inspiration
    - Cardiovascular: tachycardia, mild hypertension, arrhythmias, hypotension, cyanosis, cool, and clammy skin
    - Central nervous system: apprehension, restlessness, irritability, confusion, lethargy, combativeness, and coma
    - Other: diaphoresis, decreased urine output, and fatigue

Therapeutic Nursing Management

- **Assess/Monitor**:
    - Fluid and electrolyte status
    - Respiratory status
    - Gastrointestinal status (presence of vomiting, diarrhea)
    - Arterial blood gases, CBC, complete metabolic profile, or other laboratory data as ordered
- **Nursing Activities**:
    - Administer oxygen as prescribed.
    - Change ventilator settings per orders or notify respiratory therapy.
    - Perform the Allen test prior to arterial puncture to assess radial and ulnar arterial circulation.
    - Collect blood into heparinized syringe.
    - Maintain direct pressure over arterial puncture site for five minutes after drawing ABG (arterial blood gas).
    - If client is on anticoagulants, maintain pressure for 20 minutes or longer until bleeding stops.
    - Place the capped syringe in a basin of crushed ice and water to preserve the gas and pH levels of the specimen.
    - Avoid oxygen contamination of arterial specimen.
    - Report results of ABGs (arterial blood gases) to practitioner as soon as they are available.

Complications

- Arterial blockage
- Loss of limb
- Cardiovascular collapse
- Death

Age–Related Changes—Gerontological Considerations

- The normal PaO_2 decreases with advancing age: approximately 10 mmHg per decade beyond age 60.
- Age related changes in the respiratory system can be divided into alterations in structure, defense mechanisms, and respiratory control.

- Structural alterations include a decrease in elastic recoil of the lung and decrease in chest wall compliance, anteroposterior diameter of the thoracic cage increases. Within the lung there is a decrease in the number of functional alveoli. As a consequence, more inspired air is distributed to the lung apices and ventilation is less well-matched to perfusion causing a lowering of the PaO_2.
- Respiratory defense mechanisms are less effective because of a decline in cell-mediated immunity and formation of antibodies. The alveolar macrophages are less effective at phagocytosis. An elderly client has a less forceful cough and fewer and less functional cilia. Formation of IgA, an important mechanism in neutralizing the effect of viruses, is diminished.
- Respiratory control is altered, resulting in a more gradual response to changes in blood oxygen or carbon dioxide level. The PaO_2 drops to a lower level and the $PaCO_2$ rises to a higher level before the respiratory rate changes.
- Blood gas sampling may be challenging in some elderly persons due to changes in the vascular integrity. Veins tend to roll with venipuncture, or may be difficult to puncture without extravasation. It is particularly important to perform arterial aspiration with proficiency because altered circulation occurs in many elderly persons.
- A higher prevalence of COPD (chronic obstructive pulmonary disease) occurs in older adults, often due to prolonged exposure to tobacco, chemical, or environmental irritants. Blood gas values are altered depending on the underlying disease process.
  - Clients with chronic bronchitis commonly have a persistent cough, copious sputum production, wheezing, and increased work breathing. The ABG (arterial blood gas) typically shows hypercarbia. Hypoxemia is often present to some degree, depending on the severity of pulmonary resistance and edema in the airways.
  - Clients with emphysema are typically short of breath, particularly on exertion. The ABG (arterial blood gas) findings typically show low or normal CO_2 levels until end stage disease. Hypoxemia is the prevailing blood gas alteration.
  - Clients with asthma experience impaired exhalation and ineffective airway clearance. The nurse is likely to assess pursed lip breathing, use of accessory muscles, dyspnea, wheezing, and coughing. With untreated asthma, the blood gas findings show hypercarbia, hypoxemia, and respiratory acidosis.
- Many elderly persons experience less effective coughing, which can lead to an accumulation of secretions. The reduced airway clearance may result in accumulation of carbon dioxide and reduced oxygen exchange.

Critical Thinking Exercise: Nursing Management of the Client with Arterial Blood Gas (ABG) Abnormalities

Situation: The nurse has just received the ABG (arterial blood gas) analysis report on a client with pneumonia.

1. When assisting with drawing an arterial blood gas, it is important for the nurse to perform which actions?

_____ Administer oxygen.

_____ Assess radial and ulnar arterial circulation.

_____ Maintain direct pressure over arterial puncture site for two minutes after drawing ABG.

_____ Avoid oxygen contamination of arterial specimen.

_____ Report drawing of specimen to practitioner as soon as possible.

2. Which of the following findings are normal/abnormal?

ABGs (arterial blood gases)			Normal	Abnormal
Blood pH	7.38	pH		
PaCO$_2$	58	mmHg		
PaO$_2$	56	mmHg		
HCO$_3$	18	mEq/L		
SaO$_2$	96	%		

3. Determine the primary type of acid-base imbalance in the arterial blood sample.

	Samples				
	1	2	3	4	5
pH	7.50	7.53	7.45	7.28	7.24
PaCO$_2$	29	43	43	54	45
PaO2	91	84	63	88	102
HCO$_3$	25	31	23	26	34

Sample 1:

Sample 2:

Sample 3:

Sample 4:

Sample 5:

4. List a possible etiology for the following ABG abnormalities.

Respiratory alkalosis:

Metabolic alkalosis:

Hypoxemia:

Respiratory acidosis:

Metabolic alkalosis:

Nursing Management of the Client Undergoing a Bronchoscopy Procedure

Key Points

- Bronchoscopy is an invasive diagnostic and treatment modality, used to visualize the larynx, trachea, and bronchi.
- Bronchoscope examination includes observations of the tracheobronchial tree to assess for abnormalities and for diagnosing such conditions as localized atelectasis, bronchial obstruction, tumors, and lung abscess.
- The procedure may also be used to obtain biopsy specimen, fluid, or sputum collection for cytology or bacteriological studies or to remove mucus plugs or foreign bodies.
- Bronchoscopy can be performed as an outpatient procedure, in a surgical suite under general anesthesia, or at the bedside under local anesthesia and conscious sedation.
- Goals of collaborative management:
    - Prevent complications (bleeding, infection, pneumothorax, and hypoxia).
    - Restore and maintain oxygenation.
    - Obtain sputum/specimens for diagnostic purposes.
- Important nursing diagnoses (actual or potential):
    - Impaired gas exchange
    - Ineffective airway clearance
    - Risk for infection
    - Risk for injury
    - Knowledge deficit
    - Anxiety and fear
    - Impaired circulation related to hypoxia and/or dysrhythmias
- **Key Terms/Concepts:** Mucous plug, pneumothorax, bronchial washing, bronchoalveolar lavage (BAL)

Overview

Bronchoscopy is the visual examination of the trachea and bronchial tree by way of a narrow, flexible fiberoptic scope. Bronchoscopy may be used for examination of tumors, to assess changes resulting from treatment, to obtain biopsy specimens, and to remove foreign bodies or mucus plugs. If a tumor cannot be visualized, a saline solution can be used to flush the airways (bronchial washing), and cells obtained in this manner are sent for cytologic examination. After the nasal pharynx and oral pharynx are anesthetized with local anesthetic, the bronchoscope is coated with lidocaine (Xylocaine) and inserted, usually through the nose, and threaded down into the airways. Bronchoscopy can also be performed on mechanically ventilated clients by inserting the scope through the endotracheal tube.

Risk Factors

- Foreign object lodged in trachea or bronchi
- Difficulty breathing from unknown origin
- Thick secretions
- Mucous plug
- Suspected malignancy

Signs and Symptoms

- Anxiety
- Sore throat from bronchoscope placement after procedure
- Absence of gag reflex from local anesthetic

Therapeutic Nursing Management

- **Prevent:**
  - Aspiration following bronchoscopy procedure by checking for return of gag reflex
- **Assess/Monitor:**
  - For allergies to iodine, local anesthetics, or other medications that may be used
  - Client's respiratory status and skin color during and after the procedure
  - Airway and respiratory status following examination
- **Nursing Activities:**
  - Provide explanation about the effects of the anesthetic agent to help decrease anxiety.
  - Obtain informed consent/signed permit.
  - Maintain NPO (nothing by mouth) for 6-12 hours prior to procedure as prescribed.
  - Remove dentures prior to performing procedure.
  - Administer diazepam (if ordered by physician), atropine, or other medications (as ordered) such as midazolam and propofol.
  - Withhold oral fluids and food until gag response returns.
  - Administer oxygen if needed.
  - After procedure, monitor for signs/symptoms of hemorrhage/hemoptysis and pneumothorax.
  - Monitor vital signs every 15 minutes until stable.
  - Discourage smoking, talking, and coughing for several hours after procedure.

Pharmacology

- Atropine (to dry secretions)
- Sedatives
- Anesthetics
- Topical anesthetics (benzocaine, tetracaine, lidocaine)
- General anesthesia

Complications

- Respiratory distress
- Hypoxia
- Interruption of gag reflex
- Bleeding
- Infection
- Pneumothorax
- Perforation

Age-Related Changes—Gerontological Considerations

- Sedation given to older adults with respiratory insufficiency may precipitate respiratory arrest.
- Contact lenses, dentures, and other dental appliances need to be removed prior to the procedure. Injury may occur if left in place.
- The cough reflex may be slower to return in the elderly client receiving local anesthesia due to impaired laryngeal reflex.
- Increased risk of respiratory infection and pneumonia in the elderly due to decreased cough effectiveness and decrease in secretion clearance. Respiratory infections may be more severe and last longer in the elderly.
- Retained secretions, excessive sedation, or positioning that impairs chest expansion may substantially alter PaO_2 or SpO_2 values.
- The nurse must assess for confusion and lethargy in the elderly due to the anesthetizing effects of large doses of lidocaine given during the bronchoscopy.

Critical Thinking Exercise: Nursing Management of the Client Undergoing a Bronchoscopy Procedure

Situation: A young female client, who has a chronic cough and low-grade fever, is about to undergo a diagnostic bronchoscopy. She is unfamiliar with the procedure and is anxious.

1. Complete the sentences regarding teaching of clients undergoing bronchoscopy.

   a. You will be given a mild _____ prior to the procedure.

   b. The back of your _____ will be _____.

   c. A long, _____ _____ will be inserted into your _____ and _____.

   d. The procedure allows your _____ to be _____ and _____ obtained.

   e. You will _____ feel any _____ during the procedure.

   f. Your throat may be _____ immediately _____ the procedure.

   g. You will _____ be allowed to _____ or _____ until your _____ reflex returns.

2. Why does the client need to be NPO (nothing by mouth) for 6-8 hours preceding the bronchoscopy?

3. Which assessments are essential following a bronchoscopy?

   _____ Pupillary reaction   _____ Heart rate   _____ Blood pressure

   _____ Bowel sounds   _____ Respiratory rate   _____ Skin color

   _____ Lung sounds   _____ Temperature   _____ Pedal pulses

Nursing Management of the Client with a Tracheostomy

Key Points

- Tracheotomy is a sterile surgical incision into the trachea for the purpose of establishing an airway.
  - Tracheostomy is the stoma, or opening, that results from the tracheotomy.
  - A tracheostomy can be performed as an emergency procedure or as a scheduled surgical procedure; it can be permanent or temporary.
  - The procedure should be performed by a health care provider who is thoroughly trained in the technique.
  - The double lumen tracheostomy tube has three major parts:
    - Outer cannula: fits into the stoma and keeps the airway open; the faceplate indicates the size and type of tube and has small holes on both sides for securing the tube with tracheostomy ties
    - Inner cannula: disposable or reusable; fits snugly into the outer cannula and locks into place
    - Obturator: during insertion of the tube, the obturator is placed inside the outer cannula with its rounded tip protruding from the end of the tube to ease insertion; it is removed immediately after tube placement and is always kept with the client and at the bedside in case of accidental decannulation
- Tracheostomy tubes are classified as cuffed or uncuffed.
  - Cuffed tracheostomy tubes protect the lower airway by producing a seal between the upper and lower airway. Cuff inflation pressures should not exceed 20 mmHg because higher pressures may compress tracheal capillaries, limit blood flow, and predispose to tracheal necrosis. A cuffed tube is used in clients receiving mechanical ventilation and is designed to use a high volume of air while maintaining a low pressure on the tracheal mucosa.
  - There are two methods of cuff inflation: the minimal leak technique (for cuffs without pressure relief valves) and the occlusive technique (for cuffs with pressure relief valves).
  - A cuffless tracheostomy tube is used when the client can protect the airway from aspiration and does not require mechanical ventilation.
- Other types of tracheostomy tubes include:
  - Single-lumen tube: long tube used for clients with long or extra-thick necks
  - Tracheostomy tube with cuff and pilot balloon: low-pressure, high-volume cuff distributes cuff pressure over large area, minimizing pressure on tracheal wall
  - Fenestrated tracheostomy tube: has openings on the surface of the outer cannula that permit air from the lungs to flow over the vocal cords; allows

the client to breathe spontaneously through the larynx, speak, and cough up secretions while the tracheostomy remains in place, often used to wean the client from a tracheostomy by ensuring that the client can tolerate breathing through his/her natural airway before the entire tube is removed.

- Cuffed fenestrated tracheostomy tube: facilitates mechanical ventilation and speech. Often used for clients with spinal cord paralysis or neuromuscular disease who do not require ventilation all the time. When not on the ventilator, the client can have the cuff deflated and the tube capped for speech.
- Metal tracheostomy tube: used for permanent tracheostomy. It is a cuffless double-lumen tube and can be cleaned and reused indefinitely.
- Talking/speaking tracheostomy tube: has two pigtail tubings. One tubing connects to the cuff and is used for cuff inflation, and the second connects to an opening just above the cuff. When the second tubing is connected to a low-flow air source, sufficient air moves up over the vocal cords to permit speech. The client can then speak, although the cuff is inflated.
- Tracheostomy tube foam-filled cuff: cuff is filled with plastic foam. Before insertion, cuff is deflated. After insertion, cuff is allowed to fill passively with air, pilot tubing is not capped, and no cuff pressure monitoring is required.

- Goals of collaborative management:
  - Re-establish and maintain a patent airway.
  - Prevent dislodgment of the tracheostomy tube after insertion.
  - Provide long-term mechanical ventilation via the tube if necessary.
  - Provide adequate nutrition and hydration.
  - Help the client communicate.
  - Prevent injury.
  - Prevent bacterial contamination of the airway during suctioning.
  - Prevent respiratory and cardiovascular complications from suctioning.
  - Teach the client and family how to care for the tracheostomy at home if necessary.
- Important nursing diagnoses (actual or potential):
  - Impaired gas exchange
  - Ineffective airway clearance
  - Ineffective breathing pattern
  - Risk for injury
  - Impaired swallowing
  - Impaired nutrition, less than body requirements
  - Impaired verbal communication
  - Constipation and other bowel dysfunction
  - Body image disturbance
  - Anxiety and fear
  - Potential for ineffective management of therapeutic program.
- **Key Terms/Concepts:** Trachea, tracheal obstruction, tracheotomy, endotracheal intubation, endotracheal suctioning, cannula, obturator, cuffed, uncuffed fenestrated tracheostomy tube, decannulation, pilot balloon, speaking

tracheostomy tube (Portex, National), face plate or flange, minimal leak technique, occlusive technique

Overview

Tracheostomy is the stoma or opening that results from the tracheotomy: the surgical incision into the trachea through the neck, with insertion of a cannula, for the purpose of establishing an airway. Indications for a tracheotomy are to bypass an upper airway obstruction, facilitate removal of secretions, permit long-term mechanical ventilation, protect the airway after head and neck surgery, provide airway reconstruction after laryngeal trauma or laryngeal cancer surgery, treat for obstructive sleep apnea refractory to conventional therapy, and to permit oral intake and speech in the client who requires long-term mechanical ventilation. Several advantages make tracheostomy a better option for long-term care, namely, less risk of long-term damage to the airway, increased client comfort because no tube is present in the mouth, the client can eat with a tracheostomy because the tube enters lower in the airway. If the tracheostomy cuff can be deflated or a speaking tube is used, the client can talk with a tracheostomy in place and mobility may be increased because the tracheostomy tube is more secure. Retention sutures are often placed in the tracheal cartilage when the tracheostomy is performed. The free ends should be taped to the skin in a place and manner that leaves them accessible if the tube is dislodged. Both cuffed and uncuffed tracheostomy tubes are available. A tracheostomy tube with an inflated cuff is used if the client is at risk of aspiration or requires mechanical ventilation. Because movement of breathing and swallowing moves the tube, a cuffed tube is not protective against aspiration. When the client can adequately exchange air and expectorate secretions, the tracheostomy tube can be removed.

Risk Factors

Tracheostomy is necessary when the airway is obstructed due to:

- Aspiration of a foreign object
- Aspiration of stomach contents
- Upper airway bleeding
- Cancer of the larynx
- Tracheal tumors
- Tracheal strictures
- Enlarged thyroid
- Oropharyngeal tumor
- Mediastinal tumors
- Excess mucous in airway
- Vocal cord paralysis
- Laryngeal edema
- Epiglottitis
- Severe obstructive sleep apnea
- Need for continuous mechanical ventilation

Signs and Symptoms Necessitating Tracheostomy

- Choking/aspiration of food or a foreign body
- Complete or partial airway obstruction
- Severe obstructive sleep apnea
- Respiratory failure
- Laryngeal edema
- Laryngeal or tracheal stenosis
- Neurological depression
- Use of accessory muscles
- Suprasternal and intercostals retractions
- Wheezing
- Restlessness
- Tachycardia
- Cyanosis
- Wet, gurgling noise due to excess mucous
- Diminished breath sounds
- Difficulty swallowing
- Severe dyspnea
- Tachypnea

Diagnostic and Laboratory Tests

- Fiberoptic bronchoscopy
- Chest x-ray
- ABG (arterial blood gas) values
- Pulse oximetry
- Diagnostic tests for specific tumors (thyroid, laryngeal, oropharynx, mediastinal)

Therapeutic Nursing Management

- **Prevention of Complications from Tracheostomy**:
    - Properly secure tracheostomy tube.
    - Do not over-inflate the cuff.
    - Do not allow the tracheostomy tube to become occluded with excessive or dried secretions.
    - Prevent complications from endotracheal suctioning.
    - Prevent infection by using sterile technique during suctioning and tracheostomy care.
- **Assess/Monitor**:
    - Preoperative nursing care focuses on the client's:
        - Knowledge deficits

- Communication
- Speech

- Immediate postoperative care focuses on:
  - Ensuring a patent airway
  - Confirming the presence of bilateral breath sounds
  - Recovering the client from anesthesia
  - Assessing for complications from the procedure
- For signs of hemorrhage and shock
- Vital signs
- For dyspnea, stridor, inspiratory effort, and signs of hypoxia
- For excessive mucous in airway
- Thickness, quantity, odor, and color of mucous secretions
- Stoma and skin surrounding stoma for signs of inflammation or infection
- Client's ability to cooperate with tracheostomy care and suctioning
- For tracheoesophageal fistula before feeding orally
- Oral mucosa for dryness
- ABG (arterial blood gas) values and other lab values (CBC with differential, chemistries)

- **Nursing Activities**:
  - Provide adequate humidification.
  - Provide adequate hydration.
  - Use careful suctioning technique to prevent tracheal trauma and possible infection.
  - Provide the client with an emergency call system as well as a call light.
  - Make certain the staff knows that the client cannot speak due to the tracheostomy.
  - Provide the client with paper and pen to communicate with the staff.
  - Provide emotional support to client and family.

- **Tracheostomy Care**:
  - Explain procedure and purpose of the procedure to the client and family.
  - Assemble the necessary equipment.
  - Wash hands, maintain standard precautions.
  - Suction the tracheostomy tube if necessary, using sterile suctioning supplies.
  - Remove old dressings and excess secretions.
  - Set up a sterile field.
  - Remove and clean the inner cannula (use half-strength hydrogen peroxide to clean the cannula and sterile saline to rinse it).
  - Clean the stoma site and then the tracheostomy plate with half-strength hydrogen peroxide followed by sterile saline.
  - Change tracheostomy ties if they are soiled. Secure new ties in place before removing soiled ones to prevent accidental decannulation. If a knot is needed, tie a square knot that is visible on the side of the neck. One or two fingers should be able to be placed between the tie tape and the neck.

- Document the type and amount of secretions and the general condition of the stoma and surrounding skin.
- Document the client's response to the procedure and any teaching or learning that occurred.
- The tracheostomy tube should be changed every 6-8 weeks or per hospital protocol.
- Reposition the client every two hours.
- Provide oral hygiene every two hours.
- Minimize dust in client's room; do not shake bedding.
- If a tracheoesophageal (TE) fistula is not present, offer the client foods and fluids that are easy to swallow, as per orders.
  - Position the client in an upright position to eat.
  - Enable swallowing by tipping the client's chin to chest.
- In event of accidental extubation, call for help immediately.
- When discharging the client, explain home tracheostomy care if tracheostomy is still in place.
- Discuss signs and symptoms that client should immediately report to health care provider (e.g., signs of infection, copious secretions).
- Refer client to a home health care agency and community support groups.

Pharmacology

- Supplemental oxygen
- Anti-inflammatory drugs (if swelling of soft tissues is present) (methylprednisolone, dexamethasone)
- Antibiotics
- Humidification
- Parenteral fluids
- Aerosolized medication (bronchodilators to relieve bronchospasm)
- Mucous liquefying agents (guaifenesin)
- Laxatives (bisacodyl) to prevent vagal stimulation
- Stool softeners (docusate sodium)
- Lip balms or water soluble jelly to prevent cracked lips

Complications

- Tracheostomy
  - Tube obstruction with secretions
  - Postoperative bleeding
  - Bacterial contamination and infection
  - Subcutaneous emphysema
  - Tracheoesophageal (TE) fistula
  - Tracheal stenosis
  - Malposition of tracheostomy tube

- Trachea-innominate artery fistula (a malpositioned tube causes necrosis and erosion of the innominate artery. This is a medical emergency.
- Tracheomalacia
- Pneumothorax
- Cuff inflation problems
- Cardiac arrest
- Loss of airway due to accidental dislodgement (decannulation)
- Tissue damage (where inflated cuff presses against the tracheal mucosa)
- Endotracheal suctioning
  - Trauma to mucosal lining of airway from suction catheter
  - Hypoxemia from prolonged suctioning
  - Infection (catheter introduced bacteria)
  - Vagal stimulation
  - Alveolar collapse
  - Cardiac arrhythmias

Age-Related Changes—Gerontological Considerations

- There is an increased risk of respiratory infection and pneumonia in the elderly due to the decrease in cough effectiveness and secretion clearance. Respiratory infections may be more severe and last longer in the elderly. Retained secretions, excessive sedation, or positioning can impair chest expansion and consequently impair gas exchange, substantially altering $PaO2$ (reduce), $PaCO_2$ (increase), or SpO_2 (reduce) values. Older persons may be at risk for dehydration (due to limited mobility, decrease in appetite, medications) contributing to thick, dried secretions which can occlude the airways.
- Maintaining good hydration in the elderly, as well as providing humidification (as ordered), is important to reduce the viscosity of secretions.

Critical Thinking Exercise: Nursing Management of the Client with a Tracheostomy

Situation: A 62-year-old male client who has undergone a total laryngectomy for laryngeal cancer is being cared for on the surgical unit. He has a tracheostomy tube in place. In addition to providing tracheostomy care, the nurse it also trying to help the client communicate his needs to the staff, as he is unable to speak.

1. Why is it so important for the client with a tracheostomy to be adequately hydrated?

2. By what means can the client with a tracheostomy communicate his needs to the staff?

3. Why must the client with a tracheostomy take laxatives and stool softeners?

4. If accidental extubation occurs, what can the nurse do while waiting for emergency help to arrive?

Nursing Management of the Client with a Thoracentesis

Key Points

- Thoracenteses is an invasive procedure in which fluid (or air) is removed from the pleural space with a needle.
- Thoracentesis is the treatment of choice when pleural effusion is significant and interferes with respirations.
- Thoracentesis may be performed at the client's bedside, in a procedure room or in the physician's office.
- Thoracentesis is usually performed under local anesthesia using a large-bore needle and generally requires less than 30 minutes to complete.
- Percussion, auscultation, radiography, or ultrasonography is used to locate the effusion and needle insertion site.
- The amount of fluid removed is limited to 1200 to 1500 mL at one time to prevent cardiovascular collapse.
- Goals of collaborative management:
  - Relieve symptoms of respiratory distress.
  - Prevent complications.
  - Obtain fluid for diagnostic purposes.
  - Treat the underlying condition to prevent further fluid accumulation.
- Important nursing diagnoses (actual or potential):
  - Pain management
  - High risk for infection
  - High risk for impaired gas exchange
  - Anxiety and fear
  - Risk for injury
  - Ineffective breathing pattern
  - Activity intolerance
- **Key Terms/Concepts**: Pleural effusion

Overview

Thoracentesis is the surgical perforation of the chest wall and pleural space with a needle to obtain specimens for diagnostic evaluation, to instill medication into the pleural space, and for the removal of fluid or air from the pleural space. Aspirated fluid is analyzed for general appearance, cell counts, protein and glucose content, the presence of enzymes such as LDH and amylase, abnormal cells, and culture. The client is positioned sitting upright with elbows on an over bed table. Feet and legs should be well supported. The skin is cleaned and a local anesthetic is instilled subcutaneously. After the procedure, the client is positioned on the unaffected side and the specimen is labeled and sent immediately to the laboratory per physician's orders. As an alternative to repeated thoracentesis, a chest tube may be inserted to permit further drainage of fluid.

Risk Factors/Indications for Thoracentesis

- Pleural effusion, i.e. pneumonia
- Empyema
- Lung cancer
- Tuberculosis
- Biopsy of the pleura
- Removal of fluid for diagnostic purposes
- Instillation of medications

Signs and Symptoms Requiring Thoracentesis

- Respiratory distress
- Dyspnea
- Shortness of breath
- Cough
- Hemoptysis
- Pleuritic pain

Diagnostic and Laboratory Tests

- History and physical exam
- Ultrasonography
- Chest x-ray:
- Prior to procedure to locate pleural effusion and needle insertion site
- Post-procedure to check for pneumothorax
- Laboratory analysis of fluid (WBC, RBC, protein, glucose, presence of enzymes, abnormal cells, culture)

Therapeutic Nursing Management

Nursing care is directed toward supporting respiratory function, assisting with the procedure, and preventing complications.

- **Pre-procedure:**
  - Have client sign informed consent.
  - Provide additional explanation to the client as indicated.
  - Gather all needed supplies.
  - Position the client as indicated for the procedure.
  - Instruct client to remain absolutely still during procedure and not to cough or talk.

- Assist the primary care provider with the procedure.
- Measure and record the amount of fluid removed from the chest.
- Label and send the fluid specimen to the laboratory.
- **Post-procedure**:
  - Monitor vital signs during the first several hours after the thoracentesis, including respiratory status (lung sounds, rate, and signs of dyspnea).
  - Assess for signs of possible complication (cough or hemoptysis, puncture site for bleeding or presence of crepitus, dizziness, tachycardia, dyspnea, chest pain, nausea, pallor, cyanosis, weakness, and diaphoresis).
- **Nursing Activities**:
  - Provide emotional support.
  - Apply a dressing over the puncture site and position the client on the unaffected side for one hour.
  - Obtain pre-and post-procedure chest x-ray
  - Instruct client and family on manifestations of recurrent effusion or complications following a thoracentesis.
  - Instruct the client to report increasing dyspnea or shortness of breath, cough, and hemoptysis.

Pharmacology

- Local anesthetic (lidocaine)
- Sedative (benzodiazepines)
- Cytotoxic agents may be inserted into pleural space if malignancy present
- Analgesic

Complications

- Shock
- Pneumothorax
- Infection
- Bleeding
- Subcutaneous emphysema
- Cardiovascular collapse (intravascular shift)
- Pulmonary edema

Age-Related Changes—Gerontological Considerations

- Older clients with painful conditions or those who are confused may find it difficult to remain still during the procedure or refrain from coughing or talking.
- Frequent assessment is important in the elderly to detect possible complications of thoracentesis, such as pneumothorax, hemoptysis. A high risk of impaired gas exchange is a priority nursing diagnosis during the initial period following the procedure.

Critical Thinking Exercise: Nursing Management of the Client with a Thoracentesis

Situation: A 73-year-old male client who has been experiencing severe dyspnea is scheduled to undergo a thoracentesis for diagnostic purposes and also to relieve lung compression due to an accumulation of fluid in the pleural space. The client has arthritis and finds it very difficult to remain still during the procedure. To assist the client, the nurse holds the client and encourages him to remain quiet, particularly as the needle is being inserted. The thoracentesis takes approximately 15 minutes to perform. A chest x-ray is performed following the procedure.

1. Prioritize the client's nursing diagnoses immediately following the thoracentesis, with "1" representing the most important diagnosis.

   _____ Pain

   _____ Risk for infection

   _____ Risk for ineffective breathing pattern

2. What is the rationale for each of the nurse's actions related to the thoracentesis:

   a. Positioning the client in an upright position prior to the procedure.

   b. Holding the client and helping him to remain absolutely still during the procedure.

   c. Turning the client to the unaffected side following the procedure.

3. Which are potential complications associated with thoracentesis?

   _____ Acute myocardial infarction   _____ Shock

   _____ Pneumothorax   _____ Pulmonary embolism

   _____ Infection   _____ Bleeding

   _____ Bradycardia   _____ Subcutaneous emphysema

4. Why did the physician order a chest x-ray following the procedure?

Nursing Management of the Client with a Chest Tube Placement

Key Points

- The treatment of choice for a pneumothorax, hemothorax, or hemopneumothorax is the placement of a chest tube with water-seal drainage and suction.
- Chest tubes with attached drainage systems are placed in the pleural cavity to drain fluid, blood, or air from the pleural cavity and to re-establish a negative pressure that will facilitate expansion of the lung, restoring normal intrapleural pressure.
- Chest tubes can be inserted in the emergency department or at the client's bedside by placing the client in a sitting or lying position, or in the operating room via a thoracotomy incision.
- The chest tube may be positioned anteriorly through the second intercostal space to remove air.
- A second tube may be positioned posteriorly through the 8th or 9th intercostal space to remove serosanguineous fluid or purulent exudate.
- The tubes are sutured to the chest wall, and an airtight dressing is placed over the puncture wound.
- The tubes are then attached to drainage tubing that leads to a collection bottle or device placed several feet below the chest and tubing.
- There are four types of drainage systems:
  - One-bottle system consists of a water seal and collection of drainage in same bottle.
  - Two-bottle system is a water seal and collection of drainage in separate bottles.
  - Three-bottle system is made up of a water seal, collection of drainage, and suction control in separate bottles.
  - Disposable single units work the same as a three-bottle system (Pleurevac, Atrium, Thoraseal).
- Chest tubes are removed when the lungs have re-expanded and/or there is no more fluid drainage.
- It usually takes two to three postoperative days of chest drainage for lungs to fully expand.
- Goals of collaborative management:
  - Evacuate blood and fluid from pleural space.
  - Prevent contamination of pleural space.
  - Re-expand the collapsed lung.

- Re-establish a satisfactory ventilation-perfusion ratio.
- Prevent accidental removal of chest tubes.
- Control client's discomfort and anxiety.
- Maintain oxygenation and tissue perfusion.
- Important nursing diagnoses (actual or potential):
  - Impaired gas exchange
  - Ineffective breathing pattern
  - Anxiety and fear
  - Risk for injury
  - Risk for infection
  - Impaired mobility
- **Key Terms/Concepts:** Pneumothorax; hemothorax; thoracotomy; intrapleural space; serosanguineous fluid, water seal system; negative pressure; one-, two-, and three-bottle systems; self-contained system

Overview

Chest tubes are inserted into the intrapleural space to remove air and fluid and to re-establish negative intrapleural pressure. If intrapleural pressure becomes equal to atmospheric pressure, the lungs will collapse (pneumothorax). Air can enter the intrapleural space by a variety of mechanisms including traumatic chest injury (e.g., gunshot wound, fractured rib), thoracotomy, and spontaneous pneumothorax. Excess fluid accumulation can occur in the pleural space as a result of impaired lymphatic drainage or changes in the colloid osmotic pressure. Empyema is purulent pleural fluid, which may be associated with lung abscesses or pneumonia. When chest tube drainage is initiated to remove air or fluid, chest tubes are connected to a closed drainage system. A two-liter clear glass bottle may be used or other commercial devices. The end of the drainage system has a "water-seal" that prevents air from entering the chest cavity during inspiration and allows air to escape during expiration. Applying a low level of suction to the system helps re-establish negative pressure in the pleural space, allowing the lung to re-expand.

Risk Factors/Indications for Thoracentesis

- Blunt, crushing or penetrating chest injuries
- Tension pneumothorax
- Hemothorax
- Hemopneumothorax
- Thoracic surgery
- Pleural effusion
- Empyema
- Pneumonia
- Invasive thoracic procedures, such as lung and/or cardiac surgery
- Blunt chest trauma

Signs and Symptoms Necessitating Chest Tubes

- Dyspnea
- Agitation
- Hypotension
- Tachycardia
- Severe diaphoresis
- Absence or diminished breath sounds on affected side
- Tracheal deviation (tension pneumothorax)
- Mediastinal shift to unaffected side
- Cyanosis

Diagnostic and Laboratory Tests

- History and physical exam
- ABG (arterial blood gas) analysis
- Chest x-rays before placing and following removal of chest tube
- CT (computerized tomography)
- Pleural fluid analysis

Therapeutic Nursing Management

- **Assess/Monitor**:
  - Proper system function
  - Ensure that the water in the water-seal chamber fluctuates when suction is applied; there should not be any bubbling in the water seal (indicates air leak).
  - For blockage of drainage system
  - Potential atelectasis resulting from hypoventilation
  - For increased dyspnea
  - Vital signs
  - Breath sounds
  - Chest wall for unusual chest movements
  - Oxygen saturations
  - Complication of infection
  - Chest tube insertion site for redness, pain, infection, and crepitus
  - Wound for excessive drainage or signs of infection following chest tube removal
  - Client for signs of recurrent pneumothorax
- **Nursing Activities**:
  - Assist physician with insertion of chest tubes and set-up of drainage system.
  - Keep all tubing straight and coiled loosely. Do not let tubing lie below the top of the drainage system.

- Prevent client from lying on tubing, position client on the unaffected side to keep the tube from becoming kinked.
- Make certain that connections between the chest tubes, drainage tubing, and drainage collection bottles are tight, tape connections and tops of bottles to prevent air leaks.
- Milk the chest tubes if necessary to increase the amount of negative pressure to pleural space.
- Do not empty drainage bottles unless overflowing.
- Never clamp chest tubes without a physician's order.
- Refill the water chamber if the fluid is low.
- Encourage ambulation (ensure water-seal bottle remains below the level of the client's chest).
- Facilitate coughing and deep-breathing every two hours.
- Auscultate breath sounds frequently.
- Document the amount and characteristics of pleural fluid drainage by marking and documenting the date, hour, and drainage level on the container at the end of each shift.
- Provide pain medication one-half hour before removing chest tubes.
- After removal of chest tubes, apply airtight sterile petroleum jelly gauze dressing.
- Order chest x-rays as needed following removal of chest tubes.

Pharmacology

- Antiseptic solution to prepare site for chest tubes
- Local anesthetic (lidocaine)
- Sterile petroleum jelly gauze dressing following chest tube removal
- Pain medication (morphine, meperidine, or other)
- Antibiotics (if bacterial infection present)

Complications

- Infection
- Recurrent or new pneumothorax
- Respiratory failure
- Dislodgement of the chest tube
- Incomplete expansion of the lung
- Kinking or obstruction of the tubing leading to change in inter-thoracic pressure and possible cardiovascular compromise

Age-Related Changes—Gerontological Considerations

- Changes in fat deposition in many elderly persons may make it difficult for the physician to identify the landmarks for insertion of the chest tube.
- Proper positioning for thoracotomy may be difficult for the older person with impaired mobility or range of motion.

Critical Thinking Exercise: Nursing Management of the Client with a Chest Tube Placement

Situation: A 65-year-old-female, who has undergone a pneumonectomy for lung cancer, is receiving care in the ICU (Intensive Care Unit). Chest tubes were inserted in surgery and attached to a disposable Pleur-evac unit. The nurse carefully assesses the client's respiratory function chest tube insertion site, chest drainage, and monitors the closed chest drainage system.

1. Which are primary functions of closed chest drainage following thoracotomy?

   _____ To keep the lung collapsed until healing occurs

   _____ To remove air and serosanguineous fluid from the pleural space

   _____ To help re-expand the remaining lung tissue

   _____ To prevent hemothorax

   _____ To prevent mediastinal shift

2. Which is the primary sign/symptom of an air leak in a water seal drainage system?

   _____ Continuous bubbling in the water seal chamber during inspiration

   _____ Intermittent bubbling in the water seal chamber during expiration

   _____ Continuous bubbling in the water seal chamber during inspiration and expiration

   _____ Intermittent bubbling in the water seal chamber during inspiration and expiration

3. What should the nurse do if an air leak is suspected in a water seal drainage system?

4. Which nursing interventions are appropriate for the client with closed chest drainage?

_____ Place the drainage system two to three feet below the client's chest.

_____ Place the drainage system on the top of the bed when transporting the client.

_____ Clamp the chest tube off when ambulating the client.

_____ Record the amount of drainage for each shift.

_____ Encourage the client to lie quietly whenever possible.

Nursing Management of the Client with Peptic Ulcers

Key Points

- Peptic ulcers may occur in the stomach, pylorus, duodenum, or esophagus.
- Helicobacter pylori are the bacterium responsible for the majority of gastric and pyloric ulcers.
- Stress, corticosteroids, and NSAIDs (nonsteroidal anti-inflammatory drugs) are exacerbating factors.
- Smoking increases gastric acid secretion, increasing the occurrence and also recurrence of ulcers.
- Goals of collaborative management:
  - Eliminate *H. pylori bacteria*.
  - Reduce gastric acidity.
  - Reduce or eliminate exacerbating factors.
  - Prevent complications (hemorrhage, perforation).
- Important nursing diagnoses (actual or potential):
  - Pain management
  - Anxiety and fear
  - Ineffective individual coping
  - Ineffective individual management of therapeutic regimen
  - Potential complications of peptic ulcer
- **Key Terms/Concepts:** Pylorus, acute, chronic, perforation, exacerbation, cytoprotective

Overview

A peptic ulcer is an erosion of the mucous membrane of the stomach, pylorus, duodenum, or esophagus. The erosion may extend into the deep layers of the structure exposing tissue to gastric secretions. Peptic ulcers are four times more likely to occur in the duodenal bulb and be termed duodenal ulcers or DU. Gastri ulcers (GU) are the next most common type of peptic ulcer, commonly occurring along the lesser curvature of the antrum and in the pre-pyloric area. The majority of gastric and pyloric ulcers are associated with **Helicobacter pylori** (*H. pylori*) bacterial infection and so must be treated in order to be cured. Ulcers are seen most frequently in middle adulthood and affect men more often than women.

Risk Factors

- Infection with *H. pylori*
- High serum gastrin levels

- Rapid gastric emptying
- Gastric hyperacidity
- Chronic use of aspirin and/or NSAIDs (nonsteroidal anti-inflammatory drugs)
- Cigarette smoking
- Chronic gastritis
- Stress
- Alcohol ingestion
- Genetic predisposition
- Zollinger-Ellison syndrome (gastric hyperacidity, duodenal ulcer, gastrinomas)

Signs and Symptoms

- Duodenal ulcer
- Intermittent, dull, gnawing pain or burning in mid-epigastrium or back; usually 1-3 hours after meals
- Pain in the middle of the night that will awaken client
- Epigastric pain that is not associated with meals; may be described as discomfort, cramping, hunger pangs
- Up to one-third of clients over the age of 60 do not have abdominal pain
- Symptoms may wax and wane
- Pain relieved by eating or taking alkali products
- Epigastric tenderness
- Pyrosis (heartburn)
- Perforation: sudden, sever mid-epigastric pain with radiation to right shoulder
- Hemorrhage: dizzy, hematemesis, melena (black tarry stools)
- Gastric Ulcer
- Similar symptoms to DU but rare that there will be epigastric pain following a meal
- Associated more with NSAID (nonsteroidal anti-inflammatory drug) use and so may be silent until present with hematemesis, dizziness, and possible shock
- Either Location
- Early satiety
- Weight loss

Diagnostic and Laboratory Tests

- History and physical examination
- Upper gastrointestinal x-rays that utilize contrast medium to visualize the lower esophagus, stomach, and duodenum. These X-rays detect gastric ulcers, esophageal disorders, strictures, and tumors.
- Flexible endoscopic exams allow the passage of a lighted, flexible, fiberoptic tube or instrument through a body opening into the lumen of the gastrointestinal tract. This procedure allows direct visualization of abdominal

organs and tissues and is much more accurate than x-ray. Common gastrointestinal endoscopic procedures include:

- Esophagogastroduodenoscopy (EGD)
- Colonoscopy
- Flexible sigmoidoscopy

- Explain procedure to client, including the use of sedation and required positioning.
- Have client sign consent form with witness present.
- Instruct client to take nothing by mouth (NPO), including liquids, for a specified time depending on the procedure.
- Have the client arrange for transportation to and from the facility if procedure is to be performed on an outpatient basis.
- Following endoscopic procedures instruct the client to:
  - Avoid driving for at least 12 hours.
  - Remain NPO following an EGD until the gag reflex completely returns.
  - Observe for and immediately report any signs of perforation to the primary care provider.
- Radioimmune assays of gastrin levels
- Stool for occult blood and possible passing of nasogastric tube in emergency room to check for blood in upper gastrointestinal tract
- Carbon-14-urea breath test (also called "C-14-urea breath test" and "PY test") breath test for Helicobacter pylori - test of choice in stable clients
- Gastric secretory studies
- Biopsy
- CBC
- Clients over 50 years old with new onset ulcer symptoms, or those with anemia, weight loss, or other evidence of bleeding, should have endoscopy.

Therapeutic Nursing Management

- **Assess/Monitor**:
  - For tarry stools
  - For signs of anemia (hemoglobin, hematocrit)
  - Nutritional status
  - Weight
  - For complications (perforation, anemia, shock)
  - Pain status
  - Effectiveness of pain relief measures
  - Effectiveness of pharmacological interventions
- **Nursing Activities**:
  - Encourage smoking cessation. Smoking increases the secretion of hydrochloric acid.
  - Teach client to avoid the intake of caffeine, alcohol, spicy or fried foods, high-fat foods, and cream.

- Administer prescribed pain medications.
- Administer, normally, a triple regimen of two antibiotics (most commonly clarithromycin and amoxicillin) and a PPI (proton pump inhibitor) or histamine-2 blocker and bismuth if culprit is H. pylori. If client's ulcer is due to NSAID alone, treatment is usually with a PPI only.
- Teach client regarding medication actions and side effects.
- Teach relaxation techniques for stress reduction as appropriate.
- Provide emotional support for client and family.
- Prepare client for surgery if indicated.
- Teach client to eat small meals at regular intervals throughout the day.
- Instruct client that follow-up H. pylori testing, to confirm eradication, cannot be done via the urea breath test for at least 4 weeks after treatment, or via stool antigen test for 8 weeks after treatment, to avoid false negative results.

Pharmacology

- H2-receptor blockers or antagonists (cimetidine [Tagamet], famotidine [Pepcid], nizatidine [Axid], ranitidine [Zantac])
- Antibiotics (metronidazole, tetracycline, amoxicillin, clarithromycin)
- Cytoprotective agents (sucralfate [Carafate])
- Proton pump inhibitors (omeprazole [Prilosec], Lansoprazole [Prevacid], etc.)
- Synthetic prostaglandins (misoprostol [Cytotec])
- Bismuth (in combination with other agents to treat or prevent recurrence of H. pylori infection)
- Blood (if required for bleeding)

Complications

- Hemorrhage
- Perforation
- Pyloric obstruction
- Cancer

Age-Related Changes—Gerontological Considerations

- Increased incidence of peptic ulcers is related to delayed gastric emptying and increased use of NSAIDs (nonsteroidal anti-inflammatory drugs) among older adults.

Critical Thinking Exercise: Nursing Management of the Client with Peptic Ulcers

Situation: A 39-year-old man visits his health provider with complaints of burning, epigastric pain occurring about two hours after he eats. He consistently feels bloated and obtains little or no relief from OTC antacids. His past medical history reveals cigarette smoking, stressful job, and chronic use of NSAIDs (Non-steroidal anti-inflammatory drugs) for low back pain.

1. What are the client's risk factors for peptic ulcer disease? Which is the most serious risk factor and why?

2. Why is smoking contraindicated for clients with peptic ulcer disease?

3. Which nursing diagnoses are supported by the client's data?

_____ Alteration in nutrition: less than body requirements

_____ Pain

_____ Anxiety

_____ Ineffective individual coping

_____ Ineffective individual management of therapeutic regimen

_____ Altered elimination: tarry stools

4. What is the primary reason the practitioner prescribed these medications for the client?

a. H₂-receptor antagonist

b. Antibiotic

c. Cytoprotective agent

Nursing Management of the Client with Gastrectomy

Key Points

- Gastric surgery is indicated for treatment of intractable ulcers, perforation, hemorrhage, or obstruction.
- Goals of collaborative management:
  - Correct the underlying problem/disease.
  - Maintain gastric function.
  - Prevent complications (hemorrhage, infection, dumping syndrome, pernicious anemia, and vitamin B_{12} deficiency).
- Important nursing diagnoses (actual or potential):
  - Pain and management
  - Potential complications of gastrectomy
  - Altered nutrition: less than body requirements
  - Knowledge deficit
  - Nausea and vomiting
  - Risk for infection
- **Key Terms/Concepts:** Resection, perforation, gastroscopy

Overview

Gastrectomy refers to partial or total resection of the stomach in order to eliminate disease. Indications include gastric ulcers that do not respond to medical management, are complicated by hemorrhage or perforation, and malignant tumors.

Risk Factors/Indications

- Ineffective drug or lifestyle management of peptic ulcers
- Perforation
- Hemorrhage
- Cancer

Signs and Symptoms Indicating Need for Gastrectomy

- Sudden acute epigastric pain
- Rigid abdomen
- Vomiting blood
- Severe anemia
- Shock

Diagnostic and Laboratory Tests

- History and physical examination
- Gastroscopy

Therapeutic Nursing Management Post-Gastrectomy

- **Assess/Monitor:**
    - Postoperative pain status
    - Patency of nasogastric tube
    - Quality and quantity of drainage
    - Effectiveness of prescribed analgesics
    - For signs of anemia, and vitamin and mineral deficiencies
    - Bowel sounds, respiratory status, urinary status and cardiac status postoperatively
- **Nursing Activities:**
    - Maintain patency of nasogastric tube until removed.
    - Teach client to eat small, frequent meals high in protein and low in carbohydrates.
    - Encourage client to drink fluids between meals, rather than with meals.
    - Teach client that vitamin B_{12} injections will be needed for remainder of lifetime.
    - Administer medications as prescribed.

Pharmacology

- Antacids (Mylanta, Maalox)
- H2-receptor antagonists (cimetidine [Tagamet], famotidine [Pepcid], nizatidine [Axid], ranitidine [Zantac])
- Proton pump inhibitors (omeprazole, lansoprazole, esomeprazole, pantoprazole, rabeprazole)
- Antibiotics (for surgical prophylaxis)
- Vitamin B_{12} injections (cyanocobalamin)

Complications

- Pernicious anemia - vitamin B_{12} deficiency, with irreversible neurological changes
- Dumping syndrome
- Infection

Age-Related Changes—Gerontological Considerations

- Increased risk for surgical complications is related to the presence of chronic illness, heart disease, or fluid and electrolyte imbalances.

Critical Thinking Exercise: Nursing Management of the Client with Gastrectomy

Situation: A 44-year-old woman is first day postoperative subtotal gastrectomy for stomach cancer. Her vital signs are stable, and she has been up to the side of the bed one time. She has a nasogastric tube in place, which is connected to low intermittent suction.

1. Which nursing diagnoses are appropriate for the client during this phase of her surgery?

   _____ Pain

   _____ Altered nutrition: less than body requirements

   _____ Knowledge deficit regarding home care

   _____ Nausea

   _____ Risk for infection

   _____ Risk for fluid volume deficit

2. What is the etiology of each of the nursing diagnoses you selected?

3. What is dumping syndrome and how can it be reduced or prevented?

Nursing Management of the Client with Dumping Syndrome

Key Points

- Gastrojejunostomy (Billroth's II procedure) greatly reduces the reservoir capacity of the stomach.
- One-third to one-half of clients experience dumping syndrome after gastric surgery.
- Dumping syndrome most commonly develops following the Billroth's II surgical procedure.
- Symptoms usually subside after 6 to 12 months.
- Goals of collaborative management:
  - Prevent symptoms.
  - Set up a dietary therapeutic program.
  - Use surgical intervention if symptoms persist.
- Important nursing diagnoses (actual or potential):
  - Anxiety and fear
  - Nausea and vomiting
  - Ineffective management of therapeutic regime
  - Altered nutrition: less than body requirements
- **Key Terms/Concepts:** Gastric emptying, gastrojejunostomy, Billroth I procedure, Billroth II procedure, blood sugar

Overview

Dumping syndrome is characterized by rapid emptying (dumping) of the stomach contents into the small intestine of the client, after a gastrojejunostomy. Dumping syndrome is a result of changes that occur in the function related to storage in the stomach and/or to pyloric emptying, usually as a result of surgery for peptic ulcer disease. Normally after eating, food is stored in the stomach to be acted upon by digestive acids and proteases before transfer to the gastric antrum, where food becomes very fine particles for easy passing into the pylorus, where a sort-of-gate keeper controls the particles reaching the duodenum. Accelerated emptying or "dumping" of liquids from the stomach into the duodenum is a critical step in dumping syndrome. Sweating and weakness, which characterize the rapid emptying of the stomach after eating, are two of the symptoms of the dumping syndrome.

Risk Factors

- Peptic ulcer disease
- Gastrojejunostomy (Billroth II procedure)

- Eating large meals
- Drinking fluids with meals

Signs and Symptoms

- Weakness
- Diaphoresis
- Tachycardia
- Syncope
- Epigastric fullness
- Abdominal distention and discomfort
- Abdominal cramping
- Nausea
- Borborygmi (stomach/intestinal rumbling)
- Headache
- Flushing
- Diarrhea

Diagnostic and Laboratory Tests

- History and physical exam
- Fasting blood glucose (FBG), also called fasting blood sugar (FBS)
- 2-hour postprandial blood sugar (PPBS)
- OGTT (oral glucose tolerance test) can bring on signs and symptoms
- Positive hydrogen breath test after indigestion of glucose
- Endoscopy, possible

Therapeutic Nursing Management

- **Prevention:**
    - Avoid meals with a hyperosmolar composition.
    - Eat low carbohydrate and high protein meals.
    - Eat frequent small meals without fluids.
    - Avoid very hot or very cold foods.
    - Avoid fluids for 1 hour before and 2 hours following meals.
    - Lie down after eating and when symptoms occur.
    - Use recumbent position during eating if tolerated.
- **Assess/Monitor:**
    - Vital signs
    - Intake of food and fluid
    - Gastric and abdominal symptoms
- **Nursing Activities:**
    - Arrange for client to see a dietitian.

- Place client on a high-fat, high-protein, and low-carbohydrate diet.
- Have client limit roughage and avoid milk, sweets, and sugars.
- Report to physician if symptoms continue despite dietary regime.

Pharmacology

- Sedation (benzodiazepines)
- Octreotide subcutaneous
- Pectin/guar gum
- Acarbose helps delay absorption of carbohydrates and so may slow dumping process.
- Antispasmodic agents (dicyclomine [Bentyl], glycopyrrolate [Robinul], hyoscyamine [Levsin], Donnatal)

Complications

- Postprandial hypoglycemia
- Malnutrition
- Fluid and electrolyte imbalances

Age-Related Changes—Gerontological Considerations

- Elderly clients who live alone may not be aware of their symptoms of hypoglycemia.

Critical Thinking Exercise: Nursing Management of the Client with Dumping Syndrome

Situation: A 45-year-old client with peptic ulcer disease who has undergone a Billroth II surgical procedure has been discharged home and has developed dumping syndrome. During her first postoperative visit to the clinic, the client tells the nurse practitioner she experiences weakness, diaphoresis, tachycardia, faintness, and abdominal distention 15-30 minutes after every meal. The client also mentions that two or three hours after eating she experiences the symptoms of a hypoglycemic reaction: sweating, mental confusion, anxiety, weakness and tachycardia. The nurse practitioner provides the client with a Teaching Guide, which lists dietary regulations and restrictions for people with dumping syndrome. She also advises the client to lie down following meals.

1. What causes the symptoms associated with dumping syndrome?

2. What type of diet is recommended for clients experiencing dumping syndrome? Why?

3. Why is it important for clients with dumping syndrome to lie down after a meal?

4. Why does postprandial hypoglycemia occur 2-3 hours after eating in clients with dumping syndrome?

Nursing Management of the Client with Cirrhosis

| Key Points |

- Cirrhosis of the liver can occur from alcohol abuse, acute viral hepatitis, or chronic biliary disease.
- Some cases of cirrhosis are inherited, such as hemochromatosis, Wilson disease, and alpha-antitrypsin deficiency.
- Prevention is an important part of treatment, especially for alcohol-induced cirrhosis.
- Goals of collaborative management:
  - Maintain adequacy of nutrition.
  - Control pain.
  - Maintain fluid and electrolyte status.
- Important nursing diagnoses (actual or potential) are:
  - Pain management
  - Ineffective individual coping
  - Activity intolerance
  - Altered nutrition: less than body requirements
  - Risk for injury
  - Fear and anxiety
  - Impaired skin integrity
  - Fluid volume excess
  - Electrolyte imbalance
  - Potential for bleeding
  - Confusion and misunderstanding
- **Key Terms/Concepts**: Irreversible, degenerative, hepatic encephalopathy, autoimmune, paracentesis

Overview

Cirrhosis is an irreversible, degenerative disease characterized by replacement of normal liver tissue with diffuse fibrotic tissue that disrupts liver structure and function. Symptoms produced by cirrhosis are related to the liver's inability to detoxify substances, produce proteins, regulate glucose, and clot blood. Alcohol-related cirrhosis is termed Laennec's cirrhosis. There is no cure for cirrhosis other than liver transplantation. Treatment is aimed at minimizing gastric distress and gastric bleeding, improving nutritional status, and reducing the risk for injury related to hepatic encephalopathy.

Risk Factors

- Alcohol and Hepatitis C are responsible for 60% of the cases.
- Chronic biliary obstruction
- Biliary cirrhosis
- Hemochromatosis
- Chronic, excessive alcohol intake
- Hepatitis B
- Progressive fatty liver
- Drugs or environmental toxins
- Starvation
- CHF (congestive heart failure)
- Genetic predisposition

Signs and Symptoms

- Liver enlargement
- Ascites
- Chronic dyspepsia
- Anorexia, nausea
- Jaundice and itching
- Fatigue
- Weight loss
- Abdominal pain
- Asterixis
- Spider telangiectases
- Nose bleeds or bruising (ecchymosis)
- Dilated abdominal veins
- Varices or hemorrhoids, possible hematemesis or melena
- Hypoglycemia, or possible hyperglycemia
- Irritability
- Constipation or diarrhea
- Peripheral edema
- Amenorrhea or irregular menses

Diagnostic and Laboratory Tests

- History and physical examination
- Liver function:
  - ALP (alkaline phosphatase); also called ALK Phos, an enzyme found in the liver, bones, and placenta
  - ALT (alanine aminotransferase); also called (SGPT) serum glutamic pyruvic transaminase, an enzyme found primarily in liver cells

- AST (aspartate aminotransferase); also called (SGOT) serum glutamic oxaloacetic transaminase, an enzyme found in the liver, and elsewhere in the body
- GGTP (gamma-glutamyl transpeptidase); also called (GGT or Gamma GT), an enzyme present in the liver, pancreas, and kidneys
- Bilirubin (a waste product formed by the breakdown of red blood cells)
- Albumin (a protein synthesized by the liver)
- Total cholesterol (a substance stored in the liver)
- Total protein (a nutrient normally broken down by the liver and its enzymes)
- LDH (lactic acid dehydrogenase) an enzyme found in the liver
- PT (Prothrombin time) tests the blood's ability to clot
- Liver biopsy
- Serum electrolytes
- CBC (complete blood count)
  - Platelet count
- Coagulation studies, prothrombin time, bleeding time
- Serum ammonia levels
- MRI (magnetic resonance imaging)
- Radioisotopic liver scan
- Ultrasound

Therapeutic Nursing Management

- **Assess/Monitor:**
  - Dietary intake
  - Fluid and electrolyte status
  - Urinary input and output, and weight
  - Abdominal girth measurements
  - For overt or occult bleeding
  - Mental status
  - Effectiveness (and side effects) of prescribed medications
- **Nursing Activities:**
  - Provide a well-balanced diet of small, frequent meals; generally high protein of 1-1.5 gm protein/kg body weight, salt limit.
  - Supplement meals with vitamins and folic acid as prescribed.
  - Restrict protein intake if client demonstrates signs of coma.
  - Encourage cessation of alcohol use.
  - Assist with paracentesis if indicated, may be required every 2 weeks or more often.
  - Administer infusions of albumin as prescribed.
  - Apply prolonged pressure to injection sites.
  - Avoid giving opiates or sedatives, NSAIDs (including aspirin).

- Provide adequate rest.
- Prepare for balloon tamponade of esophageal varices if indicated or preparation for endoscopic ligation. TIPS (transjugular intrahepatic shunt) and possible liver transplantation.
- Administer TPN (total parenteral nutrition) as prescribed.
- Provide emotional support for the client and family.
- Observe client for signs and symptoms of alcohol withdrawal (tachycardia, hypertension, tremors, and delusions).

Pharmacology

- Antacids (Mylanta, Maalox)
- Vitamins (folic acid, thiamine/vitamin B_1, vitamin B_{12}, pyridoxine/vitamin B_6, riboflavin)
- Nutritional supplements
- Diuretics (spironolactone with furosemide or torsemide) to treat ascites
- Laxatives (bisacodyl, milk of magnesia)
- Lactulose to reduce ammonia levels with encephalopathy
- Colchicine may help treat primary biliary cirrhosis via its anti-inflammatory activity.
- Propanolol to decrease blood pressure and control bleeding
- Immunize for Hepatitis A & B, pneumonia, and yearly influenza
- Hepatitis C is treated with C-PEG-alpha-interferon and ribavirin
- Hepatitis B is treated with lamivudine or PEG-alpha-interferon
- Autoimmune causes – prednisone
- Milkweed thistle
- Recombinant factor Vlla for bleeding problems

Complications

- Splenomegaly
- Ascites
- Gastrointestinal hemorrhage
- Portal hypertension
- Hepatic encephalopathy
- Esophageal varices
- Anemia
- Hepatic coma
- Hyper-, hypoglycemia
- Death

Age-Related Changes—Gerontological Considerations

- Older adults who chronically ingest excessive amounts of alcohol are at an increased risk for Laennec's cirrhosis. Long-standing alcohol consumption, especially in the absence of good nutrition and a genetic predisposition for the disease, cause more damage to the liver over time.

- Due to aging, the underlying liver function is reduced; therefore, predisposing the elderly person to the hepatotoxic effects of alcohol and causing liver damage.

- Many older adults take multiple medications for a variety of health conditions. Drug metabolism commonly occurs in the liver, and thus, may result in hepatotoxicity. The client with liver impairment secondary to cirrhosis has a reduced ability to tolerate adverse drug effects. Drugs with known hepatotoxicity should be removed from the treatment regime.

- Advanced cirrhosis of the liver can involve encephalopathy. The confusion and dementia associated with neurologic involvement of the disease may be difficult to differentiate from the alterations in mentation associated with Alzheimer's disease, which is more common in the elderly population.

Critical Thinking Exercise: Nursing Management of the Client with Cirrhosis

Situation: A 65-year old male has a history of alcohol abuse. He is hospitalized because he began vomiting blood after eating tacos. Assessment data reveal: pallor, jaundice with petechiae and ecchymotic areas on his arms and legs, and a tight, protuberant abdomen. He also has pedal edema and hepatomegaly. His admission diagnosis is bleeding esophageal varices related to cirrhosis. He is receiving IV Aldactone and Lasix.

1. List all of the nursing diagnoses that may apply to this client. Which nursing diagnoses requires immediate attention?

Nursing Diagnosis	Requires Immediate Attention

Situation: The client is experiencing respiratory distress related to the ascites and the physician performs an abdominal paracentesis, withdrawing 3 L of fluid. The nurse makes the diagnoses of risk for fluid volume deficit.

2. What is the rationale for this diagnosis?

3. What nursing interventions are most appropriate for the client diagnosed with fluid volume deficit after paracentesis?

Lab values are drawn. They are:	
Platelet count	50,000/mm3
Serum ammonia	96mcg/dL
RBC	3.8million/mm3
WBC (white blood cell)	5,000/mm3
PT	40 seconds
Hgb	10.1g/dL
Hct	30%

4. Based on the client's lab values, what is the priority problem?

5. What nursing interventions are most appropriate related to the priority problem noted above?

Nursing Management of the Client with an Abdominal Paracentesis

Key Points

- To remove a specimen of ascitic fluid for laboratory analysis, the physician uses needle aspiration.
- To drain fluid that has accumulated in the abdomen, the physician makes a small incision below the umbilicus and inserts a trocar.
- Paracentesis may result in the drainage of several liters of fluid.
- In some cases, paracentesis includes lavage with normal saline or Ringer's lactate.
- Goals of collaborative management:
  - Relieve symptoms of abdominal fullness and respiratory distress.
  - Prevent infection.
  - Prevent shock.
  - Obtain ascitic fluid for diagnostic purposes.
- Important nursing diagnoses (actual or potential):
  - High risk for infection
  - Anxiety and fear
  - High risk for impaired tissue integrity
  - Altered tissue perfusion
- **Key Terms/Concepts:** Needle aspiration, peritoneal fluid, ascites, lavage

Overview

An abdominal paracentesis is a sterile, invasive procedure that involves the removal of fluid from the peritoneal cavity. The abnormal accumulation of peritoneal fluid is called ascites.

Risk Factors/Conditions Necessitating Paracentesis

- Cirrhosis of the liver
- Heart failure
- Abdominal cancer
- Metastatic carcinoma
- Bacterial peritonitis

Signs and Symptoms Requiring Paracentesis

- Abdominal discomfort and pressure
- Respiratory distress

Diagnostic and Laboratory Tests
- History and physical exam
- Peritoneal fluid analysis

Therapeutic Nursing Management
- **Prevention of complications:**
  - Use meticulous sterile technique.
  - If necessary, remind physician that fluid needs to be withdrawn slowly.
- **Assess/Monitor:**
  - Vital signs
  - For signs of shock during and following procedure
- **Nursing Activities:**
  - Provide emotional support.
  - Have client void before procedure; place urinary catheter if necessary.
  - Position client on side of bed with feet on a stool and supportive pillows at his back.
  - Assist the physician with the procedure.
  - Measure and record the amount of fluid removed from the abdomen.
  - Record the appearance, color, and odor of the fluid.
  - Dress the puncture site and monitor for fluid leakage.
  - Label and send the fluid specimens to the laboratory.

Pharmacology
- Local anesthetic (lidocaine)
- Albumin infusions
- Potassium supplements if client undergoes multiple paracenteses

Complications
- Shock (resulting from too rapid a withdrawal of fluid from the abdomen)
- Infection
- Peritonitis
- Bleeding
- Hepatic encephalopathy

Age-Related Changes—Gerontological Considerations
- Older clients have an increased susceptibility to irritation or trauma of the gastrointestinal mucosa, and are thus more susceptible to infection.
- Older people may overuse alcohol as a self-prescribed sleep-aid and pain medication, which can eventually damage the liver.
- Use of acetaminophen can cause insidious damage to the liver, as well, and is commonly used for pain management in the elderly.

Critical Thinking Exercise: Nursing Management of the Client with an Abdominal Paracentesis

Situation: A 68-year-old male client who has been hospitalized with cirrhosis of the liver is scheduled to have an abdominal paracentesis. The client has been experiencing abdominal discomfort and dyspnea due to the accumulation of a large amount of ascitic fluid in his abdomen.

1. In what order will the nurse perform these activities prior to the abdominal paracentesis, with "1" representing the first activity?

   _____ Place the client in a high-Fowler's position.

   _____ Obtain the client's weight.

   _____ Measures the client's abdominal girth.

   _____ Ask the client to void.

2. What is the rationale for:
   a. Asking the client to void just prior to the paracentesis?
   b. Positioning the client in an upright or high-Fowler's position?
   c. Administering prescribed albumin infusions following the paracentesis?

3. Which are complications that can occur during or after an abdominal paracentesis?

   __✓__ Shock   _____ Fluid overload

   _____ Hypertension   __✓__ Infection

   __✓__ Peritonitis   __✓__ Bleeding

   _____ Bradycardia   __✓__ Hepatic encephalopathy

Nursing Management of the Client with Esophageal Varices

Key Points

- Hemorrhage is a life-threatening complication of esophageal varices.
- Esophageal varices are a complication of end-stage cirrhosis.
- Recurrence is common following successful treatment.
- Goals of collaborative management:
  - Prevent rupture and subsequent hemorrhage.
  - Control hemorrhage.
  - Replace fluid volume deficit.
  - Prevent recurrence.
- Important nursing diagnoses (actual or potential):
  - Fear and anxiety
  - Fluid volume deficit
  - Altered cardiac output
  - Ineffective airway clearance
  - Powerlessness and hopelessness
  - Ineffective individual coping
  - Nausea and vomiting
  - Self-care deficit
- **Key Terms/Concepts**: Tortuous veins, portal hypertension, hematemesis, melena, exsanguination

Overview

Esophageal varices are dilated, tortuous veins that are caused by portal hypertension secondary to cirrhosis. Hemorrhage from esophageal varices is a major cause of death in clients with end-stage cirrhosis.

Risk Factors

- Cirrhosis
- Hepatitis
- Alcohol abuse
- Congenital abnormality of the splenic vein or superior vena cava
- Chronic salicylate use
- Straining at defecation, coughing, sneezing, vomiting

Signs and Symptoms

- Hematemesis
- Bloody stools (melena)
- Massive bleeding from rupture

Diagnostic and Laboratory Tests

- History and physical examination
- Hemoglobin and hematocrit
- Endoscopy (gastroscopy)
- Barium swallow
- Ultrasound
  - 2D (2-Dimensional)
  - 3D (3-Dimensional)
  - Doppler
- CT (computed tomography)/CAT (computed axial tomography) scan
- Angiography
- Liver function:
  - Alkaline phosphatase (ALP); also called ALK Phos (an enzyme found in the liver, bones and placenta)
  - Alanine aminotransferase (ALT); also called serum glutamic pyruvic transaminase (SGPT) (an enzyme found primarily in liver cells)
  - Aspartate aminotransferase (AST); also called serum glutamic oxaloacetic transaminase (SGOT) (an enzyme found in the liver and elsewhere in the body)
  - Gamma-glutamyl transpeptidase (GGTP); also called GGT or Gamma GT (an enzyme present in the liver, pancreas and kidneys)
  - Bilirubin (a waste product formed by the breakdown of red blood cells)
  - Albumin (a protein synthesized by the liver)
  - Total cholesterol (a substance stored in the liver)
  - Total protein (a nutrient normally broken down by the liver and its enzymes)
  - Lactic acid dehydrogenase (LDH) (an enzyme found in the liver)
  - Prothrombin time (PT) tests the blood's ability to clot

Therapeutic Nursing Management

- **Prevent:**
  - Aspiration
- **Assess/Monitor:**
  - For signs of active bleeding
  - Vital signs
  - Nutritional status
  - For indications of hepatic encephalopathy (drowsiness to coma)

- For complications (hypovolemic shock, hepatic encephalopathy, electrolyte imbalance, acid-base imbalance, seizures, alcohol withdrawal)
- For esophageal perforation related to endoscopic procedures
- **Nursing Activities**:
  - Establish intravenous access immediately.
  - Prepare client for nonsurgical treatment procedures if indicated (balloon tamponade, saline lavage, endoscopic sclerotherapy, esophageal banding therapy, variceal band ligation, transjugular intrahepatic portosystemic shunt).
  - Prepare client for surgery if indicated (devascularization and transection, portacaval shunt, splenorenal shunt), possible eventual liver transplantation.
  - Provide soft, fiber-free diet or TPN (total parenteral nutrition) as prescribed.
  - Administer blood and medications as prescribed.
  - Teach client to avoid straining at defecation or other activities that involve Valsalva maneuver (coughing, sneezing).
  - Provide a quiet, calm environment.
  - Offer reassurance and emotional support to client and family.

Pharmacology

- Vasoconstriction of splanchnic vessels (somatostatin or octreotide [Sandostatin] to control bleeding in order to do upper endoscopy. If not successful in controlling bleeding, then vasopressin and spironolactone.)
- Beta-adrenergic blocking agents (propranolol) helps reduce hepatic blood flow and portal pressure
- Vitamin K if prothrombin time is prolonged
- Sclerotherapy (Theolin, Scleromate, Sotradecol)
- Antibiotic possible during bleeding to prevent peritonitis

Complications

- Rupture of varices
- Death by exsanguination

Age-Related Changes—Gerontological Considerations

- Older adults who chronically ingest excessive amounts of alcohol are at an increased risk for esophageal varices. The collateral veins in the esophagus develop to bypass the scarring in the liver and portal hypertension. Esophageal varices can rupture and lead to hemorrhage and death. Elderly persons have reduced reserves to tolerate blood loss and may suffer more serious consequences as a result of reduced circulatory volume.

Critical Thinking Exercise: Nursing Management of the Client with Esophageal Varices

Situation: A 50-year-old man, with a 22-year history of alcohol abuse, developed a cough a few days ago. Upon arising this morning, he started coughing up blood, which prompted him to go to the emergency department. During the assessment, the client started coughing again, this time coughing up copious amounts of bright red blood.

1. Prioritize nursing actions for the client in regard to his bleeding, with "1" representing the most important action.

   _____ Administer oxygen.

   _____ Assess vital signs.

   _____ Initiate intravenous access.

   _____ Establish airway.

   _____ Prepare client for surgery.

2. Which are risk factors for esophageal varices?

   _____ Pancreatitis   _____ Cirrhosis

   _____ Esophageal cancer   _____ Gallbladder disease

   _____ Alcohol abuse   _____ Chronic acetaminophen use

   _____ Hepatitis   _____ Congenital splenic vein abnormality

3. Which are the two most important nursing diagnoses for the client at this time?

   _____ Risk for infection

   _____ Risk for altered nutrition

   _____ Risk for fluid volume deficit

   _____ Anxiety

   _____ Self-care deficit

Nursing Management of the Client with Cholecystitis/ Cholelithiasis and Pancreatitis

Key Points

- Cholecystitis may present as an acute or chronic disease of the gallbladder.
- Cholecystitis is often an acute complication of cholelithiasis (gallstones).
- Cholelithiasis may consist of large stones within the gallbladder or small, gravel type stones that can occlude the common bile duct.
- Pancreatitis is an acute or chronic inflammation of the pancreas.
- Acute pancreatitis is a life-threatening inflammatory process that is characterized by necrosis, hemorrhage, tissue death, and gangrene of the pancreas.
- Chronic pancreatitis is a progressive disease of the pancreas that is characterized by remissions and exacerbations due to the formation of scar tissue in the pancreas.
- Currently, there is no cure for pancreatitis.
- Goals of collaborative management:
  - Reduce the incidence of acute pain episodes.
  - Restore fluid and electrolyte balance.
  - Maintain nutritional status.
  - Remove the gall bladder as deemed necessary.
  - Remove part, or all, of the pancreas in clients with chronic pancreatitis if indicated.
  - Prevent complications (respiratory distress syndrome, hemorrhage, sepsis, bleeding abnormalities, liver failure and diabetes mellitus).
- Important nursing diagnoses (actual or potential) are:
  - Pain management
  - Nausea and vomiting
  - Altered nutrition: less than body requirements
  - Risk for infection
  - Impaired skin integrity
  - Knowledge deficit
  - Anxiety and fear
  - Fluid volume deficit
  - Impaired gas exchange related to pleural effusion (pancreatitis)
  - Potential complications of cholecystectomy (infection, hemorrhage)
  - Potential complications of pancreatitis (hemorrhage, sepsis, hyperglycemia)
- **Key Terms/Concepts:** Acute, chronic, obstruction, inflammation, infection,

hypercholesterolemia, pancreatic digestive enzymes, islets of Langerhans, exocrine tissues

Overview

- The gallbladder acts as a reservoir for bile from the liver; concentrates bile by absorbing salts and water, and releases bile to the duodenum through the sphincter of Oddi in response to the ingestion of fats.
- **Cholecystitis** is the acute or chronic inflammation of the gallbladder.
- **Cholelithiasis** is the presence of calculi (gallstones) within the gallbladder or in the biliary system.
- **Cholecystectomy** is the removal of the gall bladder.
- **Cholesterol stones**, which are more common, occur from increased production of cholesterol and inadequacy of amino acids to dissolve the cholesterol.
- **Pigment stones** contain the excess unconjugated pigments from bile.
- The pancreas is both an endocrine and an exocrine gland, and has both hormonal and digestive functions. The endocrine tissues in the islets of Langerhans secrete insulin and glucagon the hormones that regulate blood sugar. The exocrine tissue secretes digestive enzymes that break down carbohydrates, proteins, fats, and nucleic acids.
- Attacks of pancreatitis cause inflammation of pancreatic tissue due to the premature activation of pancreatic digestive enzymes. These enzymes cause autodigestion of the pancreas. Pancreatitis can also lead to insufficient insulin production, hyperglycemia, and diabetes mellitus.

Risk Factors

- **Cholecystitis/cholelithiasis:**
  - Female gender
  - Over age 40
  - Use of oral contraceptives
  - Use of estrogen
  - Multiparous status
  - Obesity
  - High-fat diet (producing hypercholesterolemia)
  - Genetic predisposition
  - Gastrointestinal disease
  - Primary bacterial infection of the gallbladder
  - Biliary parasites
  - Rapid weight loss
  - Cardiac surgery, severe trauma, burns
  - Native American, Caucasian, Hispanic ethnic origins
- **Pancreatitis:**
  - Gallstones
  - Eating fatty meals
  - Post ERCP

- Hyperglyceridemia
- Hypercalcemia
- Renal failure
- Lupus
- Sphincter of Oddi dysfunction
- Alcohol abuse (major cause of chronic pancreatitis)
- External blunt trauma
- Drug toxicities to opiates, sulfonamides, steroids, thiazides, AIDS medications, and oral contraceptives
- Infection; viral and bacterial

Signs and Symptoms

- Cholecystitis/cholelithiasis:
  - Epigastric discomfort after meals (vague upper right quadrant pain, abdominal distention, fullness, bloating)
  - Biliary colic (severe right upper gastric pain radiating to back or right shoulder)
  - Fever
  - Palpable abdominal mass (when infected)
  - Nausea, vomiting
  - Leukocytosis
  - Rebound tenderness
  - Abdominal muscle guarding
  - Jaundice (when bile duct obstructed)
  - Dark-colored urine
  - Clay-colored stools
  - Vitamins A, D, E, and K deficiencies (fat-soluble vitamins)
- Pancreatitis:
  - Severe abdominal pain (predominant symptom of acute pancreatitis)
  - Nausea and vomiting
  - Fever
  - Anorexia due to pain
  - Weight loss
  - Jaundice
  - Dark-colored urine
  - Foul smelling stools
  - Dehydration
  - Dyspnea

Diagnostic and Laboratory Tests

- History and physical examination
- Abdominal x-ray

- Serum bilirubin
- ALP (alkaline phosphatase); also called (ALK Phos)
- CBC (complete blood count) and differential
- Serum amylase, lipase, and liver enzymes
- Cholecystography
- Radionuclide imaging
- Upper gastrointestinal series
- Ultrasound – best to diagnose gallstones
  - 2D (2-Dimensional)
  - 3D (3-Dimensional)
- Computer tomography (CT)/computed axial tomography (CAT) scan, better than ultrasound to show enlargement of pancreas or to show abscess or dilation of common bile duct
- ERCP (endoscopic retrograde cholangiole pancreatotomy)
- PTC (percutaneous transhepatic cholangiography)
- HIDA scan for diagnosis of acute cholecystitis.

Therapeutic Nursing Management

- **Assess/Monitor:**
  - **Cholecystitis/cholelithiasis status post-cholecystectomy**
    - For signs of infection, bile leakage, bile drainage obstruction
    - For signs of postoperative bleeding (rigid abdomen, change in vital signs)
- **Nursing Activities:**
  - **Cholecystitis/cholelithiasis**
    - Encourage intake of low-fat, high-protein, and high-carbohydrate diet.
    - Administer nasogastric suction, analgesics, antibiotics, and intravenous fluids as prescribed.
    - Avoid administration of morphine sulfate (triggers spasm of the sphincter of Oddi).
    - Place client in low-Fowler's position for comfort.
    - Encourage client to splint abdomen to relieve pain.
    - Prepare client for surgery or lithotripsy if indicated.
    - Maintain drainage tubes and nasogastric suction following cholecystectomy if indicated.
    - Administer medications for nausea and vomiting as prescribed.
    - Encourage ambulation as permitted.
    - Provide verbal and written postoperative instructions for home care following laparoscopic cholecystectomy.
    - Teach client signs of postoperative complications (bleeding, infection).
- **Assess/Monitor:**
  - **Pancreatitis**

- For fever
- For weight loss
- For dehydration
- For dark, amber urine
- For pleural effusion
- Vital signs
- Infection
- Hyperglycemia
- Electrolyte imbalance
- Nausea and vomiting
- Triglycerides

- **Nursing Activities:**
  - **Pancreatitis**
    - Place client on nothing by mouth (NPO) during an acute attack of pancreatitis.
    - Insert a nasogastric tube and attach it to suction (usually low-intermittent).
    - Provide the client with intravenous fluids.
    - Provide the client with a bland, low-fat, low-protein diet once the acute attack subsides. With further improvement, the client may eat small portions of high-carbohydrate, high-protein foods.
    - Instruct the client to avoid alcohol, caffeine, and spicy foods. Identify other possible foods, stress, etc. that trigger chronic pancreatitis.
    - Refer clients who abuse alcohol to a recovery and support group such as Alcoholics Anonymous.
    - Prepare the client with chronic pancreatitis for a partial or complete removal of the pancreas if indicated.

Pharmacology

- **Cholecystitis/cholelithiasis**
  - Narcotic analgesics (avoid morphine sulfate)
  - Antibiotics (metronidazole, ciprofloxacin, gentamicin, ampicillin)
  - Oral bile acids (ursodiol, chenodiol)
  - Cholesterol-lowering agents (Cholestyramine)
  - Antispasmodics
  - Fluids/Hydration
- **Pancreatitis**
  - Meperidine hydrochloride (Demerol)
  - Anticholinergic agents
  - Histamine receptor antagonists
  - Antacids
  - Intravenous fluids
  - Pancreatic enzyme replacement therapy (chronic pancreatitis)

Complications

- **Cholecystitis/cholelithiasis**
    - Infection
    - Ischemia, necrosis or perforation of the gallbladder
    - Hepatic injury
    - Pancreatitis
    - Bleeding
- **Pancreatitis**
    - Respiratory distress syndrome
    - Hemorrhage
    - Sepsis
    - Bleeding abnormalities
    - Diabetes mellitus

Age-Related Changes—Gerontological Considerations

- Biliary tract surgery is the most common operative procedure performed on older adults.
- Biliary disease may be preceded or accompanied by mental changes, sepsis, hypotension, or other chronic illnesses.
- Chronic pancreatitis, which is primarily caused by chronic alcoholism, is most prevalent among people between 45 and 60 years of age.
- Increased risk for respiratory complications occurs following surgical interventions for older clients.

Critical Thinking Exercise: Nursing Management of the Client with Cholecystitis/Cholelithiasis and Pancreatitis

Situation: A 40-year-old woman has been experiencing intermittent, vague epigastric discomfort after meals for several months. This evening after eating a hamburger and french fries, the woman developed severe epigastric pain radiating to her back and right shoulder, which prompted her to go to the emergency department. Assessment reveals an obese female who is in obvious pain with tender distended abdomen, tachycardia, and tachypnea. An acute attack of cholecystitis is suspected.

1. What risk factors does the client have for cholecystitis?

2. Why is morphine sulfate contraindicated for clients with gallbladder disease?

3. What are the etiologies for each of the client's nursing diagnoses?
   a. Pain:
   b. Anxiety:
   c. Knowledge Deficit:

Nursing Management of the Client with Acute Appendicitis

Key Points

- Appendicitis is due to obstruction and infection of the appendix.
- Rupture is a serious complication that may be life threatening.
- Appendicitis is the most common cause of acute lower right quadrant pain.
- Goals of collaborative management:
  - Provide early recognition and treatment.
  - Remove the infected appendix.
  - Prevent complications (rupture, peritonitis).
  - Restore bowel function.
- Important nursing diagnoses (actual or potential):
  - Pain management
  - Risk for infection
  - Risk for injury
  - Anxiety and fear
  - Knowledge deficit
  - Potential complications of appendicitis
- **Key Terms/Concepts:** McBurney's point, Rovsing's sign, peritonitis

Overview

The appendix is a small, finger-shaped appendage attached to the cecum that empties into the colon. It is prone to obstruction because of its small lumen. When obstruction and subsequent infection occur, appendicitis is said to exist. Appendicitis is the most common reason for emergency abdominal surgery.

Risk Factors

- Male gender
- Age 10 to 30 years
- Adolescent males
- Familial tendency

Signs and Symptoms

- Abdominal pain – usually periumbilical, then moves to right lower quadrant
- Lower right quadrant pain
- Abdominal guarding
- Low-grade fever

- Nausea and vomiting
- Rebound tenderness at McBurney's point (halfway between the umbilicus and anterior iliac spine)
- Rovsing's sign – palpation of left lower quadrant produces pain in right lower quadrant
- Psoas sign – positive pain with right thigh extension
- Obturator sign – positive pain with internal rotation of flexed right thigh
- Pain lessons with flexion of right thigh
- Elevated WBC (white blood cell) count

Diagnostic and Laboratory Tests

- History and physical examination
- WBC (white blood cell) count and differential
- Abdominal and pelvic CT (computerized tomography) scan – diagnostic test of choice
- Ultrasound
  - 2-D (2-Dimensional)
  - 3-D (3-Dimensional)
- KUB (kidneys-ureter-bladder) x-ray, not usually very definitive

Therapeutic Nursing Management

- **Assess/Monitor**:
  - Pain status (onset, duration, intensity, exacerbating factors, relief measures)
  - Vital signs for changes
  - Fluid status and provide intravenous fluids, hold PO fluids if possible surgery (except for CT contrast material)
  - For indications of complications (fever, abdominal rigidity, tachycardia, elevated white blood cell count)
- **Nursing Activities**:
  - Provide emotional support to client and family.
  - Prepare client for emergency surgery.
  - Administer analgesics as prescribed.
  - Do not administer laxatives or enema preoperatively (could cause perforation).
  - Do not apply heat to the abdomen.
  - Place in semi-Fowler's position postoperatively.
  - Encourage early ambulation postoperatively, if not contraindicated.
  - Teach client regarding home care and need for follow-up care.

Pharmacology

- Antibiotics (if perforation occurs or for surgical prophylaxis)
- Analgesics (morphine, meperidine)
- Antipyretics (fever)

Complications

- Perforation
- Abscess formation
- Peritonitis
- Paralytic ileus
- Death

Age-Related Changes—Gerontological Considerations

- Symptoms may vary or may be vague or suggestive of bowel obstruction.
- Increased risk for perforation is due to vague or lacking symptoms.
- Increased incidence of perforated appendix may occur because older adults do not seek medical attention as quickly as younger adults.

Critical Thinking Exercise: Nursing Management of the Client with Acute Appendicitis

Situation: A 19-year-old college student is rushed to a near-by emergency department due to severe abdominal pain. Initial assessment reveals a well-nourished, healthy-appearing youth who is in obvious pain. He has lower right quadrant pain with rebound tenderness, complains of nausea, and a positive Rovsing's sign. Acute appendicitis is suspected.

1. Which diagnostic studies are commonly used to confirm the presence of acute appendicitis?

   _____ Ultrasound studies   _____ Physical examination

   _____ CT (computed tomography) scan   _____ Differential WBC (white blood cell)

   _____ Abdominal x-rays   _____ Barium enema

2. Why is a preoperative enema contraindicated when appendicitis is suspected?

3. What is the etiology of the client's postoperative nursing diagnoses?

   a. Pain:

   b. Risk for infection:

   c. Knowledge deficit:

   d. Risk for ineffective airway clearance:

Nursing Management of the Client with Ulcerative Colitis

Key Points

- Ulcerative colitis is primarily a disease of younger people, occurring most often in individuals 20 to 40 years of age, with a second peak in the 70s.
- Ulcerative colitis usually begins in the rectum and distal colon and spreads upward to involve the sigmoid and descending colon. Approximately 95% of clients have rectal involvement, whereas only 30% to 40% have disease extending beyond the sigmoid colon, and only 20% have pancolitis.
- Ulcerative colitis is characterized by periods of remission and exacerbation.
- Clients with ulcerative colitis for more than 10 years are at greater risk for developing colon cancer.
- Intervention is symptomatic and outcomes may be unpredictable.
- Goals of collaborative management:
    - Decrease inflammation.
    - Rest the inflamed bowel.
    - Correct nutritional deficiencies.
- Important nursing diagnoses (actual or potential):
    - Diarrhea
    - Pain, acute/chronic
    - Fluid volume deficit
    - Altered nutrition: less than body requirements
    - Coping, individual, ineffective
    - Powerlessness
- **Key Terms/Concepts**: Remission, exacerbation, inflammation, fibrosis

Overview

Ulcerative colitis is a form of inflammatory bowel disease that is characterized by diffuse inflammation of the mucosa and submucosa of the colon. The inflammatory process causes thickening and edema of the mucosa of the large intestine and rectum. Chronic inflammation can cause bleeding. Abscesses may form and become necrotic, resulting in purulent exudate and bloody stools. When the inflammatory lesions heal, the colon may become shorter and narrower due to scarring and fibrosis.

Risk Factors

- Family history
- Jewish

- Negative association with cigarette smoking
- No known risk factors regarding life-style factors
- Exposure to stressful situations

Signs and Symptoms

- Abdominal cramping
- Abdominal distention
- Left lower abdominal quadrant pain
- Rectal bleeding
- Diarrhea, up to 20 stools per day
- Blood, mucous, and sometimes pus present in diarrhea
- Weight loss
- Anorexia, nausea, and vomiting
- Fever

Diagnostic and Laboratory Tests

- History and physical examination
- CBC (complete blood count) and differential
- Serum electrolytes
- ESR (erythrocyte sedimentation rate), C-RP (C-reactive protein)
- Liver function tests
- pANCA (perinuclear antineutrophil cytoplasmic antibody) elevated in 85% of ulcerative colitis and 15% of Crohn's disease clients
- Anti-glycan antibody elevated in 75% of Crohn's and 5% ulcerative colitis clients; good diagnostic tool when used with pANCA
- Hemoglobin, hematocrit
- Stool examination for blood, mucous, and pus
- Barium enema studies
- Colonoscopy or proctosigmoidoscopy
- Biopsy and cytologic studies

Therapeutic Nursing Management

- **Prevention**:
  - No special diet, unless lactose intolerant
  - Avoid stress and anxiety.
  - Quit smoking.
  - Get adequate rest and exercise.
- **Assess/Monitor**:
  - Factors that aggravate diarrhea
  - Skin in rectal area for irritation or breakdown

- For abdominal distention, muscle guarding, and pain
- For signs of fluid and electrolyte imbalance
- Client's weight
- Client's ability to cope with stress
- **Nursing Activities**:
  - Provide bed rest.
  - Administer intravenous fluids as necessary.
  - Administer TPN (total parenteral nutrition) when indicated.
  - No special diet, unless lactose tolerant
  - Provide emotional support. and stress management, if identified as a trigger
  - Encourage regular times for bowel elimination.
  - Record amount, consistency, and frequency of stools.
  - Listen for bowel sounds.
  - Record intake, output, and hydration status.
  - Prepare client for surgery if indicated.
  - Types of surgeries include: colectomy, proctocolectomy, ileorectal anastomosis, ileal pouch-anal anastomosis, and continent ileostomy (Kock pouch).

Pharmacology

- Aminosalicylates (sulfasalazine, mesalamine, olsalazine)
- Corticosteroids (prednisone, methylprednisolone)
- Antidiarrheals/Anticholinergics (opium tincture, diphenoxylate with atropine [Lomotil])
- Immunosuppressive agents (azathioprine, 6-mercaptopurine)

Complications

- Coagulation defects
- Hemorrhage
- Nutritional deficiencies
- Fluid and electrolyte imbalances
- Bowel perforation
- Toxic megacolon
- Colon cancer
- Liver disease

Age-Related Changes—Gerontological Considerations

- Ulcerative colitis is primarily a disease of younger people.
- Cancer risk increases with advancing age.
- Older clients who require an ileostomy may have difficulty managing the equipment.

Critical Thinking Exercise: Nursing Management of the Client with Ulcerative Colitis

Situation: A 35-year-old woman is hospitalized for an exacerbation of ulcerative colitis following a stressful holiday season spent with relatives. The client is experiencing severe abdominal cramping, distention, and diarrhea, and she has signs of dehydration. The client tells the admitting nurse she has been eating a lot of high-fat holiday foods which she ordinarily avoids: rich gravies, turkey dressing made with sausage, and creamy pies. In addition, she has been drinking bourbon and several glasses of wine during dinner. The client explains she had become very upset when she allowed her mother, who was visiting, to bring up a lot of painful issues from the past, which they normally never discuss unless they are drinking.

1. How does each factor contribute to the symptoms of ulcerative colitis?

   a. Diet:

   b. Alcohol:

   c. Stress:

2. Which three nursing diagnoses are appropriate for this client?

   _____ Dehydration secondary to ulcerative colitis

   _____ Acute pain related to exacerbated ulcerative colitis

   _____ Noncompliance with therapeutic regimen secondary to stress

   _____ Knowledge deficit regarding disease process

   _____ Risk for electrolyte imbalance related to diarrhea

3. Which nursing interventions will be most helpful to the client's acute exacerbation of ulcerative colitis?

   _____ Encourage the client to remain NPO.

   _____ Provide bedrest.

   _____ Serve liquid meals for at least a week.

   _____ Provide emotional support.

   _____ Encourage client to avoid alcohol intake.

   _____ Administer 3000 mL intravenous fluids per day.

   _____ Teach client about disease process.

   _____ Administer prescribed analgesics.

Nursing Management of the Client with Crohn's Disease

Key Points

- Crohn's disease primarily affects people aged 15 to 25, with a second peak from 55 to 65, although it can occur at any age.
- Crohn's disease has a higher incidence in whites, especially Jewish people.
- Crohn's disease is characterized by periods of remission and exacerbation.
- The disease progresses slowly and involves the entire thickness of the bowel wall and particularly the submucosa.
- Etiology of Crohn's disease is unknown, but it may have a genetic basis or be an autoimmune disease.
- Goals of collaborative management:
  - Control diarrhea.
  - Manage abdominal pain and cramping.
  - Correct fluid and electrolyte imbalances.
  - Relieve stress and anxiety.
  - Promote adequate nutrition.
- Important nursing diagnoses (actual or potential):
  - Altered nutrition: less than body requirements
  - Diarrhea and other bowel dysfunctions
  - Pain: acute and chronic
  - Ineffective individual coping
- **Key Terms/Concepts:** Remission, exacerbation, inflammation, fibrosis

Overview

Crohn's disease (regional enteritis) is a form of inflammatory bowel disease that is characterized by chronic, recurrent inflammation of the mucosa of any segment of the bowel, but primarily the terminal ileum. Regional enteritis is limited to the small bowel. Lesions develop and ulcerate, resulting in abscess and fissure formation in several segments of the bowel. As the disease advances, the bowel wall becomes severely fibrosed, thickened, and narrowed.

Risk Factors

- Family history – 15% with first degree relative
- Jewish
- Caucasian
- Smoking

Signs and Symptoms

- Diarrheal stools
- Steatorrhea (fatty stools)
- Intermittent abdominal pain
- Flatulence, abdominal distention
- Borborygmus (stomach rumbling)
- Fever
- Fatigue
- Anorexia, nausea, and vomiting
- Weight loss

Diagnostic and Laboratory Tests

- History and physical exam
- CBC (complete blood count) and differential
- Serum electrolytes
- ESR (erythrocyte sedimentation rate)
- Nutrient deficiency such as Vitamin B12, folate, fat soluble vitamins
- pANCA (perinuclear antineutrophil cytoplasmic antibody) elevated in 85% of ulcerative colitis and 15% of Crohn's disease clients.
- Antiglycan antibody elevated in 75% of Crohn's disease and 5% of ulcerative colitis client; good diagnostic tool when used with pANCA
- Stool examination for blood, mucous and pus
- Barium enema studies
- Colonoscopy or proctosigmoidoscopy – colonoscopy most helpful
- Biopsy and cytologic studies
- Plain abdominal x-rays
- Abdominal CT (computerized tomography) scan

Therapeutic Nursing Management

- **Prevention**:
    - Eat a nutritious diet that includes foods that can be tolerated.
    - Avoid stress and anxiety.
    - Plan for adequate rest and exercise.
- **Assess/Monitor**:
    - Factors that aggravate diarrhea
    - Fat malabsorption
    - Weight
    - General nutrition status
    - Vitamin deficiency
    - Quality of pain

- Skin in rectal area for irritation or breakdown
- For abdominal distention, muscle guarding, and pain
- For bowel sounds
- For signs of fluid and electrolyte imbalance
- Client's ability to cope with stress
- **Nursing Activities:**
  - Provide for adequate rest.
  - Administer intravenous fluids as necessary.
  - Administer TPN (total parenteral nutrition) when indicated.
  - Provide high-calorie, high-protein, no fat, no-residue feedings after exacerbation.
  - Provide small, frequent meals.
  - Record amount, color, consistency, and frequency of stools.
  - Record intake and output and hydration status.
  - Weigh daily.
  - Provide emotional support.
  - Teach relaxation techniques.
  - Encourage regular times for bowel elimination.
  - Prepare client for surgery (if disease is intractable or complications arise); colostomy and ileostomy.

Pharmacology

- Corticosteroids (prednisone, methylprednisolone)
- Aminosalicylates (sulfasalazine, mesalamine)
- Immunosuppressive agents (azathioprine, 6-mercaptopurine, cyclosporine, methotrexate)
- Antibiotics (metronidazole)
- Antispasmodics (dicyclomine [Bentyl])
- Antidiarrheals/anticholinergics (opium tincture, diphenoxylate with atropine [Lomotil])
- Possible use of infliximab (Remicade) for healing
- Vitamin supplementation
- Fluid and electrolyte replacement
- Total parenteral nutrition

Complications

- Progression and recurrence, even after surgery
- Transient arthritis
- Fistulas
- Toxic megacolon
- Gallstones
- Osteoporosis

- Abscesses
- Perforation
- Obstruction
- Malabsorption
- Perianal fissures and abscesses

Age-Related Changes—Gerontological Considerations

- Crohn's disease is primarily a disease of younger people.
- Older clients who require an ileostomy may have difficulty managing the equipment.

Critical Thinking Exercise: Nursing Management of the Client with Crohn's Disease

Situation: A 25-year-old woman with an exacerbation of Crohn's disease is admitted to the emergency department with complaints of diarrhea, intermittent abdominal pain, flatulence, abdominal distention, and severe fatigue. The client's temperature is 102° F. The client states she has felt under stress because she recently lost her job, and has not yet secured new employment. As a result, she is very anxious about her finances.

1. Which signs/symptoms are the best indicators that the client is developing a fluid volume deficit related to diarrhea?

   _____ Hypertension

   _____ Thirst

   _____ Bradycardia

   _____ Decreased urinary output

   _____ Weight gain

   _____ Dry oral mucous membranes

   _____ Postural hypotension

   _____ Anorexia

   _____ Headache

2. List at least three dietary modifications that may reduce the client's symptoms.

3. Why are these medications commonly prescribed for clients with Crohn's disease?

   a. Corticosteroids:

   b. Antidiarrheals:

   c. Antispasmodics:

Nursing Management of the Client with Diverticular Disease

Key Points

- A diverticulum is an outpouching of the bowel mucosa.
- Diverticular disease is classified as either diverticulosis or diverticulitis. This disorder occurs most often in the sigmoid colon.
- Diverticulosis is characterized by multiple outpouchings of the bowel mucosa.
- Diverticulitis, a complication of diverticulosis, is characterized by inflammation or perforation of the diverticulum.
- Goals of collaborative management:
    - Allow the colon to rest.
    - Reduce the inflammatory process.
    - Relieve symptoms medically, if possible, and to avoid major surgery.
- Important nursing diagnoses (actual or potential) are:
    - Constipation
    - Diarrhea
    - Pain
    - Anxiety
- **Key Terms/Concepts**: Diverticula, fecolith, dietary fiber, peritonitis, bowel obstruction, colon resection

Overview

Diverticular disease develops when undigested food particles and bacteria are trapped in the diverticula, creating a hardened mass called a fecolith. The fecolith creates inflammation, which spreads to the surrounding mucosa. The resulting edema blocks off the inflamed area and restricts its blood supply. As a result, the diverticulum may bleed and perforate, while the trapped fecal contents may cause intra-abdominal perforation and peritonitis. Diverticulosis **may or may not produce symptoms.** If symptoms develop, pain is usually confined to the left lower quadrant and is related to tension in the colonic wall. Diverticulitis, which produces severe gastrointestinal symptoms, can be treated medically or surgically. **Pain from diverticulitis is usually located in the left lower quadrant but comes on more intense and abruptly than with diverticulosis and is also associated with fever and chills.** The surgery of choice for diverticulitis is a colon resection of the involved portion of the bowel. A temporary or permanent colostomy might be necessary.

Risk Factors

- Age over 40

- Stress
- Diet low in fiber ✓
- Low residue diet

Signs and Symptoms

- Changes in bowel habits
- Alternating constipation and diarrhea
- Abdominal pain, lower left quadrant
- Rebound tenderness, guarding with diverticulitis
- Abdominal pain with diverticulitis is usually sudden and intense
- Abdominal pain with diverticulosis is usually worse after eating, better after defecation or passage of flatus
- Elevated temperature and pulse
- Flatus
- Abdominal distention and tympany with diverticulitis
- Change in bowel sounds with diverticulitis depending upon if obstruction occurs
- Anorexia, nausea, and vomiting with diverticulitis
- Melena if diverticuli bleed

Diagnostic and Laboratory Tests

- History of the client's diet and bowel habits
- Physical examination
- Abdominal examination, especially of the left lower quadrant
- CBC (complete blood count) with differential
- ESR (erythrocyte sedimentation rate)
- Urinalysis
- Blood culture in disseminated cases of diverticulitis
- CT (computerized tomography) scan if diverticulitis suspected
- Sigmoidoscopy or colonoscopy : Do not perform if diverticulitis suspected or rupture with resultant peritonitis may occur.
- Ultrasonography
- Barium enema

Therapeutic Nursing Management

- **Assess/Monitor:**
  - Severity of symptoms
  - Character, frequency and presence of blood in the stool
  - Intravenous infusions
  - Diet
  - Activity level

- **Nursing Activities:**
  - Place clients who have severe symptoms on an NPO status and provide intravenous infusions to supply fluids and nutrients.
  - Insert a nasogastric tube and attach to suction to relieve nausea, vomiting, and gastric distention.
  - Provide clients with clear liquids and then solids once symptoms resolve.
  - Instruct clients to introduce high-fiber foods such as whole grain cereals, fruits, and vegetables very slowly into the diet.
  - Encourage clients to rest.
  - Instruct the client to avoid lifting, straining, coughing, and bending. These activities increase intra-abdominal pressure.
  - Prepare the client for surgery if medical measures fail to relieve the symptoms.
  - Administer antibiotics to clients with diverticulitis.
  - Administer fiber supplements to clients with diverticulosis.
  - Administer analgesics

Pharmacology

- Broad-spectrum antibiotics to control infection
- Anticholinergics/Antispasmodics to control bowel contractions
- Vasopressin for diverticular bleeding
- Pain medications for severe discomfort
- Bulk-forming laxatives to reduce constipation
- Stool softeners

Complications

- Partial or complete bowel obstruction
- Perforation of the bowel
- Peritonitis
- Fistula formation
- Hemorrhage

Age–Related Changes—Gerontological Considerations

- Over half the population who are 40 years of age and older have diverticula.
- The risk for developing diverticular disease increases as people age.

Critical Thinking Exercise: Nursing Management of the Client with Diverticular Disease

Situation: A 65-year-old woman is being admitted to the hospital for diagnostic tests and to be evaluated for diverticulitis. The client is experiencing fever, severe abdominal pain, nausea, vomiting and abdominal distention.

1. What diagnostic tests are usually ordered for clients with possible diverticulitis?

   CBC   ESR   blood culture

2. What interventions do you expect to be performed to relieve this client's severe symptoms?

3. What complications could this client develop as a result of diverticulitis?

4. If the client has diverticulitis and fails to respond to medical interventions, what surgical procedure will need to be performed?

Nursing Management of the Client with Colorectal Cancer

| Key Points |

- Colon cancer is the second most frequent cause of cancer deaths in the United States.
- Colon cancer is primarily treated surgically, depending upon the location, type, and stage of the tumor.
- Types of surgeries include:
    - Colon resection with end-to-end anastomosis
    - Colon resection with a permanent or temporary colostomy
    - Abdominal-perineal resection with a permanent or end-colostomy
- Radiation therapy may be administered prior to surgery, and isotopes may be implanted into the tumor area following surgery, if the tumor cannot be entirely removed.
- Chemotherapy is used following surgery to treat metastasis.
- Approximately 50% of clients with a localized malignancy survive for five years.
- Goals of collaborative management:
    - Remove the malignant tumor and administer radiation and/or chemotherapy.
    - Prevent complications (anemia, infection, stoma necrosis, peritonitis).
    - Teach client to care for ostomy.
    - Establish a bowel program.
    - Provide emotional support.
- Important nursing diagnoses (actual or potential):
    - Diarrhea
    - Constipation
    - Altered nutrition: less than body requirements
    - Fatigue
    - Body image disturbance
    - Impaired social interaction
    - Risk for sexual dysfunction
    - Altered skin integrity
    - Impaired tissue integrity
    - Pain management
    - Ineffective individual coping
    - Fluid volume deficit
    - Self-care deficit

- • Anticipatory grieving
- • Anxiety and fear
- • Ineffective management of therapeutic program
- **Key Terms/Concepts**: Bowel habits, high-fat diet, rectal bleeding, stool guaiac, abdominal-perineal resection, permanent or temporary colostomy, ostomy care

Overview

Colorectal cancer is a malignant tumor that involves the colon or rectum. The most frequent site is the rectosigmoid. Liver metastases are common.

Risk Factors

- • Family history of colorectal cancer
- • History of ulcerative colitis
- • Male gender
- • Older than age 50, peak incidence in 70s
- • Polyposis syndrome
- • Adenomatous polyps
- • High-fat, low-residue diet
- • Residence in highly industrialized region in Western part of world

Signs and Symptoms

- • Vague signs and symptoms in early stages
- • Change in bowel habits (especially cancer of left side of colon)
- • Weakness
- • Fatigue
- • Anemia
- • Weight loss
- • Presence of blood on tissue wipes
- • Bloody stools
- • Rectal bleeding
- • Abdominal tenderness and pain
- • Abdominal masses

Diagnostic and Laboratory Tests

- • History and physical examination
- • History of bowel habits
- • Diet history
- • Auscultation of bowel sounds
- • DRE (digital rectal examination)
- • CEA (carcinoembryonic antigen)
- • Stool guaiac

- Colonoscopy or proctosigmoidoscopy – colonoscopy is screening of choice

Therapeutic Nursing Management

- **Prevention:**
    - Instruct clients concerning the importance of a nutritious, low-fat diet.
    - Instruct clients to report changes in bowel habits.
    - Annual cancer screening examinations
    - Annual DRE (digital rectal examination) for clients over 40 years old
    - Annual stool guaiac tests for clients over 50 years old- send packet of three home with client, along with instructions on how to obtain.
- **Assess/Monitor:**
    - Vital signs
    - Laboratory reports
    - Nutritional status
    - Fluid intake, output, hydration, and electrolyte status
    - Body weight
    - For signs of bowel obstruction (distention and/or rigidity, absence of bowel sounds, abdominal pain)
    - Client's preoperative acceptance of need for colostomy
    - For postoperative complications following surgical removal of tumor
    - For pain related to surgery
    - For return of bowel sounds
    - Incision and dressing for bleeding and drainage
    - Stoma for color and hydration
    - Colostomy output
    - Following abdominal-perineal resection:
        - The character and odor of drainage from perineal drains
        - For postoperative phlebitis
    - Activity tolerance following surgery
    - For side effects resulting from chemotherapy
    - For side effects resulting from radiation therapy
- **Nursing Activities:**
    - Encourage a low-residue diet that is high in protein, carbohydrates, and calories.
    - Provide information to client and family regarding:
        - Diagnostic tests
        - Type of surgery, immediate postoperative period, and expected outcomes
        - The purpose and care of an ostomy
    - Provide emotional support to the client and family prior to the surgery.
    - Encourage verbalization of fears and concerns.
    - During the preoperative period:
        - Provide a low-residue or liquid diet.

- Administer cathartics, enemas, and antibiotics as ordered.
- Administer blood transfusions as ordered to correct anemia.
- During the postoperative period:
  - Administer routine postoperative care.
  - Maintain nasogastric suction.
  - Keep stoma site clean and dry.
  - Empty ostomy appliance as required.
- Following abdominal-perineal resection:
  - Encourage a side-lying position.
  - Change rectal dressings.
  - Provide sitz baths three to four times daily.
- Instruct client concerning care of stoma, application and emptying of pouch, colostomy irrigation, and odor control measures.
- Arrange for home health visits following discharge.
- Teach client signs and symptoms of complications that should be reported to primary care provider or home health care nurse.
- Refer client to ostomy support groups and American Cancer Society.

Pharmacology

- Pain medications as necessary (opioid)
- Chemotherapy (fluorouracil, irinotecan)
- Antibiotics (if bacterial infection present or for surgical prophylaxis)
- Blood transfusions
- Antiemetics (ondansetron, granisetron, dolasetron)
- Cathartics (Colyte)
- Enemas (Fleets)
- Implanted isotopes

Complications

- Anemia
- Bowel obstruction
- Fluid and electrolyte imbalance
- Infection
- Skin breakdown around stoma site
- Stoma necrosis, prolapse, or retraction
- Depression
- Sexual dysfunction

Age-Related Changes—Gerontological Considerations

- Colorectal cancer primarily develops in older adults who are 50 to 60 years old.
- Older clients tend to overuse laxatives and enemas.

- Older clients may not make the effort to prepare foods that are nutritious and low in fat.
- Older clients may experience problems managing ostomy care at home due to poor vision, confusion, and arthritis of the hands.

Critical Thinking Exercise: Nursing Management of the Client with Colorectal Cancer

Situation: A 60-year-old married male client has had an abdominal-perineal resection for colorectal cancer. The nurse is preparing him for discharge home.

1. Following abdominal-perineal resection, why is it important to assess the client for signs of postoperative phlebitis and how can it be prevented?

2. Prior to discharge, what instructions does the nurse give to the client and family about colostomy irrigation?

3. The client is concerned about the effect of the surgery and colostomy on his sexual relationship with his wife. What actions should be taken to help lessen concerns?

Nursing Management of the Client with a Colostomy/Ileostomy

Key Points

- Ostomies are performed to relieve small and large bowel obstructions.
- Ostomies may be temporary or permanent.
- Stomas are constructed for the majority of ostomies.
- Goals of collaborative management:
  - Relieve the obstruction.
  - Restore bowel function.
  - Prevent complications (stoma necrosis, peritonitis, infection).
- Important nursing diagnoses (actual or potential) are:
  - Body image disturbance
  - Altered skin integrity
  - Pain management
  - Ineffective individual coping
  - Potential complications of surgery/colostomy
  - Self-care deficit
  - Fluid volume deficit
- **Key Terms/Concepts**: Stoma, colostomy, ileostomy, ostomy appliance, temporary colostomy

Overview

An ostomy is a surgical opening made through the abdomen into the colon or ileum for the excretion of wastes. The location of the ostomy within the intestine determines the consistency of the excreted stool. Colostomies and ileostomies are most commonly performed to relieve large and small bowel obstructions.

Risk Factors

- Small bowel obstruction
- Large bowel obstruction
- Colon cancer
- Inflammatory bowel disease (ulcerative colitis, regional enteritis)
- Abdominal trauma

Diagnostic Tests

- Flat and upright abdominal x-rays
- Colonoscopy

- Barium studies may be contraindicated with bowel obstructions
- MRI (magnetic resonance imaging)
- CT/CAT (computer tomography/computed axial tomography) scan
- Ultrasound
  - 2-D (2-Dimensional)
  - 3-D (3-Dimensional)

Therapeutic Nursing Management

- **Assess/Monitor:**
  - For signs of obstruction (distention and/or rigidity, absence of bowel sounds, pain)
  - Fluid status
  - Urinary output
  - Stoma for color and hydration (beefy red initially, then pink)
  - Client's willingness and ability to assume self-care
- **Nursing Activities:**
  - Provide emotional support to client and family preoperatively.
  - Administer prescribed antiemetics to prevent nausea/vomiting.
  - Keep stoma site clean and dry.
  - Empty ostomy appliance frequently.
  - Encourage the client to look at and touch the stoma.
  - Teach client regarding appearance of stoma, care of stoma, changing and cleaning of appliances, and odor control measures.
  - Teach client to avoid gas-producing foods in order to control odor.
  - Encourage verbalization of fears and concerns.
  - Provide supportive environment to promote client's adaptation to change in body image.
  - Refer client and family to communicate support groups if available.
  - Teach client signs and symptoms that need to be reported if complications develop.

Pharmacology

- Skin barriers

Complications

- Skin breakdown around the stoma site
- Stoma necrosis, prolapse or retraction
- Infection
- Constipation
- Fluid and electrolyte imbalance
- Body image disturbance

Age–Related Changes—Gerontological Considerations

- Bowel abnormalities may occur due to age-related decreases in gastrointestinal mobility, muscle tone, and digestive enzymes.
- Constipation is common and related to inadequate intake of fiber.
- Laxative overuse is common among older adults.
- The increased incidence of colorectal cancer is due to a decrease in immune function.
- The elderly client with diarrhea is at increased risk for dehydration and electrolyte imbalance.
- Altered home management (ostomy care and appliance care) is possibly related to decreased vision, confusion, or arthritis deformities of the hands.

Critical Thinking Exercise: Nursing Management of the Client with a Colostomy/Ileostomy

Situation: It is the second postoperative day for a 62-year-old male who underwent bowel resection and colostomy construction as treatment for a bowel obstruction secondary to rectal cancer. His vital signs are stable, he has ambulated about in his room, and his dressing is dry and intact. His stoma is beefy red in appearance and feces and gas are draining into his pouch.

1. What is the etiology of the client's nursing diagnoses?

    a. Risk for body image disturbance:

    b. Risk for altered skin integrity:

    c. Risk for ineffective individual coping:

2. What client behaviors indicate that he is ready to participate in his own care?

    ____ Informing the nurse when the appliance needs to be changed

    ____ Asking questions about the stoma and its care

    ____ Looking at the stoma when the appliance is changed

    ____ Stating that he will care for the stoma when he gets home

3. The client is concerned about odor from the pouch. What suggestions can the nurse offer to decrease or eliminate this problem?

Nursing Management of the Client with Gastroesophageal Reflux Disease (GERD)

Key Points

- Gastroesophageal reflux disease, or GERD, is a common condition characterized by the backflow of contents from the stomach or duodenum into the esophagus, without vomiting.
- Symptoms of GERD develop when an inflammatory response is initiated.
- The severity of the inflammatory response is related to the amount of acid in the refluxed material.
- Worldwide, approximately 5% to 7% of the population experience GERD.
- Over 60 million Americans develop symptoms of GERD, and around 17.5 million Americans experience symptoms of GERD on a daily basis.
- GERD is primarily treated with drugs, lifestyle changes, and dietary modifications.
- GERD may be a predisposing factor for ear infections, sinus infections and asthma exacerbations.
- GERD symptoms may not include heartburn, but may be more specific, such as earache, headache, chronic cough, laryngitis, and chest pain.
- Left untreated, GERD can lead to erosive esophagitis and possible cancer (Barrett's esophagitis).
- Goals of collaborative management:
- Relieve symptoms.
- Encourage client to make lifestyle changes.
- Educate client about dietary changes.
- Important nursing diagnoses (actual or potential):
- Pain related to acid reflux
- Anxiety
- Knowledge deficit
- **Key Terms/Concepts**: Gastrointestinal contents, lower esophageal sphincter, acid reflux

Overview

Gastroesophageal reflux disease or GERD involves the backward flow of gastrointestinal contents into the esophagus, via inappropriate relaxation of the lower esophageal sphincter (LES). This backflow of gastrointestinal contents can irritate the mucosa of the esophagus, causing inflammation and breakdown. GERD is normally treated with medications, diet, and modifications in lifestyle. Surgery is not the treatment of choice for GERD. Surgery is performed on clients who fail to respond to aggressive medical interventions and lifestyle changes.

Risk Factors

- Cigarette smoking
- Excessive ingestion of fatty foods, chocolate, cola drinks, coffee, tea, milk, peppermint, yellow onions, spicy tomato drinks, citrus fruits, and alcohol
- Hiatal hernia
- Chronic belching
- Eradication of h. pylori infection
- Obesity
- Pregnancy
- Drugs that lower LES pressure including theophylline, anticholinergics, progesterone, alpha-adrenergic agents, benzodiazepines, calcium channel blockers, and narcotics

Signs and Symptoms

- Dyspepsia (heartburn)
- Regurgitation of a warm fluid into the throat causing soreness or a bitter taste in the mouth
- Belching
- Bloated feeling after eating
- Dysphagia or difficulty swallowing
- "Water brash" due to hypersalivation
- Chest pain (from esophageal spasms)
- Bleeding related to breakdown of esophageal tissues
- Laryngitis
- Chronic cough
- Bronchospasm
- Frequent sinus or ear infections
- Loss of dental enamel
- Headache

Diagnostic Laboratory Tests

- Barium swallow
- Radionuclide scintigraphy
- Endoscopy
- Esophagoscopy with or without biopsy
- Esophageal manometry
- Measurement of esophageal acidity (pH) monitoring every hour for 24 hours
- Empiric trial of PPI (proton pump inhibitor)

Therapeutic Nursing Management

- **Assess/Monitor**:
  - Symptoms of GERD
  - Client's food diary
  - Client's weight
  - Client's response to medications
- **Nursing Activities**:
  - Administer medications as prescribed to relieve the symptoms of GERD.
  - Encourage client to keep a diary and monitor which foods precipitate attacks.
  - Instruct the client to elevate the head of the bed (via the frame on blocks) 8 to 12 inches to prevent reflux symptoms at night. Teach the client not to use pillows for elevation at night, as this rounds the back, bringing the stomach contents up closer to the chest.
  - Suggest a weight loss program if client is obese.
  - Treatment based on stepped approach:

    Phase I – Lifestyle and diet modifications puts antacids or OTC H_2 (histamine) blockers

    Phase ll – Prescription H2 blockers, PPIs (proton pump inhibitors)

    Phase lll – PPIs or high-dose H2 blockers; or H2 blocker or PPIs plus promotility agent

    Phase lV – Surgery
  - Instruct the client to:
    - Eat small frequent meals rather than large meals.
    - Avoid evening snacks or eating before bedtime. Do not eat at least 2 to 3 hours before bedtime.
    - Eat slowly and chew foods thoroughly.
    - Quit smoking.
    - Avoid eating fatty foods and chocolate.
    - Avoid drinking carbonated beverages, coffee, tea, and alcohol.
    - Avoid wearing tight-fitting garments.
    - Assure pregnant clients that their symptoms are likely to resolve after delivery.

Pharmacology

- Antacids to neutralize acids and relieve heartburn: aluminum hydroxide (Mylanta)
- Histamine2 receptor antagonists (blockers) to reduce the secretion of acids and relieve symptoms: ranitidine (Zantac), famotidine (Pepcid), nizatidine (Axid). Note: cimetidine is also possible, but it interacts with over 60 other medications and has a higher risk profile in the elderly, so since other, safer choices are available, it should not be considered first-line.
- Proton pump inhibitors to reduce the secretion of acids: pantoprazole (Protonix), omeprazole (Prilosec), rabeprazole (AcipHex), esomeprazole

(Nexium), lansoprazole (Prevacid)

- Gastrointestinal motility agents to accelerate gastric emptying without stimulating the release of gastric acid: metoclopramide (Reglan). Note: cisapride or Propulsid are now only available via limited access due to complications.

Complications

- Aspiration pneumonia
- Esophageal strictures
- Perforation of the esophagus
- Cancer of the esophagus, Barrett's adenocarcinoma
- Asthma exacerbations
- Upper respiratory infections

Critical Thinking Exercise: Nursing Management of the Client with Gastroesophageal Reflux Disease (GERD)

Situation: A 25-year-old woman who has been diagnosed with gastroesophageal reflux disease (GERD) is meeting with the nurse practitioner to discuss her condition. The client, who is overweight, has been experiencing dyspepsia, belching, bloating after meals, dysphagia, and chest pain.

1. What pathophysiologic problem is causing this client to experience chest pain?

2. What instructions should the nurse practitioner provide this client in regard to diet?

3. What classifications of medications will help to relieve the symptoms of GERD that result from the reflux of gastrointestinal contents containing acid?

Nursing Management of the Client with Salmonellosis

Key Points

- Salmonellosis is a preventable, contagious disease transmitted via contaminated foods.
- Goals of collaborative management:
  - Prevent transmission of the Salmonella bacteria.
  - Eradicate the Salmonella bacteria.
  - Restore normal bowel function.
  - Prevent complications (electrolyte imbalance, hypovolemia).
- Important nursing diagnoses (actual or potential):
  - Diarrhea and other bowel dysfunctions
  - Nausea and vomiting
  - Pain management
  - Fluid volume deficit
  - Knowledge deficit
  - Altered skin integrity
  - Altered nutrition: less than body requirements
  - Potential complications of salmonellosis
- **Key Terms/Concepts**: Transmission, contagious

Overview

Salmonellosis is a mild to severe form of gastroenteritis caused by the Salmonella bacteria. Commonly known as food poisoning, it is transmitted by ingestion of raw or improperly cooked meat, poultry, eggs, and dairy products contaminated with the Salmonella bacteria. It may also be transmitted via intake of contaminated water or contact with infected animals such as pet turtles, reptiles, or animal water sources including cats, dogs, mice, guinea pigs, and hamsters. Direct transmission from person-to-person is less common than with other modes of transmission previously mentioned. (fecal-oral route)

Risk Factors

- Contaminated raw meat, fish, poultry, eggs
- Unrefrigerated foods containing mayonnaise, cream; especially unpasteurized milk products
- Improper hand washing
- Improper food storage and preparation
- Older adults and infants

- Immune suppression or immunodeficiency, including cancers
- Impaired gastric acidity via use of histamine2 blockers, antacids, proton pump inhibitors, surgery
- Hemolytic anemias

Signs and Symptoms

- Mild-to-severe diarrhea
- Abdominal cramping
- Nausea, vomiting
- Fever
- Chills
- Weakness
- Occult and gross blood in watery diarrhea

Diagnostic and Laboratory Tests

- History and physical examination
- Stool specimen for culture, presence of white blood cells
- Gram stain of vomitus
- Blood culture
- CBC (complete blood count) with differential

Therapeutic Nursing Management

- **Assess/Monitor:**
  - Intake and output
  - Serum electrolytes
  - For signs of dehydration/hypovolemia
- **Nursing Activities:**
  - Offer clear fluids only until diarrhea subsides.
  - Administer fluid replacement orally or intravenously as prescribed.
  - Institute enteric precautions.
  - Educate client/family regarding food storage and preparation.

Pharmacology

- Fluid, electrolyte replacement
- Antimicrobials (if infection disseminates beyond the gastrointestinal [GI] tract)

Complications

- Dehydration
- Hypovolemia
- Electrolyte imbalance
- Cardiac dysrhythmias

- Death

Age-Related Changes—Gerontological Considerations

- Increased risk for fluid and electrolyte imbalance (dehydration, hypernatremia) is due to age-related decreases in total body water content and inadequate fluid intake.

Critical Thinking Exercise: Nursing Management of the Client with Salmonellosis

Situation: An older adult woman is being treated for abdominal cramping, nausea, vomiting and severe, watery diarrhea. Her symptoms began after attending an all day picnic on a hot day at a family reunion. Stool examination confirms the presence of salmonellosis.

1. Why are older adults and infants more susceptible to development of salmonellosis than other age groups?

2. Which are the two most important nursing diagnoses for the older adult client with salmonellosis?

_____ Risk for infection

_____ Risk for fluid volume deficit

_____ Risk for altered nutrition

_____ Risk for electrolyte imbalance

_____ Risk for altered skin integrity

3. Which collaborative care measures are appropriate for the client with salmonellosis?

____ Initiating protective isolation precautions

____ Replacing fluids and electrolytes

____ Encouraging a full liquid diet

____ Administering anti-diarrheal medication

____ Administering antimicrobial therapy

Nursing Management of the Client with Constipation and Diarrhea

Key Points

- Patterns of bowel elimination vary from person to person.
- Frequency of bowel movements in healthy people may vary from 2 to 3 bowel movements per day to 2 bowel movements per week.
- A decrease in the number of bowel movements and a change in the consistency of bowel movements from what is "normal" for an individual are significant.
- Constipation is a general term for bowel movements that are unusually small, hard, dry, difficult to pass or infrequent.
- Fecal impaction is a serious complication of constipation. A fecal impaction is a mass of hardened feces that collects in the rectum and prevents the passage of normal stools.
- Diarrhea is a general term for an increase in the number, amount, or liquid content of bowel movements, as compared with the usual pattern for a particular person. Diarrhea is not a disease in itself, but it is usually a symptom of another medical condition.
- Goals of collaborative management:
  - Remove the precipitating factors for constipation.
  - Set up a dietary program that promotes a return to normal bowel elimination.
  - Set up a routine for bowel elimination.
  - Remove precipitating factors for diarrhea.
  - Stop the diarrhea.
  - Avoid or treat fluid and electrolyte imbalances.
- Important nursing diagnoses (actual or potential):
  - Constipation
  - Diarrhea
  - Pain management
  - Fluid volume deficit
  - Anxiety
  - Impaired skin integrity (diarrhea)
- **Key Terms/Concepts:** Dietary program, bowel management program, fecal impaction, inflammatory bowel disease, liquid stools, fluid and electrolyte imbalances, metabolic acidosis

Overview

Constipation is a change in normal bowel habits, which is characterized by the infrequent passage of stool, or difficulty in passing dry, hard stools. Types of constipation include:

- **Atonic:** due to weakness of the muscles of the colon and rectum
- **Colonic:** due to delayed passage of feces through the colon, resulting in hard stools
- **Dyschezia:** painful defecation caused by dependence on laxatives
- **Obstructive:** due to an intestinal obstruction that may require surgery
- **Rectal:** due to habitually delaying stool elimination when the urge arises

Diarrhea develops when intestinal motility increases, and intestinal contents are propelled rapidly through the colon, with little time for absorption of water and other substances. The result is an urgent need to expel the loose, runny, or watery stool. Many people experience abdominal pain or intestinal cramping with diarrhea.

- **Osmotic:** Substances that are poorly absorbed cause a change in the osmotic gradient to occur, puling water into the intestine. Examples are lactose intolerance, sorbitol, certain antacids, fat-blocking agents in food, etc.
- **Secretory:** Reduced absorption via the small intestine or increased secretions of the small intestine. Examples include cholera, Escherichia coli, as well as non-infectious causes.
- **Exudative:** Occurs when the intestinal mucosa is inflamed leading to leakage of pus, blood, and mucous. Can be caused by inflammatory bowel disease or infections of the small and/or large intestine.
- **Mobility disturbances:** Transit time through the bowel is hastened, not allowing for fluid to be reabsorbed. Irritable bowel disease and certain medications are examples.

Risk Factors

- Constipation
  - Inadequate fluid intake
  - Inadequate bulk in diet
  - Sedentary lifestyle, immobilization, spinal cord injury
  - Irritable bowel syndrome
  - Poor bowel habits
  - Immobilization due to illness or injury
  - Medications that promote constipation
  - Overuse of laxatives
- Diarrhea
  - Overuse of laxatives
  - Inflammatory bowel diseases such as ulcerative colitis, Crohn's disease, and irritable bowel syndrome
  - Malabsorption problems, i.e. Celiac disease

- Eating very spicy foods, fatty foods, milk products, etc., in sensitive clients
- Recent travel to area where water or food is contaminated with bacteria, or food/water contamination here at home
- Use of antibiotics, especially frequent use
- Intestinal infections due to Escherichia coli or Vibrio cholerae
- Food intolerances

Signs and Symptoms

- **Constipation**
  - Straining at defecation
  - Abdominal bloating
  - Abdominal discomfort
  - Feeling of rectal fullness
  - Diarrhea if impaction present
  - Red flags (indicate that something else is going on): abdominal pain, nausea and vomiting, melena, rectal pain, fever, and weight loss
- **Diarrhea**
  - Loose, runny or watery stools
  - Sudden and urgent need to expel stools
  - Intestinal pain or cramping

Diagnostic and Laboratory Tests

- History and physical exam
- Orthostatic blood pressure and pulse in the presence of diarrhea to assess dehydration
- Hemoccult stools as appropriate
- DRE (digital rectal examination) for impaction, masses or other lesions
- Stool cultures
- Examination of stools for WBC, mucus, pus, and parasites
- Electrolyte panel, as appropriate
- Liver function tests, as appropriate
- CBC (complete blood count) with differential, as appropriate
- Celiac disease work-up and intestinal biopsy, if suspected
- Intestinal biopsies, if irritable bowel disease suspected

Therapeutic Nursing Management

- **Prevention of Constipation**:
  - Eat a diet high in fiber, bulk, fruits, and vegetables.
  - Drink at least 6 to 8 glasses of water per day.
  - Defecate immediately when urge arises.
  - Increase activity level.
  - Avoid overuse of laxatives.

- **Prevention of Diarrhea:**
  - Avoid overuse of laxatives.
  - Avoid foods that cause allergic reactions.
  - Drink only bottled beverages in countries where water is likely to be contaminated.
- **Assess/Monitor:**
  - For constipation
  - For signs of impaction
  - For factors that may cause constipation or diarrhea
  - Frequency, shape, color, character, and volume of stools (measure liquid stools), presence of blood, mucus, pus, floats vs sinks
  - Bowel sounds
  - Abdominal pain or distention
  - Vital signs
  - Daily weight (especially for client with diarrhea)
  - Skin around perianal area for irritation from diarrhea stools
- **Nursing Activities:**
  - **Constipation**
    - Remove impaction if present.
    - Administer laxatives, suppositories, or enemas if indicated.
    - Provide a private environment.
    - Instruct client to maintain a food diary.
    - Instruct client to keep an intake and output record.
    - Assist client in setting up a bowel management program.
  - **Diarrhea**
    - Instruct client to eliminate foods that are irritating the colon (example: spicy or fried foods).
    - Ask the client to keep a food diary if uncertain which food is causing the diarrhea.
    - Provide a liquid diet for at least 8 hours to rest the bowel. Encourage fluid intake, including electrolyte replacement (commercially available sports drinks are okay).
    - Encourage frequent small feedings of high-protein, high-carbohydrate, and low-residue foods such as steamed chicken without skin. The BRAT diet (bananas, rice, applesauce and toast) is no longer recommended, due to insufficient calories.
    - Remind client to avoid foods high in fat, milk, spices/seasoning, alcohol, citrus, chocolate/caffeine, and red meat. Add fiber back into the diet, slowly.
    - Wash and gently dry the perianal area to prevent skin excoriation or skin breakdown. Apply a medicated ointment that contains vitamins A & D or zinc oxide to the area.
    - Provide the hospitalized client with privacy when using a bedpan or commode.

Pharmacology

- Constipation
  - Stool softeners (docusate)
  - Bulk producing-laxatives (psyllium [Metamucil], methylcellulose, polycarbophil)
  - Osmotic laxatives, short-term use only (milk of magnesia, magnesium citrate, phosphate of soda, lactulose, sorbitol, alumina-magnesium, polyethylene glycol)
  - Stimulant laxatives (cascara, senna), use very cautiously
  - Suppositories, only if necessary
  - Enemas, only if necessary
- Diarrhea
  - Antibiotics for diarrhea of bacterial origin, only in severe/toxic cases.
  - Administer antidiarrheal medications: loperamide hydrochloride, kaolin-pectin and bismuth subsalicylate. These products should be used no longer than 3 days and only in clients with no contraindications.
  - Administer codeine, an opiate, for severe diarrhea.
  - Intravenous solutions as prescribed for dehydrated clients
  - Vitamins A & D or zinc oxide ointment

Complications

- Constipation
  - Fecal impaction
  - Dependence on laxatives and enemas
  - Straining at defecation employs the Valsalva maneuver (can cause angina pectoris, or even cardiac arrest in clients with heart disease)
  - Hemorrhoids
  - Rectal fissure
  - Fluid and electrolyte imbalance caused by laxative use
- Diarrhea
  - Fluid and electrolyte imbalances
  - Severe dehydration
  - Metabolic acidosis, because the client loses base via diarrhea
  - Skin breakdown around anal area

Age-Related Changes—Gerontological Considerations

- Older clients who have decreased activity may be more prone to constipation.
- Aging causes slower peristalsis, which results in increased water absorption from feces.
- Older clients may tend to overuse laxatives, which can result in either constipation or diarrhea.

Critical Thinking Exercise: Nursing Management of the Client with Constipation and Diarrhea

Situation: A 75-year-old man with congestive heart failure (CHF) is being admitted to a long-term care facility. The client develops fatigue and dyspnea upon exertion, and consequently tends to severely limit his activities. The client experienced chronic constipation when at home which, at one point, resulted in an impaction that had to be manually removed by a home health nurse. During admission, the client's daughter told the nurse her father had not had a bowel movement in several days, and had been straining at defecation without results.

1. Why is the client at increased risk for these complications related to his chronic constipation?
   a. Fecal impaction:
   b. Hemorrhoids:
   c. Exacerbated angina pectoris:

2. What procedure will the nurse use to determine if the client has a fecal impaction?

3. What nursing activities will help keep the client free of constipation on a long-term basis?
   ____ Administer daily laxatives
   ____ Institute a bowel management program
   ____ Encourage increased fluid intake
   ____ Perform a daily DRE (digital rectal exam)
   ____ Encourage bedrest
   ____ Increase daily physical activities
   ____ Increase dietary fiber
   ____ Administer weekly enemas

Nursing Management of the Client with Hypernatremia

Key Points

- Sodium is the major electrolyte found in extracellular fluid. _q̄_ .
- Sodium is essential for maintenance of acid-base balance, active and passive transport mechanisms, and intracellular metabolism.
- Hypernatremia occurs with fluid volume deficits or sodium excess.
- The thirst mechanism helps guard against development of hypernatremia.
- Goals of collaborative management:
  - Prevent fluid imbalances.
  - Provide early recognition and treatment.
  - Restore fluid and sodium balance.
- Important nursing diagnoses (actual or potential):
  - Fluid volume deficit
  - Impaired skin integrity
  - Risk for injury
  - Altered urinary elimination
- When the solute concentration in the blood increases, the hypothalamus triggers the thirst mechanism.
- The average person is able to drink adequate amounts of water to correct the problem, but there are some individuals who cannot.
- Antidiuretic hormone (ADH) is secreted by the posterior pituitary to help maintain this sodium balance.
- Antidiuretic hormone (ADH) allows water to be retained, which helps lower serum sodium levels.
- **Key Terms/Concepts**: Intravascular compartment, intracellular space, extracellular fluid, hyperreflexia, anti-diuretic hormone (ADH), hypothalamus

Overview

Hypernatremia exists when the serum sodium level exceeds 145 mEq/L. The ___. condition is related to an excess of sodium or a depletion of water in the intravascular compartment. When the serum sodium is elevated, fluid is pulled out of the cell and into the intravascular compartment by the process of osmosis, ultimately leading to cellular dehydration.

Risk Factors

- Excessive dietary sodium intake
- Excessive intravenous sodium intake

- Diaphoresis
- Fluid loss related to burns or other causes
- Diabetes insipidus
- Osmotic diuresis (diabetes mellitus)
- Cushing's syndrome
- Hyperaldosteronism
- Infants
- Elderly
- Drugs (anabolic steroids, corticosteroids, antibiotics, laxatives, methyldopa, estrogens, oral contraceptives)
- Antacids
- Salt tablets

Signs and Symptoms

- Thirst
- Fever
- Tachycardia
- Dry mucous membranes
- Restlessness, agitation
- Convulsions
- Hyperreflexia
- Twitching
- Weakness
- Confusion
- Lethargy
- Coma
- Flushed Skin
- Oliguria, anuria
- Hyperventilation

Diagnostic and Laboratory Tests

- History and physical examination
- Serum sodium
- Hematocrit
- Plasma protein levels
- Urine osmolality
- Urine specific gravity
- Antidiuretic hormone
- ABG (arterial blood gas)
- Electrolytes
- Plasma glucose

Therapeutic Nursing Management

- **Assess/Monitor:**
  - Blood pressure and pulse
  - Intake and output, weight
  - Dietary sodium intake
  - Capillary refill
  - Skin turgor
  - Neurological status
- **Nursing Activities:**
  - Administer IV isotonic salt-free solution (e.g., 5% dextrose in H2O, Ringer's Lactate) as prescribed.
  - Prepare for possible dialysis if sodium extremely elevated (>200 mEq/L)
  - Protect client safety.

Pharmacology

- IV isotonic salt-free solution (e.g., 5% dextrose in H2O)
- Diuretics
- Calcium – may need to give as sodium is corrected
- Sodium bicarbonate – may need to be given for severe metabolic acidosis

Complications

- Convulsions
- Death
- Permanent neurological damage

Age-Related Changes—Gerontological Consideration

- Total body water content is decreased in older adults.
- An increased risk for dehydration and hypernatremia is related to inadequate fluid intake.
- Hypernatremia in adults is often associated with an underlying illness.

Critical Thinking Exercise: Nursing Management of the Client with Hypernatremia

Situation: A 47-year-old woman has a rapid heart rate, dry oral mucous membranes, poor skin turgor, and fever of 101.3° F orally. Her serum sodium level is 163 mEq/L.

1. Which are risk factors for hypernatremia?

_____ Diaphoresis

_____ Nasogastric suctioning

_____ Diuretics

_____ Diabetes mellitus

_____ Cushing's syndrome

_____ Vomiting

_____ Diarrhea

_____ Burns

2. Which clinical manifestations are most supportive of the presence of hypernatremia?

_____ Lethargy

_____ Dry oral mucous membranes

_____ Fever

_____ Confusion

_____ Stupor or coma

_____ Tachycardia

_____ Muscle weakness

_____ Thirst

3. Prioritize the client's nursing diagnoses, with "1" representing the most important diagnosis.

_____ Impaired skin integrity

_____ Risk for injury

_____ Altered nutrition

_____ Fluid volume deficit

Nursing Management of the Client with Hyponatremia

| Key Points |

- Sodium is the major electrolyte found in extracellular fluid.
- Sodium is essential for maintenance of acid-base balance, active and passive transport mechanisms, and intracellular metabolism.
- Hyponatremia occurs with fluid volume deficits in which both fluid and sodium are lost from the body or from fluid volume excess.
- Goals of collaborative management:
  - Prevent fluid imbalances.
  - Provide early recognition and treatment.
  - Restore fluid and sodium balance.
- Important nursing diagnoses (actual or potential):
  - Fluid volume excess
  - Fluid volume deficit
  - Pain management
  - Nausea and vomiting
  - Fatigue and restlessness
  - Risk for injury
- Hyponatremia occurs when the blood vessels contain more water and less sodium.
- **Key Terms/Concepts**: Intravascular compartment, intracellular space, extracellular fluid, third-spacing, hypertension, weight gain, rapid pounding pulse

Overview

Hyponatremia exists when the serum sodium level drops below 135mEq/ L. Hyponatremia results from a loss of sodium or an excess of water in the intravascular compartment.

Risk Factors

- Excessive oral water intake
- Deficient dietary sodium intake
- Vomiting or diarrhea
- Nasogastric suctioning
- Diuretics
- Underlying disease (chronic renal insufficiency; adrenal insufficiency; syndrome of inappropriate ADH [antidiuretic hormone] secretion; CHF [congestive heart failure])

- Third-spacing (abnormal fluid shift into a third space) - peripheral edema, bowel obstruction, ascites

Signs and Symptoms

- Lethargy
- Confusion, disorientation
- Stupor or coma
- Muscle weakness
- Anorexia, nausea, vomiting
- Headache
- Abdominal cramping
- Decreased deep tendon reflexes
- Hypothermia
- Orthostatic hypotension
- Seizures

Diagnostic Tests

- Serum sodium
- Hematocrit
- Plasma protein levels
- Urine-specific gravity
- Urine osmolality
- BUN (blood urea nitrogen) and creatinine

Therapeutic Nursing Management

- **Assess/Monitor:**
  - Daily weight
  - Intake and output
  - Blood pressure
  - Pulse
  - Orthostatic blood pressure and pulse
  - Skin turgor
  - Neurological status
- **Nursing Activities:**
  - Administer oral or IV sodium solutions as prescribed.
  - Institute seizure precautions.
  - Restrict water intake.
  - Encourage foods and fluids high in sodium (broth).

Pharmacology

- 0.9% sodium chloride solution, 3% hypertonic, sodium chloride solution in severe cases
- Lactated Ringer's solution

Complications

- Seizures
- Coma
- Respiratory arrest

Age-Related Changes—Gerontological Consideration

- Increased risk of hyponatremia in older adults is due to higher incidence of chronic illnesses, diuretic use, and insufficient sodium intake.

Critical Thinking Exercise: Nursing Management of the Client with Hyponatremia

Situation: An 87-year-old man was admitted to the acute care facility for gastroenteritis of two days duration. He is vomiting, has severe, watery diarrhea, and is complaining of abdominal cramping. His serum electrolytes are consistent with hyponatremia related to excessive sodium loss.

1. Why does hyponatremia result from vomiting and diarrhea?

2. Which clinical manifestations support the diagnosis of hyponatremia?

____ Lethargy

____ Poor skin turgor

____ Hyperreflexia

____ Convulsions

____ Agitation

____ Headache

3. Which collaborative interventions will help reduce or eliminate the client's hyponatremia?

____ Administer Lactated Ringer's solution.

____ Encourage fluid intake.

____ Weigh daily.

____ Encourage foods high in sodium.

Nursing Management of the Client with Hyperkalemia

Key Points

- **Alert!** Tall, tented (peaked) T-waves are classic signs of hyperkalemia.
- The intracellular spaces contain the majority of potassium in the body.
- Potassium directly affects the excitability of muscles and nerves.
- Potassium excess is associated with acid excess (acidosis).
- Severe hyperkalemia is a life-threatening emergency.
- Hyperkalemia occurs infrequently in persons with normal renal function.
- Goals of collaborative management:
  - Identify persons at risk for hyperkalemia.
  - Provide early recognition and treatment.
  - Eliminate excess potassium.
  - Restore normal potassium balance.
- Important nursing diagnoses (actual or potential):
  - Nausea and vomiting
  - Diarrhea and other bowel dysfunctions
  - Risk for injury
  - Activity intolerance
  - Decreased cardiac output
  - Altered urinary elimination
- **Key Terms/Concepts**: Intravascular compartment, intracellular space, extracellular fluid

Overview

Hyperkalemia exists when the serum potassium level exceeds 5 mEq/L. Hyperkalemia is caused by excessive intake, decreased excretion, or movement of potassium out of the cell in response to injury, sepsis, fever, or surgery causes hyperkalemia. Rapid increases in potassium may be lethal, whereas slow, chronic elevations are better tolerated.

Risk Factors

- Cellular damage
  - Trauma
  - Surgery
  - Acute MI (myocardial Infarction)
  - Fever

- Sepsis
- Burns
- Impaired renal function
- Metabolic acidosis
- Insulin deficiency/hyperglycemia
- Drugs:
  - Beta-blockers
  - Cyclosporine
  - NSAIDs (nonsteroidal anti-inflammatory drugs)
  - Lithium
  - Heparin
  - Too frequent use of beta2 agonists inhalers
  - Digoxin toxicity
  - Potassium-sparing diuretics
  - ACE (angiotensin-converting enzyme) inhibitors
- Addison's disease
- Overuse of potassium supplement or salt substitutes
- Severe dehydration

Signs and Symptoms

- Nausea, vomiting, diarrhea
- Paresthesias, numbness
- Muscle weakness, flaccid paralysis
- ECG (electrocardiogram) changes (peaked T-waves, widened QRS complex, prolonged PR interval, prominent U-wave)
- Dysrhythmias (ventricular fibrillation, cardiac arrest)
- Restlessness and fatigue
- Oliguria, anuria

Diagnostic and Laboratory Tests

- History and physical examination
- Serum potassium (also called K+ test)
- ECG (Electrocardiogram)
- Arterial blood gases (ABGs)
- Possible cortisol and aldosterone levels

Therapeutic Nursing Management

- **Assess/Monitor:**
  - Vital signs
  - Serum potassium levels
  - Cardiac status continually

- **Nursing Activities:**
    - Identify persons at risk.
    - Identify and correct underlying cause as prescribed.
    - Maintain safe environment.
    - Prepare client for cation-exchange (Kayexalate).
    - Administer potassium-wasting diuretics as prescribed.
    - Prepare client for hemodialysis if prescribed.
    - Administer prescribed medications.
    - Administer intravenous insulin and dextrose as an emergency measure.
    - Prepare emergency intervention in case of cardiac arrest.

Pharmacology

- Calcium gluconate (should only be used in cases with ECG changes)
- Kayexalate (cation-exchange) and sodium bicarbonate, but be careful related to possible sodium overload
- Insulin (facilitates entry of potassium into the cell)
- Sodium bicarbonate (promotes cellular uptake of potassium)
- Beta2-agonists (albuterol via nebulization - promotes cellular uptake of potassium)
- Diuretics (furosemide - enhances renal excretion of potassium)

Complications

- Ventricular fibrillation
- Cardiac arrest
- Death

Age-Related Changes—Gerontological Consideration

- Increased risk for hyperkalemia is related to the increased use of salt substitutes by older adults with chronic illnesses. Clients use salt-substitutes because they are told to cut down on salt intake, along with ACE inhibitor and potassium-sparing diuretic for blood pressure.

Critical Thinking Exercise: Nursing Management of the Client with Hyperkalemia

Situation: An elderly client with a medical history of type 2 NIDDM (non-insulin-dependent diabetes mellitus) complicated by nephropathy, CHF (congestive heart failure), and rheumatoid arthritis comes to the emergency department because of chest palpitations. She describes a feeling of fatigue and nausea without vomiting. The client's medication record is shown in the table below, left. The primary care provider orders an ECG (electrocardiogram), chest x-ray, CBC (complete blood count), serum electrolytes, BUN (blood urea nitrogen), and creatinine. The electrolyte panel results are shown in the table below.

Medication Record	
Generic Name	**Brand name**
Spironolactone	Aldactone
Digoxin	Lanoxin
Metformin	Glucophage
Magnesium hydroxide	Milk of Magnesia
Calcium carbonate	Tums

Electrolyte Panel		
Na	139	mEq/L
K	5.8	mEq/L
Cl	102	mEq/L
CO_2	28	mEq/L
BUN	25	Mg/100mL
Creatinine	1.3	mg/dL

1. Should the health care provider be concerned about the client's serum potassium level? Why or why not?

2. Which clinical manifestations are associated with hyperkalemia?

_____ Headache

_____ Thirst

_____ Cardiac dysrhythmias

_____ Muscular twitching

_____ Vomiting

_____ Paresthesia

3. Which nursing diagnoses apply to the client with hyperkalemia?

    ____ Risk for fluid volume deficit

    ____ Risk for injury

    ____ Activity intolerance

    ____ Risk for decreased cardiac output

Nursing Management of the Client with Hypokalemia

| Key Points |

- **Alert!** Never give potassium by IV push or as a bolus. It can cause death by increasing the potassium level too rapidly.
- Symptoms are diminished deep tendon reflexes, paresthesias, dysrhythmias (such as frequent, premature, ventricular contractions and cardiac arrest), or paralytic ileus.
- The intracellular spaces contain the majority of potassium in the body.
- Potassium directly affects the excitability of muscles and nerves.
- Potassium deficit is associated with excess alkalinity (alkalosis).
- Whenever sodium is retained in the body, potassium is excreted.
- Severe hypokalemia can produce potentially life-threatening dysrhythmias.
- Goals of collaborative management:
  - Identify persons at risk for hypokalemia.
  - Provide early recognition and treatment.
  - Restore potassium balance.
- Important nursing diagnoses (actual or potential):
  - Pain management
  - Nausea and vomiting
  - Fatigue and restlessness
  - Activity intolerance
  - Risk for injury
  - Key Trems/Concepts: Impaired gas exchange, intracellular space, extracellular fluid, and atony

Overview

Hypokalemia exists when serum potassium levels drop below 3.5mEq/L. When serum potassium levels are too low, cells become less excitable, resulting in muscle weakness and atony.

Risk Factors

- Metabolic alkalosis
- Insulin excess
- Reduced intake of potassium
- Failure to replace potassium losses
- Gastrointestinal losses (vomiting, diarrhea, nasogastric suctioning)
- Renal disorders, liver disease

- Prolonged administration of non-electrolyte-containing intravenous solutions
- Excessive use of laxatives
- Non-potassium sparing diuretics
- Corticosteroids
- Starvation
- Nasogastric suction, vomiting

Signs and Symptoms

- Lethargy, diminished deep-tendon reflexes, faint pulse
- Confusion, mental depression
- Weakness, flaccid paralysis, respiratory muscle weakness
- Cardiac dysrhythmias: PVCs, bradycardia, blocks, ventricular tachycardia
- Anorexia, nausea, vomiting
- Abdominal distention, paralytic ileus
- ECG (Electrocardiogram) changes (flattened or inverted T-waves, ST segment depression, prominent U-wave)
- Increased output of dilute urine
- Polyuria, polydipsia
- Hypotension

Diagnostic and Laboratory Tests

- History and physical examination
- Serum potassium
- ECG (electrocardiogram)
- Arterial blood gas (ABG), possible
- Plasma glucose, possible

Therapeutic Nursing Management

- **Assess/Monitor:**
    - Vital signs
    - Intake and output, weight
    - For cardiac dysrhythmias
    - Bowel sounds and abdominal distention
- **Nursing Activities:**
    - Identify clients at risk.
    - Identify and correct underlying cause as prescribed.
    - Encourage intake of foods high in potassium.
    - Administer oral potassium as prescribed.
    - Administer intravenous potassium as prescribed (using infusion control device).

Pharmacology

- K (potassium) oral and intravenous

Complications

- Respiratory arrest
- Cardiac arrest
- Death

Age-Related Changes—Gerontological Considerations

- An increased risk of hypokalemia is related to the increased intake of diuretics and laxatives by older adults.

Critical Thinking Exercise: Nursing Management of the Client with Hypokalemia

Situation: A 69-year-old man has a medical history of congestive heart failure (CHF) controlled by digitalis and furosemide drug therapy. Two weeks ago he developed diarrhea, which has persisted in spite of his taking OTC antidiarrheal medications. His heart rate is 86 bpm, respirations 10 bpm, blood pressure 102/56 mmHg, and he is lethargic and confused.

1. Which client data supports the presence of hypokalemia?

2. Prioritize interventions for the client, with "1" representing the most important intervention.

_____ Identify and correct underlying cause as prescribed.

_____ Encourage intake of foods high in potassium.

_____ Administer oral potassium as prescribed.

_____ Administer intravenous potassium as prescribed.

_____ Assess vital signs.

3. After his diarrhea is controlled, which foods should the client is advised to eat since they are high in potassium?

_____ Beets

_____ Cantaloupe

_____ Lettuce

_____ Powdered milk

_____ Corn

_____ Dried beans

_____ Raw mushrooms

_____ Winter squash

_____ Carrots

Nursing Management of the Client with Acid-Base Imbalance

Key Points

- Acid-base imbalance is not a disease, but rather a biochemical abnormality.
- Acid-base balance represents homeostasis of H^+ (hydrogen) ion concentration in body fluids.
- A stable level of H^+ (hydrogen) ions needs to be maintained in order to have normal cellular function.
- Minor changes in H^+ (hydrogen) ion concentration have major effects on enzymatic activities.
- The kidneys, respiratory system, and chemical buffers regulate acid-base balance.
- Compensation by the lungs or kidneys is an effort to maintain the normal 20:1 ratio between HCO_3^- (bicarbonate) and H_2CO_3 (carbonic acid) which maintains the blood pH in its normal range.
- Note: Both equations move in both directions.

Respiratory Compensation   **Metabolic Compensation**

$$H_2O + CO_2 \longleftrightarrow H_2CO_3 \longleftrightarrow H^+ + HCO_3^-$$

Water   Carbon   Carbonic   Hydrogen   Bicarbonate
    dioxide   acid   ion

    Expelled   Expelled
    by lungs   by kidneys

- pH is always the result of the respiratory and metabolic compensation functions.
- H^+ (hydrogen) ions shift from the extracellular to the intracellular compartment or vice versa in order to compensate for acid-base abnormalities.
- Arterial blood gasses (ABGs) include:
  - pH (norm 7.35 – 7.45)
  - PaO_2 (norm 80 – 100 mmHg)
  - $PaCO_2$ (norm 35 – 45 mmHg)
  - HCO_3 (norm 22 – 26 mEq/L)
  - BE Base Excess (norm –2 to +2 mEq/L)
  - SaO_2 O_2 saturation (norm 95% – 100%)
- Goals of collaborative management:
  - Identify persons at risk for acid-base imbalance.
  - Correct acid-base imbalances.
  - Maintain acid-base balance.

- Important nursing diagnoses (actual or potential):
  - Impaired gas exchange
  - Metabolic imbalances
  - Anxiety and fear
  - Altered thought processes
  - Risk for injury
- **Key Terms/Concepts**: Acidosis, alkalosis, uncompensated, partially compensated, compensated, extracellular compartment, intracellular compartment, homeostasis

Overview

Acid-base balance represents homeostasis of H+ (hydrogen) ion concentration in body fluids.

- **Acidosis** exists when the pH of arterial blood falls below 7.35.
- **Alkalosis** exists when the pH of arterial blood exceeds 7.45.

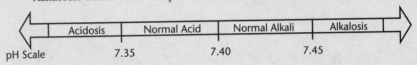

- **Metabolic acidosis** occurs when HCO_3- (bicarbonate) is lost or excess organic acids are added to body fluids.
- **Metabolic alkalosis** occurs when there is an excess of HCO_3- (bicarbonate) or lactate, or when excessive amounts of acid and H+ (hydrogen) ions are lost from the body.
- **Respiratory acidosis** occurs from hypoventilation, which increases the presence of dissolved CO_2 (carbon dioxide), H_2CO_3 (carbonic acid), and H+ (hydrogen) ions in arterial blood.
- **Respiratory alkalosis** is due to excessive pulmonary ventilation (hyperventilation), decreasing the presence of dissolved CO_2, etc., in arterial blood.

To determine presence and type of imbalance, follow these steps:

Step 1   Look at pH. If < 7.35, diagnose as acidosis.
                        If > 7.45, diagnose as alkalosis.

Step 2   Look at $PaCO_2$ and HCO_3- simultaneously.
          Determine which one is in its normal range.
          Then, conclude that the other is indicator of imbalance.
          Diagnose < 35 or > 45 $PaCO_2$ as respiratory in origin.
          Diagnose < 22 or >26 HCO_3- as metabolic in origin.

Step 3   Combine diagnoses of Step 1 with Step 2 to name the type of imbalance.

The following are the 5 classic types of ABG (arterial blood gas) results demonstrating balance and imbalance. (Other results are possible.)

	Step 1		Step 2		Step 3
	If		Determine which is in the normal range		Combine Names
Type	pH		$PaCO_2$	HCO_3^-	Diagnosis
1	7.35-7.45		35-45	22-26	Homeostasis
2	< 7.35		> 45	22-26	Respiratory Acidosis
3	< 7.35		35-45	< 22	Metabolic Acidosis
4	> 7.45		< 35	22-26	Respiratory Alkalosis
5	> 7.45		35-45	>26	Metabolic Acidosis

Step 4   Evaluate the PaO_2 and SaO_2
If the results are below the normal range, the client is hypoxic.

Step 5   Determine compensation as follows:

Uncompensated - the pH will be abnormal and either the HCO_3 or $PaCO_2$ will be abnormal.

Partially compensated - pH, HCO_3, and $PaCO_2$ will all be abnormal.

Fully compensated - pH will be normal but the $PaCO_2$ and HCO_3 will both be abnormal. Then, looking back at the pH will give you a clue as to which system initiated the problem; respiratory or metabolic. If the pH is < 7.4, think "acidosis" and determine which system has the acidosis value. If the pH is >7.4, think "alkalosis" and determine which system has the alkalosis value. Finding pH levels exactly at 7.40 is rare, fortunately, because you would need to know the real "nitty-gritty" which is beyond the scope of this text!

Risk Factors

Metabolic acidosis

- DKA (diabetic ketoacidosis)
- Renal failure
- Shock
- Diarrhea
- Adrenal insufficiency
- Excessive salicylate ingestion
- Starvation

Metabolic alkalosis

- Gastric suctioning
- Vomiting

- Excessive intake of antacids
- Cushing's syndrome
- Hyperaldosteronism
- Excessive intake of licorice
- Potassium deficiency
- Antacids
- Potassium-wasting diuretics

Respiratory acidosis

- Respiratory center depression (narcotics, head injury, anesthetics)
- Atelectasis, pneumothorax
- Disease (polio, Guillain-Barré syndrome, amyotrophic lateral sclerosis)
- COPD, should be compensated
- Sleep apnea
- Inappropriate mechanical ventilator settings
- Respiratory problems such as respiratory distress with asthma, pneumonia, pulmonary embolism, etc.

Respiratory alkalosis

- Hyperventilation
- Fever
- Hypoxia
- Medications that stimulate the respiratory system
- Respiratory complications such as asthma, pneumonia, pulmonary embolism, etc.
- Inappropriate ventilator settings

Signs and Symptoms

Metabolic acidosis

- Anorexia, nausea, vomiting, diarrhea
- Headache, lethargy
- Kussmaul's respirations
- Abdominal pain
- Weakness
- Bradycardia
- Coma
- Potassium excess

Metabolic alkalosis

- Tachycardia
- Confusion, dizziness
- Numbness, tingling
- Tetany

- Convulsions
- Potassium deficit

Respiratory acidosis

- Hyperpnea
- Tachycardia
- Headache, visual disturbances
- Drowsiness
- Confusion
- Coma

Respiratory alkalosis

- Lightheadedness
- Sweating
- Palpitations
- Tetany
- Convulsions

Diagnostic and Laboratory Tests

- History and physical examination
- ABG (arterial blood gas) analysis
- Electrolytes including potassium, sodium and chloride, also, BUN (blood urea nitrogen), creatinine, and plasma glucose
- Anion Gap

Therapeutic Nursing Management

- **Assess/Monitor:**
  - Respiratory status
  - Cardiac status
  - ABGs (arterial blood gases)
  - Electrolyte profile
- **Nursing Activities:**
  - Identify and correct underlying problem as indicated.
  - Initiate intravenous access for emergency medications.
  - Support respirations as indicated.
  - Maintain client safety.
  - Administer medications as prescribed.
  - Replenish electrolytes, fluids, and sugar as indicated.

Pharmacology

- $NaHCO_3$ (sodium bicarbonate) — antacid
- Bronchodilators (to correct respiratory disorders), possibly
- Electrolyte replacement

- Diuretics (acetazolamide)
- Lactated Ringer's solution

Complications

- Convulsions
- Respiratory depression
- Coma
- Death

Age-Related Changes—Gerontological Considerations

- Increased risk for acid-base imbalance is related to the presence of dehydration or chronic illness.
- An increased risk for altered skin integrity is due to fragile arteries, veins, and skin, which makes arterial access and venous access difficult.

Critical Thinking Exercise: Nursing Management of the Client with Acid–Base Imbalance

Situation: Acid-base imbalances can be precipitated by a variety of causes in people who are healthy as well as those with illnesses. Interpret each of the ABG (arterial blood gas) findings, and identify common clinical manifestations with acid-base abnormalities.

1. Which ABG (arterial blood gas) findings need to be reported because they are abnormal?

Lab Results		Normal	Abnormal
Blood	7.38 pH		
PaCO$_2$	52 mmHg		
HCO$_3$	30 mEq/L		
PaO$_2$	62 mmHg		

2. Match the clinical manifestation with the correct acid-base abnormality. (Hint: A manifestation may appear in more than one type of imbalance.)

Clinical Manifestation	Type of Acid-Base Imbalance			
	Metabolic Acidosis	Metabolic Alkalosis	Respiratory Acidosis	Respiratory Alkalosis
Tetany				
Headache				
Diaphoresis				
Coma				
Convulsions				
Confusion				
Kussmaul's respirations				
Hyperpnea				
Bradycardia				
Visual disturbances				

3. Which acid-base imbalance should the nurse be prepared to encounter when caring for clients with:

Diagnosis	Type of Acid-Base Imbalance			
	Metabolic Acidosis	Metabolic Alkalosis	Respiratory Acidosis	Respiratory Alkalosis
Fever				
Cushing's Syndrome				
Head injury				
Gastric suctioning				
Renal failure				
Anesthetics				
Diabetes mellitus				
Vomiting				

Nursing Management of the Client with Extracellular Fluid Volume Deficit—Dehydration

Key Points

- **Alert!** When replacing IV fluids, give gradually to avoid causing swelling of the cells in the brain or potentially causing pulmonary edema.
- There are two types of extracellular fluid volume deficit (ECFVD):
  - Hyperosmolar fluid volume deficit, where the fluid loss is greater than the solute (sodium) loss.
  - Iso-osmolar fluid volume deficit, where there is an equal proportion of fluid and solute loss.
- Fluid flows across cell membranes by active or passive processes.
- Water moves from an area of high concentration to low concentration across cell membranes (osmosis).
- Water will continue to flow until the osmolarity between two compartments are equal.
- Disease, trauma, and other pathological states can affect osmolarity and cell membrane permeability to water.
- Changes in extracellular fluid volume are often related to changes in sodium balance.
- Fluid volume deficit may occur with sodium excess or sodium loss.
- Vascular volume loss (hypovolemia) can be caused by fluid deprivation, blood or fluid being sequestered in the pleura, peritoneal or pericardial cavities, or injection of a hypertonic solution.
- ECFVD can result in an intracellular fluid volume deficit (ICFVD).
- Thirst and weight loss are prominent signs of fluid deficit.
- ECFVD is particularly dangerous in babies, young children, and elderly people.
- Goals of collaborative management:
  - Restore fluid balance.
  - Prevent complications related to dehydration and therapy.
  - Provide information on how to prevent dehydration in the future.
- Important nursing diagnoses (actual or potential):
  - Fluid volume deficit
  - Risk for fluid volume imbalance
  - Altered oral mucous membranes
  - Risk for injury
  - Risk for altered body temperature
  - Constipation

- Risk for impaired skin integrity
- **Key Terms/Concepts**: Fluid volume deficit, osmolarity, mucous membranes, skin turgor, tenting, thirst, neck veins, hypotension, intracellular, extracellular, dehydration

Overview

Extracellular fluid volume deficit (ECFVD), or dehydration as it is commonly called, is the excessive loss of intravascular and interstitial fluids, which occurs when fluid output exceeds fluid intake.

Risk Factors

- Inadequate fluid intake
- Very young age
- Very old age
- Diarrhea
- Severe vomiting
- Profuse diaphoresis
- Excessive blood loss
- Third space fluid shifts
- Fever
- Nasogastric suctioning
- Burns
- Ileostomy
- Dysphagia
- Fistula
- Use of diuretics
- Hyperventilation
- Ulcerative colitis
- DKA (diabetic ketoacidosis)
- Diabetes insipidus

Signs and Symptoms

- **Early findings**
  - Dry mucous membranes
  - Dry, cracked lips
  - Thirst
  - Poor skin turgor
  - Constipation
  - Increased small vein filling time
  - Postural/orthostatic hypotension
  - Dark, concentrated urine with high specific gravity
  - Oliguria

- Fatigue
- Dizziness
- Rapid weight loss
- Electrolyte imbalance
- Muscle weakness
- Low-grade fever
- Tachycardia, mild
- **Late findings**
  - Longitudinal furrows in the tongue
  - Decreased pulse volume
  - Narrow pulse pressure
  - Tachycardia
  - Weak, thready pulse
  - Sunken eyeballs
  - Anxiety
  - Neck veins flat in supine position
  - Altered level of consciousness
  - Hypotension

Diagnostic and Laboratory Tests

- History and physical examination
- CBC (complete blood count)
- Electrolytes along with BUN (blood urea nitrogen) and creatinine
- Serum osmolarity
- Urine SG (specific gravity)
- Central venous pressure (CVP) measurements
- Orthostatic blood pressure and pulse measurements

Therapeutic Nursing Management

- **Prevention of ECFVD:**
  - Adequate oral fluid intake that includes some sodium (not just tap water), if indicated
  - Early treatment of severe diarrhea, vomiting, or a fever
  - Avoidance of strenuous exercise in a hot, humid climate
  - Supervised fluid intake for elderly clients
- **Assess/Monitor:**
  - Vital signs
  - Body temperature
  - Laboratory findings
  - Intake and output
  - Daily weights
  - Skin turgor

- Mucous membranes
- Neck veins
- CVP
- Small vein filling time
- Level of cerebral function
- For signs of fluid overload from therapy
- **Nursing Activities:**
  - Provide oral fluids that contain some sodium and electrolytes (bouillon, juice, Gatorade).
  - Administer intravenous fluids if ordered.
  - Provide oral hygiene every two hours.
  - Provide small amounts of fluid every 15 to 30 minutes if client is vomiting.
  - Institute safety measures such as elevated side rails, low bed position, and night-lights.
  - Dangle prior to ambulating.
  - Keep call light near by for assistance with ambulation.

Pharmacology

- Intravenous infusions as indicated (0.45% sodium chloride, D_s 1/2 NS, 0.9 % sodium chloride, Ringer's lactate)
- Antidiarrheal drugs as indicated (loperamide, diphenoxylate)
- Antiemetics as indicated (meclizine, prochlorperazine)
- Electrolyte replacement therapy as indicated
- Oral electrolyte solutions (Pedialyte, Gatorade)

Complications

- Acute tubular necrosis
- Orthostatic hypotension
- Hypovolemic shock
- From fluid replacement therapy:
  - Fluid overload
  - Cerebral edema
  - CHF (congestive heart failure)
  - Pulmonary edema
- Coma

Age-Related Changes—Gerontological Considerations

- Older clients are more at risk for fluid and electrolyte imbalances than younger clients, with the exception of babies and young children.
- Thirst mechanism may be depressed in elderly clients.
- The increased use of diuretics and laxatives may lead to dehydration in the elderly population.

Critical Thinking Exercise: Nursing Management of the Client with Extracellular Fluid Volume Deficit—Dehydration

Situation: A 45-year-old female client, who had prolonged vomiting and diarrhea due to an episode of flu, is being seen in the emergency department. The woman complains of thirst, has cracked dry lips, poor skin turgor, a pulse rate of 110, a temperature of 101° F, and a blood pressure of 80/50. The client's urinary elimination is <30 mL per hour, and her urine is dark and concentrated. When in a supine position, the client's neck veins are flat. The client is seriously dehydrated and the physician orders the administration of 2 L of normal saline IV. Prior to discharge, the nurse talks with the client about methods for replacing her fluids once she goes home.

1. How do the symptoms of dehydration differ between younger clients and elderly clients?

2. When the client is being treated for dehydration with IV infusions, what can the nurse do to prevent a fluid volume overload?

3. How can the client continue to replenish her fluid losses once she is discharged home?

Nursing Management of the Client with Fluid Volume Excess

Key Points

- Fluid flows across cell membranes by active or passive processes.
- Water moves from an area of high concentration to low concentration across cell membranes (osmosis).
- Water will continue to flow until the osmolarity between two compartments are equal.
- Disease, trauma, and other pathological states can affect osmolarity and cell membrane permeability to water.
- Changes in extracellular fluid volume are often related to changes in sodium balance.
- Fluid volume excess may occur from excessive sodium intake, overhydration, or failure of renal or hormonal regulatory mechanisms.
- Rapidly-occurring weight gain, peripheral edema, and circulatory overload are manifestations of hyperosmolar overhydration.
- Goals of collaborative management:
  - Identify persons at increased risk for development of fluid volume excess.
  - Provide early recognition and treatment.
  - Eliminate excess fluid volume.
  - Prevent complications (pulmonary edema, coma).
  - Maintain fluid balance.
- Important nursing diagnoses (actual or potential):
  - Impaired gas exchange
  - Altered cardiac output
  - Anxiety and fear
  - Altered thought processes
  - Risk for injury
  - Pain management
  - Impaired skin integrity
- **Key Trems/Concepts:** Homeostasis, osmolarity, extracellular, intracellular, hypervolemia, overload, pitting edema, pulmonary edema

Overview

Fluid volume excess (hypervolemia) occurs when water and sodium are retained in the same proportions.

Risk Factors

- Excessive water intake
- Excessive sodium intake
- Malnutrition (decreased plasma proteins)
- ARF (acute renal failure) or CRF (chronic renal failure)
- CHF (congestive heart failure)
- Liver disease
- Inappropriate secretion of ADH (antidiuretic hormone)
- Excessive intravenous fluid intake

Signs and Symptoms

- Weight gain
- Edema
- Lung crackles, dyspnea
- Ascites
- Confusion
- Weakness
- Headache
- Weight gain of >2 pounds in 24 hours
- Bounding pulse
- Increased pulse pressure
- Decreased hematocrit

Diagnostic and Laboratory Tests

- History and physical examination
- Serum sodium
- Hematocrit
- Serum osmolarity
- Serum albumin and proteins
- Chest x-ray and arterial blood gases

Therapeutic Nursing Management

- Assess/Monitor:
  - Vital signs for indications of fluid overload (hypertension, bounding pulse)
  - Daily weights
  - Intake and output
  - Serum electrolytes
  - Respiratory status
- Nursing Activities:
  - Restrict fluid intake.
  - Administer diuretics as prescribed.

Pharmacology

- Diuretics
  - Thiazide
  - Potassium-sparing
  - Osmotic
  - Loop (refers to loop of Henle, a structure of the kidney involved in reabsorbing water)
- Electrolyte replacement as necessary
- Albumin replacement as necessary
- Oxygen

Complications

- Pulmonary edema
- Coma
- Death

Age-Related Changes—Gerontological Considerations

- Increased risk for fluid volume excess is related to changes in cardiac function and decreased cardiac output.

Critical Thinking Exercise: Nursing Management of the Client with Fluid Volume Excess

Situation: An older client with CHF (congestive heart failure) is readmitted to the acute care facility with dyspnea, weakness, weight gain, 3+ pitting edema of both lower extremities, and bilateral crackles in the bases of his lungs. The client has a bounding pulse and elevated blood pressure.

1. Which findings, in addition to those exhibited by the client, are supportive of fluid volume excess?

_____ Decreased pulse pressure   _____ Ascites

_____ Headache   _____ Postural hypotension

_____ Confusion   _____ Decreased hematocrit

2. Prioritize the goals of medical management for clients with fluid volume excess, with "1" representing the most important goal.

_____ Preventing complications (pulmonary edema, coma)

_____ Early recognition and treatment

_____ Identifying persons at risk

_____ Eliminating excess fluid volume

3. Which statements are true about fluid volume excess? Correct false statements.

   a. Osmosis refers to the flow of particles from an area of high to low concentration.

   b. Changes in intracellular fluid volume are often related to changes in potassium balance.

   c. Fluid volume excess most often occurs from inadequate sodium intake.

   d. Disease can affect osmolarity and cell permeability to water.

Nursing Management of the Client Requiring Total Parenteral Nutrition (TPN)

Key Points

- **Alert!** Do not allow the same bag of TPN to hang over 24 hours.
- **Alert!** Continuously assess for signs of inflammation and infection.
- Total parenteral nutrition (TPN) provides essential nutrients to support wound healing, anabolism, and weight gain or maintenance.
- All TPN solutions contain protein, fat, carbohydrates, vitamins, trace elements, and water.
- TPN solutions are tailored to meet the individual needs of the client.
- The high glucose content of TPN is an excellent media for bacterial growth.
- TPN may cause transient hyperglycemia and osmotic diuresis initially.
- Rapidly discontinuing TPN may produce hypoglycemia.
- Goals of collaborative management:
  - Maintain metabolic balance.
  - Maintain fluid and electrolyte balance.
  - Prevent infection.
  - Prevent hyperglycemia/hypoglycemia.
- Important nursing diagnoses (actual or potential):
  - Fatigue and restlessness
  - Fluid volume deficit/excess
  - Risk for infection
  - Nutrition: less than body requirements
  - Self-care deficit
  - Impaired skin integrity
- **Key Terms/Concepts:** Hyperglycemia, hypoglycemia, osmolarity, extravasation, fluid volume deficit, fluid volume excess

Overview

Total parenteral nutrition (TPN) is a hypertonic intravenous solution that provides fluids, dextrose, vitamins, electrolytes, and trace minerals to clients who are unable to ingest food or fluid. TPN and lipids (essential fatty acids) are generally administered through a central venous access site into a large vein, such as the superior vena cava. Due to the high osmolality of the TPN solution, the risk for tissue injury and necrosis with extravasation is great.

Risk Factors /Indications for Use

- Clients unable to absorb nutrients (bowel obstruction or surgery, regional enteritis, ulcerative colitis)
- Clients receiving chemotherapy, radiation, or bone marrow transplant
- Pancreatitis
- Malnutrition
- Hyperemesis during pregnancy
- Burns
- Anorexia
- Prolonged recovery following surgery, trauma, disease

Signs and Symptoms of TPN Effectiveness

- Weight gain or stabilization
- Healing skin or incision
- Normal serum electrolytes
- Normal serum glucose
- Normal urinary output

Diagnostic Tests

- Electrolytes (baseline and periodic)
- FBG (fasting blood glucose); also called (FBS) fasting blood sugar (baseline and periodic)
- Creatinine
- Phosphorus
- Albumin
- Cholesterol
- CBC (complete blood count) with differential
- Liver enzymes:
  - Alkaline phosphatase (ALP); also called ALK Phos, an enzyme found in the liver, bones and placenta
  - Alanine aminotransferase (ALT); also called serum glutamic pyruvic transaminase (SGPT); an enzyme found primarily in liver cells
  - Aspartate aminotransferase (AST); also called serum glutamic oxaloacetic transaminase (SGOT); an enzyme found in the liver and elsewhere in the body
  - Gamma-glutamyl transpeptidase (GGTP); also called GGT or Gamma GT, an enzyme present in the liver, pancreas and kidneys
  - Lactic acid dehydrogenase (LDH), an enzyme found in the liver

Therapeutic Nursing Management

- **Assess/Monitor:**
  - Venous access site for signs of infection

- Serum glucose levels qid
- For signs of fluid overload or fluid deficit
- **Nursing Activities:**
  - Administer TPN as prescribed.
  - Maintain absolute asepsis of venous access site.
  - Change intravenous access site dressing according to facility protocol.
  - Maintain patency of venous access site.
  - Change intravenous tubing and TPN bag at least daily.
  - Offer emotional support to client and family.

Pharmacology

- Parenteral nutrition (water, amino acids, dextrose, electrolytes, vitamins, trace elements)
- Lipids
- Insulin (for hyperglycemia)

Complications

- Incorrect catheter placement
- Pneumothorax
- Local or systemic infection
- Fluid overload
- Fluid volume deficit (osmotic diuresis)
- Hyperglycemia

Age-Related Changes—Gerontological Considerations

- Increased risk for serum glucose fluctuations occurs with the prolonged use or high concentrations of glucose in TPN.

Critical Thinking Exercise: Nursing Management of the Client Requiring Total Parenteral Nutrition (TPN)

Situation: A 54-year-old man with pancreatitis is unable to tolerate oral food or fluids due to pain, nausea and vomiting. He is in a severely weakened state, has lost 12 pounds, and has a fever of 101.5° F. Following assessment of the client, the practitioner prescribes TPN (total parenteral nutrition) Subsequently, a central line is placed and TPN is initiated, which contains 50% dextrose.

1. What health care condition might a client have that would necessitate the use of TPN?

2. Which nursing diagnoses are appropriate for this client, based on the data given?

_____ Fatigue

_____ Risk for fluid volume deficit/excess

_____ Infection

_____ Nutrition: less than body requirements

_____ Impaired skin integrity

3. Which findings support the effectiveness of TPN?

_____ Weight gain or stabilization

_____ Reduced pain

_____ Serum sodium of 139 mEq/L

_____ Serum glucose of 80 mg/dL

_____ Urinary output >30 cc/hour

Nursing Management of the Client with a Urinary Tract Infection (UTI)—Cystitis

| Key Points |

- Urinary tract infections (UTIs) are a significant reason for health care provider visits and hospitalizations.
- Untreated UTIs are significant in the development of chronic renal failure.
- Women are at greater risk for development of UTIs than men.
- Goals of collaborative management:
  - Identify persons at increased risk for development of UTI.
  - Provide early recognition and treatment.
  - Eliminate offending pathogen.
  - Prevent recurrence.
  - Prevent complications (chronic renal failure, urosepsis, bacteremia).
- Important nursing diagnoses (actual or potential):
  - Altered urinary elimination
  - Risk for injury
  - Anxiety and fear
  - Pain management
  - Risk for infection
  - Knowledge deficit
- **Key Terms and Concepts:** Cystitis, sexually transmitted pathogen, urethritis, urosepsis, bacteremia, asymptomatic, dysuria

Overview

A urinary tract infection (UTI, cystitis) exists when the urinary bladder becomes inflamed from an ascending bacterial infection with organisms such as *Escherichia coli*, *Enterobacter*, *Pseudomonas*, or *Serratia*. *Escherichia coli* is the most common cause of UTI in women. The same organisms or sexually transmitted pathogens can also cause urethritis, which is inflammation of the urethra. Women have a higher incidence of UTIs and urethritis than men due to a shortened urethra that is in close proximity to the rectum. **Urosepsis** is a gram-negative bacteremia originating from a urinary tract infection that can, if not aggressively treated, lead to septic shock and death. Urosepsis is more common in elderly women. As women age and estrogen is lost, the urethral opening atrophies toward the rectum. Additionally, infection is more likely because of pH changes.

Risk Factors

- Sexual intercourse
- Premature infants
- Prepubertal children
- Older age
- Indwelling urinary catheters
- Stool incontinence
- Urinary tract anomalies
- Bladder distention
- Urinary stasis
- Urinary calculi

Females

- Use of feminine hygiene sprays, perfumed toilet paper, sanitary napkins, spermicidal jellies
- Pregnancy
- Inadequate toilet hygiene
- Poorly-fitting diaphragms
- Hormonal influences on vaginal flora
- Synthetic underwear and pantyhose
- Wet bathing suits
- Submersion into water such as baths and hot tubs
- Possible genetic link in high-risk, frequent UTI women
- Residual urine in postmenopausal women due to bladder or uterine prolapse, pH changes, etc.

Males

- Bacteria found in prostatic secretions

Signs and Symptoms

- May be asymptomatic
- Urinary frequency and urgency
- Burning on urination (dysuria)
- Voiding in small amounts
- Difficulty initiating urine stream
- Cloudy, foul-smelling urine
- Hematuria
- Low back or lower abdominal discomfort
- Fever
- Nocturia
- Bacterial growth in urine culture

Diagnostic and Laboratory Tests

- History and physical examination
- Urinalysis
- Urine culture
- WBC count, and differential for urosepsis
- Blood culture for urosepsis

Therapeutic Nursing Management

- **Prevent by Teaching:**
  - Young females to wipe from urethra to perineum
  - Sexually active women to void after intercourse or submersion into baths, pools, etc.
  - Females to avoid use of feminine hygiene sprays, bubble baths, and perfumed toilet paper
  - Females to avoid wearing pantyhose with slacks or tight clothes
  - Females to avoid sitting in wet swimming suits
  - Menopausal women to use estrogen vaginal creams to restore vaginal pH
  - Double voiding
- **Assess/Monitor:**
  - Pain status
  - Urinary output (color, volume)
  - Temperature (for fever)
- **Nursing Activities:**
  - Collect clean or catheterized, sterile urine for culture and sensitivity testing prior to initiating antibiotic therapy.
  - Encourage increased fluid intake (up to 3000 mL/day, depending on BMI, and if not contraindicated).
  - Encourage the intake of acid-containing foods or fluids (cranberries, cranberry juice).
  - Avoid the use of indwelling catheters when possible.
  - Maintain asepsis when placing an indwelling urinary catheter.
  - Teach client to take medications as prescribed and complete the entire antibiotic regimen.
  - Discourage the intake of coffee, tea, or colas.
  - Teach client to take sitz bath or use heat to the abdomen to control discomfort.

Pharmacology

- Antibiotics (dependent upon organism)
- Urinary anti-infective (nitrofurantoin [Macrobid], fosfomycin [Monurol])
- Urinary analgesics (phenazopyridine [Pyridium], pentosan polysulfate sodium [Elmiron])

Complications

- Urethral obstruction
- Pyelonephritis
- Chronic renal failure (CRF)
- Urosepsis
- Death

Age-Related Changes—Gerontological Considerations

- Renal complications may occur as related to reduced numbers of functioning nephrons.
- An increased risk for urinary disorders is related to decreased fluid intake and increased incidence of stool incontinence.
- The elderly or debilitated adult requiring an indwelling urinary catheter is at risk for developing urinary tract infections. Clients in   this group have decreased resistance to infection because of reduced immune function.
- Older women may be more at risk for incontinence of stool and urine due to changes in urine pH and relaxation of the pelvic floor.

Critical Thinking Exercise: Nursing Management of the Client with a Urinary Tract Infection (UTI)—Cystitis

Situation: A 23-year-old client visits her health practitioner stating she thinks she has a UTI (urinary tract infection). She has a low-grade fever of 100.6° F, and lower abdominal tenderness on palpation.

1. What other symptoms are commonly associated with UTI (urinary tract infection)?

_____ Frequency   _____ Polyuria

_____ Urgency   _____ Low back pain

_____ Increased blood pressure   _____ Dizziness

_____ Dysuria   _____ Anuria

_____ Foul smell   _____ Nocturia

2. Why are women at greater risk for UTI than men?

3. What is the most common and important cause of UTI in older adults, and why?

Nursing Management of the Client with Renal Calculi

Key Points

- The majority of renal calculi (also known as kidney stones) is composed of calcium salts, blood, pus, and sloughed tissue.
- More than half the renal calculi that occur are idiopathic (have no known cause).
- Pain is the most significant clinical manifestation of renal calculi.
- Goals of collaborative management:
  - Relieve pain.
  - Provide early recognition and treatment.
  - Eradicate renal calculi.
  - Prevent complications (hydronephrosis, renal failure).
  - Prevent recurrence.
- Important nursing diagnoses (actual or potential):
  - Acute pain
  - Risk for infection
  - Altered urinary elimination
  - Anxiety and fear
  - Ineffective therapeutic regimen management
- **Key Terms/Concepts:** Hydronephrosis, pyuria, renal colic, lithotripsy

Overview

Renal calculi (urolithiasis) are stones that form within the kidney or urinary tract. They may be composed of calcium phosphate or oxalate, uric acid, struvite or cystine. Calculi can occlude the ureter and block the flow of urine. If the obstruction is not removed, infection or hydronephrosis of the affected kidney can lead to permanent renal damage.

Risk Factors

- UTI (urinary tract infection)
- Urinary retention or stasis, low urine output
- Strenuous work
- Extended periods of immobilization
- Hypercalcemia, hyperparathyroidism
- Excessive intake of purine-rich foods (such as anchovies, organ meats, poultry, red meats, and shellfish).

- Diets high in vitamins A, C & D, protein, oxalate (such as spinach), alkali, or uric acid
- Dehydration
- Medications: triamterene, ritonavir, indinavir, some sulfa drugs, carbonic anhydrase inhibitors, some anti-seizure medications, corticosteroids, acetazolamide
- Prolonged urinary catheterization
- Elevated uric acid levels (gout, cancer chemotherapy)
- High urine acidity or alkalinity
- Family history of renal calculi

Signs and Symptoms

- Sudden onset, severe pain radiating down the flank to the pubic area (renal colic)
- Frequency and urgency of urination
- Pallor
- Diaphoresis
- Nausea, vomiting
- Low-grade fever
- Hematuria
- Pyuria if infection is present

Diagnostic and Laboratory Tests

- History and physical examination
- Urinalysis
- CBC (complete blood count)
- Serum calcium, phosphate, and uric acid levels; parathyroid hormone if calcium elevated
- 24-hour urine sample for recurrent episodes
- Stone analysis
- Fluoroscopic exam of urinary tract
- MRI (magnetic resonance imaging)
- KUB (kidneys, ureter, bladder) x-ray
- IVP (intravenous pyelogram)
- Helical CT (computerized tomography) procedure of choice if available
- Cystoscopy
- Ultrasound
  - 2-D (2-dimensional)
  - 3-D (3-dimensional)
  - Doppler

Therapeutic Nursing Management

- Assess:
    - Fluid intake
    - Urinary output
    - Burning on urination, dysuria, blood passage of stone – catch and strain all urine
    - Vital signs
    - Acute, colicky pain in flank, back, abdomen, groin, or genitalia
    - For indications of infection
- **Nursing Activities:**
    - Initiate pain relief measures.
        - Alternative and complementary therapy
        - Administer opioid analgesics, spasmolytic agents, NSAID such as ketorolac (Toradol) as prescribed.
    - Encourage fluid intake (to 3000 mL/day).
    - Monitor I & O (intake and output).
    - Check urine pH.
    - Strain urine for stones.
    - Send stones for lab analysis.
    - Prepare client for lithotripsy, stent placement, or surgery if indicated.
    - Administer routine postoperative care.
    - If the client has an indwelling catheter, keep the drainage bottle below the level of the bladder.
    - Teach client to alter intake of foods that enhance stone formation (depends on stone composition), noting that restriction of calcium is not recommended (normal daily intake of calcium 1,000 – 1,500 mg/day does not enhance calcium stone formation).
    - Administer intravenous fluids as prescribed.
    - Encourage client ambulation to enhance stone passage.

Pharmacology

- Narcotic analgesics (morphine)
- Thiazides (hydrochlorothiazide), to increase calcium reabsorption in cases of hypercalciuria with calcium-containing stones
- Antispasmodics/Anticholinergics (propantheline [Pro-Banthine])
- Indomethacin for uric acid maintenance with allopurinol
- Antibiotics (if infection)
- Alkalinizing agents (Polycitra, Shohl's solution) and allopurinol in case of uric acid stones
- Allopurinol (Zyloprim) and vitamin B_6 (pyridoxine), in cases of hyperoxaluria and oxalate-containing stones
- Alphamerkaptopropionylglycine (aMPG) and captopril (Capoten), in cases of cystine containing stones when hydration and alkalization are ineffective

Complications

- Irreversible renal damage
- Ruptured ureter
- Infection

Age-Related Changes—Gerontological Considerations

- An increased risk for renal complications is related to reduced numbers of functioning nephrons.
- An increased risk for stone formation is related to decreased fluid intake and increased incidence of dehydration.

Cultural Considerations

- Increased incidence in Southeastern U.S., Japan, and Western Europe
- Uncommon in African-Americans

Critical Thinking Exercise: Nursing Management of the Client with Renal Calculi

Situation: While working at his desk, a 46-year-old male suddenly develops severe back pain, nausea, and diaphoresis. He is rushed to the emergency department where urinalysis is positive for hematuria. Diagnostic tests indicate the presence of a renal calculus in the lower right ureter.

1. Prioritize nursing activities for the client, with "1" representing the most important activity.

_____ Strain his urine.

_____ Take vital signs.

_____ Administer prescribed pain medication.

_____ Obtain a brief history.

2. Which nursing diagnoses are appropriate for the client at this time?

_____ Infection

_____ Altered urinary elimination

_____ Anxiety/fear

_____ Knowledge deficit

3. What is extracorporeal lithotripsy and how is the client prepared for the procedure?

Nursing Management of the Client with Urinary Incontinence

Key Points

- Urinary incontinence is not a normal physiological change of aging.
- Urinary incontinence can be prevented in the majority of clients.
- Embarrassment is a significant complication of urinary incontinence.
- Some forms of urinary incontinence are related to disease states.
- Eighty percent of clients with incontinence can be cured or the condition or significantly improved.
- Goals of collaborative management:
  - Identify the underlying cause of urinary incontinence.
  - Correct the underlying cause of urinary incontinence.
  - Restore normal urinary patterns and function.
  - Prevent complications.
  - Prevent recurrence.
- Important nursing diagnoses (actual or potential):
  - Incontinence (functional, overflow, reflex, stress, urge, overactive bladder, or mixed)
  - Altered urinary elimination
  - Anxiety and fear
  - Disturbed body image
  - Ineffective individual coping
  - Impaired skin integrity
- **Key Terms/Concepts**: Functional incontinence, overflow incontinence, reflex incontinence, stress incontinence, total incontinence, urge incontinence, Kegel exercises, urodynamic

Overview

Urinary incontinence (UI) refers to the involuntary loss of urine from the bladder. It occurs most frequently in older women and may be caused by infection, disease, or trauma. There are several types of urinary incontinence.

- **Stress incontinence** (outlet incompetence) is the loss of urine that occurs from a sudden increase in intra-abdominal pressure (coughing, sneezing, laughing, lifting, or jumping).
- **Urge incontinence** (detrusor instability or overactivity) is the loss of urine following a strong feeling of the desire need to urinate.

- **Overflow incontinence** is related to a hypotonic or atonic bladder or obstructed urinary outflow. These result in reduced urinary stream, incomplete bladder emptying, and urinary dribbling.
- **Reflex incontinence** is the loss of urine when a specific bladder volume has been reached due to neurological impairment.
- **Functional incontinence** occurs when an otherwise continent person is unable to reach the toilet due to physical or cognitive problems.
- **Total incontinence** is the involuntary, unpredictable loss of urine that does not generally respond to treatment.
- **Overactive bladder** includes urge along with urgency, frequency, dysuria, and nocturia.
- **Mixed incontinence** is a combination of stress incontinence and overactive bladder.

Risk Factors

- Aging
- History of multiple pregnancies and vaginal childbirths
- Renal disease, urinary bladder spasm, or chronic urinary retention
- Neurological disease (Parkinson's, stroke, multiple sclerosis, spinal cord injury)
- Drug therapy (diuretics, anticholinergics, sedative/hypnotics, narcotics, alpha-adrenergic antagonists, calcium channel blockers)
- Confusion/dementia
- Immobility
- Lack of motivation/depression
- Sphincter weakness or damage
- Urethral deformity
- Diabetes mellitus
- Infection
- Estrogen deficiency
- Obesity
- Hysterectomy

Signs and Symptoms

- Voiding before reaching an appropriate receptacle
- Loss of urine upon laughing, coughing or sneezing
- Enuresis (bed-wetting)
- Bladder spasms
- Urinary retention
- Frequency, urgency, nocturia

Diagnostic and Laboratory Tests

- History and physical examination
- Bladder log or voiding schedule
- Urinalysis and urine culture
- Post-void residual volumes
- BUN (blood urea nitrogen)
- Creatinine
- Urodynamic testing
- Cystometry
- Uroflow
- Urethral pressure studies
- IVP (intravenous pyelogram)
- VCU (voiding cystourethrogram)
- Ultrasound
  - 2-D (2-dimensional)
  - 3-D (3-dimensional)
  - Doppler

Therapeutic Nursing Management

- **Assess/Monitor:**
  - Intake and output
  - Lower abdomen for suprapubic fullness
  - Residual urine volumes (bladder scan with pelvis ultrasonographic scanner or post-void catheterization)
  - Urinary patterns
  - Skin integrity
  - Symptoms of urinary incontinence
  - Environmental and other barriers to toileting
  - Possible signs of urinary tract infection
- **Nursing activities:**
  - Establish and maintain an appropriate toileting schedule.
  - Teach smoking cessation.
  - Avoid or manage constipation.
  - Remove or control environmental or other barriers to toileting.
  - Provide or suggest the use of incontinence garments.
  - Encourage client to evenly space fluid during the day and decrease fluid intake prior to napping or bedtime.
  - Teach client to keep an incontinence diary.
  - Initiate bladder training or for cognitively impaired client habit training.
  - Teach and encourage use of Kegel exercises.

- Teach bladder compression techniques (Credé, Valsalva, double-voiding, splinting).
- Teach biofeedback and monitor use of vaginal sensors if ordered.
- Apply and monitor electrical stimulation of pelvic floor muscles (stress, urge, or mixed UI) if ordered.
- Teach regarding vaginal cone therapy if ordered.
- Teach client to avoid caffeine and alcohol consumption.
- Prepare client for surgery if indicated (colporrhaphy, retropubic suspension, needle bladder beck suspension, pubovaginal sling or bolsters, artificial sphincters, periurethral collagen or silicone injection).
- Apply an external catheter for males.
- Avoid the use of indwelling urinary catheters.
- Teach client regarding use of prescribed medications and possible side effects.
- Teach intermittent self-catheterization.
- If suprapubic catheter is in place, teach site and tube care.

Pharmacology

- Alpha-adrenergic agonists (Phenylpropanolamine)
- Alpha-adrenergic antagonists (doxazosin [Cardura], terazosin [Hytrin], tamsulosin [Flomax])
- Calcium channel blockers (nifedipine [Adalat], diltiazem [Cardizem], verapamil [Calan, Isoptin])
- HRT (hormone replacement therapy [Premarin cream])
- Urinary antispasmodic/anticholinergic agents (oxybutynin [Ditropan], tolterodine [Detrol], propantheline [Pro-Banthine], flavoxate [Urispas])
- Tricyclic antidepressants (imipramine [Tofranil], desipramine [Norpramin], nortriptyline [Pamelor])
- Antibiotics when urinary tract infection present

Complications

- Skin breakdown
- Altered body image
- UTI (urinary tract infection)
- Social isolation

Age-Related Changes—Gerontological Considerations

- There is increased incidence of incontinence in older adults, which may be related to decreased mobility, vision, and hearing impairment, illness, or cognitive deficits.
- Incontinence may be related to polypharmacy, especially medications that may induce urinary incontinence.

- Urinary incontinence is associated with increased number of falls, pressure ulcers, urinary tract infections, and depression.
- There is increased risk for renal complications related to decreased number of functioning nephrons, decreased muscle control, decreased hormone production, and increased incidence of chronic illness and/or physical and cognitive deficits.
- Because of change in sensation, estrogen, cognition, etc., typical symptoms associated with UTIs may not be present in elderly women; rule out UTI when incontinence begins or worsens.

Critical Thinking Exercise: Nursing Management of the Client with Urinary Incontinence

Situation: A 54-year-old woman visits her health provider because she is embarrassed about losing urine when she coughs, laughs, or sneezes.

1. The client is describing what kind of urinary incontinence?

2. Match the types of incontinence with the correct descriptors. Use the first letter of each type of incontinence as the form of answer.

F = Functional	Related to obstructed urinary outflow
O = Overflow	Involuntary, unpredictable loss of urine
R = Reflex	Related to over-activity of urinary bladder
S = Stress	Not generally responsive to treatment
T = Total	Loss of urine due to neurological dysfunction
U = Urge	Occurs with strong feeling of need to urinate
	Results in incomplete emptying of the bladder
	Urine loss follows increased intra-abdominal pressure

3. Explain Kegel exercises to the client.

4. Why are indwelling urinary catheters contraindicated for control of urinary incontinence in older adults?

Nursing Management of the Client with Acute or Chronic Glomerulonephritis

Key Points

- The glomerulus is a network of capillaries that is surrounded by a Bowman's capsule, which is part of the renal corpuscle.
- Bowman's capsule acts as a filter during urine formation.
- Glomerulonephritis may be acute or chronic.
- Most causes of acute glomerulonephritis (AGN) are post infectious or related to other systemic diseases.
- Glomerulonephritis is an inflammatory disorder of the glomerulus that develops secondary to the formation of antigen-antibody complexes elsewhere in the body; usually in response to an infection; bacterial, viral, fungal, parasitic.
- Systemic causes include Wagener granulomatosis, hypersensitivity vasculitis, systemic lupus erythematosus, polyarteritis, Henoch-Schönlein purpura, Goodpasture syndrome, and certain renal diseases.
- The most common form of acute glomerulonephritis is caused by a primary group A beta streptococcal infection.
- Acute post-streptococcal glomerulonephritis (APSGN) may occur during or shortly following a beta-hemolytic streptococcal infection; it most commonly occurs in children aged 2-12 years; only 10% of cases occur in client's over the age of 40 years. Males are affected more frequently.
- Acute poststreptococcal glomerulonephritis (APSGN) may also develop during or within 21 days following a group A beta-hemolytic streptococcal infection or the respiratory system or skin. Early onset may suggest pre-existing renal disease.
- 95% of clients with AGN improve rapidly or recover completely.
- 1% to 2% of clients with AGN will develop ESRD (end-stage renal disease), requiring dialysis or kidney transplant.
- AGN can slowly progress over 30 years to chronic glomerulonephritis in 5% to 15% of clients.
- Chronic glomerulonephritis is an autoimmune disorder that has a wide span of deterioration.
- Some clients show little sign of deterioration, while others progressively lose glomerular function to the point that they develop end-stage renal disease.
- Goals of collaborative management:
  - Prevent or control streptococcal infections.
  - Prevent or control bacterial, viral, or parasitic infections.
  - Control inflammation of the glomeruli.

- Prevent kidney damage and other complications.
- Prevent progression of acute disease to chronic glomerulonephritis.
- Important nursing diagnoses (actual or potential):
  - Fluid volume excess
  - Pain
  - Anxiety and fear
  - Impaired physical mobility
  - Risk for infection
  - Risk for impaired skin integrity
  - Altered nutrition: less than body requirements
  - Diversional activity deficit
- **Key Terms/Concepts**: Glomerulus, streptococcal infection, immunologic disorder, acute post-streptococcal glomerulonephritis (APSGN), chronic glomerulonephritis

Overview

Acute glomerulonephritis (AGN) (also called acute nephritic syndrome) is the term for a group of renal disorders characterized by inflammation of the glomeruli. This is an immune disorder affecting the function of both kidneys. The cause may be endogenous (SLE [systemic lupus erythematosus], diabetes mellitus, hypertension), or exogenous (poststreptococcal infection). Acting as antigens, streptococci stimulate the release of antibodies, which injure the glomeruli, causing inflammation of the kidney. Intervention includes the administration of anti-infective agents such as penicillin, erythromycin, or azithromycin (Zithromax). However, treatment of streptococcal infections with appropriate antibiotics may not prevent acute glomerulonephritis.

Chronic glomerulonephritis (also called chronic nephritic syndrome) may develop over 20 to 30 years. The exact cause is unknown. Possible etiological factors include the effects of hypertension, intermittent or recurrent infections, inflammation, and altered metabolism. There is no specific treatment for chronic glomerulonephritis. Clients during acute exacerbations are treated the same as clients with AGN. This disease may progress to end-stage renal disease (ESRD) where the client may require dialysis or renal transplantation.

Risk Factors

- Upper respiratory or skin infections, especially beta-hemolytic streptococcal infections
- History of systemic lupus erythematosus
- History of bacterial endocarditis
- History of vasculitis (e.g., polyarteritis nodosa)
- Exposure to nephrotoxic drugs
- High-protein diet
- High-sodium diet
- Excessive physical activity
- History of renal or urologic problems

Signs and Symptoms

- **Acute Glomerulonephritis**
  - Sudden development of hematuria and proteinuria
  - Red cell casts in the urine
  - Fever (rare)
  - Generalized edema
  - Shortness of breath or exertion related to cardiac failure and/or pulmonary edema
  - Confusion, from hypertension
  - Arthralgias (with Henoch-Schönlein purpura or systemic lupus erythematosus)
  - Hemoptysis (Goodpasture syndrome or idiopathic)
  - Skin rashes (hypersensitivity vasculitis or systemic lupus erythematosus)
  - Pharyngitis
  - Respiratory infection
  - Impetigo
  - Abdominal or flank pain
  - Rusty, or tea-colored urine
  - Nausea
  - Constipation
  - Headache, possibly related to hypertension
  - Hypertension
  - Anorexia
  - Back pain
  - Pallor
  - Oliguria and anuria in advanced cases
  - Weight gain from fluid retention
- **Chronic Glomerulonephritis**
  - Pruritus
  - Vague symptoms of anorexia, weakness, and lethargy
  - Early morning nausea and vomiting
  - Peripheral neuropathy
  - Seizures, tremors
  - Hypertension
  - Fixed specific gravity
  - Yellow color to skin, ecchymosis, and rashes
  - Edema
  - Fine to coarse crackles in lungs, dyspnea
  - Engorgement of neck veins

Diagnostic and Laboratory Tests

- History and physical examination
- CBC (complete blood count)
- Urinalysis for blood, protein, cells, casts, sediment assay
- Electrolytes
- Serum blood urea nitrogen (BUN) and creatinine
- Serum complement (C3, C4), antinuclear antibodies (ANA) and immune complex levels
- 24-hour creatinine clearance test and protein excretion
- Antistreptolysin O (ASO) titer
- Blood, skin, and throat cultures
- Renal ultrasound if chronic case suspected
- Renal biopsy

Therapeutic Nursing Management

- **Prevention:**
  - Avoid exposure to infectious agents. Clients are considered infectious until they have been on the antibiotic therapy for 24 hours.
  - Receive and complete treatment as prescribed for positive group A beta hemolytic streptococcal pharyngitis and skin infections. Early treatment does not prevent the development of poststreptococcal glomerulonephritis. Prophylaxis treatment of high-risk individuals does not prevent occurrence either.
  - Use good personal hygiene to avoid skin infections.
  - Avoid fluid volume overload.
  - Avoid overconsumption of high protein foods and liquids.
  - Avoid high sodium foods and liquids.
- **Assess/Monitor:**
  - Intake and output (I & O)
  - Daily weight
  - BUN and serum creatinine levels, electrolytes
  - Vital signs every four hours
  - Skin color and presence of ecchymosis and rashes (chronic glomerulonephritis)
  - For complications
- **Nursing Activities:**
  - Maintain bedrest during acute phase.
  - Manage energy levels.
  - Change client's position regularly.
  - Measure edematous areas daily.
  - Restrict fluids.

- Administer medications as ordered. In chronic glomerulonephritis blood pressure control may be paramount.
- Instruct client to eat a high-calorie, high-carbohydrate, and low-sodium and potassium diet and provide nutrition counseling.
- Adjust dietary protein intake to level of proteinuria and uremia.
- Provide hard candies and ice chips to lessen thirst.
- Provide skin care.
- Instruct client to report any signs of urinary tract infection immediately.
- Instruct client to report any signs of renal failure immediately.
- Teach regarding at home daily weight and blood pressure measurements and reporting abnormalities.
- Instruct client to set up appointments for laboratory studies, urinalysis, and blood pressure measurement.
- Prepare the client with chronic glomerulonephritis and severe renal disease for renal dialysis.

Pharmacology

- Plasmapheresis (Goodpasture syndrome) combined with immunosuppression
- Corticosteroids: prednisone (Meticorten), methylprednisolone (Medrol)
- Immunosuppressive therapy with cytotoxic/chemotherapeutic agents: cyclophosphamide (Cytoxan), chlorambucil (Leukeran)
- Antihypertensives: hydralazine (Apresoline), calcium channel blockers, ACE (angiotensin-converting enzyme) inhibitors, etc.
- Diuretics: (loop diuretics)
- Antibiotic therapy: penicillin, amoxicillin, clotrimazole, erythromycin, azithromycin
- Pharmacological treatment is dependent upon etiology!

Complications

- Hypertension
- CHF (congestive heart failure)
- Pulmonary edema
- Renal failure
- Increased intracranial pressure
- Need for emergent dialysis, especially with chronic glomerulonephritis, indications:
- Metabolic acidosis
- Pulmonary edema
- Pericarditis
- Encephalopathy
- Gastrointestinal bleeding
- Uremic neuropathy

- Sever anemia
- Severe hypocalcemia
- Hyperkalemia

Age-Related Changes—Gerontological Considerations

- Older clients may be at greater risk for renal complications because the aging process can impair kidney function; however, their chance of contracting acute glomerulonephritis, especially from group A beta hemolytic streptococci, is negligible.

- Older clients with renal disease may also have concurrent hypertension, diabetes, or pre-existing renal disease which complicates treatment and slows recovery.

- Fluid volume overload is a dominant sign of AGN in the older client and is easily confused with heart failure.

Critical Thinking Exercise: Nursing Management of the Client with Acute or Chronic Glomerulonephritis

Situation: A 55-year-old female client has been admitted to the medical unit with fever, chills generalized edema, ascites, tenderness of the CVA (costovertebral angle), and flank pain. She also has smoky urine that contains red cell casts and traces of blood. Around 21 days prior to this hospitalization, the client was diagnosed with a beta-hemolytic streptococcal infection of the respiratory system. The client's physician has now confirmed she has developed AGN (acute glomerulonephritis).

1. What are the three "classic" clinical manifestations of AGN?

2. Explain why beta-hemolytic streptococcal infections of the throat predispose clients to AGN?

3. What is plasmapheresis and why is it beneficial to clients with AGN?

4. Match the following drugs with the reason they are prescribed for clients with AGN.

Corticosteroids	a. Hypertension
Diuretics	b. Reduce inflammation
Antibiotics	c. Inhibit immune response
Immunosuppressants	d. Relieve edema
Antihypertensives	e. Eradicate strep infection

Nursing Management of the Client with Acute Renal Failure (ARF)

Key Points

- The kidneys regulate fluid, acid-base, and electrolyte balance and eliminate wastes from the body.
- Acute renal failure (ARF) occurs when renal flow to the kidneys is significantly compromised.
- Volume depletion, pre-renal failure, is the most common cause of acute renal deterioration and is usually reversible with prompt intervention.
- ARF is a leading cause of mortality among hospitalized clients, 50% of which is due to an iatrogenic cause.
- Goals of collaborative management:
  - Identify persons at increased risk for development of acute renal failure.
  - Provide early recognition and treatment.
  - Restore blood flow to the kidneys.
  - Prevent complications (permanent renal injury, pulmonary edema, heart failure, anemia, encephalopathy, etc.).
  - Prevent recurrence.
- Important nursing diagnoses (actual or potential):
  - Potential complications of ARF (electrolyte imbalance, dysrhythmias, fluid overload, metabolic acidosis, secondary   infection)
  - Fluid volume excess
  - Imbalanced nutrition
  - Risk for infection
  - Impaired skin integrity
  - Activity intolerance
  - Self-care deficit
  - Decreased cardiac output
  - Impaired gas exchange
  - Altered oral mucous membranes
  - Disturbed thought processes
  - Knowledge deficit
- **Key Terms/Concepts:** Uremia, azotemia, oliguria, anuria, diuresis, nephrotoxic, hypovolemia, septicemia

Overview

Acute renal failure (ARF) is the sudden, abrupt cessation of renal function related to trauma, stress, drugs, or anything that decreases blood flow to the kidneys. The three phases of acute renal failure are:

- **Phase 1**: oliguria, which begins with the renal insult and lasts for three weeks
- **Phase 2**: diuresis, which begins when the kidneys start to recover and lasts from 7 to 14 days
- **Phase 3**: recovery, which continues until renal function is fully restored and requires three to 12 months

Acute renal failure is divided into pre-renal, intra-renal (renal), or post-renal failure depending upon which portion of the kidney the failure is affecting.

- **Pre-renal**: before the kidney; dehydration, congestive heart failure, cirrhosis, nephrotic syndrome, sepsis
- **Intra-renal**: **acute tubular necrosis** – nephrotoxic drugs or other nephrotoxic agents, infections; **glomerular** – pregnancy, systemic lupus erythematosus; **vascular** – renal artery stenosis
- **Post-renal**: obstruction such as renal calculi

Risk Factors

- Hypovolemia (hemorrhage, dehydration, burns, osmotic diuresis)
- Septicemia
- Nephrotoxic drugs or chemicals (specific antibiotics, NSAIDs, organic solvents, contrast dye, heavy metals)
- Hemolytic transfusion reactions
- Shock (cardiogenic, septic, anaphylactic, hypovolemic)
- Glomerular disease
- Urinary tract obstruction
- Debilitating or serious illness
- Decreased renal perfusion from acute myocardial infarction (MI), heart failure, disseminated intravascular coagulation (DIC), sepsis

Signs and Symptoms

- Sudden onset of oliguria progressing to anuria
- Hypertension
- Restlessness, twitching, convulsions
- Headache
- Nausea, vomiting
- Weight gain
- Peripheral edema, lung crackles
- Ammonia odor to breath
- Deep, rapid respirations

Diagnostic and Laboratory Tests

- History and physical examination
- Urinalysis
- Urine specific gravity
- BUN (blood urea nitrogen) and creatinine
- Serum electrolytes
- CBC (complete blood count)
- Renal ultrasound, KUB (kidneys-ureter-bladder), x-rays, CT (computerized tomography), aortorenal angiography, cystoscopy, retrograde pyelography, renal biopsy

Therapeutic Nursing Management

- **Prevent by**:
  - Identifying and assisting with correction of underlying cause
  - Controlling nephrotoxic drug use and exposure to industrial chemicals
  - Preventing prolonged episodes of hypotension and hypovolemia
  - Monitoring renal laboratory values (serum creatinine, serum electrolytes, BUN, urine specific gravity, and urine electrolytes)
- **Assess/Monitor**:
  - Intake and output
  - Daily weight
  - ECG (electrocardiogram)
  - Serum electrolytes
  - For fluid overload:
    - Periorbital edema
    - Peripheral edema
    - Lung crackles
    - Dyspnea
    - Distended neck veins
    - Hypertension
  - For signs of fluid volume deficit during diuretic phase
- **Nursing Activities**:
  - Maintain complete bed rest if critically ill.
  - Prepare for fluid challenge and diuretics during prerenal azotemia if client is showing signs of fluid volume deficit.
  - Restrict fluid intake during oliguric phase.
  - For client not requiring dialysis, restrict dietary intake of protein, sodium, and potassium during oliguric phase.
  - Provide diet high in carbohydrates and moderate in fat (critically ill client may require total parenteral nutrition [TPN]).
  - Administer calcium as prescribed to prevent bone demineralization.
  - Prepare client for hemodialysis, peritoneal dialysis, or hemofiltration.

- Administer loop diuretics or osmotic diuretics as prescribed.
- Provide emotional support for client and family.
- Provide skin care to prevent breakdown.
- Maintain client safety.
- Teach client the importance of follow-up care.
- Teach client signs and symptoms of recurrent renal failure.
- Prepare for possible hemodynamic monitoring of CVP or pulmonary artery pressures.

Pharmacology

- Intravenous isotonic fluids and plasma expanders, hypovolemia
- Dopamine (in low doses to promote renal perfusion)
- Loop or osmotic diuretics (furosemide, etc., mannitol) to decrease fluid retention
- Kayexalate, insulin, etc. (to treat elevated potassium)
- Calcium (to prevent bone demineralization)
- Antihypertensives if hypertension present (clonidine)
- Calcium channel blockers in ARF caused from nephrotoxic acute tubular necrosis (ATN)

Complications

- Hyperkalemia
- Hypertension
- Hemorrhage
- Seizures
- Cardiac dysrhythmias
- Pulmonary edema
- Infection
- Metabolic acidosis
- Uremia

Age-Related Changes—Gerontological Considerations

- Older persons are at increased risk for acute renal failure related to decreased number of functioning nephrons, decreased GFR (glomerular filtration rate), and water and sodium-conserving and compensating mechanisms.
- Increased risk for dehydration is related to inadequate fluid intake.
- Symptoms may be missed or confused with other chronic illnesses until extensive renal damage has occurred.
- The older adult generally has a poorer prognosis after an episode of ARF than a younger person.
- There is a 5% to 25% increased mortality rate from ARF in the older adult.

Critical Thinking Exercise: Nursing Management of the Client with Acute Renal Failure (ARF)

Situation: A 39-year-old man was admitted to the critical care unit following an automobile accident in which he suffered multiple injuries, blood loss and hypovolemic shock. He has been diagnosed with ARF (acute renal failure) in spite of aggressive fluid resuscitation.

1. What risk factor(s) does the client have for ARF (acute renal failure)?

2. Match the phases of acute renal failure with their correct descriptors. Use the numbers 1, 2, and 3 as the form of answer.

1 = Phase 1	Nocturia
2 = Phase 2	Lasts 3-12 months
3 = Phase 3	Period of oliguria
	Begins when the kidneys start to recover
	May last 1-3 weeks
	Renal function is fully restored
	Lasts 7-14 days
	Period of diuresis

3. Which five assessments are essential for the client who is in acute renal failure?

Cardiac enzymes	Blood pressure	Urine output
Blood glucose	Serum creatinine	RBC (red blood cell) count
Serum sodium	Lung sounds	ABGs (arterial blood gases)

4. Prioritize the client's nursing diagnoses, with "1" representing the most important diagnosis.

_____ Risk for Infection

_____ Impaired skin integrity

_____ Pain

_____ Knowledge deficit

_____ Fluid volume excess

Nursing Management of the Client with Chronic Renal Failure (CRF)

Key Points

- The kidneys regulate fluid, acid-base, and electrolyte balance and eliminate wastes from the body.
- Chronic renal failure (CRF) is progressive, irreversible kidney disease.
- End-stage renal failure exists when 90% of functioning nephrons have been destroyed and are no longer able to maintain fluid, electrolyte, or acid-base homeostasis.
- Diabetes mellitus, hypertension, HIV-associated, and chronic glomerulonephritis are leading causes of CRF.
- Medicare benefits began covering the costs of dialysis in 1973.
- Goals of collaborative management:
    - Identify persons at increased risk for development of chronic renal failure.
    - Recognize and treat contributing diseases early.
    - Maintain effective dialysis procedures to restore fluid, electrolyte, and acid-base balance.
    - Prevent complications (anemia, infection, congestive heart failure [CHF], pulmonary edema).
    - Transplant, when appropriate.
    - Control or manage symptoms.
- Important nursing diagnoses (actual or potential):
    - Potential complications of CRF (electrolyte imbalance, fluid overload, metabolic acidosis, secondary infection, anemia)
    - Fluid volume excess
    - Imbalanced nutrition
    - Risk for infection
    - Impaired skin integrity
    - Activity intolerance/fatigue
    - Self-care deficit
    - Decreased cardiac output
    - Impaired gas exchange
    - Altered oral mucous membranes
    - Altered thought processes
    - Knowledge deficit
    - Powerlessness and hopelessness
    - Ineffective management of therapeutic regimen

- Noncompliance and potential risk
- Risk for injury
- Caregiver role strain
- Ineffective individual/family coping
- Anticipatory grieving
- **Key Terms/Concepts**: Uremia, azotemia, oliguria, anuria, hypervolemia, hemodialysis, peritoneal dialysis, uremic lung, uremic frost

Overview

Chronic renal failure (CRF) refers to the progressive and irreversible loss of renal function that results in accumulation of waste products and the inability to maintain fluid and electrolyte balance. The five stages of CRF are:

- **Stage 1**: Minimal kidney damage with normal or increased GFR
- **Stage 2**: Kidney damage with mildly decreased GFR
- **Stage 3**: Moderate kidney damage with moderate decrease in GFR
- **Stage 4**: Sever kidney damage with sever decrease if GFR (chronic renal failure)
- **Stage 5**: Kidney failure, end-stage renal disease (ESRD), GFR continues to decline

Risk Factors

- Acute renal failure (ARF)
- Diabetes mellitus
- Chronic glomerulonephritis
- Nephrotoxic drugs or chemicals
- Hypertension, especially if African American
- Autoimmune disorders (systemic lupus erythematosus [SLE])
- Polycystic kidney
- Pyelonephrosis
- Renal artery stenosis
- Recurrent infections

Signs and Symptoms

- May be asymptomatic except during periods of stress (infection, surgery, trauma)
- Fatigue
- Nausea
- Anorexia
- Nocturia, polyuria
- Pruritus
- Erectile dysfunction
- Restless leg syndrome

- Insomnia
- Confusion
- Changes in taste, especially acquiring a metallic taste
- Osteomalacia
- Edema
- Ascites, congestive heart failure, pericardial effusion
- Asterixis
- Lethargy
- Encephalopathy
- Stomatitis
- Depression
- Intractable hiccups
- Muscle cramping, twitching
- Orthostatic hypotension
- Hyperesthesia, paresthesia – neuropathy
- Anemia
- Shortness of breath
- Chest pain
- Vomiting
- Anuria
- Marked azotemia
- Severe fluid overload
- Pulmonary edema, uremic lung
- Uremic frost
- Seizures, coma

Diagnostic and Laboratory Tests

- History and physical examination
- Urinalysis, including osmolality
- Serum creatinine and BUN
- Serum electrolytes (sodium, potassium, calcium, phosphate, bicarbonate, liver function, etc.)
- CBC (complete blood count) and differential
- Serum glucose and lipids
- Ultrasound
  - 2-D (2-dimensional)
  - 3-D (3-dimensional)
  - Doppler
- IVP (intravenous pyelogram)
- Renal biopsy

- MRI (magnetic resonance imaging)
- CT/CAT (computer tomography/computed axial tomography) scan
- 24-hour Urine Creatinine Clearance Test: A measure of the volume of plasma that is cleared of creatinine in a fixed time period (mL /min). Because of the unique properties of creatinine (stable plasma concentrations, freely filtered, not reabsorbed, and minimally secreted by the kidneys), creatinine clearance is used to estimate the glomerular filtration rate (GFR). The GFR, in turn, is the standard by which kidney function is assessed.
- Glomerular filtration rate (GFR)
- Urinary protein excretion over 24 hours

Therapeutic Nursing Management

- **Assess/Monitor:**
  - Urinary elimination patterns (amount, color, odor, consistency)
  - Vital signs
  - Weight (1 kg daily weight increase is approximately 1 L of fluid retained)
  - Energy level
  - For signs of bruising or bleeding
  - BUN (blood urea nitrogen), serum creatinine, and electrolytes
  - Serum Hgb (hemoglobin) and Hct (hematocrit)
  - Acid-base status
  - Urinary specific gravity, protein, and hematuria
  - Neurological status
  - Respiratory status
  - Psychological status
  - For signs of infection
  - For signs of fluid overload
  - For cardiac dysrhythmias, signs of heart failure
  - Renal osteodystrophy (skeletal bone loss), osteoporosis
  - Hyperlipidemia
  - Uremic halitosis and stomatitis (mouth inflammation)
  - Anorexia, nausea, vomiting, hiccups
  - Vascular access or peritoneal dialysis insertion site
- **Nursing Activities:**
  - Obtain detailed drug and herb history.
  - Provide high-carbohydrate and moderate-fat content in the diet.
  - Restrict intake of fluids (based on urinary output).
  - Control protein intake based on stage of renal failure and type of dialysis.
  - Provide high biological value protein (milk, eggs, meat).
  - Restrict dietary sodium, potassium, phosphorous, and magnesium in late stages of CRF.
  - Administer vitamin and mineral supplements.

- Balance activity and rest.
- Prepare to administer Kayexalate to decrease serum potassium levels.
- Prepare client for hemodialysis, peritoneal dialysis, and hemofiltration.
- Administer antihypertensive agents and diuretics as prescribed; often used are ACE (angiotensin-converting enzyme) inhibitors.
- Administer aluminum hydroxide as prescribed (to prevent bone demineralization), vitamin D, and calcium supplements.
- Provide skin care to increase comfort and prevent breakdown.
- Administer erythropoietin alfa or darbepoetin alfa as prescribed to stimulate red blood cell production, as well as ferrous sulfate, folic acid, and vitamin B_{12}.
- Possibly administer growth hormone.
- Teach client home blood pressure and weight measurement and recording.
- Teach client to avoid antacids containing magnesium.
- Teach client home care of dialysis access site.
- Teach client signs and symptoms that require immediate reporting.
- Protect client from injury.
- Provide emotional support to client and family.
- Encourage client to ask questions and discuss fears.
- Refer to community resource or support groups.
- Refer to smoking cessation support and counseling if needed.
- Encourage strict blood glucose control in diabetics.
- Encourage client to obtain yearly influenza vaccine and to get the pneumococcal vaccine.
- Encourage diet, exercise, and medication control of hyperlipidemia.

Pharmacology

- Antihypertensives (ACE inhibitors, calcium channel blockers [avoid dihydropyridine as monotherapy], alpha-adrenergic and beta- adrenergic blockers, and vasodilators)
- Iron supplements
- Folic acid
- Kayexalate
- Erythropoietin alfa (Epogen, Procrit)
- Alkalizers (sodium bicarbonate)
- Phosphate binders
  - Aluminum hydroxide
  - Calcium carbonate or acetate
  - Sevelamer hydrochloride (Renagel)
- Vitamin D supplements, calcium supplements
- Stool softeners (docusate)
- Diuretics (except in ESRD)

- Note: Many medications that clients with CRF are taking for other conditions may need to be adjusted based on renal function!

Complications

- Pulmonary edema
- CHF (congestive heart failure)
- Metabolic acidosis
- Seizures
- Cardiac dysrhythmias
- Peripheral neuropathies
- Pericarditis
- Pericardial effusion
- Uremic encephalopathy
- Bone demineralization, osteoporosis
- Depression
- Anemia
- Bleeding
- Malnutrition
- Electrolyte imbalances
- Access site infection
- Access site clotting
- Coma
- Death

Age-Related Changes—Gerontological Considerations

- There is a greater occurrence of ESRD in individuals 65 to 69 years of age.
- An increased incidence for chronic renal failure may be related to the prevalence of diabetes mellitus, hypertension, and use of NSAIDs (non-steroidal antiinflammatory drugs) in the older adult.
- The increased risk for renal failure is related to the decreased number of functioning nephrons, decreased GFR (glomerular filtration rate), and water- and sodium-conserving mechanisms.
- Dehydration may occur, due to inadequate fluid intake.
- Symptoms may be missed or confused with other chronic illnesses until extensive renal damage has occurred.

Cultural Considerations

- African-Americans, Native Americans, and Asians have the highest incidence of ESRD.
- Caucasians have the lowest incidence of ESRD.

Critical Thinking Exercise: Nursing Management of the Client with Chronic Renal Failure (CRF)

Situation: A 55-year-old woman is admitted to the acute care facility for weight gain, pedal edema, hypertension, and decreased urine output. Her past history reveals chronic use of NSAIDs (Nonsteroidal anti-inflammatory drugs) for low back pain and type 2 diabetes mellitus of twelve years duration. Her family history is positive for coronary artery disease and diabetes mellitus.

1. What risk factors does the client have for CRF?

2. How does chronic renal failure differ from acute renal failure?

3. Match the characteristics with the correct stage of chronic renal failure. Use the Stage number as your response for each answer.

Stage 1: Decreased renal reserve	Nocturia
Stage 2: Renal insufficiency	Anemia
Stage 3: Renal failure	Normal BUN (blood urea nitrogen)
Stage 4: End stage renal failureuremia	CHF (congestive heart failure)
	Headache
	Anuria
	Polydipsia
	Metabolic acidosis
	Normal serum creatinine
	Marked azotemia

4. Prioritize nursing activities for the client, with "1" representing the most important activity.

_____ Monitor serum potassium levels.

_____ Turn every two hours.

_____ Offer emotional support to family.

_____ Assess lung sounds.

5. Which are the two most important collaborative interventions for the client at this time?

_____ Providing adequate pain control

_____ Preventing complications

_____ Correcting electrolyte imbalance

_____ Teaching the client about dialysis

Nursing Management of the Client Requiring Hemodialysis/ Peritoneal Dialysis

Key Points

- Dialysis is performed to rid the body of excess fluid and electrolytes, achieve acid-base balance, and eliminate waste products.
- Dialysis involves the movement of fluid and particles across a semi-permeable membrane to restore internal homeostasis (osmosis, diffusion, and ultrafiltration).
- Dialysis can sustain life for clients with both acute and chronic renal failure.
- Dialysis does not replace the hormonal functions of the kidney.
- Hemodialysis involves shunting the client's blood from the body through a dialyzer and back into the client's circulation via an external or internal access device.
- Peritoneal dialysis involves instillation of fluid into the peritoneal cavity where the peritoneum serves as the filtration membrane.
- Goals of collaborative management:
  - Select the best source of dialysis for the individual client.
  - Evaluate the effectiveness of dialysis.
  - Maintain internal homeostasis and remove waste products.
  - Prevent complications.
- Important nursing diagnoses (actual or potential):
  - Potential complications of hemodialysis (access clotting, infection, hemorrhage, hypovolemia)
  - Potential complications of peritoneal dialysis (peritonitis, outflow obstruction, insertion site infection, hyperglycemia)
  - Fluid volume excess/deficit
  - Impaired skin integrity
  - Activity intolerance
  - Decreased cardiac output
  - Impaired gas exchange
  - Knowledge deficit
  - Powerlessness and hopelessness
  - Ineffective management of therapeutic regimen
  - Noncompliance and potential risk
  - Caregiver role strain
  - Ineffective individual/family coping
- **Key Terms/Concepts:** Dialysate, dialyzer, arteriovenous shunt, arteriovenous graft, homeostasis, dwell time

Overview

When diet and medications can no longer compensate for deteriorating renal function, hemodialysis or peritoneal dialysis is required.

Hemodialysis (HD) is achieved by filtering blood, which has been accessed using the subclavian internal jugular, or femoral veins, arteriovenous fistula, or arteriovenous graft, through an artificial kidney (dialyzer) and returning it to the body. Hemodialysis restores acid/base and electrolyte balance, cleans the blood of accumulated waste products, removes the by-products of protein metabolism, and removes excess water.

Peritoneal dialysis (PD) is achieved by placing a siliconized rubber catheter into the abdominal (peritoneal) cavity through which dialysate solution is infused. Following a prescribed dwell time, the fluid is drained from the abdominal cavity by gravity. Peritoneal dialysis removes waste products and excess water by the processes of diffusion and osmosis. Many types of PD are available, including continuous ambulatory PD, multiple continuous ambulatory PD, automated PD, intermittent PD, and continuous cycle PD.

Risk Factors/Indications

- Renal insufficiency
- ARF (acute renal failure)
- CRF (chronic renal failure)
- Drug overdose

Diagnostic and Laboratory Tests

- History and physical examination
- CBC (complete blood count)
- BUN (blood urea nitrogen)
- Serum creatinine
- Serum electrolytes
- FBG (fasting blood glucose); also called fasting blood sugar (FBS)

Therapeutic Nursing Management

Hemodialysis

- Assess/Monitor:
  - BUN (blood urea nitrogen), serum creatinine, electrolytes, and hematocrit prior to and after hemodialysis
  - Vital signs before, during, and after hemodialysis
  - Weight before and after hemodialysis
  - For patency of access site (presence of bruit, distal pulses, and circulation)
  - For complications (hypotension, access clotting, headache, muscle cramps, bleeding, disequilibrium syndrome, hepatitis)
  - Access site for indications of bleeding, infection
  - For nausea, vomiting and level of consciousness

- For signs of hypovolemia following dialysis
- **Nursing Activities:**
    - Discuss with health care provider any medications to be withheld until after dialysis.
    - Provide emotional support prior, during, and after procedure.
    - Teach client to avoid lifting heavy objects with access-site arm or carrying objects that compress the extremity.
    - Avoid taking blood pressure, administering injections or venipunctures, or starting IV lines on arm with access site.
    - Elevate extremity following surgical development of AV fistula.
    - Teach hand exercises to promote fistula maturation.
    - Instruct client to avoid sleeping with body weight on top of extremity with access device.
    - Avoid invasive procedures for 4 to 6 hours after dialysis.

Peritoneal dialysis

- **Assess/Monitor:**
    - Vital signs before, every 24 hours during, and after peritoneal dialysis
    - Serum electrolytes, creatinine, BUN
    - Blood glucose level before peritoneal dialysis and daily during PD
    - Weight before and after procedure
    - Color and amount of outflow (clear, light yellow is expected)
    - For signs of infection (fever, bloody, cloudy, or frothy dialysate return, drainage at access site)
    - For complications (respiratory distress, abdominal pain, insufficient outflow, discolored (red, brown, etc.) outflow)
- **Nursing Activities:**
    - Warm dialysate prior to instilling; avoid use of microwaves which cause uneven heating.
    - Check abdominal dressing for wetness.
    - Follow specified amounts and times for infusion, dwell, and outflow ordered by health care provider.
    - Maintain asepsis of catheter insertion site.
    - Maintain sterile technique when accessing the PD catheter.
    - Keep outflow bag lower than client's abdomen.
    - Reposition client if inflow or outflow is inadequate.
    - Carefully milk PD catheter if fibrin clot has formed.
    - Teach client home care of access site.
    - Provide emotional support to client and family.

Complications

- Peritonitis (the major complication of PD)
- Clotting of access site
- Infection at access site

- Disequilibrium syndrome
- Dialysis encephalopathy
- Hypotension
- Anemia
- Bleeding/hemorrhage
- Peritonitis
- Hyperglycemia

Age–Related Changes—Gerontological Considerations

- There is an increased risk for access site complications related to chronic illnesses and/or fragile veins, both of which are present in the elderly.
- Older adults may be unable to care for a peritoneal access site due to cognitive or physical deficits.
- Clients over age 65 are at increased risk for dialysis-induced hypotension.
- The most common cause of death in the elderly receiving dialysis is cardiovascular disease followed by withdrawal for dialysis treatment.
- The increasing number of elderly, debilitated clients receiving dialysis for ESRD has raised ethical concerns about the use of scarce resources in a population with a limited life expectancy.

Critical Thinking Exercise: Nursing Management of the Client Requiring Hemodialysis/Peritoneal Dialysis

Situation: A 35-year-old male has received hemodialysis for renal failure or end-stage renal disease (ESRD) for the past seven years due to diabetes mellitus. While awaiting renal transplant, he receives hemodialysis three times each week via an arteriovenous fistula created in his left arm.

1. Which nursing interventions are most important to perform immediately prior to initiating the client's hemodialysis?

    _____ Determine current medications being taken by client.

    _____ Assess AV fistula for bruit.

    _____ Calculate total urine output for the night.

    _____ Assess dietary intake.

    _____ Obtain blood glucose level.

    _____ Obtain a current weight.

    _____ Assess hydration status.

    _____ Draw serum electrolytes.

    _____ Obtain a current blood pressure reading.

2. Which nursing interventions need to be implemented following the client's hemodialysis procedure?

    _____ Obtain BUN (blood urea nitrogen) and serum creatinine.

    _____ Assess for headache and/or confusion.

    _____ Obtain blood glucose level.

    _____ Administer antihypertensive medication for hypertension.

    _____ Obtain serum electrolytes.

    _____ Assess access site for indications of bleeding.

3. Provide rationale for the client's nursing diagnoses.

    a. Risk for fluid volume deficit:

    b. Risk for injury:

    c. Risk for activity intolerance:

    d. Risk for ineffective breathing pattern:

Nursing Management of the Client with a Renal Transplant

Key Points

- Donors for renal transplantation are selected on the basis of blood type (ABO) compatibility, histocompatibility, human leukocytic antigen (HLA), white blood cell cross match, and mixed lymphocyte culture and reaction.
- The size of the donor kidney is seldom a problem.
- The donor kidney is placed in the anterior iliac fossa with the renal artery anteriorly, and the renal vein posteriorly.
- Renal transplant clients face the possibility of organ rejection immediately after transplantation (hyperacute rejection), one to two weeks following transplantation (acute rejection), or months-to-years following transplantation (chronic rejection).
- Public Law 92-603 (End-Stage Renal Disease Act), passed in 1972, made it easier for elderly, poor, and minority clients to obtain renal transplants or dialysis.
- Renal transplantation is more cost-effective than dialysis treatments administered over a nine-year period.
- Goals of collaborative management:
  - Prepare the preoperative client for post-transplantation lifestyle changes.
  - Prevent organ rejection.
  - Prevent other postoperative complications.
  - Promote compliance with procedures following surgery and follow-up appointments.
- Important nursing diagnoses (actual or potential):
  - Risk for fluid volume excess
  - Risk for fluid volume deficit
  - Risk for constipation
  - Body image disturbance
  - Risk for infection
  - Fear and anxiety
  - Altered thought processes
  - Altered nutrition: less than body requirements
  - Noncompliance
- **Key Terms/Concepts**: End-stage renal disease (ESRD), donor kidney, immunosuppression, organ rejection, dialysis

Overview

Renal transplantation is the replacement of a diseased kidney with a surgically-implanted donor organ from a living donor, non-heart-beating donor, or cadaver.

The purpose of renal transplantation is to sustain life in a client with end-stage renal disease (ESRD) rather than utilizing dialysis.

Risk Factors

Poor Candidates for Renal Transplantation

- Age younger than four years
- Age older than 70 years
- Advanced, untreatable cardiac disease
- Malignancies
- Active vasculitis
- Extreme obesity
- Severe psychiatric disorders
- History of intravenous drug use
- Chronic infectious or systemic diseases
- Coagulopathies and certain immune disorders

Signs and Symptoms of ESRD

Necessitating Renal Transplantation

- Anuria
- Marked azotemia
- Severe electrolyte imbalances
- Pulmonary edema
- Uremic lung
- Uremic frost
- Pruritus
- Proteinuria
- Heart failure

Diagnostic and Laboratory Tests

- History and physical exam
- CBC (complete blood count) and differential
- Urinalysis
- Serum electrolytes
- Urine specific gravity
- BUN (blood urea nitrogen)
- Creatinine
- **Creatinine clearance** — A measure of the volume of plasma that is cleared of creatinine in a fixed time period (mL/min). Because of the unique properties of creatinine (stable plasma concentrations, freely-filtered, not reabsorbed, and minimally secreted by the kidneys), creatinine clearance is used to estimate the glomerular filtration rate (GFR). The GFR, in turn, is the standard by which kidney function is assessed.

- Glomerular filtration rate (GFR)
- 24-hour urinary protein excretion
- MRI (magnetic resonance imaging)
- Computer tomography (CT)/computed axial tomography (CAT) scan
- Radionuclide renal scans
- Renal biopsy if indicated

Therapeutic Nursing Management

- **Preoperative Care (in addition to routine care):**
  - Schedule preoperative assessment routines several weeks ahead of the transplantation surgery, because it is difficult to predict exactly when a donor kidney will be available.
  - Prepare the client mentally and emotionally for the procedure.
  - Advise the client to immediately stop smoking.
  - Advise the client that compliance with the post-transplant procedures and appointments is crucial to the success of the transplantation.
  - Review laboratory values for acceptable levels.
- **Assess/Monitor (Postoperative Period):**
  - Vital signs continually
  - Intake and output at least hourly
  - Urine appearance and odor hourly (initially pink and bloody gradually returning to normal in a few days to several weeks)
  - If continuous bladder irrigation is ordered, evaluate that urine output is at least greater than 30 mL/hr plus amount of solution instilled.
  - Laboratory values
  - Daily urine tests, including urinalysis and glucose determinations
  - Renal function continually
  - For fluid and electrolyte imbalances
  - For signs of respiratory infection
  - For side effects from immunosuppressive drugs
  - For signs of organ rejection
- **Nursing Activities (Postoperative):**
  - Administer intravenous fluids.
  - Help client to turn, cough, and deep breathe.
  - Attach urinary catheter to bedside drainage.
  - Provide daily catheter care.
  - Remove urinary catheter once risk of urinary retention is over.
  - Reinsert catheter if client is unable to void.
  - Administer oral fluids and discontinue IVs once bowel functions return.
  - Weigh the client daily.
  - Administer immunosuppressive drugs.
  - Educate the client and family about the increased risk for infection during immuno-suppressant therapy.

- Immediately notify the surgeon if any signs of organ rejection appear.
- Administer stool softeners.
- Report signs of paranoia or psychosis and arrange for psychiatric evaluation if necessary.
- Continue postoperative dialysis until kidney function is satisfactory.
- Arrange for post-transplant follow-up appointments and procedures.
- Arrange for counseling for clients and family if necessary.

Pharmacology

- Intravenous fluids
- Diuretics and osmotic agents, such as mannitol, if oliguria occurs
- Immunosuppressive drugs (prednisone, cyclosporin, azathioprine)
- Pain medications (opioid and nonopioid)
- Stool softeners (docusate)

Complications

- Organ rejection
- Acute tubular necrosis
- Renal artery stenosis
- Thrombosis or vascular leakage
- Infection, most common cause of first transplant year morbidity and mortality
- Psychosis and paranoia
- Constipation
- Hypokalemia
- Hyponatremia
- Hypovolemia
- Fluid overload
- Genitourinary, including kinked ureter, ureteral leakage, fistula, obstruction, calculus, bladder neck stricture, scrotal swelling, and graft rupture
- Noninfectious hepatitis
- Chronic liver failure, cirrhosis
- Peptic ulcer disease
- Hypertension
- Osteoporosis
- Myopathy
- Malignancy – colon, lung bladder, skin, kidney, non-Hodgkin lymphoma, genital, etc.
- Cyclosporin toxicity
- Hypertension
- Cardiovascular disease

Age-Related Changes—Gerontological Considerations

- Clients older than 70 years of age are poor candidates for renal transplantation.
- Older clients are more likely to have advanced heart disease and malignancies, which make them poor candidates for renal transplantation surgery.

Critical Thinking Exercise: Nursing Management of the Client with a Renal Transplant

Situation: A 40-year-old male client with failing renal function has undergone a renal transplant and is four days postoperative. He is being treated on the surgical unit. The urinary catheter has been removed, and the client is able to void. The client is still receiving intravenous infusions with electrolyte replacements, but will be started on oral fluids today. Thus far, the client has not had any signs of transplant rejection.

1. Which fluid and electrolyte imbalances is the client at greatest risk for?

_____ Hypokalemia   _____ Hypercalcemia

_____ Hyponatremia   _____ Hypomagnesemia

_____ Fluid overload   _____ Hypovolemia

2. Which are the four priority nursing diagnoses during the early postoperative phase following organ transplantation?

_____ Risk for fluid volume deficit   _____ Risk for constipation

_____ Body image disturbance   _____ Risk for infection

_____ Fear and anxiety   _____ Altered nutrition: less than body requirements

_____ Noncompliance with therapeutic regimen

3. Which are clinical manifestations of organ rejection?

_____ Malaise   _____ Elevated serum creatinine

_____ Bradycardia   _____ Tender kidney

_____ Weight gain   _____ Hypotension

_____ Decreased serum BUN (blood urea nitrogen)   _____ Headache

_____ Fever   _____ Oliguria

4. Why is the client undergoing organ transplantation at greater risk for infection than other surgical clients?

Nursing Management of the Client with Nephrotic Syndrome

Key Points

- Nephrotic syndrome is a complex of signs and symptoms rather than a disease entity.
- Nephrosis (nephrotic syndrome) includes edema, proteinuria, hypoalbuminemia, hyperlipidemia, lipiduria, increased coagulation, and hypertension.
- The majority of adults with nephrotic syndrome develop chronic renal failure within five years.
- Many clients experience periods of exacerbation and remission.
- Goals of collaborative management:
  - Reduce albuminuria.
  - Control edema.
  - Cure or control the primary disease.
  - Prevent complications (chronic renal failure).
- Important nursing diagnoses (actual or potential):
  - Fluid volume excess
  - Risk for infection
  - Altered nutrition: less than body requirements
  - Impaired skin integrity
  - Knowledge deficit
  - Anxiety and fear
  - Altered body image
  - Ineffective individual coping
- **Key Terms/Concepts**: Syndrome, proteinuria, hypoalbuminemia, hyperlipidemia, lipuria

Overview

Nephrotic syndrome is said to exist when diffuse glomerular injury results in severe proteinuria greater than 3.5 grams of protein in 24 hours. It is most often seen in children and older adults.

Risk Factors

- Hyperlipidemia
- Systemic diseases (diabetes mellitus, SLE [systemic lupus erythematosus])
- Systemic infections
- Adverse drug reaction

- Allergic reactions
- Neoplasms
- Vascular disorders
- Inherited nephritic disease
- Numerous disorders
- Drug addiction
- Hepatitis B, C, and HIV

Signs and Symptoms

- Hematuria
- Edema
- Irritability
- Malaise
- Anorexia
- Abnormal menses
- Amenorrhea
- Hypertension
- Waxy appearance of skin
- Anemia

Diagnostic and Laboratory Tests

- History and physical examination
- Serum triglycerides, phospholipids, and cholesterol
- Urinalysis – proteinuria, hematuria, glycosuria, lipiduria, casts, foamy, etc.
- 24-hour urine protein levels
- Urine specific gravity
- Azotemia

Therapeutic Nursing Management

- **Assess/Monitor**:
  - Vital signs
  - Daily weight
  - Intake and output
  - For signs of edema
  - For signs of fluid volume deficit
  - For effects of diuretic therapy
  - For anorexia
- **Nursing Activities**:
  - Maintain bed rest when edema is severe.
  - Measure abdominal girth or extremity size.

- Provide low-fat diet with increased carbohydrates.
- Decrease dietary protein if glomerular filtration rate (GFR) is decreased. If GFR is normal, proteins in the diet should contain all essential amino acids.
- Limit sodium intake as prescribed.
- Limit potassium intake if serum potassium is elevated.
- Administer medications as prescribed.
- Provide skin care to prevent breakdown.
- Cleanse edematous extremities carefully.
- Provide emotional support for client and family.
- Encourage client to receive the pneumococcal vaccine and yearly influenza vaccine.
- Teach client to avoid excessive sunlight.

Pharmacology

- Diuretics (furosemide, torsemide) to control edema
- Corticosteroids (prednisone)
- Lipid-lowering agents (colestipol, lovastatin)
- Erythropoietin or darbepoetin for anemia
- Antihypertensives if indicated
- Cytoxic agents for immunosuppression (cyclophosphamide or chlorambucil)
- Plasma volume expanders (albumin, plasma, dextran)
- Anticoagulants (heparin, warfarin)
- Antibiotics, if infection present

Complications

- ARF (acute renal failure)
- Renal vein thrombosis
- Thromboembolism
- Skin breakdown
- Shock
- Death

Age-Related Changes—Gerontological Considerations

- Increased incidence of diabetes mellitus, hyperlipidemia, and other chronic diseases occur in older adults with nephrotic syndrome.
- Increased risk for decreased protein levels is related to inadequate dietary intake of protein.

Critical Thinking Exercise: Nursing Management of the Client with Nephrotic Syndrome

Situation: An older man with a 30-year history of diabetes mellitus is experiencing excessive protein wasting, edema, and hypertension. Based on the client's clinical manifestations and proteinuria of 3.7 g/day, the client is diagnosed with nephrotic syndrome.

1. Which areas of the client's body will the nurse assess to determine the presence of edema related to nephrotic syndrome?

   _____ Posterior neck   _____ Hands   _____ Buttocks

   _____ Sacrum   _____ Elbow   _____ Ankles

2. Which statements are true about the client's condition? Correct false statements.
   a. Nephrotic syndrome is a disease that causes edema and proteinuria.
   b. Hypoalbuminemia, hyperlipidemia, and lipuria are consequences of nephrotic syndrome.
   c. Nephrotic syndrome is a reversible condition when diagnosed and treated early.
   d. Periods of exacerbation and remission are common in clients with nephrotic syndrome.
   e. Nephrotic syndrome is related to glomerular disease or injury.

3. Prioritize nursing activities for this client, with "1" representing the most important activity.
   _____ Encourage bedrest.
   _____ Limit potassium intake.
   _____ Teach regarding exacerbating factors.
   _____ Provide low-protein, high-carbohydrate diet.

Nursing Management of the Client with Prostate Cancer

| Key Points |

- Prostatic carcinomas are slow growing tumors, with the most frequent cell type being adenocarcinoma.
- Prostate cancer and benign prostatic hypertrophy (BPH) are the most common conditions diagnosed in male clients 50 years of age and older; the mean age of diagnosis is 71 years old.
- It is crucial to diagnostically differentiate prostate cancer from BPH as soon as possible.
- Prostate cancer is spread via the lymphatic system to pelvic region and bones.
- Prostate cancer may be asymptomatic until well advanced.
- By the time of diagnosis, most prostatic cancers have metastasized to adjacent structures.
- Conservative management of prostate cancer involves deferring treatment or "watchful waiting."
- Early stage prostate cancer is generally curable.
- If serious problems develop, prostate cancer is treated with surgery, chemotherapy, radiation therapy, hormone replacement therapy, and androgen suppressing agents.
- Surgical procedures include prostatectomy, prostatectomy with pelvic lymphadenectomy, radical prostatectomy, cryosurgical ablation, and bilateral orchiectomy.
- Goals of collaborative management:
  - Provide early recognition and treatment.
  - Remove the existing cancer surgically.
  - Initiate appropriate chemotherapy and/or radiation therapy and pharmacologic therapy.
  - Prevent recurrence.
  - Support dying client and family.
- Important nursing diagnoses (actual or potential):
  - Altered urinary elimination
  - Pain
  - Anxiety and fear
  - Knowledge deficit
  - Potential complications of chemotherapy/radiation therapy
  - Sexual dysfunction

- Body image disturbance
- Decisional conflict
- **Key Terms/Concepts:** Adenocarcinoma, lymphadenopathy, cancer staging, asymptomatic, PSA (prostate specific antigen), digital rectal examination (DRE), prostatic biopsy, "watchful waiting," prostatectomy, hormone therapy

Overview

Cancer of the prostate is the most common malignancy occurring in men over the age of 50. The majority of prostate cancers are adenocarcinomas, which originate in the posterior of the prostate gland. Prostate cancer rarely produces symptoms until it is well advanced. This form of cancer generally grows slowly.

Risk Factors

- Genetic predisposition
- Environmental and dietary carcinogens
- STD (sexually transmitted disease)
- Advanced age - 50 years and older
- African-American heritage
- High-fat diet

Signs and Symptoms

- May be asymptomatic
- Difficulty initiating urinary stream, hesitancy, incomplete emptying of bladder
- Dysuria
- Nocturia
- Gross, painless hematuria - rare
- Anemia
- Obstruction of urethra or bowel
- Weight loss
- Pain in lower back or leg
- Painful ejaculation
- Unexplained cystitis
- Lymphadenopathy (advanced cancer)
- Bone pain (advanced cancer)
- Spinal cord compression (advanced cancer)

Diagnostic and Laboratory Tests

- History and physical examination
- Digital rectal examination (DRE)
- Prostatic biopsy
- Magnetic resonance imaging (MRI)

- Computer tomography (CT)/computed axial tomography (CAT) scan
- Prostate specific antigen (PSA); also called Total PSA or Free PSA, reliably predicts the extent of neoplastic disease and recurrence after prostatectomy.
- Ultrasound
  - 2-D (2-dimensional)
  - 3-D (3-dimensional)
  - Doppler
- Prostatic acid phosphatase (PAP), also called: serum acid phosphatase test
- Excretory urography
- ProstaScint scan or single-photon emission computed tomography (SPECT) is used to detect the spread of prostate cancer to pelvic lymph nodes.

Therapeutic Nursing Management

- **Assess/Monitor:**
  - Intake and urinary output
  - Client's ability to urinate and empty bladder preoperatively
  - For indications of urethral stricture (dysuria, straining to urinate, decreased force of urine stream)
  - For postoperative blood loss
  - Postoperative pain level
  - For indications of deep vein thrombosis and pulmonary embolism
- **Nursing Activities:**
  - Prepare client for surgery, radiation, or chemotherapy if indicated.
  - Provide emotional support to client and family, especially when prognosis is unfavorable.
  - Encourage client to verbalize feelings regarding possible surgical outcomes (incontinence, impotence).
  - Administer pain medications as prescribed.
  - Maintain strict asepsis of indwelling urinary catheter.
  - Encourage fluid intake after surgery.
  - Perform bladder irrigation postoperatively as prescribed.
  - Provide skin care to protect from breakdown.
  - Encourage perineal exercises within 24 to 48 hours after surgery.
  - Avoid rectal temperatures.
  - Instruct client not to strain during a bowel movement.
  - Teach client regarding side effects of hormonal therapy if prescribed (gynecomastia, fluid retention, nausea, and thrombophlebitis).
  - Administer bisphosphonates to clients with advanced prostate cancer who are at risk of bone metastases.
  - Teach client how to care for urinary catheter and drainage bag when discharged home.
  - Teach client who develops urinary incontinence after prostatectomy to perform Kegel exercises after every urination, decrease or eliminate the consumption of caffeine, and stop smoking.

- Refer client to community cancer support group.
- Refer client for sexual counseling as appropriate.

Pharmacology

- Estrogen replacement therapy
- Testosterone ablating agents to cause androgen deprivation: finasteride, dutasteride; (turosteride, flutamide, and leuprolide rarely used)
- Luteinizing hormone-releasing hormone (LH-RN) agonists: leuprolide (Lupron), goserelin (Zoladex)
- Chemotherapy: vinblastine (Velban), mitomycin (Mutamycin)
- Radiation therapy
- Radioactive seed implants (brachytherapy)
- Bisphosphonates: zoledronate (Zomax), risedronate (Actonel)

Complications

- Incontinence
- Impotence
- Metastasis
- Spinal compression
- Fractures due to bone metastases
- Hemorrhage
- Death

Age-Related Changes—Gerontological Considerations

- There is an increased risk for cancer with advanced age.
- The symptoms of prostate metastasis can mimic other disorders, which makes it difficult to monitor the progression of the cancer.

Critical Thinking Exercise: Nursing Management of the Client with Prostate Cancer

Situation: A 70-year-old man is scheduled for a radical prostatectomy for prostate cancer. The client has been experiencing back pain, difficulty initiating his urinary stream, and bloody urine. Both his PSA (prostate specific antigen) and PAP (prostatic acid phosphate) were positive.

1. Why are the client's laboratory findings (PSA and PAP) important?

2. What is the difference between a radical perineal prostatectomy and a TURP (transurethral resection of the prostate)?

3. Which nursing activities will be most effective in reducing the client's anxiety over his diagnosis and impending surgery?

_____ Explaining the pathophysiology of prostate cancer

_____ Establishing a trusting relationship

_____ Encouraging the client to verbalize his concerns

_____ Encouraging the client to not worry unnecessarily

_____ Answering the client's questions simply but honestly

_____ Including the client in all care planning

Nursing Management of the Client with Benign Prostatic Hypertrophy (BPH)

Key Points

- Benign prostatic hypertrophy (BPH) is the most common benign tumor developing in older men.
- BPH develops to some degree in all elderly men.
- Conservative management of BPH involves deferring treatment or "watchful waiting." If symptoms worsen, the client may undergo drug therapy or surgery.
- More than 300,000 surgical procedures for BPH are performed yearly in the U.S.
- The goal of surgical procedures for BPH is to remove excess prostate tissue and thus eliminate symptoms.
- The four major surgical procedures for BPH are:
  - Transurethral resection of the prostate (TURP)
  - Suprapubic or transvesical prostatectomy
  - Retropubic or retrovesical prostatectomy
  - Perineal prostatectomy
- Newer surgical procedures include transurethral needle ablation (TUNA), balloon dilation of the prostate, transurethral microwave thermotherapy (TUMT) of the prostate, transurethral laser incision, transurethral electrovaporization of the prostate (TUVP), and insertion of prostatic stents.
- The prognosis for men undergoing surgery for BPH is excellent.
- Goals of collaborative management:
  - Reduce or eliminate symptoms.
  - Prevent urinary obstruction and retention.
  - Prevent infection.
  - Restore normal urinary function.
  - Prevent and treat complications of treatment.
  - Help client to re-establish normal sexual relationships.
- Important nursing diagnoses (actual or potential):
  - Altered urinary elimination
  - Risk for fluid volume deficit
  - Risk for infection
  - Pain
  - Fear/anxiety
  - Hemorrhage
  - Ineffective therapeutic regimen management

- **Key Terms/Concepts**: Urgency, dysuria, prostate specific antigen (PSA), transurethral resection of the prostate (TURP), suprapubic prostatectomy, retropubic prostatectomy, perineal prostatectomy, alpha-adrenergic blockers, testosterone ablating agents

Overview

Benign prostatic hypertrophy (BPH) or hyperplasia is a benign enlargement of the prostate due to abnormal growth of prostate tissue. If symptoms worsen after "watchful waiting", the client will be treated with medications and surgery. Treatment has a high success rate.

Risk Factors

- Male gender
- Age over 50 years, 50%; age over 70 years, 80%
- Family history (particularly first-degree relatives)
- Western cultural heritage
- Diet high in zinc, butter, and margarine, possible
- Caucasian

Signs and Symptoms

- Nocturia
- Urgency
- Difficulty initiating urination
- Urination that starts and stops
- Diminished size and force of urinary stream
- Straining with urination
- Post-void dribbling
- Feeling that urine is being retained after urination
- Hematuria
- Dysuria
- Incontinence

Diagnostic and Laboratory Tests

- History and physical examination
- Digital rectal examination (DRE)
- Urinalysis with culture
- Serum creatinine and other renal function tests
- Prostate specific antigen (PSA)
- Post-void residual
- Uroflowmetry
- Transrectal ultrasound (TRUS)
- Cystourethroscopy

- Preoperative blood work and urinalysis
- Electrolyte panel

Therapeutic Nursing Management

- **Prevention:**
  - Because gender and aging are primary risk factors, BPH cannot be prevented.
  - A diet low in butter and margarine and high in fruit intake may help lower risk.
- **Assess/Monitor:**
  - Assess for bladder distention after voiding.
  - Monitor for acute urinary retention.
  - Monitor intake and output.
  - Assess for signs of infection.
  - Monitor general postoperative condition if client undergoes surgery. Monitor:
    - Vital signs
    - Drains and wound packing for bleeding
    - Acute pain
    - Cloudy, foul-smelling urine and elevated temperature which indicate urinary tract infection
    - Hemoglobin and hematocrit levels for anemia due to blood loss
    - Urinary catheter drainage for blood and clots
    - Urinary catheter for kinking or obstruction
    - Continuous bladder irrigation
    - For hyponatremia as a result of absorption of bladder irrigating fluid
    - For urinary retention following catheter removal
  - Monitor for postoperative complications (infection, deep vein thrombosis, pulmonary embolism, hemorrhage).
  - Assess for anxiety and fear about effects of surgery or medications on sexual functioning.
- **Nursing Activities:**
  - Encourage client to void when urge occurs.
  - Instruct client to drink 2500-3000 mL of fluid a day or as directed by physician.
  - Instruct client to avoid drinking large quantities of fluid over a short time period.
  - Discuss alternative/complementary therapies with client if appropriate. Advise client to speak with primary care provider before trying alternative treatments.
  - Educate client to use alcohol, caffeinated beverages, and spicy foods in moderation.
  - Teach client to avoid medications that can cause urinary retention, such as anticholinergics, antihistamines, and decongestants.

- Insert urinary catheter to drain bladder if ordered.
- Provide routine preoperative and postoperative care if surgery is performed.
  - Maintain urinary drainage system following surgery.
  - If bleeding occurs, arrange for blood component therapy as ordered.
  - Remind client to keep his leg straight if catheter is taped to his thigh.
  - Remove indwelling catheter when ordered.
- Make appointments for follow-up visit with primary care provider or nurse practitioner.
- Advise client to contact primary health care provider if urine appears bloody.
- Advise client to avoid strenuous activities, driving, working, prolonged periods of travel, stair climbing, and sexual activity until surgeon approves these activities.
- Advise client not to strain while having bowel movements and to take stool softeners as ordered.
- Teach client to perform Kegel exercises to establish urinary control.
- Suggest sexual counseling if the client experiences erectile dysfunction and disruptions of sexual activities.

Pharmacology

- Alpha-adrenergic blockers to decrease muscle tone and improve voiding: prazosin, terazosin, tamsulosin, doxazosin, alfuzosin – contraindicated with clients using vardenafil for erectile dysfunction!
- Testosterone ablating agents to cause androgen deprivation: finasteride, dutasteride; (turosteride, flutamide, leuprolide are rarely used)
- Androgen inhibitors which reduce the size of the prostate gland: finasteride (Proscar)
- Antispasmodics for bladder spasms
- Pain medications: opioid and nonopioid
- Stool softeners: docusate (Colace)
- Antibiotics: clotrimazole (Mycelex)
- Extract of saw palmetto (Serenoa repens) which is an alternative antiandrogen herb, similar to finasteride in efficacy
- Laser therapy
- Microwave hyperthermia
- Cryotherapy

Complications

- Acute urinary retention
- Urinary reflux
- Infection
- Dilation of the ureters and kidney

- Postoperative complications
- Sexual dysfunction

Age-Related Changes—Gerontological Considerations

- 50% of males develop some degree of BPH by age 60.
- 90% of males develop microscopic evidence of BPH by age 85.
- 25% of males in the U.S. will have symptoms severe enough to require intervention by age 80.
- When caring for elderly client who may be disoriented, reorient the client frequently and remind the client not to pull on the catheter.
- Ask family to provide client with a family picture that he can hold on to for a feeling of security.
- Avoid restraining disoriented elderly clients if possible.
- Monitor older clients for signs of infection following surgery because existing conditions may compromise their immune system and lower resistance to microorganisms.
- Assess older clients following surgery for pneumonia and other complications of immobility. Have client turn, cough, deep breathe, and ambulate as soon as possible.

Critical Thinking Exercise: Nursing Management of the Client with Benign Prostatic Hypertrophy (BPH)

Situation: A 70-year-old male is being admitted to the surgical unit to undergo a TURP (transurethral resection of the prostate). The client has been experiencing dysuria, urgency, and nocturia for over a year.

1. What is the most common surgery for BPH and how is it performed?

2. Describe the other major surgeries for BPH.

   Suprapubic prostatectomy:

   Retropubic prostatectomy:

   Preinial prostatecomy:

3. Why are alpha-blocking agents administered to clients with BPH?

4. As the prostate enlarges, there is a danger of complete urinary obstruction and retention. What are the precipitating factors that may lead to retention?

Nursing Management of the Client with a Transurethral Resection of the Prostate (TURP)

Key Points

- Transurethral resection of the prostate (TURP) does not involve an external incision and results in fewer complications.
- A TURP is performed by inserting a resectoscope through the urethra in order to remove a small amount of prostate tissue.
- TURP is the procedure of choice for debilitated clients who are poor risks for major surgery.
- TURP is a relatively low-risk procedure, and the outcome is excellent for 80% to 90% of clients.
- Goals of collaborative management:
  - Re-establish urinary function.
  - Prevent bladder spasms.
  - Prevent bleeding or hemorrhage.
  - Promote fluid and electrolyte balance.
  - Prevent postoperative complications.
  - Teach home catheter care if client is discharged with catheter in place.
- Important nursing diagnoses (actual or potential):
  - Pain management
  - Urinary retention
  - Altered urinary elimination
  - Urge incontinence
  - Risk of infection
  - Impaired skin integrity
  - Ineffective management of therapeutic regimen
  - Anxiety
- **Key Terms/Concepts:** Benign prostatic hyperplasia, urinary function, urinary retention, urethral obstruction, indwelling catheter, urinary drainage system, catheter traction, bladder spasms, urinary bleeding and clots, Kegel exercises

Overview

Transurethral resection of the prostate (TURP) is indicated for small, well-defined tumors; benign tumors of the prostate; and benign prostatic hypertrophy (BPH) or hyperplasia. The surgery involves the removal of only the tissue that is causing bladder neck obstruction and blocking the urethra.

Risk Factors

- BPH (benign prostatic hypertrophy)
- Bladder neck obstruction
- Obstruction of urethra
- Impeded urinary outflow
- Urinary reflux

Signs and Symptoms Necessitating Surgery

- Difficulty initiating urinary stream
- Hesitancy
- Straining to urinate
- Dysuria
- Incomplete emptying of bladder
- Decreased force of urine stream

Diagnostic and Laboratory Tests

- History and physical examination
- Complete blood count (CBC) and differential
- Urinalysis
- Urine culture
- Digital rectal examination (DRE)
- Blood urea nitrogen (BUN)
- Creatinine
- Prostatic acid phosphatase (PAP); also called: serum acid phosphatase
- Prostate specific antigen (PSA); also called: Total PSA or Free PSA
- Urodynamic flow studies
- X-ray studies of the kidneys, ureters, and bladder (KUB)
- Intravenous pyelography (IVP)
- Ultrasound
  - 2-D (2-Dimensional)
  - 3-D (3-Dimensional)
  - Doppler
- Excretory urography

Therapeutic Nursing Management

- Prevention of BPH Symptoms:
  - Teach client to void immediately upon feeling the urge.
  - Instruct client to avoid the diuretic effects of alcohol.
  - Instruct client to avoid forcing a lot of fluids all at once.
  - Instruct client to avoid medications that can cause urinary retention such as anticholinergics, antihistamines, and decongestants.

- Encourage client to seek immediate treatment for urinary tract infections.
- Assess/Monitor (Postoperative Period):
  - Intake and output
  - Electrolyte levels
  - Vital signs
  - Lung sounds
  - Body temperature every 4 hours
  - Color and amount of urine every 2 hours
  - Three-way indwelling catheter and drainage system
  - Traction that surgeon may have applied to the catheter when first taped to client's thigh or abdomen
  - Continuous bladder irrigation (CBI)
  - Patency of the catheter
  - Urinary drainage for blood or clots
  - For urinary tract infection
  - For signs of deep vein thrombosis
  - Client following removal of catheter
- Nursing Activities (Postoperative Period):
  - Administer pain medications as prescribed.
  - Administer antispasmodic medications as prescribed for bladder spasms.
  - Perform bladder irrigation as prescribed.
  - Adjust the bladder irrigation flow rate to maintain a colorless or light pink drainage.
  - Notify the surgeon if color of the drainage is bright red with numerous clots, as this may signify arterial bleeding. The CBI rate may require adjustment.
  - Notify surgeon if color of the drainage is burgundy as this may signify venous bleeding.
  - Assist the surgeon with adjusting the traction on the catheter if necessary.
  - Keep catheter tubing from kinking or obstructing urine flow.
  - Notify the surgeon immediately if the catheter appears to be obstructed and the obstruction does not resolve with manual irrigation.
  - Encourage fluids.
  - Maintain strict asepsis of indwelling urinary catheter.
  - Encourage perineal or Kegel exercises.
  - Teach client who is being discharged with an indwelling catheter appropriate catheter care. Instruct the client to:
    - Thoroughly wash hands before initiating catheter care.
    - Use aseptic technique.
    - Monitor and record fluid intake and output.
    - Cleanse skin around the catheter gently.
    - Change the urinary drainage bag.
    - Report a fever or cloudy urine as these symptoms may indicate infection.

- Following catheter removal, palpate bladder post-voiding for urinary retention and for client's ability to fully empty the bladder.
- Instruct client at discharge to:
    - Not lift anything heavier than 10 pounds.
    - Limit stair climbing.
    - Avoid driving until given permission by primary care physician.
    - Not strain when trying to have a bowel movement.
    - Take stool softeners daily.
    - Increase dietary fiber.
    - Drink between 2000 and 3000 mL of fluid every day, unless contraindicated.
    - Avoid sexual activity until surgeon gives permission.
    - Limit alcohol and caffeinated beverages.
    - Observe for blood in the urine, and to notify surgeon if bleeding continues.

Pharmacology

- Pain medications (opioids)
- Intravenous infusion
- Antibiotics (for surgical prophylaxis)
- Antispasmodics (flavoxate, propantheline)
- Stool softeners (docusate sodium)

Complications

- Infection
- Urinary strictures
- Urinary retention
- Urinary obstruction
- Bleeding or hemorrhage

Age-Related Changes—Gerontological Considerations

- Aging increases the risk of developing BPH.
- TURP is primarily used to treat BPH in older clients.
- Following TURP, remind elderly clients to not disturb catheter or other tubing.
- Older clients with renal disease or congestive heart failure may not be able to tolerate a large daily fluid intake, and fluid requirements will need to be lowered.

Critical Thinking Exercise: Nursing Management of the Client with a Transurethral Resection of the Prostate (TURP)

Situation: A 70-year-old client with BPH has been discharged home with an indwelling catheter following a TURP. Prior to discharge, the nurse carefully instructed the client and his wife on the way to care for the catheter and drainage system.

1. Which important points does the nurse need to teach the client and his wife about home catheter care?

   _____ Wash hands thoroughly prior to caring for the catheter.

   _____ Use clean technique when caring for the catheter.

   _____ Securely tape the catheter to his penis.

   _____ How to irrigate the catheter

   _____ How to change the catheter

   _____ Monitor and record fluid intake and output.

   _____ Keep the area around the catheter clean.

2. Which instructions should the client be given about his surgery and recovery?

   _____ He should avoid heavy lifting (> 10 lb or 4.5 kg).

   _____ He can take car trips no further than 500 miles.

   _____ Stair climbing and driving short distances are okay.

   _____ Sexual activity should be avoided until approved by the physician.

   _____ Take a daily stool softener.

3. Which two complications is the client most at risk for developing within the first week postoperatively?

4. What is the rationale for advising the client to increase his intake of fiber and drink 2000-3000 mL of fluid per day?

Nursing Management of the Client with a Radical Prostatectomy

Key Points

- Radical prostatectomy is performed using either a suprapubic, perineal, or retropubic incision.
- Radical prostatectomy has a 50% to 90% chance of resulting in erectile dysfunction.
- Radical prostatectomy may be followed by bilateral orchiectomy.
- Best candidates for radical prostatectomy have a discrete tumor involving less than one lobe (e.g., stage B-1), and a life expectancy of at least 10 years.
- Surgical removal of the prostate is also usually performed with a favorable prognosis in males having stage B-2 or C tumors.
- Use of the perineal approach during radical prostatectomy is associated with a high risk of impotency.
- For younger clients, a nerve-sparing procedure may be used to try to prevent erectile dysfunction.
- Artificial urinary sphincters (AUS) may be implanted in clients with refractory postoperative urinary incontinence.
- An AUS is a fluid-filled system composed of a silicone rubber cuff that encircles the urethra, and a synthetic pump implanted into the scrotum via an abdominal incision.
- Goals of collaborative management:
  - Prepare the client for possibility of erectile dysfunction.
  - Prepare client for some degree of urinary incontinence following surgery.
  - Remove the existing cancer.
  - Control pain.
  - Prevent skin breakdown.
  - Prevent postoperative complications.
  - Emotionally support the client and family.
  - Correct fluid volume disturbances.
  - Prevent recurrence of cancer.
  - Prepare the client for the possibility of infertility following surgery and refer the client to counseling if necessary.
- Important nursing diagnoses (actual or potential):
  - Pain management
  - Risk of infection
  - Urinary retention

- Altered urinary elimination
- Impaired skin integrity
- Anxiety and fear
- Ineffective individual or family coping
- Altered sexuality patterns
- Sexual dysfunction
- **Key Terms/Concepts:** Prostate gland, seminal vesicles, regional pelvic lymph nodes, perineal approach, erectile dysfunction, sexual dysfunction, incontinence, artificial urinary sphincter (AUS)

Overview

Radical prostatectomy, which is indicated for prostate cancer, involves the complete removal of the prostate gland, seminal vesicles, and regional pelvic lymph nodes. Prostate cancer rarely produces symptoms until it is well advanced.

Risk Factors/Indications for Surgery

- Cancer of the prostate gland
- Cancer not controlled by hormonal therapy, radiotherapy, or chemotherapy

Signs and Symptoms Indicating Need for Surgery

- Stony, hard, fixed lesion in substance of gland or in posterior lobe
- Weight loss
- Dysuria
- Urinary retention
- Decreased size and force of urinary stream
- Rectal pressure or obstruction
- Pain in lower back or leg (due to metastases)
- Painful ejaculation

Diagnostic and Laboratory Tests

- History and physical examination
- History of urinary function
- Digital rectal examination (DRE)
- Complete blood count (CBC) and differential
- Urinalysis
- Biopsy of prostate gland
- Magnetic resonance imaging (MRI)
- Computer tomography (CT)/computed axial tomography (CAT) scan
- Ultrasound (transrectal)
  - 2-D (2-dimensional)
  - 3-D (3-dimensional)
  - Doppler

- Prostatic acid phosphatase (PAP); also called: serum acid phosphatase
- Prostate specific antigen (PSA); also called: Total PSA or Free PSA
- Alkaline phosphatase (ALP); also called: ALK Phos
- Excretory urography

Therapeutic Nursing Management

- **Prevention of Postoperative Complications and Problems:**
  - Reduce anxiety prior to surgery.
  - Explain surgical procedure and urinary drainage system.
  - Prepare client and significant other for possibility of sexual dysfunction following surgery.
  - Provide emotional support to client and family, especially when prognosis is unfavorable.
  - Encourage client to verbalize feelings regarding possible surgical outcomes (incontinence, impotence).
  - Explain that client may require an artificial urinary sphincter (AUS) for refractory postoperative urinary incontinence.
  - Encourage client to discuss feelings and concerns prior to surgery.
- **Assess/Monitor (Postoperative Period):**
  - Intake and output
  - Vital signs
  - For blood loss
  - Catheter drainage for bleeding or clots
  - For urinary tract infection
  - For epididymitis
  - For deep vein thrombosis and pulmonary embolism
- **Nursing Activities (Postoperative Period):**
  - Administer pain medications as prescribed.
  - Apply antiembolism stockings or pneumatic hose or other antithrombotic devices.
  - Maintain strict asepsis of indwelling urinary catheter.
  - Force fluids.
  - Perform bladder irrigation as prescribed.
  - Provide skin care to prevent breakdown.
  - Change dressing as needed using aseptic technique.
  - Clean area thoroughly after bowel movements if client has a perineal incision.
  - Use double-tailed T-binder or mesh pants to secure dressing for perineal incision.
  - Encourage perineal exercises within 24 to 48 hours after surgery.
  - Teach client who is being discharged with an indwelling catheter appropriate care.
  - Do not take rectal temperatures or give enemas.

- Instruct client regarding hormonal therapy following surgery.
- Instruct client to not sit for prolonged periods of time.
- Emphasize that client should not use Valsalva's maneuver as it increases venous pressure and can cause bleeding.
- Advise client to avoid long car trips and high-impact exercise.
- Advise client to drink sufficient amounts of water.
- Refer client to community cancer support group.
- Refer client for sexual counseling if needed.
- Encourage client who continues to be incontinent to discuss implantation of an artificial urinary sphincter (AUS) with the surgeon.

Pharmacology

- Estrogen replacement therapy
- Testosterone ablating agents to cause androgen deprivation: finasteride, dutasteride; (turosteride, flutamide, leuprolide are rarely used)
- Chemotherapy: vinblastine (Velban), mitomycin (Mutamycin)
- Radiation therapy

Complications

- Erectile dysfunction
- Impotence
- Incontinence
- Hemorrhage
- Infection
- Catheter obstruction
- Metastasis to bone, lymph nodes, brain, and lungs
- Mechanical failures
- Erosion of the urethra

Age-Related Changes—Gerontological Considerations

- Elderly males are at an increased risk for prostatic cancer.
- Elderly clients are at increased risk of postoperative complications following radical prostatectomy.

Critical Thinking Exercise: Nursing Management of the Client with a Radical Prostatectomy

Situation: A 65-year-old male client who was diagnosed with a grade C prostate tumor has undergone a radical prostatectomy using a perineal approach. The client is now being prepared for discharge from the hospital. The client is concerned about erectile dysfunction. The client also has some degree of urinary incontinence. If urinary incontinence continues, the client will be evaluated for implantation of an AUS (artificial urinary sphincter).

1. The perineal approach to radical prostatectomy places the client at increased risk for which complications?

   _____ Infection   _____ Impotency   _____ Fecal incontinence

   _____ Urinary incontinence   _____ Erectile dysfunction   _____ Hemorrhage

2. Prioritize nursing activities for this client, with "1" representing the most important activity.

   _____ Instruct client regarding hormonal therapy.

   _____ Change dressing when soiled.

   _____ Provide skin care to prevent breakdown.

   _____ Administer pain medication as prescribed.

3. Why is the client taught to avoid these activities for the first two months following radical prostatectomy?

   a. Valsalva maneuver during bowel movements:

   b. Strenuous activities:

   c. Long motor trips or prolonged sitting:

4. What is an AUS (artificial urinary sphincter), and why is it used?

Nursing Management of the Menopausal Client Receiving Hormone Replacement Therapy (HRT)

| Key Points |

- HRT can only be recommended on an individual basis, generally less than 5 years, and contraindicated in certain situations. HRT is not indicated for prophylaxis of heart disease and generally is not prescribed for women at high risk for heart disease.

- Hormone replacement therapy (HRT) is prescribed to help control symptoms associated with menopause.

- Menopause is defined as the cessation of menses and the following twelve months. The average age of menopause is 51.3 years, although perimenopausal symptoms can occur over ten or more years.

- Estrogen replacement therapy (ERT) may also be prescribed following a hysterectomy; however, cautious use is indicated for those with cardiac disease. ERT is used to treat male clients with prostate cancer.

- HRT might be recommended for women with moderately severe to severe peri- or postmenopausal symptoms. It is suggested that women with severe genitourinary symptoms use topical estrogen, rather than oral compounds. Women who are at significant risk for osteoporosis, and in whom non-hormonal treatments are inappropriate or contraindicated, commonly utilize HRT for osteoporosis.

- HRT can increase the risk of venous thrombosis, heart disease (including risk of myocardial infarction in the first year of therapy), stroke, pulmonary embolism, and breast cancer.

- In women with an intact uterus, estrogen is typically prescribed with a progestin or progesterone in order to prevent endometrial hyperplasia and possible uterine cancer.

- HRT can be prescribed cyclically (mimicking a woman's monthly cycle) or continuously. Some women prefer not to have menses and thus, prefer continuous therapy.

- Bio-identical hormone replacement therapy or natural hormone replacement therapy use plant-based estrogen, progesterone, DHEA, and testosterone hormones in an attempt to fine-tune a woman's hormonal issues. Unlike synthetic hormones, or those derived from horse urine, these plant-based hormones are manipulated to be the exact same molecular configuration as the woman's endogenous hormones. Female estrogens; estriol, estradiol, and estrone, can be replaced in varying amounts. Some women are choosing this form of treatment to reduce the severity and/or duration of perimenopausal symptoms. However, it should be noted more prospective studies regarding efficacy of this treatment are indicated.

- Goals of collaborative management:
  - Carefully screen and select clients who will benefit from HRT; where the benefit ratio outweighs the risk ratio.
  - Identify clients for whom HRT is contraindicated.
  - Educate client about the advantages and disadvantages of HRT.
  - Prevent complications from HRT.
- Important nursing diagnoses (actual or potential) are:
  - Ineffective management of therapeutic program
- **Key Terms/Concepts:** Menopause, estrogen, progesterone, estrogen implant, vaginal rings, depot injections, estrogen patches, bio-identical hormones (troches, gels, suppositories, micronized capsules), atrophic vaginitis, atherosclerosis, uterine cancer, osteoporosis, venous thrombosis

Overview

Hormone replacement therapy (HRT), in the broadest sense, is the administration of a natural or synthetic hormone to treat a hormone deficiency.

Menopause is the stage of a gradual biological process during which the ovaries reduce their production of the female hormones estrogen and progesterone. This stage starts about 3 to 5 years before the final menstrual period. This transitional phase is called perimenopause. Menopause is considered complete when a woman has been without periods for one year, which usually occurs around 51.3 years. Many women experience menopause around the same age as their mothers did.

Risk Factors (Contraindications for HRT)

- Heart disease or at high risk for heart disease
- Cancer of the breast
- Cancer of the uterus
- Heavy smoking
- Stroke
- Liver disease
- Severe hypertension
- History of thrombophlebitis
- Pregnancy
- Gallbladder disease
- Undiagnosed abnormal vaginal bleeding

Signs and Symptoms (Side Effects of HRT)

- Breast tenderness and enlargement
- Edema
- Bloating
- Vaginal bleeding
- Leg cramps

- Nausea
- Fatigue
- Chest pain
- Severe headache
- Visual disturbances
- Chloasma (pigmented skin discolorations)
- Venous thrombosis, especially during the first year of therapy
- Myocardial infarction, especially during the first year of therapy
- Heart disease
- Stroke
- Pulmonary embolism
- Breast cancer

Diagnostic and Laboratory Tests

- History and physical exam
- Weight
- Blood pressure checks
- Pelvic examination with PAP smear
- Breast examination with mammogram
- Biopsy of uterine lining in cases of undiagnosed abnormal uterine bleeding in a woman over 40 years old or in whom menses has stopped for a year, and bleeding begins again
- FSH, if needed to confirm menopause
- Blood, urine, saliva hormone levels (estrogens, progesterone, DHEA-S, testosterone)
- Bone mass measurements to confirm the presence of osteopenia/osteoporosis

Therapeutic Nursing Management

- **Prevention of Age-Related Problems**:
    - Osteoporosis
    - Atrophic vaginitis which is characterized by vaginal burning and bleeding, pruritus, and painful intercourse
    - Atherosclerosis
- **Assess/Monitor**:
    - Side effects from HRT
    - For increased blood pressure
    - For increased weight due to fluid retention
    - For breast lumps or abnormalities
    - For vaginal bleeding
    - For venous thrombosis
    - For symptoms of heart or cerebrovascular disease

- **Nursing Activities:**
  - Instruct client in advantages and disadvantages of HRT.
  - Instruct client in self-administration of HRT.
  - Advise client to immediately quit smoking.
  - Teach the client how to prevent and assess the development of venous thrombosis.
    - Avoid wearing constricting socks.
    - Avoid wearing knee-high stockings.
    - Note and report symptoms of leg pain.
    - Note and report unilateral leg edema.
    - Note and report whether skin of affected extremity is warm, red, or tender.
    - Avoid sitting for long periods of time.
    - Take short walks throughout the day to promote circulation.
    - Do frequent ankle pumps and move and stretch legs.
  - Schedule annual physical, pelvic examinations, and mammograms.
  - Schedule bone density tests when ordered.
  - Instruct client on atypical presentation of myocardial infarction signs and symptoms in women, such as abdominal pain, vague chest symptoms, arm pain, leg swelling, etc. and to seek assistance immediately.
  - If using vaginal creams or suppositories of estrogen compounds, be sure to refrain from inserting prior to intercourse, or partner may absorb some of product.

Pharmacology

- Estrogen
  - Conjugated from horse urine, synthetic, bio-identical
  - Estradiol, estriol, estrone
  - Forms: oral tablets, vaginal creams and suppositories, vaginal rings, intramuscular depots, transdermal gels, transdermal patches, micronized capsules
- Progesterone
  - Synthetic and bio-identical. Note that Prometrium (micronized progesterone) is made form peanuts, so women with peanut allergies should not use.
  - Only synthetic progesterone is found in combination with estrogen product (Estratest).
  - Bio-identical in forms via same as progesterone and only available via a compounding pharmacy.
- Combination drugs

Complications

- Myocardial infarction
- Stroke

- Pulmonary embolism
- Breast cancer
- Uterine cancer
- Venous thrombosis

Age-Related Changes—Gerontological Considerations

- Based on current findings, most women are not candidates for HRT or should only consider HRT during the first 5 years of menopause (the early 50s) to help erase moderately severe to severe symptoms, such as hot flashes.
- Older clients can also decrease the risk of osteoporosis by performing regular weight-bearing exercises, increasing intake of high-protein and high-calcium foods, avoiding alcohol, caffeine, and tobacco, and taking calcium with vitamin D supplements.

Critical Thinking Exercise: Nursing Management of the Menopausal Client Receiving Hormone Replacement Therapy (HRT)

Situation: A 45-year-old client has been experiencing irregular menstrual periods, hot flashes, and night sweats. After a thorough history and physical, the primary care provider recommends HRT. First, the primary care provider schedules the client for a conference with the nurse practitioner who discusses the advantages and disadvantages of HRT.

1. What are the major advantages of HRT?

2. What are the major disadvantages of HRT?

3. What are the causes and symptoms of atrophic vaginitis, and how is it treated?

Nursing Management of the Client with a Cystocele and/or Rectocele

Key Points

- A cystocele or rectocele develops when structures that support the bladder or rectum are injured, usually during vaginal childbirth.
- The exact incidence of cystocele and rectocele is unknown, although the majority of women who have had vaginal birth experience these defects to some degree.
- Cystocele and rectocele may also develop in women who have never experienced childbirth.
- A non-surgical option for treatment of cystocele is a pessary.
- A pessary is a doughnut-shaped object, which the client inserts into her vagina to help hold the bladder in place.
- Surgery for severe cystocele is called anterior colporrhaphy or anterior repair.
- Surgery for severe rectocele is called posterior colporrhaphy or posterior repair.
- Surgery for combined cystocele and rectocele is called an anterior/posterior repair.
- Goals of collaborative management:
    - Treat with conservative medical interventions initially.
    - Perform surgical repair if conservative measures fail.
    - Prevent infection and other complications of surgery.
    - Instruct clients in self-care following surgery.
- Important nursing diagnoses (actual or potential):
    - Risk for infection
    - Constipation
    - Bowel and/or bladder incontinence
    - Altered urinary elimination
    - Stress incontinence
    - Urinary retention
    - Pain
    - Impaired tissue integrity
- **Key Terms/Concepts:** Hormone replacement therapy, pessary, anterior colporrhaphy, anterior repair, posterior colporrhaphy, posterior repair, anterior/posterior repair

Overview

Cystocele is the protrusion or herniation of the bladder downward through the vaginal wall.

Rectocele is the protrusion or herniation of the rectum through the vaginal wall.

Risk Factors

- Vaginal childbirth
- Multiple births
- Difficult childbirth with lacerations
- Obesity
- Over 35 years of age
- Congenital defects of supporting tissues
- Loss of estrogen after menopause
- Atrophic vaginitis
- Chronic constipation
- Large fibroid tumors
- Chronic lung conditions that result in excessive coughing (e.g., chronic bronchitis)

Signs and Symptoms

- Asymptomatic for many clients
- Low backache
- Difficult sexual intercourse
- Cystocele
    - Urinary frequency
    - Difficulty voiding
    - Urinary retention
    - Urinary incontinence
    - Urinary tract infection (UTI) with burning and frequency
    - Feeling of vaginal fullness
    - Urinary leakage
    - Difficult sexual intercourse
    - Bladder protrudes down into vagina or outside of vagina
- Rectocele
    - Constipation
    - Low back pain
    - Flatus
    - Fecal incontinence
    - Feeling of rectal fullness
    - Feeling of vaginal fullness
    - Difficulty evacuating bowels

Diagnostic and Laboratory Tests

- History and physical examination
- Pelvic examination
- Ultrasound

- 2-D (2-dimensional)
- 3-D (3-dimensional)
- Catheterization for residual urine

Therapeutic Nursing Management

- **Prevention**:
  - Avoid traumatic vaginal childbirth with an early and adequate episiotomy.
  - Encourage routine pelvic and physical examinations.
  - Inform client of advantages and risks to prevent atrophic vaginitis and prolapse.
  - Advise clients at risk to lose weight if obese.
  - Instruct clients to eat a high-fiber diet and drink adequate fluids to prevent constipation.
- **Assess/Monitor**:
  - For urinary retention
  - For urinary incontinence
  - For constipation
  - For fecal incontinence
  - For pain
  - For signs of urinary tract infection
  - Postoperative status
  - Vital signs following surgery
  - Intake and output following surgery
  - For postoperative complications (shock, hemorrhage, pulmonary complications)
  - Indwelling catheter patency and drainage
  - Client's ability to perform CISC (clean intermittent self-catheterization)
  - For complications related to catheterization (urinary tract infection, retention, obstruction, and trauma)
  - For constipation or straining at stool following surgery
- **Nursing Actions**:
  - Explain the cause of a cystocele or rectocele.
  - Instruct the client how to insert and care for a pessary.
  - Arrange for an appointment with the health care provider 3 days following initial insertion of a pessary, and then make appointments for re-examination every 6 weeks thereafter.
  - Instruct client with a pessary to report vaginal discomfort, vaginal itching, changes in the amount, color, or consistency of vaginal discharge, or if the pessary falls out.
  - Teach the client how to perform Kegel exercises to strengthen the urinary sphincter. Instruct the client to squeeze the muscles that control defecation and urination together, hold for 5 seconds, and repeat this exercise throughout the day.

- Explain electrostimulation therapy, which is used to stimulate pelvic floor muscle contractions.
- Instruct the client with a rectocele to eat a high-fiber diet.
- Provide routine postoperative care following an anterior/posterior repair.
- Administer analgesics as needed.
- Administer antibiotics as ordered.
- Provide perineal care at least twice daily following surgery, and after every urination or bowel movement.
- Apply an ice pack to the perineal area to relieve pain and swelling.
- Provide a liquid diet immediately following surgery followed by a low-residue diet until normal bowel function returns.
- Instruct the client in how to care for an indwelling catheter at home following surgery.
- Remind client to thoroughly wash her hands before and after handling the catheter and to remove any crust or debris that has collected around the catheter.
- Recommend that the client drink at least 2000 mL of fluid daily, unless contraindicated.
- Following removal of the catheter, instruct client to void every 2 to 3 hours to prevent a full bladder and stress on stitches.
- Teach the client how to perform clean intermittent self-catheterization (CISC) techniques in the event that the client is unable to void.
- Instruct the client to:
  - Assume a comfortable position.
  - Separate the labial folds with the thumb and mid-finger of the nondominant hand.
  - Wash perineal area from front toward the anus.
  - Keep labial folds separated and insert catheter into the urinary meatus.
  - Allow urine to flow until flow stops.
  - Remove catheter slowly.
- Instruct the client to keep catheter clean, wash it carefully, and store it in a clean container after each use.
- Remind the client that CISC is only a temporary measure while she heals following surgery.
- Caution client to avoid straining at defecation, sneezing, coughing, lifting, and prolonged sitting, walking or standing following surgery.
- Instruct client to tighten and support pelvic muscle when coughing or sneezing.
- Advice client to avoid sexual intercourse until surgeon gives permission.
- Suggest that the client take frequent warm sitz baths to sooth the perineal area.
- Arrange for home care visits for the first 7 to 10 days following surgery as ordered.
- Schedule follow-up appointments with primary care provider or nurse practitioner.

Pharmacology

- Stool softeners: docusate sodium
- Laxatives: bisacodyl, or bulk-forming
- Vaginal cream
- Pessary
- Analgesics: (opiate and non-opiate)
- Antibiotics (for surgical prophylaxis and post-operative infections)

Complications

- Recurrent cystitis
- Fecal impaction
- Bowel obstruction
- Infection related to pessary
- Complications of surgery
- Wound infection
- Loss of vaginal sensation, which may last for several months
- Urinary tract infection (UTI) related to:
  - Foley catheter
  - Clean intermittent self-catheterization (CISC)
- Urinary retention

Age-Related Changes—Gerontological Considerations

- Cystocele and rectocele develop in older female clients, usually following menopause.
- Older clients tend to overuse laxatives and enemas for the relief of constipation.
- Older clients are at greater risk of complications following surgery.

Critical Thinking Exercise: Nursing Management of the Client with a Cystocele and/or Rectocele

Situation: A 65-year-old woman diagnosed with serious cystocele and rectocele is being discharged home with an indwelling catheter following an anterior/posterior repair. If the client has difficulty voiding following removal of the catheter, she will need to perform CISC (clean intermittent self-catheterization). For the two years previous to the surgery, the client attempted to control symptoms with the use of a pessary and Kegel exercises.

1. What instructions should the nurse provide the client who is wearing a pessary?

2. What instructions should the nurse provide to the client concerning Kegel exercises?

3. What measures can the client take to prevent UTI (urinary tract infection) related to the use of an indwelling catheter?

4. What instructions should the nurse provide to the client concerning CISC (clean intermittent self-catheterization)?

Nursing Management of the Client with a Hysterectomy

Key Points

- Hysterectomies are one of the most common surgeries experienced by women over the age of 50.
- Disorders that warrant surgical removal of the uterus (and other reproductive organs) include abnormal uterine bleeding; endometriosis; fibroid tumors; prolapse of the pelvic structures; or cancer of the uterus, cervix, fallopian tubes, or ovaries.
- Hysterectomies may be performed vaginally or abdominally through an incision.
- A vaginal hysterectomy may be performed with laparoscopic assistance, which reduces postoperative complications and recovery time.
- An abdominal hysterectomy is used for most malignant conditions or for more complex or larger benign tumors.
- A hysterectomy may be total, including removal of the ovaries; or partial, where the ovaries remain intact.
- Goals of collaborative management:
    - Correct underlying disease/problem that precipitated the need for hysterectomy.
    - Prevent complications such as infection, bleeding, urinary incontinence, paralytic ileus, and thromboembolism.
    - Prevent body image disturbances or relationship problems due to altered sexuality.
- Important nursing diagnoses (actual or potential):
    - Pain management
    - Activity intolerance
    - Knowledge deficit
    - Altered body image
    - Sexual dysfunction
    - Fear and anxiety
    - Risk for situational low self-esteem
    - Fatigue and restlessness
    - Ineffective individual coping
    - Decisional conflict
- **Key Terms/Concepts:** Dysfunctional uterine bleeding, vaginal hysterectomy, total abdominal hysterectomy, sterilization, Papanicolaou (PAP) test, hormone replacement therapy (HRT)

Overview

A hysterectomy is the surgical removal of the uterus and cervix, most often performed for cancer of the endometrium (uterus) or dysfunctional uterine bleeding. A total abdominal hysterectomy (TAH) involves removal of the uterus through a surgical opening in the abdomen. A vaginal hysterectomy involves removal of the uterus through the vagina. The recovery time following a vaginal hysterectomy is generally shorter than from an abdominal excision.

Risk Factors/Indications

- Dysfunctional uterine bleeding
- Uterine or cervical cancer
- Endometriosis
- Fibroid tumors
- Uterine rupture
- Uterine prolapse

Signs and Symptoms

- Symptoms of disorder indicating need for hysterectomy
- Anxiety related to impending surgery
- Fear of loss of self-worth, femininity, and/or ability to bear children
- Feelings of guilt, anger, or embarrassment regarding need for surgery

Diagnostic and Laboratory Tests

- History and physical examination
- Papanicolaou test (PAP) test (also called Pap smear)
- Colposcopy
- Endometrial or cervical biopsy
- Ultrasound
  - 2-D (2-dimensional)
  - 3-D (3-dimensional)
- Magnetic resonance imaging (MRI)
- Computer tomography (CT)/computed axial tomography (CAT) scan

Therapeutic Nursing Management

- Assess/Monitor:
  - Surgical dressing or vaginal packing for indications of postoperative bleeding
  - Intake and output
  - For pain
  - For decreased or absence of bowel sounds indicating intestinal obstruction and paralytic ileus
  - For abdominal distention

- For ability to urinate following removal of indwelling urinary catheter
- For urinary incontinence following removal of indwelling urinary catheter
- For Homans' sign, which is a rare diagnostic finding of venous thrombosis of the deep veins of the calf
- For anxiety or restlessness
- For signs of postoperative depression
- **Nursing Activities:**
  - Explore the client's feelings about the hysterectomy and possible sexual problems prior to surgery.
  - Suggest that the client discuss worries and concerns with the surgeon prior to the surgery.
  - Provide pain medication following surgery as prescribed.
  - Encourage deep breathing and frequent use of the incentive spirometer to prevent pneumonia following abdominal hysterectomy.
  - Teach client to splint the abdominal incision when coughing and deep breathing.
  - Insert a rectal tube if necessary to relief gastric distention and abdominal discomfort.
  - Provide emotional support to client and family.
  - Encourage verbalization of fears and concerns regarding hysterectomy.
  - Encourage ambulation and frequent changes of position to prevent thrombophlebitis.
  - Initiate leg exercises, antiembolism stockings, and early ambulation as prescribed.
  - Teach client regarding cessation of menstruation, to avoid sexual intercourse for 4 to 6 weeks, and to avoid heavy lifting for 6 to 8 weeks as prescribed.
  - Instruct client to report signs of urinary tract infection or urinary incontinence.
  - Advise the client to take her temperature daily for at least a week following discharge, and report any elevation in temperature over 100° F (37.8° C).
  - Encourage the client to perform Kegel exercises to increase pelvic floor muscle strength.
  - Teach client how to perform self-catheterization if indicated.
  - Remind client to drink adequate fluids and to add fiber to her diet to prevent constipation.
  - Refer the client to community support groups or sexual counseling as appropriate.
  - If the client is premenopausal and the ovaries have been removed and HRT is not expected, instruct the client regarding signs and symptoms of menopause and prevention or complications such as osteoporosis.

Pharmacology

- Hormone replacement therapy (HRT): estrogen replacement only – may not be recommended. Refer to chapter on hormone replacement therapy.

- Analgesics: (opiate and non-opiate)
- Antibiotics (for surgical prophylaxis or post-operative infection)

Complications

- Paralytic ileus
- Thrombophlebitis and pulmonary embolism
- Pneumonia
- Abdominal wound infection
- Urinary tract infection
- Urinary incontinence
- Constipation
- Body image disturbance
- Altered sexuality
- Depression

Age-Related Changes—Gerontological Considerations

- Hysterectomies are one of the most common surgeries experienced by women over the age of 50.
- Older clients are at increased risk for surgical complications following surgery, particularly if they have chronic coronary, respiratory, gastrointestinal, or renal disorders.

Critical Thinking Exercise: Nursing Management of the Client with a Hysterectomy

Situation: A 53-year-old woman just returned from the PACU (post-anesthesia care unit) after undergoing an abdominal hysterectomy and oophorectomy. Her vital signs are stable and her dressing is dry and intact. She is able to administer her own pain medication by means of a PCA (patient-controlled analgesia) pump.

1. What other essential assessments need to be made by the nurse?

_____ Vaginal drainage	_____ Abdominal distention
_____ Pupillary response	_____ Bowel sounds
_____ Urinary output	_____ Gag reflex
_____ Homan's sign	_____ Pain status

2. List two positive and two negative effects a hysterectomy can have on a woman's self-image.

3. Prioritize nursing activities for the client at this time, with "1" representing the most important activity.

_____ Assess effectiveness of prescribed pain medication.

_____ Provide emotional support to client and family.

_____ Encourage ambulation to the chair or bathroom.

_____ Encourage active leg exercises.

_____ Teach client regarding cessation of menstruation.

Nursing Management of the Client with an Ovarian Cyst

Key Points

- Ovarian cysts are classified as follicular cysts, corpus luteum cysts, theca lutein cysts, ruptured cysts, inflammatory cysts, and polycystic ovary (Stein-Leventhal syndrome).

- Stein-Leventhal syndrome can lead to endometrial hyperplasia and carcinoma, insulin resistance, infertility and cardiovascular disease. This syndrome is associated with obesity and hirsutism. This syndrome is more commonly known as Polycystic Ovarian Syndrome (PCOS) or Polycystic Ovarian Disease (PCOD).

- Ovarian cysts can develop in women of any age, but rarely do so after menopause.

- Ovarian cysts can contain large amounts of fluid as well as semi-solid material.

- Oral contraceptives are administered to suppress ovulation and shrinks cysts.

- Follicular cysts may disappear within 60 days without treatment.

- Some ovarian cysts may have to be surgically removed due to the pain and pressure they cause; or because the pedicle may become twisted, resulting in gangrene; or because of rupture, which can lead to hemorrhage and shock.

- Cystectomy rather than oophorectomy is the surgery of choice.

- Goals of collaborative management:
  - Give an accurate differential diagnosis.
  - Relieve pain.
  - Treat cause of cyst.
  - Provide preoperative and postoperative teaching.
  - Prevent complications.
  - Prevent depression, body image disturbances, and sexual problems (Stein-Leventhal syndrome).

- Important nursing diagnoses (actual or potential):
  - Pain
  - Risk for infection
  - Risk for altered body temperature
  - Body image disturbance (Stein-Leventhal syndrome)
  - Sexual dysfunction (Stein-Leventhal syndrome)
  - Ineffective management of therapeutic program

- **Key Terms/Concepts**: Follicular cysts, corpus luteum cysts, theca lutein cysts, Stein-Leventhal syndrome, ovarian cancer, oral contraceptives, antibiotics, cystectomy

Overview

An ovarian cyst is a nonmalignant sac that develops in the ovary, and consists of one or more fluid-containing chambers. Generally, ovarian cysts occur as a result of an egg being released during ovulation. Ovarian cysts must be differentiated from ovarian cancer.

Risk Factors/Indications

- Genetic predisposition with PCOS
- Ovulating female
- Hydatidiform mole for theca lutein cysts
- Gonorrhea for inflammatory cysts
- Excessive levels of LH (luteinizing hormone)

Signs and Symptoms

- Follicular cysts: asymptomatic unless cyst ruptures; rupture causes acute, severe pain (follicular cysts)
- Corpus luteum cysts: tenderness, dull ache low in the pelvic region, amenorrhea
- Ruptured cysts: fever, severe pain, leukocytosis, possible hemorrhage
- Theca lutein cysts: feeling of pelvic fullness
- Stein-Leventhal syndrome: obesity, irregular menses, dysfunctional uterine bleeding, amenorrhea, infertility, acne, and hirsutism

Diagnostic and Laboratory Tests

- History and physical exam
- History of menstrual periods
- Pregnancy history
- Pain assessment
- Urinalysis
- Complete blood count (CBC) and differential
- Human chorionic gonadotropin (HCG) levels (also referred to as: pregnancy test)
- Papanicolaou (PAP) test
- Bimanual and rectovaginal palpation
- Ultrasound (to rule out ovarian cancer)
  - 2-D (2-Dimensional)
  - 3-D (3-Dimensional)
- Laparoscopy (to rule out ovarian cancer)
- Abdominal radiograph (to rule out ovarian cancer)
- Cystectomy (to rule out ovarian cancer)

Therapeutic Nursing Management

- **Prevention:**
  - Routine pelvic and physical examinations
  - Prompt treatment of acute infections
  - Prompt treatment of gonorrhea
- **Assess/Monitor:**
  - For pain
  - For signs of infection
  - For abdominal or pelvic masses
  - Vital signs following cystectomy
  - General postoperative condition following cystectomy
- **Nursing Activities:**
  - Administer analgesics as needed.
  - Arrange for follow-up visits to monitor cyst size.
  - Apply moist heat to vulva to relieve pain.
  - Apply dry heat to abdomen to relieve pain.
  - Teach client relaxation exercises.
  - Provide preoperative and postoperative instructions if surgery is required. May be indicated for a cyst measuring greater than 2 cm or for a rupture with associated hemorrhage
  - Arrange for follow-up visits following surgery.
  - Arrange for counseling for women with Stein-Leventhal syndrome

Pharmacology

- Oral contraceptives
- Antibiotics (for surgical prophylaxis)
- Analgesics (opioid or nonopioid)
- Anti-androgen drugs (Stein-Leventhal syndrome), insulin sensitizers
- Fertility drugs for women desiring to become pregnant

Complications

- Infection
- Rupture of a cyst
- Infertility
- Hemorrhage
- Cyst recurrence
- Gangrene
- Endometrial hyperplasia (Stein-Leventhal syndrome)
- Carcinoma (Stein-Leventhal syndrome)
- Cardiovascular disease (Stein-Leventhal syndrome)
- Type 2 diabetes mellitus (Stein-Leventhal syndrome)

Age-Related Changes—Gerontological Considerations

- Ovarian cysts may develop at any age.
- Ovarian cysts are uncommon after menopause.

Critical Thinking Exercise: Nursing Management of the Client with an Ovarian Cyst

Situation: A 25-year old woman is visiting her health care provider because she has missed several menstrual periods. The client has also been experiencing lower abdominal pain and tenderness. Upon examination, the nurse practitioner finds a palpable pelvic mass. Following diagnostic tests, the client is diagnosed with a corpus luteum ovarian cyst.

1. What is the cause of a corpus luteum ovarian cyst?

1. A suspected ovarian cyst must be differentiated from what other female reproductive disorder?

1. What diagnostic tests are used to differentiate an ovarian cyst from a neoplasm?

Nursing Management of the Client with Ovarian Cancer

Key Points

- The exact etiology of ovarian cancer is unknown; however, the number of times of ovulation in a woman's lifetime seems to be a risk factor since ovarian cancer is more predominant in women with early onset menses, late onset menopause, nulliparity, and use of infertility agents. There is also a familial tendency and an association between risk of breast cancer and ovarian cancer and their BRCA-1 and BRCA-2 genes.

- 1 out of every 56 women is at risk of developing ovarian cancer; it is the leading cause of gynecological cancer death in women.

- Epithelial cancers occur between ages 40 to 75 years and germ cells in clients less than 20 years of age.

- There is an increased risk of ovarian cancer among women who are postmenopausal.

- There is some evidence that women who have taken birth control pills, have been pregnant, and have breastfed have a decreased risk of ovarian cancer. This evidence may indicate that lowering the number of cycles of ovulation reduces the risk of ovarian cancer.

- Women who have mutations of the BRCA genes (tumor suppressor genes that inhibit tumor growth) are at greater risk of ovarian cancer.

- Ovarian tumors are usually epithelial in nature.

- The most common ovarian tumor is serous adenocarcinoma, a type of cancer that grows and spreads rapidly.

- Survival rates are low because early diagnosis is difficult; survival rate has not changed in the past 60 years.

- Ovarian cancer usually does not present symptoms at an early stage, and consequently is not detected until the tumor causes pressure on other organs.

- The Papanicolaou (PAP) test is of limited value in diagnosing ovarian cancer because it produces abnormal results in only 20% to 30% of women who have a malignancy, and thus misses the diagnosis in 70% to 80% of cases. The PAP test is much more predictive in diagnosing cervical cancer. Currently, there is no accurate screening method for diagnosing ovarian cancer.

- Metastases may occur before the primary malignancy is diagnosed.

- Staging of ovarian cancer is determined at the time of exploratory laparotomy when the tumor is removed and examined by the pathologist. There are four stages:
  - Stage I: Cancer limited to the ovaries

- Stage II: Cancer involves one or both ovaries with pelvic extension to the uterus, fallopian tubes, or other pelvic tissues; ascites may develop which also contains malignant cells.
        - Stage III: Cancer involves both ovaries, and implants are found outside of the pelvis in the peritoneal cavity.
        - Stage IV: Cancer involves both ovaries, with direct metastasis to the liver or the lungs. Pleural effusion and parenchymal liver metastases may develop.
- Primary interventions are surgery, traditional chemotherapy, intraperitoneal chemotherapy, and pelvic and abdominal irradiation.
- Ovarian cancer is surgically managed with total abdominal hysterectomy with bilateral salpingo-oophorectomy (TAH-BSO), with tumor removal, and omentectomy (removal of the peritoneal lining).
- The surgery is followed with chemotherapy for 6 to 12 months to destroy any remaining cancer cells.
- Radiation therapy may be prescribed if the tumor does invade other organs. The use of intra-abdominal radioactive colloids is increasing survival rates. This radioactive agent is injected through a catheter that has been placed in the peritoneal cavity during surgery.
- Goals of collaborative management:
    - Diagnose and treat cancer early.
    - Reduce pain and discomfort.
    - Provide emotional support.
    - Prevent complications.
    - Assist client and family with anticipatory grieving process.
- Important nursing diagnoses (actual or potential):
    - Pain management
    - Risk of infection
    - Fluid volume imbalance
    - Urinary retention
    - Risk for injury
    - Fear and anxiety
    - Sleep pattern disturbances
    - Anticipatory grieving
    - Caregiver role strain
    - Ineffective individual/family coping
    - Fatigue and restlessness
    - Knowledge deficit
    - Ineffective management of therapeutic regimen
    - Self-care deficit
    - Altered nutrition: less than body requirements
    - Impaired skin integrity
- **Key Terms/Concepts**: Metastasis, serous adenocarcinoma, staging of cancer, total abdominal hysterectomy with bilateral salpingo-oophorectomy (TAH-BSO), omentectomy, chemotherapy, radiation therapy, intra-abdominal radioactive colloids

Overview

Ovarian cancer is a malignant tumor of the ovary. It is the leading cause of death from female reproductive system cancers, and it is the second most common gynecologic cancer.

Risk Factors/Indications

- Female gender
- Over 40 years of age
- Nulliparity or first pregnancy after 30 years old
- Family history of ovarian, breast, or colon cancer
- History of dysmenorrhea or heavy bleeding
- High-fat diet, possible
- Use of baby talc (possible risk)
- Hormone replacement therapy (HRT)
- Use of infertility drugs

Signs and Symptoms

- No symptoms or mild symptoms (early stage)
- Ascites (advanced stage)
- Pelvic masses (advanced stage)
- Indigestion
- Loss of appetite
- Dyspepsia
- Abdominal pain
- Abdominal bloating
- Urinary obstruction
- Heavy menstrual flow
- Premenstrual tension
- Dysfunctional uterine bleeding
- Bowel obstruction
- Urinary frequency and urgency
- Pleural effusion
- Painful feelings of pressure as tumor grows
- Painful intercourse

Diagnostic and Laboratory Tests

- History and physical examination
- Reproductive history
- Family history
- Papanicolaou test (also called Pap smear)
- Computer tomography(CT)/computed axial tomography (CAT) scan

- Ultrasound (vaginal and abdominal)
  - 2-D (2-Dimensional)
  - 3-D (3-Dimensional)
- Cancer antigen test (CA-125 antigen), better at measuring treatment than screening for presence of disease
- Exploratory surgery to establish clinical stage of tumor
- "Second look" surgical procedure following treatment to determine if there is a residual tumor, or if the cancer has been successfully treated.

Therapeutic Nursing Management

- **Prevention and Early Diagnosis:**
  - Promote cancer screening.
  - Obtain obstetric history and family history of breast/ovarian cancer to potentially identify those at risk.
  - Schedule routine pelvic examinations.
  - Schedule routine bimanual rectovaginal examinations, especially in women over 40.
  - Evaluate women over 40 years old with persistent gastrointestinal symptoms for ovarian cancer.
  - Encourage a low-fat diet.
- **Assess/Monitor:**
  - Nutritional status
  - Weight
  - Pain status
  - Laboratory data
  - Urinary frequency and urgency
  - Signs of urinary obstruction
  - Signs of bowel obstruction
  - Emotional status of client and family
  - Postoperative status
  - Vital signs
  - Abdominal incision
  - Postoperative complications: shock, hemorrhage, pulmonary complications
  - Infection
  - Side effects and toxic effects of chemotherapy
  - Side effects and toxic effects of radiation therapy
- **Nursing Actions:**
  - Promote adequate food and fluid intake.
  - Provide pain control.
  - Teach client regarding diagnostic tests.
  - Provide preoperative teaching and care.
  - Provide routine postoperative care.

- Change abdominal dressings as ordered.
- Provide pain relief as ordered.
- Prepare client for chemotherapy and radiation therapy.
- Prepare the client for the injection of an intra-abdominal radioactive agent into her abdomen through a catheter if prescribed. Advise the client that she will be turned in different positions - to the right, left, feet down, head down, prone, then supine - so that the radioactive agent is distributed throughout the peritoneal cavity.
- Relieve unpleasant side effects due to chemotherapy and/or radiation therapy.
- Encourage client to express feelings about the cancer and fears of death.
- Help client and family to develop coping strategies.
- Monitor client's progress through the stages of grief.
- Arrange for a visit with a survivor of ovarian cancer if possible.
- Provide information about cancer support groups.
- Provide information about hospice care when appropriate.

Pharmacology

- Nutritional supplements
- Enteral feeding
- Parenteral hyperalimentation (TPN)
- External radiation therapy
- Chemotherapy (paclitaxel [Taxol], cisplatin [Platinol], cyclophosphamide [Cytoxan], doxorubicin [Rubex], etoposide [Toposar])
- Chromic phosphate P 32 (a radiopharmaceutical agent) administered via intra-abdominal route
- Possible 5-fluorouracil
- Antiemetics

Complications

- Bowel obstruction
- Pleural effusion
- Cardiovascular collapse
- Sepsis
- Metastasis
- Death

Age-Related Changes—Gerontological Considerations

- Women who develop ovarian cancer are usually over 40 years old.
- Older clients are at greater risk of complications following surgery for cancer.

Critical Thinking Exercise: Nursing Management of the Client with Ovarian Cancer

Situation: A 62-year-old female client is being evaluated for possible ovarian cancer. She has been experiencing vague gastrointestinal symptoms and urinary urgency for several months. The physician has discovered a small pelvic mass and has ordered a group of diagnostic studies.

1. Why is a PAP (Papanicolaou) test of limited value in diagnosing ovarian cancer?

2. What is the purpose of exploratory surgery?

3. What are the stages of ovarian cancer?

4. What is the treatment of choice for clients with ovarian cancer?

Nursing Management of the Client with Cervical Cancer

Key Points

- The incidence of cervical cancer in situ is increasing and affecting a younger population than in the past.
- The mortality rate from cervical cancer has declined significantly with the widespread use of the Papanicolaou (PAP) test, especially with use of liquid-based preparations rather than fixed-slides and HPV (human papilloma virus) identification.
- Papanicolaou (PAP) tests are an effective screening tool for detecting the earliest changes associated with cervical cancer.
- Early detection of cervical cancer is crucial.
- Early cervical cancer is generally asymptomatic. Symptoms do not develop until the cancer has become invasive.
- Findings of a PAP smear are usually classified according to the Bethesda System of 2001 as follows:
  - Satisfactory for evaluation
  - Unsatisfactory for evaluation
  - Interpretation
    - Negative for intraepithelial lesion or malignancy
    - Other
    - Epithelial cell abnormalities
    - Squamous cell
    - Atypical squamous cells
    - Of undetermined significance (ASC-US)
    - Cannot exclude HSIL (ASC-H)
    - Low grade squamous intraepithelial lesion (LSIL) (HPV/mild dysplasia/ CIN 1)
    - High grade squamous intraepithelial lesion (HSIL) (moderate and severe dysplasia, CIS/CIN 2 and CIN 3)
    - Squamous cell carcinoma
    - Glandular cell
    - Atypical
    - Endocervical cells, NOS
    - Endometrial cells, NOS
    - Glandular cells, NOS
    - Atypical
    - Endocervical cells, favor neoplastic

- Glandular cells, favor neoplastic
- Endocervical adenocarcinoma, in situ
- Adenocarcinoma
- Endocervical
- Endometrial
- Extrauterine
- Not otherwise specified (NOS)
- Other malignant neoplasms

- The stages of cervical cancer are:

  - Stage 0 or carcinoma in situ (CIS): The cancer is present only in the top one or two layers of cells lining the cervix.
  - Stage I: The cancer is limited to the cervix, with different degrees of involvement related to depth and size of the invasion.
  - Stage II: Cancer extends beyond the cervix into the vagina and nearby areas, but is still confined to the pelvis.
  - Stage III: Cancer has extended to one or both pelvic walls, with vaginal, ureter, and/or kidney involvement.
  - Stage IV: Cancer has extended beyond the pelvis into the bladder or rectal mucosa and distant organs such as the lungs or the liver.

- Interventions that are often curative include conization, cryotherapy, laser ablations, or loop electrocautery excision procedure (LEEP).

- Conization is the surgery of choice for women who want to have children, and it is the definitive treatment for microinvasive cervical cancer. Conization is used for stage 0 cancer or carcinoma in situ.

- Cryotherapy is the freezing of abnormal tissue with nitrous oxide.

- LEEP is a procedure that can be performed in the physician's office with local anesthesia. An electrosurgical instrument is used to remove cervical tissues. Following LEEP, the pathologist can determine if surrounding tissues have been invaded by cancer cells.

- Clients with more extensive cancer may require a total abdominal hysterectomy or pelvic exenteration.

- Pelvic exenteration is a radical surgery that involves removing the uterus, ovaries, fallopian tubes, vagina, bladder, urethra, and pelvic lymph nodes. Sometimes the descending colon, rectum, and anal canal are also removed.

- Goals of collaborative management:

  - Set up screening programs for women at risk for cervical cancer.
  - Identify the cancer early.
  - Educate the client about treatment procedures and follow-up care.
  - Help the client control fears and anxieties concerning cancer and treatment.
  - Eliminate the cancer surgically.
  - Control pain.
  - Initiate chemotherapy or radiation as indicated.
  - Prevent complications (infection, bleeding).
  - Prevent and identify metastasis.

- Prevent recurrence of the cancer.
- Treat recurrences or advanced stages of cancer appropriately.
- Important nursing diagnoses (actual or potential):
  - Pain management
  - Activity intolerance
  - Knowledge deficit
  - Fatigue and restlessness
  - Fear and anxiety
  - Ineffective individual coping
  - Decisional conflict
- **Key Terms/Concepts**: Papanicolaou (PAP) test, in situ preinvasive cancer, dysplasia, staging of cancer, conization, cryotherapy, laser therapy, loop electrocautery excision procedure (LEEP), hysterectomy, pelvic exenteration

Overview

Cervical cancer is the most common carcinoma of the female reproductive system. Cervical cancer is classified according to the extent of the cancer's spread. The staging system is from Stage O, very localized and small, through Stage IV, most advanced stage with metastasis. Approximately 60% of cervical cancers are found in Stage I, 25% in Stage II, 10% in Stage III, and 5% in Stage IV.

Risk Factors

- Early sexual activity (before 18 years old)
- Multiple sexual partners, either self or male partner
- Male partner who had a female partner with cervical cancer
- Low economic status
- Hispanic, African-American, and Native American heritage
- Chronic inflammation
- Infection with human papilloma virus (HPV), associated in 90% of cases
- History of STDs (sexually transmitted diseases)
- Infection with HIV
- Cigarette smoking
- Immunosuppression
- Intrauterine exposure to DES (diethylstilbestrol) during pregnancy

Signs and Symptoms

- May be asymptomatic early in the disease process
- Postcoital spotting, vaginal discharge, spotting between periods
- Longer or heavier periods than usual
- Pain during sexual activity
- Watery, blood-tinged vaginal discharge
- Dark, foul-smelling vaginal discharge (later sign)

- Abdominal or pelvic pain
- Vaginal leakage of urine or feces
- Anorexia, weight loss
- Anemia
- Hematuria
- Rectal bleeding
- Pelvic, back, or leg pain or unilateral leg swelling (late sign)

Diagnostic and Laboratory Tests

- History and physical examination
- Papanicolaou (PAP) test (also called Pap smear)
- Internal pelvic examination and visualization of the cervix and vaginal wall using a speculum
- Colposcopy, if indicated
- Biopsy
- Endocervical curettage
- Cervical conization, if indicated
- Lymphangiography
- Cystography
- Magnetic resonance imaging (MRI)
- Computer tomography (CT)/computed axial tomography (CAT) scan
- Sigmoidoscopy
- CBC, for anemia

Therapeutic Nursing Management

- **Prevention**:
  - Avoid risk factors.
  - Schedule regular pelvic examinations that include a PAP test and are performed between menstrual periods. Clients should not use a vaginal deodorant or douche, or have sexual intercourse for 24 hours prior to the examination.
  - Start screening for cervical cancer around 3 years after initiating sexual intercourse, but no later than age 21.
  - Continue screening annually if exposed to DES before childbirth or HIV infection.
  - Schedule screening every 2 to 3 years starting at 30 years old if PAP test results are normal 3 times in a row.
- **Assess/Monitor**:
  - Intake and output
  - Vital signs
  - For bleeding and/or signs of bleeding
  - For vaginal discharge

- For pain
- For infection
- For changes in body image
- For depression
- For anxiety and concerns regarding sexual functioning
- **Nursing Activities:**
  - Treat and reverse anemia as indicated
  - Treat any pelvic, vaginal, or urinary tract infections.
  - Administer pain medications as prescribed.
  - Provide emotional support to client and family.
  - Prepare client for biopsy, cryosurgery, conization, laser therapy, loop electrocautery excision procedure (LEEP), radiation, or surgery as indicated.
  - Teach client signs and symptoms of infection.
  - Teach client regarding home care following special procedures (vaginal discharge, pain, avoiding douches, avoiding sexual intercourse, safety precautions, and post-radiation treatments).
  - Refer to community support group as appropriate.
  - Refer client to counseling if depressed or expresses concerns over sexuality.

Pharmacology

- Antineoplastic/chemotherapeutic agents: bleomycin (Blenoxane), vincristine (Oncovin), cisplatin (Platinol), mitomycin-c (Mutamycin), hydroxyurea, fluorouracil, carboplatin, etoposide, ifosfamide
- Radiation therapy
- Analgesics (opioid and nonopioid)
- Antiemetics

Complications

- Infection
- Severe bleeding
- Metastasis
- Complications from extensive surgeries, chemotherapy, or radiation therapy
- Death

Age-Related Changes—Gerontological Considerations

- Increased risk of cervical cancer occurs with advancing age
- Older clients are at an increased risk for surgical complications due to the presence of chronic heart, renal, gastrointestinal, or respiratory disorders.

Care of the Client with a Sealed Radiation Source

- Place the client in a private room with a private bath.
- Place a caution sign on the client's door.

- Organize nursing tasks to minimize exposure to the radiation source.
- Limit time to one-half hour per care provider per shift.
- Wear a shield to reduce the transmission of radiation.
- Limit visitors to one-half hour per day; visitors should be at least 6 feet from the source.
- Teach client they must stay in bed and as flat as possible to prevent dislodgement of the radioactive substance.
- Provide a room deodorizer because the destruction of cells due to the radiation may produce a foul-smelling vaginal discharge.
- Relieve symptoms of nausea, vomiting, and diarrhea if they develop.
- Teach client to select a low-residue diet to prevent abdominal distension.
- Advise client to report problems such as vaginal bleeding, cystitis, or phlebitis to the primary care physician.

Critical Thinking Exercise: Nursing Management of the Client with Cervical Cancer

Situation: A 33-year-old woman underwent a loop electrosurgical excision procedure (LEEP) for cervical cancer one week ago. Pathology reports confirmed the cancer was preinvasive and due to dysplasia. The client is greatly relieved, but understands she will have to maintain close follow-up care for the next few years.

1. Place a "**P**" in front of statements that are true for **Preinvasive** cervical carcinoma and an "**I**" in front of statements that are true for **Invasive** cervical carcinoma.

   _____ Abnormal cells within the lower third of cervical epithelium

   _____ Involves the basement membrane

   _____ Metastasis via the lymphatic system

   _____ Abnormal cells contained within full thickness epithelium

   _____ Has a 75%-90% cure rate if diagnosed and treated early

   _____ Directly spreads to adjacent pelvic structures

2. Prioritize the goals of collaborative care for the client with preinvasive cancer of the cervix, with "1" representing the most important goal.

   _____ Prevention of complications   _____ Surgical elimination of the cancer

   _____ Prevention of recurrence   _____ Absence of pain

3. Prioritize nursing activities to reduce the client's anxiety while waiting for diagnostic study results or treatment for carcinoma of the cervix, with "1" representing the most important activity.

   _____ Encourage the client to verbalize her fears and concerns.
   Verbalizing fears and concerns often reduces them.

   _____ Assess the client's feelings about having a hysterectomy.
   To determine the need for further intervention or different interventions; cannot assess the client's feelings unless the client verbalizes them.

   _____ Acknowledge the client's feelings.
   It is important to acknowledge feelings so the client will continue to share those feelings.

   _____ Establish a trusting relationship.
   Must be established before honest communication and client sharing will occur.

Nursing Management of the Client with Breast Disorders: Breast Cancer and Fibrocystic Breast Disease

Key Points

- Breast cancer is the most common cancer among women age 30 to 80, with a peak age of 45 to 65. Males, 1%, can also develop breast cancer.

- 65% of breast cancer cases occur after age 50 years. There is a 1 in 8 lifetime chance of a woman having breast cancer.

- Early detection of breast cancer is the key to effective treatment and longer survival rates.

- Some women detect breast cancers during their BSE (breast self-examinations), although there has been controversy lately about women performing BSE.

- The American Cancer Society (ACS) recommends an annual clinical breast examination (CBE) performed by a health care professional and an annual mammogram for women after age 40. From age 20-39, the ACS suggests having a CBE every 3 years and that all women over the age of 20 do BSE.

- An annual clinical breast exam and mammogram should be performed earlier for women at risk for breast cancer.

- Mammography is regarded as the primary standard for early detection of breast cancer, even before physical signs can be palpated.

- The majority of breast cancers occur in the upper, outer quadrant of the breast.

- Definitive diagnosis of breast cancer is made by biopsy of the suspected lesion.

- The hormonal receptivity of the tumor is identified from the biopsy using the estrogen and progesterone receptor assay. Postmenopausal women are more at risk for estrogen receptor positive or ER+ lesions.

- Staging of the cancer is performed to determine the best treatment approach and the prognosis.

- The stages of breast cancer are:
  - Stage I: Tumor smaller than 2 cm with 0 to 1 lymph node positive and no metastasis.
  - Stage II: Tumor 2 to 5 cm without involvement of lymph nodes.
  - Stage III: Tumor larger than 5 cm with no lymph node involvement; smaller than 2 cm with axillary node involvement; or 2 to 5 cm with supraclavicular or interclavicular node involvement.
  - Stage IV: Any size tumor with or without lymph node involvement, but presence of distant metastasis.

- The choice of treatment for cancer depends on the stage of the tumor, the size of the tumor, and nodal involvement.

- Surgical procedures for breast cancer include breast-conserving procedures like lumpectomy, wide excision or partial mastectomy, total mastectomy, modified radical mastectomy, radical mastectomy, and reconstructive surgery.
- Adjuvant radiation therapy is often prescribed following breast conservation surgery to prevent microscopic spread.
- Chemotherapy or hormonal therapy may be used after surgery, or if surgery is not an option.
- The most common sites of metastatic disease are the lungs, bones, brain, and liver.
- Fibrocystic breast disease (FBD) is a benign breast condition.
- FBD is the most common breast disorder found in women between the ages of 20 and 50.
- The symptoms of FBD often appear prior to menses and subside after a menstrual period.
- FBD generally disappears with menopause.
- Having FBD does not increase the chances of developing breast cancer.
- Goals of collaborative management:
  - Provide early recognition and treatment of breast cancer.
  - Eliminate the cancer by surgery, radiation, chemotherapy, or combination.
  - Provide management of pain.
  - Initiate chemotherapy or radiation therapy if indicated.
  - Prevent recurrence and complications (infection, bleeding, lymphedema, metastasis).
  - Prevent and treat depression and body image disturbances.
  - Provide care during breast reconstruction procedures.
  - Help client adapt to breast prosthesis if necessary.
- Control the symptoms of fibrocystic breast disease.
- Refer to resources, such as Reach to Recovery.
- Important nursing diagnoses (actual or potential):
  - Impaired skin integrity
  - Altered body image
  - Pain
  - Risk for infection
  - Decisional conflict
  - Fear and anxiety
  - Ineffective individual/family coping
  - Knowledge deficit
- **Key Terms/Concepts**: Adenocarcinoma, in situ, invasive, noninvasive, mammography, biopsy, hormonal receptivity, hormonal manipulation, staging, lumpectomy, mastectomy, reconstructive surgery, chemotherapy, radiation therapy, lymphedema, metastasis, breast prosthesis

Overview

Breast cancer is the abnormal proliferation of cells within the breast. There are several classifications of breast cancers based on location and histological appearance.

- **Adenocarcinoma** arises from epithelial cells. This term refers to any malignant tumor that originates in glandular tissue.
- **Infiltrating ductal carcinoma** involves breast parenchymal tissue. It is the most common type of breast cancer. This form of carcinoma develops in the epithelial cells that line the mammary ducts.
- **Intraductal carcinoma or Paget's disease** develops within the breast ducts. This condition is different from Paget's disease of the bone.
- **Noninvasive ductal carcinoma** develops and remains in the mammary ducts.
- **Ductal carcinoma** in situ is the most common type of noninvasive ductal carcinoma. It is usually detected through mammography, and is considered stage 0 breast cancer.
- **Invasive ductal carcinoma** develops in the intermediate ducts. This cancer can be palpated as a hard mass and it often infiltrates the axillary nodes.
- **Infiltrating lobular carcinoma** is a tumor that originates in the milk-producing glands or lobules of the breast, and invades the breast tissue. It accounts for around 10% of invasive breast cancers, and is more difficult to detect by mammogram than the ductal type.
- **Lobular carcinoma in situ** is rarely associated with invasive disease. It involves tumors of the glandular tissue lobes.
- Inflammatory carcinoma of the breast is a rare, rapidly growing tumor. The breast is painful, tender, and enlarged, with nipple retraction. Also the skin is reddened. This type of tumor spreads rapidly to other organs.

Treatment of breast cancer involves surgical removal of the cancer, chemotherapy, radiation therapy, and/or hormonal therapy. Surgical removal of breast cancer may involve the performance of a lumpectomy, simple mastectomy, and modified radical or radical mastectomy. Treatment is guided by staging of the cancer. Staging was previously described.

Fibrocystic breast disease is a benign condition that is characterized by the development of excess fibrous tissues, increased production and dilation of mammary ducts, and the formation of cysts in the breasts. Nodules and masses may develop in both breasts and are usually located in the upper, outer quadrants.

Risk Factors

- Breast Cancer
  - Female sex (less than 1% of males develop breast cancer)
  - Age over 40
  - Genetic predisposition
  - First-degree relative with breast cancer (parent, sibling, or child)

- Early menarche
- Late menopause
- First pregnancy after age 30
- Endometrial or ovarian cancer
- Early or prolonged use of oral contraceptives
- High-fat diet, possible
- Low-fiber diet, possible
- Excessive alcohol intake, possibly related to folic acid depletion
- Cigarette smoking
- Exposure to low level radiation
- Hormone replacement therapy (HRT)
- Obesity
- History of endometrial or ovarian cancer

Signs and Symptoms

- Breast Cancer
  - Lump or mass in breast
  - Asymmetry in size of breasts
  - Thickening, dimpling, edema, or ulceration around nipple
  - Nipple retraction
  - Warm or hot area of skin
  - Discharge or unusual drainage from nipple (bloody, serous, white, creamy, greenish)
  - Enlarged axillary and supraclavicular lymph nodes
  - Breast soreness or pain
  - Edema of arm
  - Pain
  - Many times masses may feel like "rocks on the side of a cliff"; rough
  - Fibrocystic Breast Disease
  - Premenstrual breast tenderness
  - Palpable bilateral nodules (1/2 - 1 cm in diameter) that are mobile and fluctuate somewhat in size with menstrual cycle
  - Fluid-filled cysts that may require aspiration
  - Many times masses may feel like "pebbles in a river"; smooth

Diagnostic and Laboratory Tests

- History and physical examination
- Breast biopsy
- Mammography
- Ultrasound
  - 2-D (2-Dimensional)
  - 3-D (3-Dimensional)

- Breast self-examination (BSE)
- Bone scan
- Computer tomography (CT)/computed axial tomography (CAT) scan
- Alkaline phosphatase (ALP); also called ALK Phos
- Hormonal receptor assay for estrogen and progesterone
- Sentinel node examination to determine spread of the cancer
- Lymphatic mapping and sentinel lymph node dissection (SLDN)
- Cell proliferation indices
- CXR (chest x-ray) – for metastasis
- CBC (complete blood count)
- LFTs (liver function tests) – for metastasis
- Estrogen and progesterone receptor determination
- S phase determination

Therapeutic Nursing Management

- **Assess/Monitor**:
  - Client's risk factors for breast cancer, especially gynecological/obstetrical, alcohol, and smoking
  - Client's family history of breast cancer
  - Client's history of breast self-examination and mammography
  - Client's understanding and expectations of treatment
  - Dressings, drains for indications of postoperative bleeding
  - Circulator status of affected arm
  - Intake and output
  - Vital signs
  - For postoperative drainage
  - For fluid collection or swelling at operative site
  - For signs of infection
  - For pain
  - For signs of altered body image
  - Need for prosthesis if client elects not to have breast reconstruction
- **Nursing Activities**:
  - Prepare client for mammogram; instruct client to not use talcum powder or deodorant before procedure.
  - Mammograms are best done in the first two weeks of the menstrual cycle so that the incidence of cystic changes is at a minimum.
  - Prepare client for surgery, radiation, or chemotherapy, as indicated.
  - Administer pain medications as prescribed.
  - Maintain surgical asepsis of dressings, incision, and drains.
  - Support arm on operative side with sling while ambulating.
  - Encourage client to lie on affected side postoperatively to relieve pain.

- Encourage early arm exercises to avoid lymphedema.
- Encourage early ambulation.
- Consult with the physical therapist and surgeon to teach the client postmastectomy exercises to regain full range of motion of the arm.
- Teach the client to decrease dietary intake of caffeine-containing products to help decrease fibrocystic breast disease.
- Teach breast self-examination.
- Encourage the client to wear a supportive bra.
- Encourage client to discuss reconstruction alternatives with the surgeon.
- Refer the client to a person certified to fit breast prosthesis if indicated.
- Avoid administering injections, taking blood pressure, or drawing blood from affected arm.
- Teach the client not to wear constrictive clothing and to avoid cuts and injuries to affected arm.
- Provide emotional support to client and family.
- Arrange for a visitor from Reach for Recovery to speak with the client.
- Refer the client to home health care services for care of drains and dressings, and for help with the activities of daily living.
- Emphasize the importance of a well-fitting breast prosthesis for a client who has had a mastectomy.
- Instruct the client to report numbness, pain, heaviness, or impaired motor function of the affected arm to the surgeon, as these are signs of lymphedema.
- Advise client to avoid a dependent arm position as this position will interfere with wound healing.
- Refer to community support group as appropriate.

Pharmacology

- Hormone treatments (block estrogen): tamoxifen (Nolvadex), toremifene (Fareston), fulvestrant (Faslodex)
- Antineoplastic/chemotherapeutic agents: doxorubicin (Adriamycin), cyclophosphamide (Cytoxan), epirubicin (Ellence), vinorelbine (Navelbine), paclitaxel (Taxol), docetaxel (Taxotere), capecitabine (Xeloda), methotrexate – in monotherapy or in combination
- Monoclonal antibody therapy: trastuzumab (Herceptin) for HER-2 positive breast cancer clients. Can be used as monotherapy or in combination with doxorubicin and cyclophosphamide.
- Aromatase inhibitors (prevent change of testosterone into estrogen): anastrozole (Arimidex), letrozole (Femara), exemestane (Aromasin) – used in postmenopausal women
- Luteinizing hormone-release hormone agonists: goserelin, leuprolide – in premenopausal women
- Other potential hormone therapy in pre- and postmenopausal women: ethinyl estradiol, fluoxymesterone
- Progesterone-like hormone: megestrol (Megace)

- Other medications: platinum, etoposide, vinblastine, fluorouracil
- Peripheral stem cell therapy
- Radiation therapy (primary radiotherapy, adjuvant radiotherapy, high-dose radiotherapy, palliative radiotherapy)
- Analgesics (opioid and nonopioid)
- Antiemetics

Complications

- Recurrence (most common complication)
- Lymphedema
- Fibrosis and cellulitis due to lymphedema of arm
- Postmastectomy pain syndrome
- Metastasis
- Infection
- Depression/body image distortion
- Death

Age-Related Changes—Gerontological Considerations

- The incidence of benign breast lumps decreases after menopause, but the risk of malignant lumps increases with age.
- From age 50 to 60, 1 out of every 35 women is at risk of a breast cancer diagnosis.
- From age 60 to 70, 1 out of every 28 women is at risk of a breast cancer diagnosis.
- By age 85, 1 in 9 American women face the risk of a breast cancer diagnosis.

Critical Thinking Exercise: Nursing Management of the Client with Breast Disorders: Breast Cancer and Fibrocystic Breast Disease

Situation: A 37-year-old female is scheduled to undergo breast biopsy for a lump she discovered in her left breast four days ago. Her history includes cigarette smoking for seventeen years, use of oral contraceptives, one child who is 4-years-old, and family history of coronary artery disease. She denies breast trauma, alcohol use, or exposure to radiation. She is 20 pounds above the desired weight for her height.

1. What are the client's risk factors for breast cancer?

2. What is the most significant screening conducted for breast cancer? Why?

3. Which statements are true regarding breast cancer? Correct false statements.
   a. Breast cancer is the most common cancer among women age 45-75.
   b. Breast cancer is the leading cause of death in women age 55-65.
   c. Women detect most breast cancers during their annual mammogram.
   d. The majority of breast cancers occur in the lower inner quadrant of the breast.
   e. An important goal of care is early recognition and treatment of breast cancer.

4. Prioritize nursing activities for the client with breast cancer, with "1" representing the most important activity.
   _____ Encourage client to lie on affected side to relieve pain.
   _____ Administer pain medications as prescribed.
   _____ Maintain surgical asepsis of dressings, incision and drains.
   _____ Support arm on operative side with sling while ambulating.
   _____ Encourage early arm exercises to avoid lymphedema.
   _____ Prepare client for surgery as indicated.

Nursing Management of the Client with a Sexually Transmitted Disease (STD)

- Sexually transmitted diseases (STDs) are preventable.
- People with STDs frequently have more than one infection.
- Goals of collaborative management:
  - Provide early recognition and treatment.
  - Eradicate the pathogenic organism.
  - Prevent transmission from one person to another.
  - Prevent recurrence.
- Important nursing diagnoses (actual or potential):
  - Pain
  - Infection management
  - Risk for injury
  - Anxiety and fear
  - Altered health maintenance
  - Knowledge deficit
- **Key Terms/Concepts**: Transmission, multiple sex partners, systemic, localized, prevention, seroconversion

Overview

A sexually transmitted disease (STD) is a viral, fungal, or bacterial infection spread through sexual contact. Most STDs occur in persons under the age of 25 years. Examples of sexually transmitted diseases include HPV (human papilloma virus) of which there are many. Genital warts is only one example, but one which also is highly correlated with cervical cancer. Other STDs include syphilis, gonorrhea, chlamydia, genital herpes, HIV, trichomoniasis, bacterial vaginosis, and Hepatitis B.

Risk Factors

- Unprotected sexual intercourse
- Multiple sex partners
- Compromised immune system
- Lesions or open sores in the genital area
- Inadequate genital hygiene
- Homosexual relations, especially male

Signs and Symptoms

Chlamydia

- Women may be asymptomatic, but many times complain of abnormal vaginal discharge, dysuria, vaginal bleeding, and pelvic pain.
- Long-term effects for women include:
  - Chronic pain
  - Increased risk of ectopic pregnancy
  - Postpartum endometriosis
  - Infertility
- Men are frequently nonsymptomatic, or may complain of penile discharge.
- Chlamydia and gonorrhea frequently occur together.

Herpes

- Many cases may be asymptomatic or very mild and unrecognized by client.
- First episode is usually the worst
- May have fever and lymphadenopathy
- Numbness, tingling, pain, and itching at site prior to eruption of vesicles
- Vesicles generally reoccur at the same site, because of multiple sexual practices, include oral and anal sex. Herpes simplex 2 (HSV 2) lesions may appear anywhere on the body just as HSV 1 lesions may appear anywhere on the body.

Genital Warts

- Most HPV infections are asymptomatic.
- Painless clusters on the vulva, vagina, cervix, anorectal, or glans penis
- May appear as large, fleshy lesion or look white and more like a cauliflower
- Visible genital warts are cause by HPV types 6 and II. There are more than 30 types of HPV currently known that can invade the genital area. The HPV types associated with cervical cancer include 16, 18, 31, 33, and 35.

Gonorrhea

- Men may experience penile discharge.
- Women experience the following symptoms:
  - Dysuria
  - Increased vaginal discharge or bleeding
  - Can cause PID (pelvic inflammatory disease)
  - If infected during menstruation or pregnancy, may cause disseminated disease which is noted by tenosynovitis, petechial or pustular skin lesion, fever, and arthralgias.

Trichomoniasis

- Frequently asymptomatic
- Vaginal discharge that is malodorous, yellow-green, and itchy
- Men usually do not have symptoms, or if they do, have a nongonococcal urethritis.

Bacterial Vaginosis

- Most common cause of vaginal discharge (fishy) and odor in women
- In women, often confused with a yeast infection and client may be frustrated that OTC anti-yeast preparations do not work
- May not be sexually transmitted, can be found in non-sexually active persons, but can be present with other STDs

Hepatitis B

- May be asymptomatic
- May have flu-like symptoms

HIV

- Flu-like symptoms, including fever, malaise, lymphadenopathy, and rash
- Diarrhea
- Weight loss
- Being prone to secondary infections
- Neuropsychiatric complications in late stage

Syphilis

- **Primary stage:**
  - Chancre at genitalia, mouth, or anus
  - Lymphadenopathy
- **Secondary stage:**
  - Maculopapular, non-pruritic rash appearing at palms and soles of feet
  - Generalized lymph enlargement
  - Mucous patches in mouth
  - Flu-like symptoms
  - Patchy hair loss
- **Latent stage:**
  - No symptoms
- **Late Stage:**
  - CNS symptoms, including mental illness, altered judgment, slurred speech, ataxia, and paralysis

Diagnostic and Laboratory Tests

- History and physical examination
- Cultures (drainage, tissue scrapings, blood)
- VDRL (venereal disease research laboratory) serological test for syphilis
- Darkfield microscopy and direct fluorescent antibody tests of exudates or tissue in early syphilis are very specific
- RPR (rapid plasma regain) serological test for syphilis
- KOH (potassium hydroxide) whiff test and presence of clue cells of wet prep of vaginal secretions for bacterial vaginosis
- Presence of flagellated protozoa on wet prep of vaginal secretions

- NAATs (nucleic acid amplification tests) for gonorrhea and chlamydia, more sensitive than culture
- Viral culture for HSV, lesion must be "unroofed" with Dacron-tipped swab
- Hepatitis B antibody screening
- CBC (complete blood count), and differential
- ELISA (Enzyme Linked Immunosorbent Assay) for HIV
- Western Blot Test if ELISA is positive (Since the Western blot test is an antibody detection test, its results will not be accurate until an HIV infected person seroconverts. Seroconversion describes the process by which the body "reacts" to the viral infection by trying to defend itself through production of antibodies. This process occurs anywhere from 2 to12 months after infection with HIV. However, most clients will seroconvert within 6 months. After an infected person has seroconverted, a positive Western blot indicates an HIV infection is present.)
- Immunofluorescent assays for serum antibody levels
- Gram stains
- CSF (cerebrospinal fluid) examination

Therapeutic Nursing Management

- **Prevent by**:
  - Educating teens and young adults about STDs and their transmission
  - Encouraging abstinence or the use of condoms to prevent disease transmission
- **Nursing Activities**:
  - Report STDs according to County Health Department policy.
  - Identify and treat sexual partners.
  - Provide instructional material regarding use of condoms and safe sex.
  - Teach client regarding drug therapy and need for medical compliance.
  - Administer medication specific to the disease as prescribed.
  - Advise client to inform sexual partners of infected status prior to engaging in sexual practices.

Pharmacology

- Antivirals: acyclovir, famciclovir, valacyclovir (genital herpes)
- Antibiotics: cefixime, ceftriaxone, ofloxacin, levofloxacin plus azithromycin or doxycycline if Chlamydia also present (gonorrhea)
- Penicillin, doxycycline in PCN allergic clients, ceftriaxone, azithromycin – treatment dependent upon stage (syphilis)
- Antibiotics: doxycycline, azithromycin, ofloxacin, erythromycin (chlamydia)
- Metronidazole for trichomoniasis and bacterial vaginosis
- Metronidazole or clindamycin (oral and intravaginally) for bacterial vaginosis
- Imiquimod 5% cream or Podofilox 0.5% solution or gel as client-applied medication for genital warts

- Liquid nitrogen, podophyllin resin 10-25% in compound tincture of benzoin, trichloroacetic acid (TCA) or bichloracetic acid (BCA) 80-90% for provider-applied treatment of genital warts
- Protease inhibitors (HIV)
- Nucleoside reverse transcriptase inhibitors (HIV)
- Nonnucleoside reverse transcriptase inhibitors (HIV)
- Immunomodulator (HIV)
- Antifungals (miconazole, terconazole, fluconazole)
- Hepatitis B: acute treatment not indicated, chronic, etc. treat as per chapter on Hepatitis A, B, C
- Analgesics (opioid or nonopioid) for HSV 2, mainly

Complications

- Systemic infection
- Infertility
- Newborn infection
- Disfigurement
- Dementia
- Death

Age–Related Changes—Gerontological Considerations

- The risk for sexually transmitted disease (STD) is related to frequency of sexual contact with infected persons. STDs affect all age groups and socioeconomic strata, and are associated with significant illness, and even death with advanced disease.
- Clients with latent syphilis may have no symptoms for two or more years after the appearance of the primary lesion. The latent stage may last up to 50 years. The majority of clients will remain in this stage without further problems, although approximately 1/4 to 1/3 of persons eventually develop the irreversible complications of late-stage disease. This stage typically occurs in the late years of adulthood and may ultimately lead to death.

Critical Thinking Exercise: Nursing Management of the Client with a Sexually Transmitted Disease (STD)

Situation: A 19-year-old college student comes to the clinic because she has developed a yellowish vaginal discharge and painful urination. The client has a history of pelvic inflammatory disease and infrequent menses.

1. Upon initial assessment, what other information does the nurse need to gather from the client?

2. Describe the types of laboratory and physical exams likely to be performed. Give the rationales for the test or exam. (Hint: Answer key lists at least six.)

Test / Exam	Rationale

After the client's lab tests are reviewed, the physician tells her she has gonorrhea and is pregnant.

3. What are the key points the client needs to know about gonorrhea and pregnancy?

Nursing Management of the Client Requiring Preoperative Care

Key Points

- Major classifications of surgery include:
    - Cosmetic
    - Curative
    - Diagnostic
    - Elective
    - Emergency
    - Palliative
    - Required
    - Restorative
- Approximately 60% of surgeries are performed on an outpatient basis.
- A major aspect of preoperative care is the assessment of surgical risk.
- It is the surgeon's responsibility to obtain permission for the surgery and to explain benefits, risks, and possible complications from the surgery.
- Preoperative care includes a thorough preoperative assessment of the client's physical, emotional, and psychosocial status prior to surgery.
- Preoperative teaching includes instructions concerning pain management, deep breathing and coughing techniques, and leg and foot exercises.
- Today, as a result of advances in surgical techniques and instrumentation, as well as anesthesia, many surgical procedures that were once performed in an inpatient setting now take place in an ambulatory or outpatient setting.
- Today many clients arrive at the hospital the morning of surgery and go home after recovering in the post-anesthesia care unit from the anesthesia.
- The use of ambulatory or same-day surgery means that clients leave the hospital sooner, which increases the need for teaching, discharge planning, preparation for self-care, and referral for home care and rehabilitation services.
- In addition to all the other preoperative teaching, clients who undergo same-day surgery must be taught when and where to report, what to bring (insurance card, list of medications, allergies), what to leave at home (jewelry, watch, medication, contact lenses) and what to wear (loose fitting, comfortable clothes and flat shoes).
- Goals of collaborative management:
    - Create an atmosphere of trust and open communication with client and family.
    - Collect pertinent assessment data.
    - Obtain the client's (or guardian's) informed consent to perform the surgery.

- Provide physical preparation.
- Acknowledge transcultural differences that could affect preoperative care.
- Provide client with clear explanations and instructions regarding the surgery.
- Review and address each item on the preoperative checklist.
- Administer preoperative medications as ordered.
- Safely transport client to operating suite with completed records.

Important nursing diagnoses (actual and potential):

- Fear and anxiety
- Knowledge deficit
- Anticipatory grieving
- Risk for infection
- Risk for injury
- Risk for pain
- Risk for fluid volume deficit
- Altered urinary elimination
- Risk for impaired skin integrity
- Risk for impaired tissue integrity
- Body image disturbance
- Risk for caregiver role strain
- Ineffective individual coping
- Impaired physical mobility
- Powerlessness
- **Key Terms/Concepts**: Surgical risk, informed consent, preoperative assessment, physical preparation, preoperative medications, preoperative checklist, preanesthesia care unit

Overview

Preoperative care begins when the surgery is planned, and ends when the client arrives in the preanesthesia care unit or operating room.

Risk Factors

- Obesity/emaciation
- Hypovolemia
- Dehydration/electrolyte imbalances
- Extremes of age
- Infection/sepsis/toxic condition
- Pregnancy
- Hepatic disorders: cirrhosis, hepatitis
- Cardiac disorders: dysrhythmias, angina, hypertension, congestive heart failure (CHF), myocardial infarction (MI)
- Respiratory disorders: pneumonia, chronic obstructive pulmonary disease, emphysema, asthma

- Neurological disorders: seizures, Alzheimer's disease
- Renal disorders: renal insufficiency, urinary tract infections, prostatic hypertrophy, dysuria, hematuria, urinary frequency
- Endocrine disorders: diabetes, hyperthyroidism, hypothyroidism, adrenal insufficiency
- Gastrointestinal disorders: peptic ulcers, ulcerative colitis, cirrhosis, hiatus hernia
- Immunologic conditions: allergies to foods, drugs, and environmental factors
- Hematologic conditions: anemia, sickle cell disease, history of excessive bleeding
- Substance abuse
- Inadequate diet and exercise
- Disorders that produce nutritional deficiencies: cancer, organ failure, chronic illness
- Musculoskeletal conditions—muscle weakness, ROM (range of motion), prostheses
- Limited mobility
- High anxiety level
- Intense fears associated with surgery
- Cultural beliefs that may adversely affect view of surgery
- Financial concerns

Signs and Symptoms

- Signs and symptoms of disorder for which surgery is being performed
- Signs and symptoms of fear and anxiety: pounding heart, difficulty breathing
- Signs and symptoms of underlying medical disorders

Diagnostic and Laboratory Tests

- History and physical examination
- Urinalysis
- Chest x-ray
- CBC (complete blood count)
- FBG (fasting blood glucose); also called: fasting blood sugar (FBS) test
- Serum electrolytes, liver function tests, renal function
- ECG (electrocardiogram)
- Tests relevant to disorder undergoing treatment with surgery

Therapeutic Nursing Management

- **Prevention of Postoperative Complications:**
  - Be aware of client's medical history, medical-surgical disorders, and genetic problems that may affect the outcomes of surgery and known allergies.

- Provide client with instruction regarding coughing and deep breathing.
- Provide client with instruction regarding leg exercises.
- Identify and address risk factors prior to surgery.
- Identify and address client's preoperative anxiety.
- Promote adequate rest and sleep prior to surgery.
- Ensure that the preoperative check list is complete and in order.

- **Assess/Monitor:**
  - Client's anxiety level
  - Overall emotional state
  - Client's and family's knowledge of impending surgery
  - Preoperative laboratory data
  - Understanding of invasive preoperative devices and procedures
  - Client's understanding of coughing, deep breathing, and leg exercises
  - Client's reactions to preoperative medications
  - Allergy to latex
  - Previous anesthetic history
  - Spiritual and cultural beliefs
  - If the client is going home the same day, assess the availability of safe transportation and verify the presence of an accompanying responsible adult.
  - Risk of postoperative complications

- **Nursing Actions:**
  - Provide preoperative teaching concerning postoperative pain management.
  - Demonstrate deep breathing and coughing exercises.
  - Discuss importance of postoperative leg and foot exercises and turning and range of motion exercises.
  - Explain invasive devices that client may return with from surgery.
  - Demonstrate use of client-controlled analgesia pump following surgery or any type of catheter that may be used for pain management.
  - Discuss postanesthesia unit.
  - Describe postoperative diet following surgery.
  - The American Society of Anesthesiologists has made a recommendation for persons undergoing elective surgery who are otherwise in healthy states. The recommendations depend on the age of the client and type of food eaten. For example, adults are advised to fast for 8 hours after eating fatty food and 4 hours after ingesting milk products. Most clients are allowed clear liquids up to 2 hours before an elective procedure.
  - Administer an enema or laxatives the night before surgery if client undergoing bowel surgery. May be repeated in the a.m. if ordered.
  - Insert an indwelling catheter if required for a lengthy surgery or have the client void immediately before going to the operating room.
  - Cleanse the skin with a mild antimicrobial soap solution night before surgery.

- Generally hair is not removed preoperatively unless the hair at or around the incision site is likely to interfere with the operation. If hair must be removed, electric clippers are used for safe hair removal immediately before the operation.
- Remove jewelry, makeup, dentures, hairpins, nail polish, glasses, and prostheses.
- Give valuables to family members or lock up in hospital safe.
- Check vital signs.
- Note last time client ate or drank.
- Verify that operative consent has been signed.
- Administer preoperative medications and raise side rails.
- Review and check-off each item on the preoperative checklists.
- Transport client to the preanesthesia care unit with all records completed.
- Share information with the preanesthesia staff.
- Answer client and family questions.
- Establish IV line.
- Verify surgical site and mark site per institutional policy.
- Obtain medication history including over-the-counter and herbal medications.
- Describe the procedure and explain sensations that the client will experience.
- Ask the client to sign the surgical consent and witness the client's signature.
- Report unexpected findings or any deviations from normal.

Pharmacology (Preoperative Medications)

- Sedative agents (benzodiazepines, barbiturates)
- Narcotic analgesics (opioids)
- Anticholinergics (atropine)
- Antiemetic agents (prochlorperazine, metoclopramide, dolasetron)
- Antacid or H2-receptor blockers (famotidine, ranitidine)
- Intravenous infusions
- Blood products
- Antibiotics for surgical prophylaxis (usually given with induction of anesthesia)

Complications (Reactions Related to Preoperative Medications)

- Sleepiness, dizziness, dryness of mouth
- Respiratory depression
- Falls due to reactions to drugs
- Severe anxiety and panic
- Cardiac dysrhythmias

Age-Related Changes—Gerontological Considerations

- Elderly clients are at greater risk of adverse reactions to preoperative medications.
- During preoperative period, inform elderly clients that pre-existing disorders can raise surgical risk.
- Elderly clients may need to have surgical consent forms signed by a legal guardian.
- Elderly clients may be more fearful due to financial concerns and lack of social support.
- The underlying principle that guides the preoperative assessment, surgical care, and postoperative care is that the elderly client has less physiologic reserve than the younger client.
- The elderly often have sensory limitations so the nurse must be alert to maintaining a safe environment.
- The mouth of the elderly needs to be assessed preoperatively for any problems that may occur during intubation, especially for disruption of teeth.
- The elderly perspire less which leads to dry, itchy skin that becomes fragile and easily abraded. Precautions need to be taken when moving the elderly clients.
- Decreased subcutaneous fat makes the elderly clients more susceptible to temperature changes so they need to be covered with lightweight cotton blankets when they are moving to and from the operating room.

Critical Thinking Exercise: Nursing Management of the Client Requiring Preoperative Care

Situation: A 55-year-old-female client is scheduled for an exploratory laparotomy. The client has been experiencing abdominal symptoms for several months. A baseline assessment of all symptoms was conducted. The client has received instructions concerning: (a) the procedure; (b) pain control following the surgery; and (c) the importance of coughing, deep-breathing, and leg exercises. The client has also signed an informed consent for the surgery. The nurse has completed the client's physical preparation for the surgery. The client is now being transported to the preanesthesia care unit with her records and the completed preoperative checklist.

1. What are the nurse's responsibilities in regard to obtaining the client's informed consent for the surgery?

2. What measures can the nurse take to reduce the client's anxiety concerning the surgery?

3. What important transcultural considerations should the nurse recognize when preparing clients for surgery?

4. What are the major items on the preoperative checklist the nurse must ensure have been carried out?

Nursing Management of the Client Requiring Postanesthesia Care

Key Points

- Postanesthesia care is usually provided in the postanesthesia care unit (PACU), where skilled nurses can closely monitor the client's recovery from anesthesia.
- Postanesthesia care involves making postoperative assessments, providing postoperative medications, managing the client's pain, preventing postoperative complications, and determining when the client is ready to be discharged from the PACU.
- During the postanesthesia stage, the client must be continually assessed for airway patency and adequate ventilation.
- Goals of collaborative management:
  - Return client to normal physiologic functioning following anesthesia.
  - Maintain asepsis.
  - Manage pain.
  - Prevent postoperative complications.
- Important nursing diagnoses (actual or potential):
  - Risk for fluid volume imbalance
  - Impaired gas exchange
  - Ineffective airway clearance
  - Ineffective breathing pattern
  - Decreased cardiac output
  - Risk for infection
  - Pain management
  - Altered tissue perfusion
  - Impaired tissue integrity
  - Altered oral mucous membranes
  - Impaired skin integrity
  - Nausea and vomiting
- Transferring the postoperative client from the operating room to PACU is the responsibility of the anesthesiologist. During transport, the anesthesia provider and a member of the surgical team remain with the client.
- **Key Terms/Concepts:** Postanesthesia care unit (PACU), airway patency, ventilation, fluid and electrolyte balance, pain management, emergency equipment and medications, postoperative complications, client-controlled analgesia (PCA), Aldrete Scoring System

Overview

Postanesthesia care is provided during the immediate stage, which is the period of 1 to 4 hours following surgery. The intermediate stage occurs 4 to 24 hours following surgery, and the extended stage is at least one to four days following surgery.

The Aldrete Scoring System is used to evaluate a client's status in the post-anesthesia period. As a part of the determination of the client's readiness for transfer from the Postanesthesia Care Unit (PACU) or discharge home, the nurse performs an assessment and documents an Aldrete Score on the client's medical record. Standard criteria for transfer or discharge should be applied. General parameters for client readiness for transfer or discharge is generally acceptable when the client's Aldrete Score is 9-10.

Aldrete Scoring System			
Criteria	Observation / Assessment	Possible Scores	Score Assigned
Activity	Able to move 4 extremities	2	
	Able to move 2 extremities	1	
	Able to move 0 extremities	0	
Consciousness	Fully awake	2	
	Arises upon calling	1	
	Unresponsive	0	
Respiration	Deeply breathes, coughs freely	2	
	Dyspnea or limited breathing	1	
	Apneic	0	
Color	Pink	2	
	Pale, dusky, blotchy, jaundiced	1	
	Cyanotic	0	
Circulation	Systolic BP < 20 mmHg of pre-procedure BP level	2	
	Systolic BP = 20 mmHg-50 mmHg of pre-procedure BP level	1	
	Systolic BP > 50 mmHg of pre-procedure BP level	0	
Total Score			

The nurse's documentation prior to transfer or discharge includes:

- Aldrete Score
- Time of transfer or discharge
- Discharge plan, including location and name of person responsible for the client's care

- Discharge instructions, including:
  - Medications
  - Activity restrictions
  - Dietary guidelines, if applicable
  - Special treatment instructions
  - Emergency contact for all clients discharged home

Risk Factors for Immediate Postoperative Complications

- Pre-existing heart, respiratory, renal, hepatic, or blood disorders
- Pre-existing neurologic disorders
- Diabetes mellitus
- Steroid therapy
- Obesity
- Poor nutrition
- History of substance abuse

Signs and Symptoms of Immediate Postoperative Complications

- Aspiration of gastric contents
- Ineffective gag reflex and swallowing
- Decreased breath sounds, decreased SaO2, tachypnea (airway obstruction)
- Crowing sounds with an incomplete spasm (laryngospasm)
- Hypoxia
- Hypoventilation
- Wheezing, dyspnea, tachypnea (bronchospasm)
- Pink and frothy sputum, dyspnea, cold skin, cyanosis (pulmonary edema)
- Decreased blood pressure and urinary output, increased heart rate, slow capillary refill (hypovolemic shock)
- Hypopharyngeal obstruction: choking, noisy irregular respirations, decreased oxygen saturation scores and cyanosis

Diagnostic and Laboratory Tests during Postanesthesia Stage

- History and physical examination
- ABGs (arterial blood gases)
- Automatic blood pressure monitoring
- Pulse oximetry
- ECG (electrocardiogram)
- CBC (complete blood count)
- Chemistries may include electrolytes, blood sugar, liver function, renal function

Therapeutic Nursing Management

- **Prevention of postoperative complications during postanesthesia stage:**
  - Be aware of client's past medical history and medical-surgical disorders.
  - Continually assess client for immediate postoperative complications.
  - Have emergency equipment and medications on hand.
- **Assess/Monitor:**
  - Continually for airway patency and adequate ventilation
  - Vital signs every 15 minutes until stable
  - Client skin color and condition
  - Mucous membranes, lips and nail beds for cyanosis
  - For hypothermia
  - For signs of fluid and electrolyte imbalance
  - For nausea and vomiting
  - Drainage tubes for patency and proper function
  - For after-effects of anesthesia
  - I&O (intake and output) every 15 minutes to hourly as directed in PACU
  - For signs of hypervolemia and hypovolemia
  - Bladder for distention
  - Urinary catheters for patency
  - Color, consistency, odor, and amount of urine
  - Surgical wound, incision site and dressing
  - For pain
  - For movement of extremities
  - Level of consciousness
  - Blood oxygen levels
  - ECG (electrocardiogram) readings
- **Nursing Activities:**
  - Position client on side if unconscious or comatose.
  - Keep an airway in place if comatose.
  - Administer humidified oxygen.
  - Assist with turning, coughing, and deep breathing.
  - Administer intravenous infusions and maintain a patent IV line.
  - Suction accumulated secretions if the client is unable to cough.
  - Elevate legs if shock develops.
  - Do not elevate legs higher than placement on a pillow if client has received spinal anesthesia.
  - A preventative approach rather than an "as needed" approach is more effective in relieving pain. With a preventative approach, the medication is administered at prescribed intervals versus when the pain becomes severe or unbearable. Monitor the client every 30 minutes for pain relief and respiratory rate.
  - Provide continuous pain relief through use of a PCA (client-controlled analgesia) pump. Epidural and intrathecal infusions are also available.

- Discourage "PCA by proxy" (family members administering PCA doses for the client).
- Ensure that the client who does not have a catheter voids at least 200 mL of urine within six hours after surgery.
- Palpate the bladder of the client following voiding to assess for bladder distention.
- Maintain client on NPO (nothing by mouth) until return of the gag reflex and peristalsis.
- Irrigate nasogastric suction tubes.
- Provide ice chips and sips of water.
- Provide frequent oral hygiene.
- Change wound dressings as required, using sterile technique.
- Use an abdominal binder for obese or debilitated clients.
- Score client on a scale such as the Aldrete Scoring System.
- Discharge client from PACU to the surgical unit or home if client's Aldrete Score is satisfactory, vital signs are stable, wound drainage is minimal or moderate, and urine output is 30 mL/hr for an adult.
- Notify surgical unit that client will be arriving from PACU.
- Complete documentation of client's care in PACU and send record with client.
- When clients undergo same day surgery, instructions should be given to both client and the adult who will accompany client home, because anesthesia clouds memory for concurrent events.
- Make referrals for home care if client is being discharged after same-day surgery.
- Apply pneumatic compression stockings or elastic stockings.

Pharmacology

- Narcotic analgesics (morphine, meperidine)
- Humidified oxygen
- Intravenous infusions
- Blood products
- Antiemetics (prochlorperazine, metoclopramide, dolasetron)
- Antibiotics for surgical prophylaxis may be continued post-op
- Narcotic antagonists, if necessary, to counteract respiratory depression from opiates (naloxone [Narcan])

Complications during Postanesthesia Phase

- Aspiration
- Airway obstruction by client's tongue
- Shock
- Hypothermia
- Pulmonary edema

- Laryngospasm
- Bronchospasm
- Atelectasis
- Pulmonary embolism
- Cardiac dysrhythmias
- Malignant hyperthermia

Age-Related Changes—Gerontological Considerations

- Elderly clients are at greater risk of postoperative complications such as fluid and electrolyte imbalances.
- Elderly clients may have pre-existing disorders that complicate recovery from the anesthesia and surgery.
- Elderly clients may have stronger adverse reactions to pain medications than younger clients.
- Elderly clients are more susceptible to hypothermia, so keep them warm.
- Postoperative confusion is common in the elderly. The confusion is aggravated by social isolation, restraints, anesthetics and analgesics, and sensory deprivation. Hypoxia can also present as confusion and restlessness.

Critical Thinking Exercise: Nursing Management of the Client Requiring Postanesthesia Care

Situation: A 55-year-old-female was admitted two hours ago to the PACU following an exploratory laparotomy. The nurse has been continually assessing the client for airway patency and adequate ventilation. The nurse has also been monitoring the client's vital signs and dressing every 15 minutes. The client is receiving an intravenous infusion of normal saline, and a PCA pump is set to administer 1 mg of morphine every 6 minutes. The client is now responding to the nurse's voice and moving her extremities. Her Aldrete Score is satisfactory.

1. Prioritize the client's nursing diagnoses while in the PACU, with "1" representing the most important diagnosis.

   _____ Risk for fluid volume imbalance

   _____ Ineffective breathing pattern

   _____ Risk for infection

   _____ Pain

   _____ Risk for impaired skin integrity

   _____ Risk for altered oral mucous membranes

2. What should the nurse do if the client's oxygen saturation levels start to drop?

3. List at least three advantages of PCA (patient-controlled analgesia).

4. The client is awake, but having difficulty voiding. What measures can the nurse take to help her void?

5. What is the Aldrete Scoring System, and what is its purpose?

Nursing Management of the Client Requiring Intermediate and Extended Postoperative Care

Key Points

- The client's response to surgery is influenced by personality, age, surgical risk, preoperative condition, and the extent and type of surgery.
- Surgery activates the stress response, lowers defenses against infection, impairs mobility, decreases sensory input, decreases awareness, may disturb body image, interferes with normal role performance, disrupts normal activities and self-care routines, and disturbs sleep patterns and comfort.
- During the intermediate and extended postoperative period, clients require continuous evaluation and reassessment of their status.
- During the intermediate postoperative period, clients remain at risk for respiratory, circulatory, or gastric problems.
- During the extended postoperative period, the wound continues healing, and the client progresses toward recovery and discharge.
- Goals of collaborative management:
  - Prevent complications of surgery.
  - Promote wound healing.
  - Promote self-care.
  - Promote rapid recovery.
  - Provide balanced nutrition.
  - Encourage early ambulation.
  - Provide emotional support.
  - Prepare the individual and family for discharge.
- Important nursing diagnoses (actual or potential):
  - Risk for infection
  - Pain management
  - Ineffective airway clearance
  - Impaired tissue integrity
  - Impaired skin integrity
  - Altered nutrition: less than body requirements
  - Altered urinary elimination
  - Nausea and vomiting
  - Activity intolerance
  - Fatigue
  - Anxiety
  - Fear

- Dysfunctional grieving
- **Key Terms/Concepts:** Surgical unit, surgical wound care, postoperative complications, postoperative exercises, incentive spirometry, ambulation, criteria for discharge

Overview

- **Intermediate postoperative phase** begins when the client is transferred from the postanesthesia care unit (PACU) to the surgical unit, or home, and it generally lasts from 48 to 72 hours. Can also include recovery and extended stay in the intensive care unit (ICU).
- **Extended postoperative phase** begins two to three days after surgery, and usually lasts for one to four days following surgery, although it may extend to 10 days.

Risk Factors

- Pre-existing heart, respiratory, renal, blood or neurologic disorders
- Diabetes mellitus
- Obesity
- Emergency surgery
- Complications from anesthesia during surgery
- Use of anesthesia for longer than three hours
- Use of an inhalant anesthesia
- Extensive blood loss during surgery
- Cardiorespiratory complications during surgery
- Cultural beliefs concerning sufficient pain relief as inappropriate
- Religious or cultural beliefs concerning blood transfusions
- Complications during the postanesthesia phase (shock, hypothermia, atelectasis, pulmonary embolism)
- Wound complications following surgery
- Anxiety and fear related to surgery

Signs and Symptoms

- **Intermediate postoperative period**
  - Pain
  - Nausea and vomiting
  - Fever
  - Abdominal discomfort and "gas pains"
  - Dyspnea
  - Altered breath sounds
  - Decreased or absent bowel sounds
  - Bladder discomfort
  - Urinary retention
  - Pooling of secretions in lungs

- Restlessness
- Sodium deficit
- Potassium deficit
- Hypovolemia
- Hypernatremia
- Signs of wound infection (redness, swelling, and tenderness at surgical site)
- Bleeding from surgical site
- Constipation
- **Extended postoperative period**
  - Weight loss
  - Decreased skin turgor
  - Venous stasis
  - Signs of UTI, (urinary tract infection) particularly if client has had indwelling catheter
  - Signs of respiratory infection
  - Signs of wound infection
  - Signs of wound dehiscence (staining or gushing of serosanguineous fluid)
  - Fatigue
  - Passivity and depression
  - Stress-related symptoms
  - Anxiety over implications of the surgery

Diagnostic and Laboratory Tests

- Physical examination
- ABGs (arterial blood gases)
- Neurological examination
- ECG (electrocardiogram)
- Urinalysis
- CBC (complete blood count) with differential
- Chemistries: electrolytes, blood sugar, renal function, liver function, cardiac enzymes, etc.
- Tests relevant to specific surgery

Therapeutic Nursing Management

- **Prevention of Postoperative Complications:**
  - Be aware of client's past medical history and medical-surgical disorders.
  - Manage postoperative pain early.
  - Continually monitor client for intermediate postoperative complications and intervene with preventative measures.
  - Continually monitor client for extended postoperative complications and intervene with preventative measures.

- **Assess/Monitor:**
    - **Intermediate period**
        - Postoperative pain (type, location, intensity, and degree of relief with analgesics)
        - For changes in vital signs
        - Fluid intake and output
        - For signs of fluid and electrolyte imbalance
        - For nausea, vomiting, and hiccups
        - Drainage tubes for patency and proper function
        - For urinary retention
        - Bladder for distention
        - Urinary catheters for patency. Report rates < than 30 cc/hr.
        - Color, consistency, odor, and amount of urine
        - The surgical wound, incision site and dressing
        - ECG (electrocardiogram) readings, laboratory, and other diagnostic findings
        - Safety of client
        - Position of client
        - Skin color and temperature
        - Mental status, orientation and level of consciousness
        - Breath sounds
        - Oxygen saturation levels
        - Patency of IV lines
        - Bowel sounds and abdominal distention
    - **Extended Postoperative Period**
        - For re-establishment of normal oxygen exchange, cardiovascular functioning, and elimination
        - For signs of thrombophlebitis
        - Pulmonary embolism
        - For signs of wound dehiscence or wound evisceration
        - Increases in physical activity and mobility
        - Surgical wound healing
        - Ability to perform self-care activities
        - Understanding of follow-up and home care procedures
        - For depression or grieving regarding loss of body part during surgery
- **Nursing Actions:**
    - **Intermediate period**
        - Receive report and client records from PACU (postanesthesia care unit) nurse.
        - Review client's records concerning the surgery, client's condition during surgery, postanesthesia recovery, and nursing and medical interventions.

- Begin a baseline assessment of client's respiratory function, cardiovascular function, neurologic and sensory function, and fluid and electrolyte balance.
- Position the client in bed comfortably.
- Notify family of client's return to the surgical unit, and discuss client's condition.
- Speak quietly with the client and allay anxiety.
- Check client's dressing and any drainage tubes.
- Regulate intravenous infusions if present.
- Provide analgesia as necessary unless client is using client-controlled analgesia.
- Keep lighting low in room to help client rest.
- Gradually increase diet from surgical liquids to solid food as tolerated.
- Encourage the client to perform deep-breathing and coughing exercises, extremity exercises, turning, and gradual ambulation.
- Apply elastic stockings, pneumatic hose, or other antithromboembolic stockings.
- Assist client with use of incentive spirometry to increase lung expansion during deep breathing.
- Splint abdominal and thoracic incisions when performing coughing exercises.
- Provide emotional support to the client and family.

- **Extended Period**
  - Encourage extremity activity and early ambulation.
  - Splint wound during vigorous coughing or movement.
  - If wound evisceration occurs, protect wound with a sterile dressing and notify surgery.
  - Assist client with increasing ambulation.
  - Promote self-care activities.
  - Provide a balanced nutritional diet.
  - Assist the client and family with depression or grieving that may result from the surgery.
  - Prepare the client and family for discharge.
  - Make home referrals when necessary.
  - Refer client to community support systems as appropriate.
  - Provide discharge teaching regarding home self-care activities.

Pharmacology

- Antiemetics (prochlorperazine, dolasetron)
- Antibiotics for surgical prophylaxis may be continued post-op or if infection present
- Analgesics (opioid and nonopioid)
- Narcotic antagonists (naloxone [Narcan])

- NSAIDs (nonsteroidal anti-inflammatory drugs) (diclofenac, ibuprofen, ketoprofen, ketorolac, naproxen)
- Transcutaneous electrical stimulation
- Laxatives (bisacodyl, senna)
- Antiarrhythmia drugs (if dysrhythmia present)
- Stool softeners
- Anticoagulants (low molecular weight heparin and low dose warfarin)

Complications

- **Intermediate Stage**
  - Acute respiratory distress syndrome
  - Atelectasis
  - Pneumonia
  - Ileus
  - Postoperative pain
  - Urinary retention
  - Wound infection
- **Extended Stage**
  - Thrombophlebitis
  - Pulmonary embolism
  - Wound dehiscence
  - Wound evisceration

Age-Related Changes—Gerontological Considerations

- Elderly clients are at greater risk of postoperative complications during the intermediate and extended postoperative phases, such as pneumonia and infection.
- Older clients may tolerate a soft diet and six small feedings better than a standard diet following surgery.
- Fluid and electrolyte imbalances are more common in elderly clients because of decreased renal blood flow and glomerular filtration rate.
- Elderly clients may have pre-existing disorders that make early ambulation and increased activity following surgery more difficult.
- Postoperative delirium, characterized by confusion, perceptual and cognitive deficits, altered attention levels, disturbed sleep patterns and impaired psychomotor skills, is a significant problem for older clients.

Critical Thinking Exercise: Nursing Management of the Client Requiring Intermediate and Extended Postoperative Care

Situation: A 55-year-old-female who has undergone an exploratory laparotomy has been discharged from the PACU and admitted to the surgical unit. The nurse reviewed the client's condition with the PACU staff, performed a baseline assessment and set-up a plan of care for the intermediate and extended postoperative period. The plan of care included preventative measures for complications that may arise during these periods.

1. During the intermediate postoperative period, what signs should alert the nurse to immediately call the surgeon?

2. What is the purpose of incentive spirometry, and what instructions should the nurse provide the client?

3. What are the manifestations of pneumonia (a complication of the intermediate period), and how can pneumonia be prevented?

Critical Thinking Exercise Answer Keys

Situation: A 42-year-old man is brought into the emergency department following a fire that destroyed the warehouse where he was working. Initial assessment reveals extensive burns covering the majority of his anterior arms, face, and anterior thorax. His burns are a mixture of intact and open blisters with reddened bases and shiny, weeping surfaces. He is awake and alert and complaining of extensive pain and sensitivity to cold air. He has singed nasal hairs, eyebrows, and eyelids; and is hoarse with a brassy cough.

1. Estimate the man's percentage of burns using the Rule of Nines.

Anterior arms	=	4.5%	x 2 =	9.0%
Anterior face	=	4.5%	=	4.5%
Anterior chest	=	18.0%	=	18.0%
				31.5% TBSA

2. Which three assessments are of greatest importance during the man's initial care?

X Serum electrolytes   **X** Airway

_____ Signs of infection   _____ Body image

X Vital signs   _____ Blood glucose

3. Which assessment findings indicate that man may have sustained an inhalation injury?

_____ Frothy urine   _____ Decreased blood pressure

X Cough   _____ Open blisters

_____ Facial pain   **X** Hoarseness

4. Match the type of burn with its clinical manifestations:

C	Deep red, black or brown in color	A. Superficial
E	< 25% TBSA, but > 15% TBSA of partial thickness	B. Partial thickness
D	No pain or blisters	C. Full thickness third-degree burn
A	Healing occurs within seven days	D. Full thickness fourth-degree burn
C, D	Grafting required	E. Moderate
B	Involves epidermis and dermis	F. Major
A	Tenderness eased with cooling	
B	Sensitivity to cold air	
C	Brown or white fat exposed	
B	Large blister formation	
D	Black, edematous lesion	
A	Skin blanches with pressure	
F	> 10% TBSA of full thickness	
C	Little pain experienced	
B	Grafting may be required	

Nursing Management of the Client with Wound Infections
Answer Key

Situation: A 39-year-old female underwent a partial bowel resection (removal of the bowel) as treatment for a malignant tumor. Prior to her surgery, she received radiation and chemotherapy in an effort to reduce the size of the tumor. She has lost a significant amount of weight over the past six months and is about twenty pounds under her ideal weight. Currently, her incision is well approximated, free of redness, tenderness or swelling.

1. If noted during wound assessment, which findings must be reported to the surgeon since they indicate the client is developing a wound infection?

    _____ Pallor   _____ Approximation

    X Swelling   **X** Erythema

    X Tenderness   _____ Serosanguineous drainage

2. Which are the risk factors that predispose this client to development of wound infection?

    X Advanced age   **X** Malignant tumor

    _____ Hyperlipidemia   **X** Chemotherapy

    X Debilitation   **X** Radiation

    X Surgery   **X** Septicemia

    _____ Hypertension

3. What is the single most important nursing intervention to protect the woman from developing a postoperative wound infection?

    Meticulous hand washing

4. List the classical clinical manifestations of system infection in a person who has wound infection.

    Fever, chills, malaise, elevated white blood cell count

Nursing Management of the Client with a Wound Dehiscence and Evisceration Answer Key

Situation: A 67-year-old client with long-standing diabetes mellitus underwent surgery to remove an abdominal tumor after being diagnosed with a partial bowel obstruction. The client relates a history of several months of abdominal pain, bloating, nausea, and weight loss. At the time of surgery, he was about 15% below his ideal body weight. The client progressed well during his postoperative period and remained free of incision infection or other complications. On his seventh postoperative day, which was the day he was to be discharged to home, the nurse removed the client's abdominal sutures as ordered by his surgeon. An hour later, the client called the nurse to his room stating when he coughed he felt something "give" at his incision. Inspection revealed a one-inch separation of the client's wound edges.

1. What factors increase the risk for would dehiscence?

   Nutritional deficit (15% below ideal weight), which results in impaired wound healing.

   Abdominal surgery due to stress placed on incision by internal organs.

   Older age, which may result in slower healing.

   Diabetes mellitus, which causes slower healing.

2. During what activities is a client most likely to experience wound dehiscence?

   Deep breathing, coughing, straining during defecation, vomiting

3. In what order will the nurse implement the following actions related to the client's wound dehisence?

   3 Have another nurse notify the surgeon while you remain with the client.

   4 Cover any protruding coils of intestine with sterile dressings moistened with sterile normal saline; if sterile supplies are not available, use clean towels or dressings.

   1 Remain calm.

   5 Document the incident.

   2 Place the client in bed in semi-Fowler's position with the knees slightly arched. If the wound has not completely opened or has not eviscerated, this position may prevent further tear.

4. How does wound dehiscence differ from wound evisceration?

Dehiscence refers to separation of wound edges.

Evisceration refers to the protrusion of an internal organ through an incision. An evisceration is a more severe complication than wound dehiscence.

Nursing Management of the Client with Pressure Ulcers
Answer Key

Situation: A 68-year-old female is in a vegetative state after suffering a traumatic brain injury in an automobile accident. She does not respond to verbal commands or pain. She receives nutrition and fluids via a gastrostomy tube. The woman is incontinent of urine and has diarrheal stools. Even though she received very good nursing care and frequent turning, she developed a Stage 3 pressure ulcer on her coccyx.

1. Which of the following statements best describes a Stage 3 pressure ulcer?

   _____ Full-thickness skin loss with extensive destruction, tissue necrosis, and damage to muscle and/or bone.

   _____ A reddened area that does not blanch with pressure and returns to normal within 15-20 minutes when pressure is relieved.

   X Full-thickness skin loss and the presence of white, gray, or yellow exudates and purulent drainage at the base of the ulcer.

2. Complete each sentence pertaining to the client's risk factors for skin breakdown.

   The client may be experiencing diarrhea as a result of the **tube feedings**.

   The nurse should take care to **reposition (or turn)** the client at least every **two** hours to prevent further skin breakdown.

   Adequate amounts of **protein** are necessary to support nutrition and aid in wound **protein**.

   Avoid **massaging** the skin over bony prominences; current evidence suggests this may be harmful.

3. Which nursing activities will help promote wound healing?

_____ Assessing the wound daily	_____ Applying a dressing to the ulcer
X Relieving pressure over the affected site	**X** Maintaining adequate nutrition
X Turning and repositioning q 2-4 hrs	_____ Administering intravenous antibiotics

Nursing Management of the Client with Skin Cancer
Answer Key

Situation: A 19-year-old college student visits the student health center because she is concerned about a small, red, nodular epidermal lesion on her arm. The woman relates a history of frequent sunbathing, participation in water sports in the summer, and use of tanning beds in the winter. She is unaware of any close relatives who have a history of skin cancer.

1. Describe the appearance of each skin cancer listed below:

   a. Basal cell

   Basal cell is a waxy-appearing nodule that is generally located on the face. Metastasis is rare.

   b. Squamous cell

   Squamous cell is a small, red, nodular lesion that usually appears on the face, or upper extremities.

   c. Malignant melanoma

   Malignant melanoma is a white, gray, black, brown, or blue lesion that may begin as a mole.

2. Which factors increase a person's risk for developing skin cancer?

   X Using tanning oils when sunbathing

   _____ Applying make-up over sunscreen

   X Routinely using a tanning bed

   X Wearing clothing that is too tight

3. What is the rationale for teaching a clients to apply SPF 15 sunscreen or higher prior to spending lengthy periods of time in the sun?

   Sunscreen with SPF factors greater than 15 protect the skin from exposure to ultraviolet light when frequently applied.

Nursing Management of the Client with a Rash Answer Key

Situation: A 25-year-old woman who has recently started employment in a fast-food restaurant is being seen for eczema (atopic dermatitis). The nurse notes patches of dry, red, and scaly skin on the backs of the client's hands and on her arms. The client has a history of eczema, and is allergic to a number of medications and cleaning products. The client states that at her new job she washes her hands frequently with hot water and an antibacterial soap.

1. What measures should the nurse instruct the client to take to avoid exacerbation of her eczema?

The nurse should instruct this client to:

- **Wash her hands in tepid water**
- **Use a very mild soap**
- **Use a light, nongreasy, unscented lotion following hand washing**
- **Avoid skin products containing alcohol**
- **Consider wearing cotton-lined gloves while working**

The nurse should also warn the client to avoid scratching the lesions as scratching can result in skin infections.

2. What nursing diagnoses apply to the care of the client with eczema?

Nursing diagnoses that apply to clients with eczema are:

- **Impaired skin integrity related to dry skin**
- **Risk for infection related to skin excoriation and to scratching of lesions**
- **Body image disturbance related to unsightly skin lesions**
- **Ineffective management of therapeutic regimen related to knowledge deficit of causes of eczema**

3. What medications will the primary care provider most likely prescribe for this client?

   The primary care provider will most likely prescribe:
   - Topical steroids
   - Systemic antihistamines
   - Topical antipruritics, such as calamine lotion
   - Antibiotics, if signs of a skin infection are present

Nursing Management of the Client with Herpes Zoster—Shingles
Answer Key

Situation: A 59-year-old man is receiving chemotherapy for colon cancer. This morning the man is experiencing pain beneath his right arm and across the right side of his back. The nurse notes the client has several draining lesions that run in a linear pattern across the right side of his back and extending beneath his right arm.

1. What signs are most indicative that the client is experiencing an outbreak of herpes zoster (shingles) rather than an allergic reaction to his chemotherapy?

    Unilateral, painful skin lesions running across his back. This pattern is consistent with inflammation of a peripheral sensory nerve of the trunk, which is different from that caused by a drug hypersensitivity reaction.

2. Which nursing activities need to be implemented in response to the client's symptoms?

    X   Monitor for infection.   **X**   Place the client on wound precautions.

    _____ Discontinue the chemotherapy.   _____ Drain the blisters.

    _____ Cover lesions with sterile dressing.   **X**   Administer prescribed pain medication.

3. Provide a rationale for each of these nursing activities related to herpes zoster.

    a. Place an air mattress on the client's bed

    An air mattress will relieve pressure on the client's painful lesions.

    b. Administer an anti-inflammatory agent

    The varicella-zoster virus produces inflammation of the dorsal root ganglia. Anti-inflammatory agents help reduce inflammation, which decreases symptoms and increases comfort.

    c. Use acetic acid compound on lesions

    Acetic acid compounds reduce localized inflammation and reduce pain.

Nursing Management of the Client with Osteoporosis Answer Key

Situation: The client is a 50-year-old secretary at a local high school. She has just been diagnosed with osteoporosis based on bone density studies that revealed approximately 30% bone demineralization.

1. List three questions appropriate for the nurse to ask the client regarding her risk factors for osteoporosis.

> **What prescribed and over-the-counter medications are you currently taking?**
>
> **Have your monthly periods ceased or are they irregular (an indication of menopause)?**
>
> **How much exercise do you engage in on a daily basis?**
>
> **Do you smoke?**
>
> **How much do you currently weigh?**
>
> **Is there a history of osteoporosis in your family?**

2. Which of the following activities is most beneficial for the client? Rank in priority with "1" representing the most beneficial.

   2 Swimming

   4 Yoga

   1 Walking

   3 Tennis

   The activities are designed to allow the client to engage in regular, weight-bearing exercise to prevent further reduction in bone density associated with osteoporosis.

3. The client asks the nurse about taking antacids since they contain calcium. What information is most important for the nurse to give the client in this regard?

   - **The calcium found in antacids does support essential bone formation, however, the extent of this benefit is unknown.**

   - **Antacids commonly recommended include Maalox, Mylanta, Rolaids, and Tums. This form of calcium requires accompanying vitamin D.**

Nursing Management of the Client with a Fracture Answer Key

Situation: A 29-year-old man was admitted to the emergency department for injuries suffered in an automobile accident. Physical examination and radiological studies reveal a fractured left femur just above his knee. The skin is broken, but there is no evidence of bone protrusion. A sterile dressing is covering the open wound.

1. Match the fractures with their correct description:

e	One part of the bone is compressed by another.	a. Complete
b	A break is partially through the bone width.	b. Incomplete
g	One side of the bone is fractured, while the other side is bent .	c. Compound
a	The bone is broken into two parts and separated.	d. Comminuted
d	The bone is broken into fragments or splintered.	e. Compression
f	A bone is fractured beneath intact skin	f. Simple
c	A bone is fractured and protrudes through the skin.	g. Greenstick

2. Mark the subjective data with an "S" and the objective data with an "O."

O	Bone protrusion	S	Impaired sensation
O	Loss of pulse distal to the fracture	S	Tenderness over affected site
O	Shortening of the extremity	S	Muscle spasms

3. Prioritize the nursing interventions for this client, with "1" representing the most important intervention.

   3   Immobilize the limb without altering its position

   1   Control bleeding if present

   5   Assess pain status

   4   Assess for other possible problems (internal injuries, head injury, etc.)

   2   Obtain vital signs

   6   Assist with preparation for cast or surgery as indicated

Nursing Management of the Client with Total Hip Replacement
Answer Key

Situation: A 72-year-old male client is being discharged home from the hospital following hip replacement surgery. In addition to the prevention of other complications, the staff has made every effort to prevent deep vein thrombosis and pulmonary embolism: the two most common causes of postoperative mortality in older clients. Prior to discharge, the nurse gives the client a list of instructions for positioning, sitting, and ambulating at home. The client is also instructed to use a walker or crutches until weight bearing is safe, and to employ adaptive devices for everyday activities. Finally, the client is advised to watch for any signs of hip prosthesis loosening or dislocation, and to call the surgeon immediately if such signs occur.

1. Which are the signs and symptoms of deep vein thrombosis?

    X Pain in the area of thrombus

    _____Fever >101.0° F

    X Swelling proximal to the site of thrombus

    _____Pallor and cool extremity

    X Positive Homan's sign

2. Which are the signs and symptoms of pulmonary embolism?

X	Hemoptysis	_____	Respiratory alkalosis
_____	Bradycardia	**X**	Apprehension
X	Dyspnea	**X**	Cough
_____	Subnormal body temperature	**X**	Diaphoresis
X	Respiratory crackles	_____	Pneumothorax
X	Pleuric pain	_____	Hyperventilation
X	Cyanosis	**X**	Hemoptysis

3. List several types of adaptive equipment useful for clients who have undergone hip replacement surgery.

    Adaptive equipment that is available for clients who have undergone hip replacement surgery include a reacher, sock donner, long-handled shoehorn, elevated toilet seat, shower chair, and a long-handled sponge for bathing.

4. Which are signs of prosthetic hip dislocation?

  X   Leg shortening

_____ Hypermobility of affected leg

  X   Abnormal rotation

  X   Malalignment

_____ Extremity numbness

5. What measures can be taken to prevent prosthetic hip dislocation?

> **To prevent dislocation, the client needs to position his leg in abduction by using abduction splints, wedge pillows, or two or three pillows between his legs.**

Nursing Management of the Client Requiring Traction Answer Key

---

Situation: An 88-year-old man fractured his right hip when he fell on his icy driveway. His right femur is stabilized with balanced suspension skeletal traction. He has a Thomas ring with Pearson attachment and 25 pounds traction on his right leg and 8 pounds of traction on the balanced suspension. The client is receiving oral codeine every 3-4 hours for pain.

---

1. What assessments does the nurse need to make in regard to each of the following:

   a. **Client: Body aligned correctly in relation to pull of the traction, appearance of pin insertion site, presence of pain, signs of pressure on Achilles tendon, circulation and sensation in affected foot**

   b. **Ropes: Freedom of movement, ensure that knots in the rope do not catch in the pulley, free of linen**

   c. **Pulleys: Proper attachment to support bars**

   d. **Weights: Hanging freely; not resting on the floor**

2. What signs will alert the nurse the client is developing a wound infection at the pin insertion site?

   Signs of infection include warmth, swelling, erythema extending for an inch or more from the pin insertion site, and purulent drainage from the site.

3. What is the etiology of the nursing diagnoses of the client?

   a. **Pain: Related to the client's fracture and/or traction**

   b. **Risk for constipation: Related to immobility and prescribed medication**

   c. **Risk for impaired skin integrity: Related to immobility and traction**

4. What can the nurse do to prevent skin alterations in any person who is immobilized due to traction?

   • **Observe all bony prominences for signs of impaired circulation and pressure (heels, hips, coccyx, shoulders).**

- Reposition at least every two hours.
- Encourage movement in bed using an overhead trapeze bar.
- Pad or protect areas of skin that are in contact with traction rope.
- Keep skin clean and dry, especially if the client experiences urine or stool incontinence.

Nursing Management of the Client with an Amputation
Answer Key

Situation: A 24-year-old male is twelve hours post-operation for a below-the-knee amputation of his right leg as treatment for osteogenic sarcoma. His stump is elevated on two pillows and the gauze and elastic dressings are dry and intact. His vital signs are stable and he is controlling his pain with morphine sulfate via a PCA (patient controlled analgesia) pump.

1. What is the rationale for:

   a. Elevating the client's stump on a pillow for the first 24 hours post op?

   Prevents and/or reduces fluid accumulation in the stump, which reduces pain from swelling and facilitates healin.

   b. Progressively applying pressure to the end of the stump after the incision has healed?

   Toughens the stump so a prosthesis can be worn

2. Which postoperative assessments does the nurse need to make at least every 2 hours over a period of 12 hours following the client's amputation?

   _____ Client's ability to participate in own care

   X Presence and amount of drainage

   _____ The presence of fever

   _____ Signs of situational depression

   X Client's response to pain medication

   X Presence of stump swelling

   X Vital signs

3. The client complains he is experiencing pain in the foot that is no longer there. What is this type of pain called, why does it occur, and what can be done to relieve the pain?

   The pain is known as phantom pain. It is pain felt in the limb that has been amputated. It is related to severed nerve pathways. The pain often mimics preoperative pain in the limb, but will subside with time. The nurse should encourage the client to use his pain medication to relieve phantom pain.

Nursing Management of the Client with Osteoarthritis— Degenerative Joint Disease Answer Key

Situation: A 57-year-old woman is being evaluated for possible total knee replacement as treatment for her chronic osteoarthritis. The client and two of her four siblings suffer from the same disease with varying degrees of pain and disability. The client is obese and leads a sedentary lifestyle because of her weight.

1. What are the most common risk factors for osteoarthritis?

   Common risk factors for osteoarthritis include genetic predisposition, obesity, sedentary lifestyle, age greater than 40 years, chronic joint stress, and poor posture.

2. Which pain characteristics are common for osteoarthritis?

X Joint stiffness	**X** Deep, aching pain
X Pain relieved by rest	____ Warm, edematous joints
____ Severe joint deformity	**X** Joint instability
____ Morning stiffness	____ Pain following exercise

3. What is the most likely etiology for each of the nursing diagnoses of the client?

   a. Pain

   Common risk factors for osteoarthritis include genetic predisposition, obesity, sedentary lifestyle, age greater than 40 years, chronic joint stress, and poor posture.

   b. Impaired mobility

   Impaired mobility related to joint pain, stiffness, and instability

   c. Risk for injury

   Risk for injury related to joint pain and instability

   d. Knowledge deficit

   Knowledge deficit related to lack of previous experience regarding disease and treatment

4. Why is it important for clients with osteoarthritis to engage in active stretching exercises?

Active stretching exercises help maintain joint mobility, prevent deformity, facilitate weight loss, and maintain straight posture.

Nursing Management of the Client with a Head Injury Answer Key

Situation: A 31-year-old woman received a closed head injury during an automobile accident approximately six hours ago. Her CT scan indicates she has sustained a contusion of moderate severity to the left side of her brain. She is unresponsive to verbal commands, but does respond to pain. Her blood pressure is 150/68; heart rate 72 bpm; her respirations are 28 per minute and mildly labored.

1. Match the following clinical manifestations with correct head injury:

		a. Nuchal rigidity
a,c,e,f	Skull fracture	b. Amnesia
b,d	Concussion	c. Cerebrospinal fluid (CSF) leakage from the ears
a,c,e,f	Hematoma	d. Hypotension
		e. Hemiparesis
		f. Fixed, dilated pupil on affected side

2. Which are common signs of increased intracranial pressure (ICP)?

X Tachypnea	_____ Decreased body temperature
X Restlessness	**X** Headache
_____ Gastric distention	**X** Paralysis
X Vomiting	_____ Tachycardia
X Seizures	_____ Narrowed pulse pressure

3. List two nursing activities for each of the client's priority nursing diagnosis.

a. High risk for ineffective airway clearance

- **Establish and maintain patent airway.**
- **Position to facilitate respirations.**
- **Elevate head of bed 30º to reduce intracranial pressure.**
- **Suction if needed.**
- **Monitor for signs of increased intracranial pressure.**

- Initiate use of Glasgow Coma Scale.
- (Other activities are possible.)

b. High risk for impaired skin integrity
- Reposition at least every two hours.
- Assess skin for signs of breakdown.
- Massage bony prominences.
- Keep skin clean and dry.
- Maintain adequate protein and fluid intake.
- Keep linens wrinkle free beneath client.
- (Other activities are possible.)

4. List a desired outcome for these nursing diagnoses:
   a. Alterations in nutrition

   Client will maintain present weight. Alternatively, client will maintain ideal body weight.

   b. Risk for complications of head injury

   Client will remain free of complications related to head injury.

Nursing Management of the Client with an Intracranial Hemorrhage Answer Key

Situation: Three clients are being cared for on the neurosurgery unit. One client has an epidural hematoma, a second has a subdural hematoma, and a third has an intracerebral hematoma. All three are semi-conscious and restless, but stable, and all are demonstrating indications of improvement.

1. Match the type of hematoma with its correct description. There is more than one answer to each type.

d.f.i	Subdural hematoma	a.	Multiple hemorrhage
b,e,h	Epidural hematoma	b.	From tear in meningeal artery
a,c,g	Intracerebral hematoma	c.	Due to closed head trauma
		d.	Forms slowly
		e.	Between dura and skull
		f.	Beneath the dura
		g.	In frontal lobe
		h.	Forms rapidly
		i.	Related to tears in veins

2. Decide if each statement is true or false. Correct false statements.
   a. Shallow, rapid respirations are associated with intracranial hemorrhage.
      False. Cheyne-Stokes respirations are associated with intracranial hemorrhage.

   b. Diabetes mellitus is a risk factor for intracranial hemorrhage.
      True.

   c. Intracranial hemorrhage seldom results in increased intracranial pressure.
      False. Intracranial hemorrhage frequently causes increased intracranial pressure.

   d. Neuro checks should be performed every four hours when intracranial pressure is suspected.
      False. Neuro checks should be performed every fifteen minutes until the client is stable when intracranial pressure is suspected.

3. All three clients have the nursing diagnosis of "risk for injury related to restlessness." List two nursing actions to protect their safety.

- Monitor for restlessness (which may be due to hypoxia) and intervene appropriately to increase oxygenation or decrease pain (morphine is contraindicated due to respiratory depression).

- Pad side rails.

- Place hands in protective mitts.

- Reduce environmental stimuli.

Nursing Management of the Client with Increased Intracranial Pressure (ICP) Answer Key

Situation: A 29-year-old male fell off the roof on which he was working three days ago and received a blunt head injury. He is unconscious, intubated, and receiving mechanical ventilation to support respirations. He has an indwelling urinary catheter and is receiving intravenous fluids and medications, which includes Mannitol and Decadron.

1. List four signs of increased intracranial pressure, other than decreased level of consciousness.

   Initially, there are subtle changes:
   - **Restlessness, complaints of headache, disorientation, and confusion**
   - **Projectile or recurrent vomiting**
   - **Changes in vital sign pattern and pupillary reactions**
   - **Progressive difficulty breathing**

2. Match each drug with the reason for its use in treating clients with increased intracranial pressure.

f	Osmotic diuretics	a.	Prevent or control seizures
d	Corticosteroids	b.	Reduce fever
a	Anticonvulsant	c.	Control blood pressure
e	Stool softeners	d.	Reduce inflammation
c	Anti-hypertensives	e.	Prevent fecal impaction
b	Antipyretics	f.	Eliminate excess fluid

3. Which is an achievable outcome for the person with increased intracranial pressure?

   _____ Client will be free of intracranial pressure within 24 hours.

   _____ Client will be turned every two hours to prevent skin breakdown.

   X Client will maintain a patent airway throughout hospitalization.

Nursing Management of the Client with a Cerebrovascular Accident (CVA)—Stroke Answer Key

Situation: A 50-year-old woman is admitted to the acute care facility after her family finds her in a confused state. Admission assessment reveals a history of hypertension and diabetes mellitus. Her vital signs are BP 190/110, respirations 16, pulse 90, rectal temperature 100.6° F, and Glasgow Coma Scale = 8. She has right-sided weakness with loss of sensory input and facial drooping. Her admitting medical diagnosis is acute brain attack or stroke (cerebrovascular bleed).

1. Which of the following nursing diagnoses are appropriate based on the client's data?

   X Risk for impaired physical mobility   **X** Risk for injury

   X Self-care deficit   _____ Altered nutrition

   X Sensory-perceptual alteration   _____ Ineffective family coping

   _____ Ineffective individual coping

2. Prioritize the following nursing interventions, with "1" representing the most important intervention.

   3 Monitor temperature.

   2 Assess neurological status.

   1 Assess respiratory status.

   4 Elevate the client's head to a 45° position (high-Fowler's position).

3. Which signs and symptoms are produced by increased intracranial pressure (ICP)?

   X Confusion   **X** Restlessness   _____ Constricted pupils

   _____ Hiccoughs   **X** Elevated temperature   _____ Narrowed pulse pressure

   X Bradycardia   _____ Increased respiratory rate   _____ Tetany

4. List three complications that can occur in a client experiencing a stroke.

   - **Constipation**
   - **Urinary incontinence**
   - **Aspiration pneumonia**

- Pressure ulcers
- Contractures
- ARDS (acute respiratory distress syndrome)
- Seizures
- Coma
- Death
- Others are possible.

Nursing Management of the Client with Pain Answer Key

Situation: A 43-year-old woman is being treated for severe and unrelenting back pain that began about three days ago after she lifted several heavy objects. Upon assessment, the client rates her pain as "8" on a scale of 1-10.

---

1. What type of pain is the client experiencing? Why?

   The client is experiencing acute pain because it is related to a specific traumatic event that occurred three days ago. If it lasts longer than six months or becomes intermittent, it will be reclassified as chronic pain.

2. What information needs to be collected from a client experiencing either acute or chronic pain?
   - **Location of the pain**
   - **Time of onset**
   - **Intensity**
   - **Quality**
   - **Patterns**
   - **Precipitating and exacerbating factors**
   - **Management techniques attempted and past effective management techniques.**

3. State the rationale for implementing each of the nursing actions for this client's pain.

   a. Encourage client to report pain before it becomes severe.

   Pain is more readily relieved when treatment measures are initiated before the pain becomes severe.

   b. Implement pain strategies that have been previously successful.

   If the client has experienced previous successes from a relief measure, it has a good chance of being successful again.

c. Instruct the client to call for assistance when getting out of bed to ambulate.

Clients receiving pain medication may become dizzy, weak, or confused, which places them at increased risk for falls and injury. Therefore, they should be assisted when ambulating.

4. Categorize each type of pain as acute or chronic:

   a. Abdominal cramping from gastroenteritis

   Acute

   b. Bone pain related to cancer

   Chronic

   c. Migraine headache

   Acute or Chronic (One headache is acute; intermittent headaches are chronic.)

   d. Toothache

   Acute

Nursing Management of the Client with a Spinal Cord Injury
Answer Key

Situation: While playing football, a 19-year-old college student suffered a 12th thoracic fracture with resulting paraplegia. He has no muscle control of his lower limbs, bowel, bladder, or genital area. He is a week postoperative from spinal stabilization surgery.

1. Which of the following are the primary goals of collaborative management during the acute phase following spinal cord injury?

   _____ Administer morphine sulfate to control pain.

   X Maintain physiological stability.

   _____ Teach client about the disease process.

   _____ Prevent alterations in nutrition.

   X Prevent further spinal cord injury.

2. The client received high dose glucocorticoid drug therapy when initially admitted to the neuro-surgery unit. Which of the following are risks associated with glucocorticoid therapy?

   X UTI (urinary tract infection)   _____ Hypoglycemia

   X Fluid retention   **X** Sodium retention

   _____ Decreased appetite   _____ Hypotension

3. What is the etiology for these client problems?

   a. Anxiety

   Anxiety related to fear of the unknown, OR uncertain prognosis, OR unknown outcome of his injuries, OR fear of changes that will need to be made in his lifestyle. Other etiologies are possible.

   b. Hopelessness

   Hopelessness related to inability to assume normal lifestyle OR inability to control current situation, OR lack of ability to fully recover from injuries. Other etiologies are possible.

   c. Powerlessness

   Powerlessness related to inability to control present situation or future. Other etiologies are possible.

4. Define autonomic dysreflexia.

Autonomic dysreflexia is the state in which a person with a spinal cord injury experiences a life-threatening uninhibited sympathetic response of the nervous system to noxious stimuli.

Nursing Management of the Client with Seizures Answer Key

Situation: A young woman with a history of epilepsy is scheduled to undergo minor outpatient surgery. Before the nurse can obtain data about the woman's seizure history during the admission process, the woman states she is going to have a seizure.

1. What should the nurse do while the client is seizing?

   The nurse should stay with the client, turn the client's head to the side, and prepare to suction if needed. Restrictive clothing should be loosened. The nurse should prepare to administer prescribed anticonvulsant medications.

2. What is the rationale for these nursing actions?

   a. Turn the client on her side.

   To prevent the client from aspirating if she vomits during the seizure

   b. Loosen restrictive clothing.

   To allow for maximum ventilation and oxygenation

   c. Minimize external stimuli.

   External stimuli can trigger a seizure or make it worse.

3. Match the type of seizure with its common sign.

b	Brief, generalized jerking	a. Tonic-Clonic
e	Localized jerking of a specific area	b. Myoclonic
a	Rigidity of muscles lasting 10-30 seconds	c. Atonic
c	Sudden, momentary loss of muscle tone	d. Absence
f	Slow, repetitive jerking of a body part	e. Simple
d	Sudden, momentary loss of muscle tone	f. Focal

4. Why is it important to administer seizure medications on time?

Seizure medications must be administered on time in order to maintain a steady state of blood levels and effectively prevent seizure activity.

Nursing Management of the Client with Alzheimer's Disease
Answer Key

Situation: A 72-year-old man is a resident in a long-term-care Alzheimer's facility. He is in very good physical health, but is unable to care for himself, recognize members of his family, or communicate his needs. An extensive evaluation of the client indicates he is in Stage 2 of the disease process.

1. Match the following characteristics of Alzheimer's disease with the correct stage of the disease process. Use "1," "2" or "3" as your answer.

	2	"Sundowning"
	3	Absent motor skills
	2	Wandering behavior
1 = Stage 1	**1**	Difficulty with depth perception
2 = Stage 2	**1**	Decreased attention span
3 = Stage 3	**2**	Impaired judgment
	3	Disoriented to time and place
	2	Irritability and agitation
	1	Subtle personality changes
	1	Mild cognitive deficits
	3	Bladder incontinence

2. If the following statement about Alzheimer's disease is not true, then make the appropriate correction.

a. Alzheimer's disease is a progressive, inflammatory neurological disorder.

   False. Alzheimer's disease is a progressive, degenerative (not inflammatory) neurological disorder.

b. Alzheimer's' disease causes severe behavioral dysfunction and changes in personality.

   True.

c. Alzheimer's disease is an uncommon form of senile dementia.

   False. Alzheimer's disease is a common form of dementia among older adults.

d. Alzheimer's disease begins suddenly with forgetfulness and progresses to total mental incapacitation.

False. Alzheimer's disease begins insidiously (not suddenly) with forgetfulness and progresses to total mental incapacitation.

3. State the etiology for each of the client's nursing diagnoses:

a. Risk for injury

   Related to:
   - **Loss of motor skills; OR**
   - **Confusion; OR**
   - **Difficulty with depth perception; OR**
   - **Inability to understand and follow directions**

b. Altered nutrition

   Related to:
   - **Inability to eat without assistance; OR**
   - **Inability to understand the need for eating; OR**
   - **Confusion; OR**
   - **Loss of appetite**

c. Self-care deficit

   Related to:
   - **Absent motor skills; OR**
   - **Inability to understand and follow directions; OR**
   - **Lack of cognitive ability necessary to care for self**

4. Complete the following sentences about clients with Alzheimer's disease:

a. Older adults with Alzheimer's disease are at increased risk for **pneumonia, dehydration,** and **malnutrition.**

b. It is important to encourage **exercise** to maintain **mobility** as long as frequent **rest periods** are also scheduled.

c. Family members may feel **powerless**; therefore, it is important for the nurse to provide **emotional** support.

Nursing Management of the Client with Parkinson's Disease
Answer Key

Situation: A 79-year-old male was diagnosed with Parkinson's disease two years ago. In spite of his condition, he is able to live independently with his partner of 59 years. He takes levodopa with carbidopa (dopamine agonist) to control his disease. The couple has two grown children who live nearby to offer assistance when needed. Due to a recent episode of pneumonia, the client is receiving home health visits.

1. Which are considered the classic signs of Parkinson's disease?

_____	Mask-like faces	**X**	Akinesia	_____	Memory loss
_____	Shuffling gait	_____	Slow speech	_____	Difficulty sleeping
X	Muscle rigidity	_____	Drooling	_____	Diaphoresis
X	Tremor				

2. Why is the client at increased risk for the development of pneumonia?

   People with Parkinson's disease experience muscle weakness, which can affect their ability to swallow, placing them at increased risk for aspiration pneumonia.

3. Correct any of the following statements which are false regarding Parkinson's disease.

   a. Drug therapy may lose its effectiveness over time.

   True.

   b. Clients with Parkinson's disease are at increased risk for malnutrition.

   True.

   c. Parkinson's disease is a common, progressive, crippling disease of the peripheral nervous system.

   False. Parkinson's disease is a common, progressive, crippling disease of the central nervous system.

   d. Parkinson's disease affects females more commonly than males.

   False. Parkinson's disease affects males more commonly than females.

   e. Levodopa is the drug of choice for treating Parkinson's disease.

   True.

Nursing Management of the Client with Myasthenia Gravis
Answer Key

Situation: A 66-year-old male is recovering from myasthenia crisis during which time he suffered respiratory distress requiring mechanical ventilation for several days. The care provider believes an earlier episode of gastroenteritis triggered the crisis.

1. Match the terms associated with myasthenia gravis with the correct definition.

a	Liberates acetylcholine	a.	Cholinergic
g	Destruction of self	b.	Anticholinergic
d	Difficulty swallowing	c.	Aspiration
e	Filtering of plasma	d.	Dysphagia
b	Blocks acetylcholine	e.	Plasmapheresis
c	Drawing in of fluid	f.	Dysarthria
f	Difficulty speaking	g.	Autoimmune

2. What is the rationale for each nursing activity?

a. Encourage semi-Fowler's position.

   To facilitate breathing and prevent choking or aspiration

b. Maintain hydration.

   To facilitate liquefaction of respiratory excretions

c. Administer medications 30 minutes before meals.

   To facilitate chewing and swallowing

d. Thicken liquids.

   To reduce the risk of choking

3. Which signs indicate the presence of a myasthenia crisis?

X	Respiratory distress	____	Unusual euphoria
X	Difficulty talking	____	Abdominal cramps
____	Muscle spasms	____	Fever
X	Tearing	**X**	Increased muscle weakness
____	Signs	**X**	Difficulty swallowing

Nursing Management of the Client with Multiple Sclerosis (MS) Answer Key

Situation: A home health care nurse is interviewing a 24-year-old client with newly diagnosed MS. The client is upset over her increasing loss of mobility, decreased visual acuity, and the severe fatigue that worsens as the day progresses. In addition, the client states she is experiencing mood swings she cannot control. As the client has a decreased libido, she is also worried about her relationship with her husband. The client tells the nurse she and her husband had planned a pregnancy, but now they have been forced to put their lives on hold.

1. What initial assessments should the home health care nurse make in regard to the client's MS?

    The nurse should assess the client's:

    - **Motor dysfunction (weakness, paralysis, spasticity, abnormal gait)**
    - **Cognitive dysfunction (changes in short-term memory, short-attention span)**
    - **Emotional ability**
    - **Sensory dysfunction (paresthesias, decreased temperature perception and proprioception, and blurred vision)**
    - **Cerebellar dysfunction (tremor, ataxia, vertigo)**
    - **Bowel and bladder dysfunction (constipation, incontinence, spastic bladder)**
    - **Sexual dysfunction**
    - **Fatigue**
    - **Ability to perform the activities of daily living (ADLs)**

2. What actions should the nurse take to help the client increase mobility and lessen fatigue?

    It is important to encourage the client to conserve her energy and increase mobility by using assistive devices such as canes, walkers, and wheelchairs. In addition, for safety, the client should wear leather-soled flat, tie shoes. The nurse should check the home environment to make certain lighting is adequate, and cords and throw rugs that could trip the client have been removed. The client needs to schedule major activities in the morning, and then plan rest periods during the afternoon. The nurse should arrange with the physical therapy and occupational therapy departments for periodic home visits.

3. What instructional materials and recommendations should the nurse leave with the client and her husband?

> The client needs to receive:
>
> - Information about MS, available community resources, and the National Multiple Sclerosis Society
> - Drug information, including side effects of prescribed medications and possible drug interactions with over-the-counter drugs
> - Menus and recipes for nutritious, well-balanced meals
> - Precautions for preventing the complications of immobility
> - As the client has expressed concern about her marital relationship, the nurse could recommend the client and her husband seek professional counseling.

Nursing Management of the Client with Meningitis Answer Key

Situation: A 21-year-old college student is being treated for bacterial meingitis. She complains of a stiff neck and severe headache. Initial assessment by the nurse reveals a positive Kernig's sign and positive Brudzinski's sign.

1. Describe a positive Kernig's sign.

   Kernig's sign is positive when the client complains of pain in the hamstring muscles after flexing the thigh upon the body and then extending the leg.

2. Describe a positive Brudzinski's sign.

   Brudzinski's sign is positive when clients flex their hips as their neck is flexed from a supine position.

3. Match the meningitis with the symptoms it produces. Use "V," or "B" as your answer.

	V	Mild, flu-like symptoms
	B	Irritability
	V,B	Headache
V = Viral Meningitis	V,B	Nuchal rigidity
B = Bacterial Meningitis	V	Drowsiness
	B	Chills and high fever
	B	Photophobia
	V,B	Seizures
	V	Low-grade fever
	B	Back and abdominal pain
	B	Twitching

4. Identify the following nursing activities as appropriate or inappropriate for the client with meningitis. Correct inappropriate nursing activities.

   a. Monitor vital signs every four hours

      Inappropriate. Vital signs should be monitored more frequently than every four hours.

   b. Initiate oxygen therapy

      Appropriate

   c. Institute seizure precautions if there is evidence of seizures

      Inappropriate. Seizure precausions should be instituted before signs of seizures occur.

   d. Initiate protective isolation

      Inappropriate. Respiratory, not protective isolation must be initiated.

   e. Obtain intravenous access for fluids and medications

      Appropriate.

Nursing Management of the Client with Eye Trauma Answer Key

Situation: A 37-year-old male accidentally caught a fishhook in his eye while casting for fish. His brother, who was with him at the time, rushed him to the emergency department to have the fishhook removed. The man is in pain and frightened he will lose his sight. His initial assessment reveals no bleeding or loss of fluid from the eye.

1. What is the rationale for each of the nurse's actions?
   a. Leaving the fishhook in place

      Prevents further damage/injury to the eye.

   b. Placing a patch on the client's uninjured eye

      Since eyes move in tandem, this will limit the motion of the uninjured eye and therefore limit the motion of the injured eye, helping reduce the likelihood of additional damage to the injured eye.

   c. Providing emotional support to the client

      Decreases anxiety and reduces fear.

2. What can the nurse do to reduce the client's fears?
   a. **Inform the client about all procedures that are being performed.**
   b. **Explain there is no loss of blood or fluid from the eye, which could cause permanent eye damage.**
   c. **Stay with the client and offer reassurance.**

3. Which are desired client outcomes for this injury? Correct any incorrect/inappropriate outcomes.
   a. Absence of infection

      Appropriate outcome.

   b. Monitoring vital signs

      Inappropriate. Monitoring vital signs is a nursing activity, not a desired outcome.

   c. Maintenance of vision

      Appropriate outcome.

Nursing Management of the Client with Cataracts Answer Key

Situation: A 62-year-old woman who has long-standing diabetes mellitus is being discharged to home following right cataract removal and intraocular lens implant. She is in stable condition and will be staying with her daughter until fully recovered.

1. Which are risk factors for the development of cataracts?

   _____ Hypertension **X** Diabetes mellitus _____ Hypothyroidism

   X Steroid therapy **X** Eye trauma _____ Infection

2. Which statements are true about cataracts? Correct false statements.

   a. Cataract formation is a pathological process that can be prevented if diagnosed early.

   False. Cataracts may occur following a pathological condition such as diabetes mellitus, but may also be related to normal aging. Cataract formation and progression cannot be prevented by early diagnosis.

   b. Older adults with cataracts are at increased risk for injury due to falls.

   True.

   c. A cataract is a clouding that begins around the inside of the lens.

   False. A cataract is a clouding that begins around the outside of the lens and progresses until the entire lens is opaque.

   d. Lenses with cataracts have a grayish, pearly appearance.

   True.

3. List the rationale for:

   a. Teaching the client to avoid coughing and lifting when she returns home

   Coughing and lifting increase intraocular pressure and may contribute to postoperative complications following cataract removal.

b. Cautioning the client about driving an automobile

Depth perception is altered and takes time to return. The client may have difficulty judging distances and should, therefore, be encouraged to avoid driving until her depth perception returns.

c. Encouraging the client to obtain a new prescription for eyeglasses

The client's vision will improve following cataract removal and lens implantation; therefore, her previous eyeglass prescription will not allow her to see clearly.

Nursing Management of the Client with Glaucoma Answer Key

Situation: A 51-year-old man suffered bilateral retinal detachments three years apart. As a result of his two retinal surgeries, he now has secondary, chronic, open-angle glaucoma. His only prescribed medication is Timoptic, a topical beta-blocking agent. He is visiting the outpatient eye clinic for his annual eye examination.

1. Which statements are true regarding glaucoma? Correct false statements.

    a. Glaucoma produces abnormally low intraocular pressure.

    False. Glaucoma produces abnormally high intraocular pressure.

    b. Glaucoma can temporarily damage the optic nerve.

    False. Glaucoma can permanently damage the optic nerve.

    c. The two most common types of glaucoma are open angle and angle closure.

    True.

    d. Untreated glaucoma results in gradual loss of vision.

    True.

2. Match the clinical manifestation with the correct type of glaucoma. Use "OA" or "AC" for your answers.

OA =	Open Angle	AC	Rapid onset
AC =	Angle Closure	OA	Mild aching in the eye
		OA	Loss of peripheral vision
		AC	Moderate pupil dilation
		AC	Photophobia
		OA	Halos around lights
		AC	Ophthalmic emergency

3. The nurse establishes teaching outcomes to determine the effectiveness of client education. Which expectations of client understanding are appropriate for the client with glaucoma?

_____ The procedure for instilling antibacterial eye ointments.

_____ The need to avoid straining at defecation.

X Signs and symptoms of increased IOP (intraocular pressure).

X How and when to use prescribed medications.

X Clinical manifestations of eye infection.

_____ Probable need for retinal surgery.

Nursing Management of the Client with Sensorineural Hearing Loss Answer Key

Situation: An 80-year-old male client has been diagnosed with sensorineural hearing loss due to presbycusis. The client is taking niacin and is learning to use a hearing aid. The nurse is also providing the client with a list of community resources for people with impaired hearing.

1. What does niacin do that may help the client with sensorineural hearing loss?

   Nicotinic acid (niacin) acts to dilate the blood vessels that supply the inner ear, thus increasing circulation to the cochlea and acoustic nerve.

2. Prioritize nursing activities for the client with sensorineural hearing loss, with "1" representing the most important activity

   4 Encourage client to have extra hearing aid batteries on hand.

   1 Protect client from injury related to dizziness and falls.

   3 Teach client how to care for his hearing aid.

   2 Facilitate communication with the client.

3. Which instructions will the nurse give the client about caring for his hearing aid?

   _____ Keep the hearing aid turned on throughout the day.

   X Open the battery compartment at night to avoid draining the battery.

   _____ Monthly cleaning is adequate for the ear mold.

   X Completely dry the ear mold before reattaching it to the receiver.

   X Avoid wearing the hearing aid if ear infection is present.

4. What should the client do if his hearing aid fails to work?

   • **Check the on-off switch.**

   • **Make sure the battery has been correctly inserted.**

- Examine the cord for breaks.
- Try replacing the battery, cords, or both.
- Check the placement of the ear mold in the ear, particularly if the hearing aid "whistles."

Nursing Management of the Client with Hypothyroidism
Answer Key

Situation: A 46-year-old client visits the outpatient clinic for symptoms of fatigue, cold intolerance, dry scaly skin, hoarseness, weight gain, and fluid retention. Based on her symptoms, thyroid studies were obtained that revealed an elevated TSH (thyroid stimulating hormone) and decreased T3 and T4 levels. The client was placed on Synthroid 0.1 mg PO daily and instructed to return to the clinic in one month.

---

1. Which other clinical manifestations are common with hypothyroidism?

   _____ Hypertension   **X** Decreased appetite   **X** Dyspnea

   X Hair loss   _____ Diarrhea   **X** Elevated cholesterol

   X Menstrual disturbances   _____ Euphoria   **X** Dulled mental processes

2. State the rationale for each nursing activity. Teaching the client:

   a. The importance of maintaining lifelong hormone replacement therapy

   Since the client's thyroid gland will not ever be able to produce an adequate amount of thyroid hormone, the client will have to take thyroid replacement medication for the rest of her life to assure normal metabolic function.

   b. Increase her intake of fluids

   Clients with hypothyroidism are at increased risk for constipation. Maintaining adequate fluid intake helps prevent constipation.

   c. The signs of thyroid over-medication

   Too much medication will affect the client adversely, causing tachycardia, nervousness, restlessness, and insomnia.

3. Which findings best indicate that the client is responding effectively to the prescribed drug therapy?

   X Reversal of signs and symptoms

   _____ Absence of drug side effects

   X Reported improved quality of life

   _____ Absence of complications

Nursing Management of the Client with Hyperthyroidism
Answer Key

Situation: A 46-year-old male client visits the outpatient clinic for new-onset symptoms of feeling as though his heart is racing, insomnia, and anxiety. Upon further questioning there has been a 10 pound weight loss over the past two weeks without the client dieting. Based on his symptoms, the nurse practitioner obtained thyroid studies, which revealed a decreased TSH (thyroid stimulating hormone) and increased T3 and T4 levels. The client is diagnosed with hyperthyroidism and is scheduled to see an endocrinologist for further evaluation and treatment. In the meantime, the client is placed on Lopressor 50 mg a day.

1. What is the usual treatment for hyperthyroidism?

    Treatment falls under one of three categories: surgery, antithyroid medications, or radioactive iodine. Surgery, once considered the gold standard, has fallen out of favor; mainly due to the potential complications of hemorrhage, hypoparathyroidism, and vocal cord paralysis. The current gold standard is radioactive iodine. Treatment goals may be to make the client euthyroid or to totally ablate the gland, leaving the client hypothyroid. Results may take 4 to 12 weeks to reach. Side effects are minimal, but thyroiditis, inflammation of the thyroid gland with release of thyroid hormone, can occur. Treatment for hyperthyroidism may be accomplished with antithyroid medications. Antithyroid medications include methimazole and propylthiouracil. These medications induce remission of the disease, but are not curative. Antithyroid medications can be used safely during pregnancy and may be the treatment option of choice for the elderly or cardiac clients before initiating radioactive iodine. They may cause agranulocytosis

2. Why did the nurse practitioner place the client of Lopressor?

    The use of beta-blockers is part of the stabilization process that should be carried out as soon as possible, before the client sees the endocrinologist for definitive treatment. Stabilization is done to decrease the potential untoward cardiac effects, such as tachycardia and atrial fibrillation that may accompany hyperthyroidism. If the client has a contraindication to beta-blocker, such as a history of asthma, then calcium channel blockers can be tried; although they are not always as effective.

3. A potential complication of hyperthyroidism is thyroid storm. What signs and symptoms might the client with thyroid storm exhibit and what would the nursing management include?

> **Thyroid storm, also called thyroid crisis or thyrotoxicosis, usually occurs with Graves' disease. The condition develops rapidly and can be life-threatening. Thyrotoxicosis is precipitated often by trauma or infection. The rapid increase in metabolic rate leads hypertension, nausea, diaphoresis, fever, and tachycardia. Priority nursing management includes:**
>
> - **Maintain a patent airway.**
> - **Offer a cooling blanket for hyperthermia.**
> - **Administer antipyretic as prescribed.**
> - **Administer supplementary oxygen therapy as prescribed.**
> - **Administer pharmacological intervention as ordered, such as propylthiouracil, methimazole, sodium iodide solution, propranolol, and glucocorticoids.**

4. Match the symptoms. Put an arrow next to the sign or symptom.

   (up arrow) = hyperthyroidism

   (down arrow) = hypothyroidism

   a. dry skin __D__

   b. heat intolerance __U__

   c. constipation __D__

   d. exophthalmos __U__

   e. palpitations __U__

   f. weight loss __U__

   g. weight gain __D__

   h. cold intolerance __D__

   i. excess perspiration __U__

   j. amenorrhea __U__

   k. low blood pressure __D__

   l. insomnia __U__

   m. bradycardia __D__

   n. increased blood pressure __U__

Nursing Management of the Client with a Thyroidectomy
Answer Key

Situation: A 25-year-old female client is being admitted to the postanesthesia care unit (PACU) following a thyroidectomy for hyperthyroidism. The nurse places the client in a semi-Fowler's position and is supporting her head and neck with pillows and sandbags. The nurse frequently checks the client's vital signs, and assesses her suture line for strain or bleeding. Once the immediate postoperative period has passed, the client will be transferred to the surgical floor where she will recuperate and learn about lifelong thyroid replacement therapy.

1. Which equipment should the nurse have available at the client's bedside?

   X   Tracheostomy set   ____ Sodium bicarbonate

   X   Endotracheal tub   ____ Thoracentesis tray

   X   Suction equipment   **X**   Calcium gluconate

   ____ Thyroxine   **X**   Laryngoscope

   ____ Defibrillator

2. Which complications is the client most at risk for immediately following thyroidectomy?

   ____ Infection   **X**   Airway obstruction

   X   Edema of glottis   **X**   Tetany

   ____ Seizures   **X**   Laryngeal nerve damage

   ____ Hemothorax   **X**   Tracheal compression

   ____ Thyroid storm

3. What is the rationale for supporting the client's head and neck with sandbags and pillows?

   Sandbags and pillows are used to immobilize the client's head and neck in order to prevent flexion and hyperextension of the neck, which could strain the suture line, resulting in disruption of the sutures and hemorrhage.

4. Which are clinical manifestations of thyroid storm?

X	Fever	_____	Hypertension
X	Tachycardia	**X**	Respiratory distress
_____	Lethargy	**X**	Confusion
X	Coma	_____	Abdominal cramping
_____	Thirst		

Nursing Management of the Client with Adrenal Disorders: Cushing's Syndrome and Addison's Disease Answer Key

Situation: A 62-year-old woman has been taking 10 mg prednisone PO for over two years to control pulmonary inflammation from COPD (chronic obstructive pulmonary disease). When assessing the client, the nurse notes she has a round-appearing puffy face, a large abdomen, and thin arms and legs. There are multiple bruises on the woman's arms and legs.

1. What is the most common risk factor for Cushing's syndrome?

   Long-term exogenous corticosteroid therapy

2. Which are common symptoms of cortisol excess (Cushing's syndrome)?

_____	Weight loss	**X**	Weakness
X	Abdominal striae	_____	Hypoglycemia
X	Electrolyte imbalance	**X**	Excessive hair growth
X	Bone demineralization	**X**	Cataracts
X	Glaucoma	_____	Hypotension

3. State the rationale for:

   a. Placing the nursing diagnosis "risk for injury: fractures" on the client's nursing care plan.

   Excessive cortisol destroys bone proteins and alters calcium metabolism, which predisposes the person to back pain, compression fractures of the vertebrae, and rib fractures.

   b. Teaching the client to avoid abruptly discontinuing her replacement medication.

   When taken for a long period of time, exogenous steroids (prednisone) suppress the adrenal gland, causing it to become non-functioning. When the drug is withdrawn, the adrenal gland cannot produce enough cortisol for bodily needs, the client will develop adrenal crisis and possibly die.

Nursing Management of the Client with Diabetes Mellitus
Answer Key

Situation: A 44-year-old female client has a 25-year history of Type 1 IDDM (insulin-dependent diabetes mellitus). She lives with her husband and two teen-aged daughters. The client has been able to adequately manage her diabetes mellitus, care for her family and work full-time as a cook at the local elementary school cafeteria, where she enjoys cooking and interacting with the children. The client's past medical history includes the usual childhood illnesses, tonsillectomy at age six, and vaginal hysterectomy at age 39 for dysfunctional uterine bleeding secondary to fibroid tumor growth. She is 5'-4" tall and weighs 143 pounds.

1. What are the similarities and differences between Type 1 and 2 diabetes mellitus?

Similarities	Differences
(Examples) **Both are metabolic diseases** **Both result in hyperglycemia** **Both are associated with increased incidence of diabetic neuropathy, atherosclerotic heart disease (ASHD)** **Both require dietary management**	(Examples) Type 1: a **Absolute insulin deficiency** b **Complete absence of insulin production due to autoimmune destruction of pancreatic beta cells within the islets of Langerhans** c **Must be treated with insulin** d **More common in young persons** Type 2: a **Decreased insulin sensitivity (resistance) or decreased production of insulin** b **Relative insulin deficiency** c **Can often be controlled with diet, exercise or oral hypoglycemic agents** d **More common in adulthood**

2. List the common clinical manifestations that occur from diabetes mellitus, noting those that occur early in the disease process, those that occur late in the disease process.

   a. Early clinical manifestations:

Polydipsia	**Blurred vision**
Polyphagia	**Weight loss**
Polyuria	**Fatigue**

b. Late clinical manifestations:

Coma	Hypertension
Diabetic retinopathy	Dyslipidemia
Diabetic foot	

3. What are the major consequences of insulin deficiency to each of the following organs/tissues, and what is the overall result of such consequences?

Organ Tissue	Consequence
Liver	Hyperglycemia (elevated serum glucose) Hypertriglyceridemia (elevated triglycerides) Excess ketone production
Skeletal Muscle	**Ineffective uptake of glucose** **Ineffective uptake of amino acids**
Adipose Tissue	**Lipolysis (fat breakdown)** **Elevated free fatty acid levels in the circulation**
Overall Result	**Progressive hyperglycemia & glycosuria**

Additional Information: The client visits her health care practitioner yearly unless she experiences problems. Two years ago she was diagnosed with hypertension secondary to her diabetes mellitus and was placed on the drug metoprolol (Lopressor) 50 mg bid and a low-salt diet to control her blood pressure. Her daily insulin dose was also adjusted because her GHb (glycosylated hemoglobin) was elevated. Other medications include 1 mg estradiol daily and over-the-counter Advil (ibuprofen) for occasional headaches.

4. What does the client's elevated GHb (glycosylated hemoglobin) level imply?

GHb (glycosylated hemoglobin) is blood glucose bound (attached) to hemoglobin for the life of the hemoglobin, or about 120 days. The amount of GHb is a reflection of the amount of glucose available and how well glucose levels have been controlled during the past 3-4 months. Since the client's GHb was elevated, it implies that her blood glucose level has not been well controlled over the past few months.

5. What is the relationship between the client's hypertension and her diabetes mellitus?

Answers may vary, but should include: Hypertension in type 1 diabetics strongly suggests the presence of renal disease. DM (especially insulin resistant) is associated with hypertriglyceridemia (high serum triglycerides), decreased HDL levels and hypercholesterolemia (high serum cholesterol), all of which are risk factors for the development of arteriosclerosis and subsequent cardiovascular disease, including hypertension.

6. Is there reason for concern about the client's combination of prescribed and over-the-counter medications? Why or why not?

Possibly. Metoprolol is an antihypertensive medication that may mask the symptoms of hypoglycemia. Increased urine glucose may be present in diabetic clients taking estrogen. Ibuprofen (Advil) may exacerbate hypertension. The client should be taught about the possible interactions of these drugs and to monitor for hypoglycemia.

Situation: The client has self-administered 35 units of NPH human insulin and 20 units of Regular human insulin at 7:30 a.m. each morning since her last visit to the clinic, which she feels is controlling her diabetes well. She inconsistently monitors her blood glucose levels because she dislikes pricking her own fingers and believes that she can "feel" when her blood glucose is not within normal limits. The client intakes between 1300 and 1400 calories each day per the American Diabetic Association exchange system, which includes an evening snack.

---

7. In regard to the client's insulin:

a. How may she mix her insulin so that she can avoid administering more than one injection?

She should draw up the regular (fast acting) insulin first, then drawing up the NPH (long acting) insulin. The fast acting insulin must remain free of long acting insulin so that if needed during an emergency, it will act quickly.

b. How does NPH insulin differ from regular insulin?

Regular insulin is clear, fast acting insulin, which has a short duration of action. NPH insulin has a slower onset of action (as does Lente and Ultralente) but has a longer duration of action.

8. While this client has self-administered her own insulin for years, many clients need to be taught the skill. Cite at least four principles a newly diagnosed diabetic should be taught about insulin and its administration.

   Examples:
   - Clear, regular insulin is fast acting; cloudy insulin is longer lasting.
   - Insulin should be stored in the refrigerator when not in use.
   - Each injection site should be placed at least one inch away from the previous site.
   - Wash hands prior to preparing or injecting insulin.
   - Cleanse the site with alcohol or soap and water before injecting insulin.
   - A smaller insulin syringe (50 units) may be useful for smaller prescribed dosages.
   - It is unsafe to bend, recap, or break needles; dispose of needles in a puncture- resistant container.
   - (Other answers are possible).

9. What is the underlying principle supporting the American Diabetes Association exchange list and how does the client use it to calculate her daily dietary intake?

   The American Diabetes Association exchange list is based on six main exchange lists: fruit, vegetable, milk, meat, bread/starch, and fat. The underlying principle is that foods, in portions specified, contain approximately the same number of calories, fats, proteins, and carbohydrates. The client is provided with a meal plan that include choices from the exchange lists based on her dietary needs and preferences. She can interchange foods on the exchange lists to provide greater mealtime variety.

10. Should the client be counseled regarding monitoring of her blood glucose levels? Why or why not?

    Yes, counseling is warranted. Clients who take insulin should self-monitor their blood glucose on a regular basis to maintain the best possible control. Clients may become accustomed to higher blood glucose levels that place them at greater risk for complications.

11. Clients with Type 1 IDDM occasionally use a sliding scale to determine their insulin needs. What is a sliding scale and what type of insulin is administered when using a sliding scale?

    The term "sliding scale" refers to the varying dosages of insulin that clients take based on their blood glucose levels. As their blood glucose levels go up or down, their insulin dose is adjusted up or down as well. Only regular insulin is administered when using a sliding scale since it is administered on a frequent basis, such as before meals and bedtime. Often clients are able to maintain more normal blood glucose levels when they use a sliding scale for their insulin dosage.

12. Cite at least five signs and symptoms that should be taught to diabetic clients and their significant others because they indicate the presence of hypoglycemia.

- Headache
- Sweating (diaphoresis)
- Rapid heart rate (tachycardia)
- Nervousness (anxiety)
- Irritability
- Trembling
- Hunger
- Double vision
- Mental confusion
- Convulsions
- Coma

13. What are the most common reasons why diabetic clients develop hypoglycemia?

- Drug over dosage
- Inconsistent or missed dietary intake
- Alcohol consumption
- Exercise without snack compensation

Nursing Management of the Client Requiring Insulin Therapy
Answer Key

Situation: A 44-year-old female client has a 25-year history of Type 1 IDDM (insulin-dependent diabetes mellitus). She lives with her husband and two teen-aged daughters. The client has been able to adequately manage her diabetes mellitus, care for her family and work full-time as a cook at the local elementary school cafeteria, where she enjoys cooking and interacting with the children. The client's past medical history includes the usual childhood illnesses, tonsillectomy at age six, and vaginal hysterectomy at age 39 for dysfunctional uterine bleeding secondary to fibroid tumor growth. She is 5' 4" tall and weighs 143 pounds.

1. What are the "classical" early manifestations commonly associated with diabetes mellitus and what other signs and symptoms does the disease produce?

Classical Early Manifestations	Other Signs and Symptoms
Polyuria	Weight Loss
Polydipsia	Fatigue
Polyphagia	Blurred Vision
	Coma

2. Cite at least three major consequences that may occur from undiagnosed diabetes mellitus that is not well controlled for long periods of time?

   Major complications:
   - Hypertension
   - Cardiovascular disease
   - Atherosclerosis
   - Renal disease (chronic renal failure)
   - Diabetic retinopathy (blindness)
   - Peripheral and sensory neuropathy (skin ulcers, paresthesia)

Additional Information: The client visits her health care practitioner quarterly unless she experiences problems. Two years ago she was diagnosed with hypertension secondary to her diabetes mellitus and was placed on the drug metoprolol (Lopressor) 50 mg bid and a low-salt diet to control her blood pressure. Her daily insulin dose was also adjusted because her GHb (glycosylated hemoglobin) was elevated. Other medications include over-the-counter acetaminophen for occasional headaches.

3. Why is it important for the client and nurse to understand the differences between NPH and regular insulin?

> NPH insulin is cloudy, has a slower onset, and a longer duration of action. Regular insulin is clear, fast acting, and has a short duration of action. It is important that the client understand that regular insulin can be given to quickly lower her blood glucose levels if needed. It is also important that the client consume her prescribed diet after administering her NPH insulin since it will be effective for a long period of time.

4. The client took her insulin at 0730 this morning and it is now 1600. At what time did her insulin take effect, when did it peak and is it still being effective?

	Insulin Type			
	Regular		**NPH**	
Type of Effect	Duration (in hours)	Time Frame as Measured on the Clock (Start & Stop)	Duration (in hours)	Time Frame as Measured on the Clock (Start & Stop)
Initial	Within -1 hour	0800-0830	Within 1-2 hours	0830-0930
Peak	2-4 hours	0930-1130	4-12 hours	1130-1930
Duration	5-7 hours	1230-1430	8-24 hours	1530-0730
Current (at 1600 hours)	None	NA	Still effective	NA

5. Is this client monitoring her blood glucose often enough? If not, how often should she be monitoring it?

> No. Clients who take insulin should self-monitor their blood glucose at least daily in order to maintain the best possible glucose control.

Situation: Four weeks ago the client's mother died following a massive stroke. She is currently responsible for handling her mother's estate and disposing of personal property. This has placed an emotional and physical burden on the client, whose husband is frequently out of town on business. The client isn't sleeping well, and doesn't feel hungry most of the time; consequently, she sometimes forgets to eat when alone.

This evening, when the client's husband returned home, he found his wife lying on the sofa. When he attempted to talk to her he noticed she was pale and sweating profusely. She mumbled something about being tired and having a headache, but her verbalizations were difficult to understand. Upon further questioning, her answers were incoherent. Uncertain about his wife's condition, the husband decided to take her to the emergency department at their local acute care facility.

6. Based on the client's clinical manifestations, what is most likely occurring and why?

> **The client's symptoms are consistent with hypoglycemia, although hyperglycemia should be ruled out. If present, hypoglycemia is most likely related to NPH insulin dose and inadequate dietary intake secondary to grief and poor appetite.**

7. How can the ED nurse best validate the presence of hyper- or hypoglycemia in this client?

> **The nurse will assess the client's blood glucose level. If it is 60 mg/dL or below, the presence of hypoglycemia is validated.**

Situation: On arrival at the emergency department, the client remained lethargic and disoriented, mumbling incoherently. Vital signs were assessed, oxygen initiated at 6 L/min per nasal cannula, intravenous access obtained with an infusion of normal saline. Physical assessment revealed:

Client Data		
Vital Signs		
Blood Pressure	128/88	mmHg
Heart Rate	100	bpm
Respirations	28	bpm
Temperature	99.6°	F oral
Electrolyte Panel		
Na	142	mEq/L
K	5.1	mEq/L
Cl	103	mEq/L
Glucose	54	mg/dL

Creatinine	1.0	mg/dL
BUN	15	mg/dL
CBC		
Hgb	12.0	g/dL
Hct	36	%

8. If noted, what signs would alert the nurse that the client's intravenous infusion had infiltrated and what action would be necessary?

   a. Signs of infiltration:

- **Swelling at site**
- **Cool to touch**
- **Pale or blanched skin**
- **No or slow infusion of fluid**

   b. Nursing Activities:

- **Stop the infusion immediately**
- **Gather equipment to restart IV infusion in another site**
- **Place a warm cloth over the IV site to enhance circulation**

Situation: Hypoglycemia was diagnosed based on the client's assessment and laboratory findings. 1 ampule of 50% dextrose was administered as ordered by the ED physician.

---

9. Mark an "x" in the box to indicate which priority nursing actions should be implemented immediately following the administration of IV dextrose and why or why not?

Priority	Nursing Action	Why or Why Not
	Insert an indwelling urinary.	Not necessary following the IV administration of dextrose.
X	Monitor for changes in the client's sensorium.	Essential recovery should occur within 1-2 minutes following IV administration of dextrose.
	Place the client in a supine, flat position.	Not necessary. The client may be more comfortable with the head of the bead elevated.
X	Monitor blood glucose levels every 15 minutes.	Essential in order to monitor the effectiveness of the IV dextrose.
X	Reassess vital signs.	Essential to detect changes in client's status.
	Monitor for irregular pulse rate.	Dextrose does not produce an irregular heartbeat.

10. Why was intravenous dextrose administered to this client rather than a fast-acting carbohydrate such as juice or candy?

> **Oral glucose should never be administered to a client who may not be able to follow directions. The client was lethargic, disoriented and mumbling incoherently, consequently, she is at increased risk for aspiration of oral food or fluid since she may not be coherent enough to follow directions regarding swallowing.**

11. What signs or symptoms help the nurse differentiate between insulin excess and diabetic coma (insulin deficiency)? What signs and symptoms are similar for both conditions and cannot, therefore, be used to differentiate between the conditions?

Insulin Excess	Insulin Deficiency	Signs and Symptoms that Occur in Both Insulin Excess and Deficiency
Diaphoresis	Polyuria	**Confusion**
Headache	Polydipsia	**Coma**
Pallor	Polyphagia	
Irritability	Lethargy	
Nervousness	Warm, flushed skin	
Tachycardia	Dry mucus membranes	
Palpitations	Poor skin turgor	
Trembling	Dehydration	
Weakness		
Seizures		

12. While this client is being treated for insulin excess, clients with diabetes mellitus are at increased risk for the development of insulin deficiency. What serious complication is associated with insulin deficiency that must be immediately treated?

> **Metabolic acidosis**

Management of the Client in Hyperglycemic Crises: Diabetic Ketoacidosis (DKA) and Hyperosmolar Hyperglycemic State (HHS) Answer Key

Situation: A 43-year-old female client has a 24-year history of Type 1 IDDM (insulin-dependent diabetes mellitus). Four weeks ago, the client's mother died, following a massive stroke. The client is currently responsible for handling her mother's estate and disposing of personal property. This has placed a serious emotional and physical burden on the client, whose husband is frequently out of town on business. Since her mother's death, the client has lost ten pounds even though she has been snacking more than usual, is not sleeping well, and is drinking more caffeinated beverages in order to combat her chronic fatigue. Her teenage daughters are supportive of their mother but are involved in numerous school and extra-curricular activities.

1. What is the relationship between stress and blood glucose levels in the diabetic client?

    Physical and/or psychological stress stimulates the sympathetic nervous system "fight or flight" response. This response results in increased production of cortisol and catecholamines, epinephrine and norepinephrine. These hormones elevate blood glucose levels, placing the client at increased risk for the development of hyperglycemia and its complications.

Situation: When the client's husband returned home from work last evening, he found the client sleeping on the sofa. One of the daughters stated that her Mom had complained of a headache and nausea and thought she would feel better if she rested for a while. About an hour later, the client's husband decided to awaken her, only to find that he could not arouse her without shaking her vigorously. The husband called 911 and the client was immediately taken to the emergency department of the local acute care facility.

2. What does the data suggest about the client's physical state?

    The client's history of physical and emotional stress, recent weight loss, snacking, fatigue, complaints of headache and nausea, and lethargy suggest the presence of DKA (diabetic ketoacidosis).

3. Describe the process of DKA (diabetic ketoacidosis) and list factors that precipitate it.

   a. Process:

   DKA occurs when there is a relative or absolute insulin deficiency coupled with an increase in insulin agonist hormones, such as catecholamines, cortisol, glucagons, and growth hormone. These hormones not only increase glucose production but also decrease glucose utilization. When this occurs, glucose utilization in the periphery decreases, fat mobilization is increased, and ketogenesis results.

   a. Precipitating Factors:

   Surgery, infection, acute myocardial infarction (MI), trauma, lack of insulin, and emotional stress

Situation: Upon initial assessment the client was very lethargic, but awoke with shaking. She was disoriented to time and place, but she did know her name. She had rapid, deep respirations, fruity breath odor, and warm, dry, flushed skin with poor skin turgor.

CLIENT DATA		
Vital Signs		
Blood Pressure	86/50	mmHg
Heart Rate	122	bpm
Respirations	28	bpm
Temperature	99.6° F	oral
Electrolyte Panel		
Na	128	mEq/L
K	5.9	mEq/L
CL	94	mEq/L
CO_2	8	mEq/L
Glucose	593	mg/dL
Creatinine	1.9	mg/dL
Blood urea nitrogen (BUN)	28	mg/dL
ABGs (on room air)		
pH	7.2	

CLIENT DATA		
PaCO$_2$	45	mmHg
PaO$_2$	82	mmHg
SaO$_2$	92	%
HCO$_3$	12	mEq/L
Base Excess	-6.2	mEq/L
CBC		
Hgb	14.2	g/dL
Hct	45	%
Other		
Serum osmolarity	330	mOsm/L
Urine osmolarity	970	mOsm/L
Urine ketones		Positive
Serum ketones		Positive

The diagnosis of DKA (diabetic ketoacidosis) is confirmed via the client's assessment and laboratory findings. The client is ordered to receive an infusion of normal saline (NS) at 1 L over the first hour, an insulin drip to run at 5 units per hour, oxygen at 100% FIO2 per non-rebreather face-mask, placement of an indwelling urinary catheter, hourly blood glucose levels, electrolyte levels, urinary output, blood gas analysis every four hours and vital signs every 15 minutes until stable.

4. The nurse will immediately initiate several essential actions. Cite at least two priority actions and explain why each action is essential at this time.

Nursing Action	Reason for Action (Rationale)
Initiate oxygen	The client's arterial blood gases (ABGs) indicated the beginning of an oxygen deficit; therefore, oxygen is essential.
Access a vein	To provide an accessible route for emergency fluids and medications.
Initiate fluid replacement	The client's condition indicates hypovolemia, so fluid is essential to prevent hypovolemic shock. Fluid replacement also enhances glucose excretion by the kidneys.
Protect client safety	Since the client is neither alert nor completely oriented, it is necessary to protect her from injury, such as falls, pulling out IV lines, etc.

5. Which of the client's clinical manifestations support the presence of fluid volume deficit and why did she develop this complication?

   a. Signs and symptoms of fluid volume deficit:

   Warm, dry, flushed skin with poor skin turgor, elevated blood urea nitrogen (BUN) and serum creatinine, elevated Hgb and Hct, decreased blood pressure, and elevated serum potassium.

   b. Factors involved in the development of fluid volume deficit:

   In the absence of insulin, two mechanisms result in hyperglycemia: the liver increases its production of glucose and the amount of glucose moved into cells is markedly reduced. The kidneys compensate by increasing the excretion of glucose, water, sodium and holding onto potassium, which is known as osmotic diuresis and is manifested by polyuria (excessive urination). Osmotic diuresis produces an average loss of 6.5 liters of fluid within 24 hours.

6. What acid-base imbalance is the client experiencing based on analysis of her arterial blood gases (ABGs) and how does this imbalance develop?

   a. Type of imbalance: **Metabolic acidosis**

   b. Compensation: Uncompensated pH 7.20 = acidosis

   $PaCO_2$ = 45 mmHg = normal (not yet compensating)

   HCO_3 = 12 mEq/L = acidosis

   In the absence of insulin, fat breaks down into free fatty acids and glycerol. In response, the liver converts fatty acids into ketone bodies (acids), which accumulate in the circulation, producing metabolic acidosis. Insulin halts this process by preventing the breakdown of fatty acids.

7. Why is normal saline (NS) the initial fluid of choice for treatment of DKA, and at what point will dextrose be added to the infusion?

   NS (normal saline) is infused in order to replace the electrolytes (sodium and chloride) depleted as a result of osmotic diuresis. 5% dextrose, as either 5% D/W or 5% D/0.45 NS, will be added when the client's blood glucose level reaches between 250-300 mg/dL to prevent a rapid drop in blood glucose.

8. Calculate the infusion rate of insulin in order to achieve the ordered 5 units per hour if the fluid bag contains 500 mL 0.9% NS and 100 units of regular insulin.

Set up a fraction representing the amount of insulin within the infusate:

$$\frac{100 \text{ units of insulin}}{500 \text{ mL of fluid}}$$

Recall how you can reduce the numerator and denominator of a fraction by dividing them both by the same number. Here we can reduce both numbers by a common factor of 100 to get:

$$\frac{1 \text{ unit of insulin.}}{5 \text{mL of fluid}}$$

This indicates 1 unit of insulin is contained in each 5 mL of fluid.

The reciprocal of that:

$$\frac{5 \text{ mL of fluid}}{1 \text{ unit of insulin}}$$

indicates that 5 mL of fluid will be delivered with each unit of insulin. Therefore, to deliver 5 units of insulin per hour, multiply the amount of fluid transporting 1 unit of insulin by 5 hours, using the following equation:

$$\frac{5 \text{ mL of fluid}}{1 \text{ unit of insulin}} \quad \text{x} \quad \frac{5 \text{ units of insulin}}{1 \text{ hour}} \quad = \quad \frac{25 \text{ mL of fluid insulin}}{1 \text{ hour of insulin}} \quad = 25 \text{ mL/hour}$$

So, delivering 25 mL of the fluid per hour will deliver the required 5 units of insulin per hour.

9. Why is it essential the nurse carefully monitor the client's serum potassium levels?

DKA produces an intracellular to extracellular shift in potassium, as evidenced by the client's 5.9 mEq potassium level. As insulin is administered, glucose will move back into the cells, taking potassium with it, and placing the client at greatly increased risk for the development of hypokalemia.

10. Why wasn't the client's acid-base imbalance immediately treated with sodium bicarbonate?

> **Moving glucose back into the cell via the administration of exogenous insulin stops the breakdown of fat and is generally sufficient to correct the imbalance. The infusion of sodium bicarbonate can cause a sudden and potentially fatal hypokalemia.**

11. Given the client's current physical status, which three nursing diagnoses take precedence at this time?

    Risk for self-care deficit related to fatigue, illness

    Altered nutrition: Less than body requirements

X   Fluid volume deficit related to osmotic diuresis secondary to hyperglycemia

X   Anxiety related to fear, loss of control

    Knowledge deficit regarding causes of diabetic acidosis

X   Risk for injury related to altered mental status

12. After the client's condition has stabilized:

    a. Which three nursing diagnoses will take precedence?

X   Risk for self-care deficit related to fatigue, illness

X   Altered nutrition: Less than body requirements

    Fluid volume deficit related to osmotic diuresis secondary to hyperglycemia

    Anxiety related to fear, loss of control

X   Knowledge deficit regarding causes of diabetic acidosis

    Risk for injury related to altered mental status

    b. Why will priorities change?

> **Collaborative management shifts from emergency or life-threatening concerns/ diagnoses (hyperglycemia, hypokalemia and ketoacidosis) to management of non-life-threatening problems such as nutrition, management of diet/insulin, recognition of stress and need for assistance as the client's condition stabilizes.**

13. Why didn't the client's practitioner suspect HHNS (hyperglycemic hyperosmolar nonketotic syndrome) rather than DKA?

> **Many of the manifestations are similar (hyperglycemia, hyperosmolarity, osmotic diuresis, etc.), however, ketosis and acidosis are not characteristics of HHS. DKA is associated with absolute insulin deficiency (Type 1 diabetes mellitus), whereas HNS is associated with**

insulin resistance (Type 2 diabetes mellitus). With HHNS, there is not enough insulin to prevent hyperglycemia, but there is enough insulin to prevent fatty acid breakdown and acidosis.

14. Which expected outcomes are most realistic for the client during the immediate recovery period following diabetic ketoacidosis and why?

X   Restoration of fluid balance

    Knowledge of pathophysiology of diabetic ketoacidosis

X   Restoration of acid-base balance

    Restoration of normal weight

X   Decreased anxiety

X   Absence of complications

X   Restoration of electrolyte balance

    Ability to care for self independently

With immediate and appropriate collaborative interventions, the client experiencing diabetic ketoacidosis can be returned to a normal state of fluid, electrolyte, and acid-base balance; avoiding complications. Clients may not be able to fully understand the complicated pathophysiology of the condition. Restoration of normal weight may take weeks to months. The client may not be able to provide self-care independently during the immediate recovery time period.

Nursing Management of the Client with Cardiac Dysrhythmias (Arrhythmias) Answer Key

Situation: The nurse is monitoring several clients in the cardiac care unit who are at risk for the development of cardiac dysrhythmias.

1. One of the clients loses consciousness and has no palpable pulse. The cardiac monitor indicates the client is experiencing ventricular fibrillation. Which action will the nurse perform first?

   _____ Document the dysrhythmia

   _____ Notify the physician

   X   Begin CPR

2. Explain why these nursing diagnoses are appropriate for clients at risk for cardiac dysrhythmias.

   a. Risk for decreased cardiac output

   When the heartbeat is irregular, the heart's ability to pump blood is compromised; therefore the client is at increased risk for decreased cardiac output.

   b. Risk for altered tissue perfusion

   Tissues will not receive enough blood and oxygen if the heart does not pump effectively and cardiac output is lowered. Persons experiencing decreased cardiac output are at increased risk for altered tissue perfusion.

   c. Anxiety

   Clients who suffer dysrhythmias experience anxiety related to fear of the unknown. They do not know if they will recover or suffer permanent heart damage.

3. What are some of the common risk factors, other than cardiac disease, for development of cardiac dysrhythmias?

> **In addition to cardiac disease, risk factors for cardiac dysrhythmias include:**
> *   Chronic renal, hepatic, or lung disease
> *   Drug use or abuse
> *   Shock
> *   Fear
> *   Electrolyte disturbances
> *   Fever
> *   Pain
> *   Anxiety
> *   Hypoxia
> *   Infection

Nursing Management of the Client Requiring an Electrocardiogram (ECG) Answer Key

Situation: As part of his yearly physical examination, a 55-year-old male client is undergoing an ECG (electrocardiogram) exercise stress test. The client is instructed to walk on a treadmill for 30 minutes while the nurse performs an ECG. Prior to the procedure, the nurse obtains the client's baseline blood pressure, pulse rate, and rhythm strip. The nurse carefully monitors the client and ECG tracings throughout the procedure. Once the procedure is over, the nurse helps the client to a resting position, and continues to monitor his ECG and vital signs until they are stable.

1. What is the purpose of ECG stress testing?

   The purpose of ECG testing is to determine how the client's cardiovascular system reacts to the challenge of increased physical activity.

2. Which conditions contraindicate the use of ECG stress testing?

   _____ Angina pectoris   **X** Heart failure

   X Myocarditis   _____ Mild hypertension

   X Bradycardia   **X** Recent acute MI

   X First-degree heart block   **X** Endocarditis

   X Severe aortic stenosis   _____ Sinus dysrhythmia

3. Which instructions should the nurse give the client prior to ECG stress testing?

   _____ Do not eat or drink for at least 12 hours prior to the test.

   X Avoid nicotine, alcohol, coffee, and tea on the test day.

   X Wear loose comfortable clothes and sturdy shoes.

   _____ Hold all prescribed medications until after the test.

   X Report any chest pain or dyspnea during and following the test.

   _____ Take a hot shower after completing the test.

4. List the clinical manifestations for which ECG testing must be stopped.

- Chest pain
- Fatigue
- Leg cramps
- Dizziness
- Severe tachycardia or sudden development of bradycardia
- Cardiac arrhythmias
- Sudden drop in blood pressure
- Severe dyspnea
- ST segment depression
- Sudden loss of coordination

Nursing Management of the Client with Angina Pectoris
Answer Key

Situation: A 42-year-old male visits the emergency department stating he developed severe chest pain radiating to his jaw while mowing his lawn. His blood pressure is 140/90, pulse 88 bpm and respirations 26 bpm. The nurse administers a prescribed sublingual nitroglycerin tablet and starts oxygen by nasal cannula at 5 L per minute. Within 30 minutes, the client states his pain is relieved.

1. Which instructions should be given to the client before he goes home?

   X   How to use nitroglycerine at home should his chest pain return

   X   To take rest periods between activities to prevent chest pain

   _____ To self administer an antiarrhythmic drug if his chest pain persists

   _____ How to take his own blood pressure and pulse

   X   The need to make immediate changes in his lifestyle

2. Match the type of angina with the clinical manifestations it produces. Use "V", "S", "U" or "I" as your answers.

V = Variant angina (Prinzmetal's)	**V**	Not relieved by conventional methods
S =Stable angina (Exertional)	**V**	Lasts for a long period of time
U = Unstable angina	**S**	Relieved by rest
I = Intractable angin	**U**	Increases in severity over time
	I	Persistent, incapacitating pain
	V,U	Occurs with exercise or stress

3. Which statements are true about angina? Correct any false statements.

   a. Angina may produce pain that radiates to the neck or arms.

   True.

b. Angina is often described as a sharp, unrelenting pain.

False. Angina is usually described as dull and aching.

c. Clients with angina are taught to take nitroglycerin every fifteen minutes for severe pain.

False. Clients with angina are taught to take nitroglycerin every five minutes for three doses for severe pain.

d. Eating a heavy meal can precipitate angina pectoris.

True.

Nursing Management of the Client with Myocardial Infarction (MI)
Answer Key

Situation: A 46-year-old man is brought to the emergency department after experiencing sudden, crushing substernal chest pain, which was unrelieved by rest or nitroglycerin. He is pale, cool, clammy, and diaphoretic. He complains of nausea and of the inability to take a deep breath. His blood pressure is 105/80, heart rate 92 bpm, and respirations 28 per minute.

---

1. What is the rationale for implementing these collaborative interventions for a client who is suffering an acute MI (myocardial infarction)?

   a. Initiate oxygen

   Providing oxygen increases the amount of oxygen supplied to the heart muscle, decreasing workload and ischemia.

   b. Obtain intravenous access

   It is essential to obtain intravenous access in the event that emergency drugs need to be rapidly delivered.

   c. Initiate continuous cardiac monitoring

   Continuous cardiac monitoring is initiated to determine heart rate and rhythm, and guide emergency drug therapy.

   d. Administer morphine sulfate

   Morphine sulfate is the drug of choice for acute myocardial infarction to decrease pain and anxiety.

2. What are the most reliable tests to determine if the client is experiencing a MI (myocardial infarction) or angina?

   X Serial electrocardiograms

   _____ Serum electrolytes

   _____ Chest x-ray

   X Serum enzyme studies

3. For which three complications is the client most at risk during this early stage of MI (myocardial infarction)?

_____ Electrolyte imbalance	**X** Sudden death
X Cardiac dysrhythmias	_____ Metabolic acidosis
X Cardiogenic shock	_____ CHF (congestive heart failure)

Nursing Management of the Client with Cardiac Arrest
Answer Key

Situation: A 60-year-old hospitalized male client who had experienced an acute MI three days earlier was in stable condition when he suddenly developed ventricular fibrillation swiftly followed by cardiac arrest. Following verification that the client had arrested, CPR was started immediately. The staff quickly responded to the emergency code, and arrived at the client's bedside with the crash cart. The attending physician defibrillated the client, while the nurse prepared and administered emergency medications via the client's intravenous line. The client responded satisfactorily to the emergency interventions. The nurses documented the event and notified the family of the client's condition.

1. For which purpose is cardiac defibrillation used?

   _____ Cardiac standstill   _____ Premature ventricular contractions

   X Ventricular fibrillation   _____ Atrial fibrillation

2. What is an AED (automated external defibrillator), and what is its primary advantage?

   The AED is an automatic defibrillator that does not require analysis of data or selection of settings by the staff. Staff members place electrodes and the machine automatically analyzes the client's rhythm, chooses an energy level, charges the machine, and shocks the client. The AED allows for faster defibrillation of the client.

3. What are the purposes of ACLS (advanced cardiac life support)?

   The purposes of ACLS (advanced cardiac life support) include:
   - **Basic life support**
   - **The use of specialized equipment and techniques for ventilating the client and reestablishing circulation**
   - **ECG (electrocardiogram) monitoring**
   - **Immediate recognition of dysrhythmias**
   - **Establishment of an intravenous line**
   - **Stabilization in the phase following cardiac arrest**
   - **Treatment of clients with suspected acute MI.**

4. What should the nurse document, following the defibrillation process?

_____ The presence of family members	**X** The client's condition prior to intervention
_____ Any known allergies	**X** The pre-procedure rhythm
_____ The number of defibrillation attempts	**X** The post-defibrillation rhythm
X Vital signs	_____ Intake and output
X Emergency drugs administered	

Nursing Management of the Client with Central Venous Pressure (CVP) Monitoring Answer Key

Situation: A 55-year-old male client with right ventricular failure is being assessed for increased CVP. During admission, a nurse estimated the client's CVP and determined it was high. The client's CVP was then measured several times over the next 24 hours. The client's CVP ranged from 12 cm H_2O to 15 cm H_2O. However, the next reading was 8 cm H_2O.

1. What does "CVP" stand for, and what does it measure?

   CVP stands for central venous pressure. It measures the pressure in the right atrium of the heart, as well as the workload on the heart's right side.

2. Clients with which of the following problems are candidates for CVP monitoring?

_____ Acute appendicitis	**X**	Hypertension
X CHF (congestive heart failure)	_____	Acute MI (myocardial infarction)
_____ ARF (acute renal failure)	_____	Tuberculosis
X Septic shock	**X**	Cardiac tamponade
X Hemorrhage		

3. What actions does the nurse perform prior to assessing a client's CVP?

   The nurse places the client in the supine position and elevates the head of the bed 45º.

4. List at least three factors that can cause a CVP measurement to differ significantly from previous readings.

   - **Incorrect positioning of the client, catheter, or manometer**
   - **Loose or disconnected tubing**

- Hemorrhage
- An obstructed catheter
- Client coughing or restlessness
- Client airway obstruction

Nursing Management of the Client with Congestive Heart Failure (CHF) Answer Key

Situation: A 72-year-old woman is admitted to the acute care facility for dyspnea, fatigue, and dizziness. She has a history of hypertension and coronary artery disease. She lives independently and reports that her diet consists primarily of canned soups and other pre-packaged foods. Assessment reveals bilateral crackles, irregular heart rate with a bounding pulse at 92 bpm, blood pressure of 190/96, and 4+ pitting edema of both ankles.

1. What risk factors does the client have for congestive heart failure?

   Older age, history of hypertension and congestive heart failure, and her intake of high sodium-containing food

2. What is the etiology for each of the client's nursing diagnoses?

   a. Fluid volume excess

   Fluid volume excess related to decreased cardiac output secondary to hypertension, cad, and high sodium intake.

   b. Impaired gas exchange

   Impaired gas exchange related to fluid in alveoli.

   c. Activity intolerance

   Activity intolerance related to fatigue and fluid in alveoli.

   d. Risk for altered skin integrity

   Risk for altered skin integrity related to peripheral edema.

3. Prioritize the following nursing interventions, with "1" representing the most important intervention.

   1 Assess breath sounds and breathing patterns.

   3 Report laboratory results.

   5 Assess capillary refill.

   4 Monitor urine output.

   2 Place client in high-Fowler's position.

4. How does the drug digitalis help to alleviate the signs and symptoms associated with congestive heart failure?

   Digitalis decreases the signs and symptoms associated with congestive heart failure by increasing the force of myocardial contraction and the refractory period of the atrioventricular (AV) node, which enhances circulation and allows the kidneys to excrete excess fluid.

5. What should the client be taught about her intake of canned soup and pre-packaged food?

   The client should be taught that canned soups and prepackaged foods generally contain excessive amounts of salt (sodium), which contribute to the development of congestive heart failure. The client should be taught to avoid the intake of high sodium-containing foods.

Nursing Management of the Client with Hypertension Answer Key

Situation: During a routine physical examination, a 55-year-old moderately obese male with a 13-year history of Type 2 NIDDM (non-insulin dependent diabetes mellitus) learns he has hypertension. The client is divorced, does not exercise on a regular basis, and has a stressful job. He controls his diabetes mellitus with a daily oral hypoglycemic agent and diet, although he admits he doesn't control his diet as well as he should.

1. Which statements are true about hypertension? Correct any false statements.

   a. Hypertension is a major risk factor for other diseases, such as renal failure.

   True.

   b. Maintaining a diastolic pressure below 80 mmHg is a goal of treatment for hypertension.

   False. Maintaining a diastolic pressure below 90 mmHg is a goal of treatment for hypertension.

   c. Moderate smoking has little effect on blood pressure.

   False. Moderate smoking produces vasoconstriction, which contributes to hypertension.

   d. Arterial plaque increases peripheral vascular resistance, producing secondary hypertension.

   True.

2. What is the difference between primary and secondary hypertension?

   Primary (essential) hypertension has no identifiable medical cause, whereas, secondary hypertension results from a specific cause, such as arterial disease, renal disease or diabetes mellitus.

3. Which risk factors for hypertension are modifiable?

_____ Hereditary predisposition	**X** Sedentary lifestyle
_____ Diabetes mellitus	_____ Gende
X Diet	_____ Race
X Tobacco use	**X** Obesity
X Stress	_____ Advancing age
_____ Arteriosclerosis	**X** Chronic illness

Nursing Management of the Client with Thrombophlebitis
Answer Key

Situation: A 43-year-old obese female underwent abdominal surgery two days ago and is now experiencing acute pain in her right calf. The pain is exacerbated by activity and not relieved by rest. The limb is obviously swollen and warm to the touch. Her peripheral pulses are palpable bilaterally. Her routine medications are birth control pills and vitamins.

---

1. What risk factors does the client have for thrombophlebitis?

   Surgery after the age of 40, obesity, and oral contraceptives

2. Prioritize the client's nursing diagnoses, with "1" representing the most important diagnosis.

   1 Altered tissue perfusion (right lower extremity)

   4 Risk for impaired skin integrity

   3 Impaired mobility

   5 Risk for activity intolerance

   2 Pain

3. What teaching needs to be done before the client is discharged to home following her recovery?

   _____ Take aspirin daily with anticoagulant therapy

   X Avoid long periods of standing or sitting

   _____ Massage the limb gently if pain occurs

   X Report blood in the urine or bleeding gums

Nursing Management of the Client with a Coronary Artery Bypass Graft (CABG) Answer Key

Situation: A 75-year-old client is home after being discharged from the surgical unit following CABG (coronary artery bypass graft) surgery for severe left main coronary artery obstruction. The client is in the process of starting his cardiac rehabilitation program. The home health nurse is giving the client general instructions for self-care following CABG. The client is learning about his medications, how to care for his support stockings, and when to call his physician should problems arise. The nurse is also scheduling the client for a home exercise rehabilitation program.

1. For which problems should the client be instructed to call his physician?

    X Elevated temperature for over 24 hours

    _____ Mild fatigue following performance of daily hygiene

    X Separation of suture line

    _____ Increased heart rate with exercise

    X Foul-smelling drainage from the suture line

    X Red, swollen suture line

    _____ Flaking skin around suture line

2. What are support stockings, how often are they worn, and how are they cared for?

    Support stockings are elastic stockings that help improve the client's circulation and prevent swelling of the limb. The stockings are worn every day; therefore, the client should have two pairs. The stockings should be washed in warm, soapy water and hung up to dry. The stockings will be damaged if placed in a clothes dryer.

3. The client is beginning an at-home exercise rehabilitation program. When and how often will the client exercise? What records will the client need to keep about his exercise and its results?

    The client will begin his exercise program as soon as he arrives home. He will gradually work toward his exercise goals. Once met, he will be advised to continue exercising at least three times weekly. The client will be asked to keep a daily log of heart rates, exercise parameters, and any problems that arise during exercise sessions.

Nursing Management of the Client with Atherosclerosis— Coronary Artery Disease (CAD) Answer Key

Situation: A 41-year-old African-American male who smokes two packs of cigarettes a day visits his health care provider because of unusual fatigue and shortness of breath when climbing stairs or exerting himself. He drives a truck for a living and works six or seven days a week. The client's health care provider suspects that the client is experiencing these symptoms due to his smoking and the presence of coronary artery disease.

1. Which statements are true about atherosclerosis? Correct false statements.

   a. Atherosclerosis ultimately leads to decreased tissue perfusion.

      True.

   b. Hypertension is a major contributing factor to the development of atherosclerosis.

      False. Atherosclerosis is a major contributing factor to the development of hypertension.

   c. Atherosclerosis is more common among older adults with chronic illnesses.

      True.

   d. It is desirable to have higher LDL levels than HDL levels.

      False. The reverse is true. It is desirable to have higher HDL levels than LDL levels.

2. Which of the client's risk factors for atherosclerosis are not modifiable?

_____ Tobacco use	**X**	Age
_____ Obesity	_____	Sedentary lifestyle
_____ Stress producing job	**X**	Race
X Gender		

3. Provide rationale for implementing these nursing interventions.

   a. Monitor blood pressure.

      CAD produces hypertension; therefore, the client's blood pressure should be monitored closely.

b. Monitor blood glucose levels.

Hyperglycemia is a primary risk factor for the development of CAD; therefore, blood glucose levels need to be monitored.

c. Help the client to identify risk factors for CAD.

Identifying and addressing risk factors that can be modified will help the client control or even reverse the progression of CAD

Nursing Management of the Client with Iron-Deficiency Anemia Answer Key

Situation: A 22-year-old woman volunteers to donate blood at her nearby community blood bank. After the nurse checks the woman's hemoglobin, the woman is informed she cannot donate blood because her hemoglobin level is too low. The client is advised to follow-up with her health care provider, who determines the client has iron-deficiency anemia most likely related to insufficient dietary intake of iron.

1. What are the most common causes of iron-deficiency anemia?

   Blood loss or inadequate intake of iron-containing foods

2. State rationale for each of the nursing interventions for iron-deficiency anemia.

   a. Provide frequent oral hygiene.

   The corners of the mouth may crack and become red and painful. This condition, called cheilosis, may be soothed with gentle oral care. It is important to avoid oral mouthwashes that contain alcohol. The nurse should provide teaching regarding the hydration and lubrication of the lips and oral mucosa.

   b. Encourage the intake of foods high in fiber.

   Increasing dietary fiber helps prevent the constipation that commonly occurs when taking iron supplements.

   c. Encourage increased fluid intake.

   Increasing fluid intake will help prevent the constipation that commonly occurs when taking iron supplements.

   d. Teach client that supplemental iron is eliminated in stool.

   This prevents the client from becoming anxious or fearful when green or black stools are observed.

   e. Teach client that liquid iron preparations should be taken through a straw.

   Iron preparations can stain the teeth; therefore, clients should be encouraged to take liquid iron supplements through a straw.

3. When the nurse advises the client to eat organ meats the client replies that she is a vegetarian and does not eat meat or poultry. What other foods can the nurse suggest to the client?

_____	Signs of infection	_____	Body image
_____	Carrots	**X**	Beans
X	Leafy green vegetables	**X**	Raisins
_____	Bananas	**X**	Molasses

Nursing Management of the Client with Abdominal Aortic Aneurysm (AAA) Answer Key

Situation: A 49-year-old man is being prepared for surgery following his admission to the emergency department for severe abdominal and back pain. He has smoked cigarettes for 34 years and has a history of hypertension controlled by medication. Assessment and radiographic studies reveal the presence of a leaking AAA (abdominal aortic aneurysm).

1. What are the client's risk factors for development of an AAA (abdominal aortic aneurysm)?

   - **Tobacco use**
   - **Male gender**
   - **Hypertension**

2. While all of these interventions are important, which four need to be implemented first, and in what order?

   1 Administering oxygen

   3 btaining intravenous access

   _____ Inserting an indwelling urinary catheter

   4 Administering pain medication

   _____ Initiating a preoperative care plan

   _____ Teaching the client about the surgery

   2 Monitoring vital signs

   _____ Providing emotional support to the family

3. The client is at increased risk for shock if his aneurysm ruptures. The nurse will, therefore, carefully monitor the client for which serious complications?

_____ Nausea		**X**	Hemorrhage
_____ Seizures		**X**	Acute renal failure
_____ Hypertensive crisis		**X**	Arterial occlusion

Nursing Management of the Client with a Femoral-Popliteal Bypass Graft Answer Key

---

Situation: A 68-year-old male client with atherosclerosis in his lower limbs has just undergone a femoral-popliteal bypass graft. Upon admission to the PACU (Postanesthesia Care Unit), the nurse monitors the client's vital signs, assesses the operative limb, takes ABI (ankle-brachial index) measurements, and monitors for signs and symptoms of bypass graft occlusion.

---

1. Which assessments are made hourly following popliteal bypass graft surgery?

   _____ Blood pressure   **X** Limb color ✓

   X Limb capillary refill ✓   _____ Oral temperature

   _____ Apical heart rate   _____ Femoral pulse

   X Limb peripheral pulses ✓ **X** Limb temperature ✓

   _____ Limb movement

2. How did the nurse calculate the client's ABI (ankle-brachial index) measurement?

   This test is done by measuring blood pressure at the ankle and in the arm while a person is at rest. Measurements are then repeated at both sites after 5 minutes of walking on a treadmill.

   By dividing the blood pressure at the ankle by the blood pressure in the arm, the ankle-brachial index (ABI) can be calculated.

   A standard ABI measurement is 1.0. ABI measurements decrease with occlusion of the bypass graft

3. What is the purpose of obtaining postoperative ABI (ankle-brachial index) measurements on clients who have undergone popliteal bypass graft surgery?

   ABI (ankle-brachial index) measurements are used to diagnose the severity of atherosclerotic disease, and to monitor the potency of bypass grafts following surgery.

4. What signs and symptoms indicate occlusion of the bypass graft?

_____ Decreasing blood pressure	**X**	Cool, operative limb
X Pallor of limb	**X**	Nonpalpable peripheral pulses
X Extremity numbness	_____	Increasing ankle-brachial index measurements
_____ Extremity twitching	**X**	Severe limb pain

Nursing Management of the Client with a Blood Transfusion
Answer Key

Situation: A 44-year-old man has hemoglobin of 7.8 g/dL due to blood loss secondary to a slowly bleeding gastric ulcer. The bleeding has been controlled and the client is stable. Two successive whole blood transfusions have been prescribed to replace his lost blood volume.

1. Prior to initiating the blood transfusion, it is important for the nurse to assess the client's **temperature, pulse, respirations** and **blood pressure.**

2. The client states he is afraid to receive a transfusion because of AIDS. How should the nurse respond to the client's concern?

> **Reassure the client the nation's blood supply is very safe and his need for the transfusion far outweighs the risks involved. If the client continues to be concerned, the health care provider should be contacted. The client has a right to refuse treatment.**

3. Match the type of blood reaction with its associated signs and symptoms.

a. Febrile	**d**	Chills
b. Anaphylactic	**a,f**	Headache
c. Mild Allergic	**b,d**	Hypotension
d. Acute hemolytic	**a**	Rapid onset fever
e. Sepsis	**c**	Itching
f. Circulatory overload	**b,d**	Dyspnea
	b,f	Cyanosis
	d,f	Tachycardia
	f	Hypertension
	e	Abdominal pain

	d	Low back pain
	b,d,e	Shock
	e	Vomiting
	d,f	Tachypnea
	a,d	Flushing

4. Prioritize nursing actions for the client who experiences a reaction to a blood transfusion, with "1" representing the first action needed.

   3   Assess vital signs

   4   Open the infusion of normal saline

   2   Notify the client's practitioner

   1   Stop the transfusion

Nursing Management of the Client with Digitalis Toxicity
Answer Key

Situation: A 67-year-old female with a history of congestive heart failure is admitted to the acute care facility due to increased shortness of breath and peripheral edema. Her usual dose of 0.125 mg of oral digitalis has been increased to 0.25 mg PO each morning and evening.

---

1. Prior to administering the fifth dose of digitalis, the nurse assesses the client's apical heart, which is 54 and irregular. What should the nurse do?

   Hold the digitalis, note the client's cardiac rate and rhythm on her cardiac monitor, and report the findings to the client's health care provider.

2. Which signs should alert the nurse to the presence of digitalis toxicity?

   _____ Constipation   **X** Bradycardia _~low breathing_

   X Yellow vision   **X** Nausea ✓

   _____ Hypertension   _____ Leg cramps

   X Vomiting ✓   **X** Diarrhea ✓

   X Heart block ✓

3. Which tests most accurately demonstrate the presence of digitalis toxicity?

   X ECG (electrocardiogram)   _____ Serum electrolytes

   _____ BUN (blood urea nitrogen)   **X** Serum digitalis level

Nursing Management of the Client with HIV/AIDS Answer Key

Situation: A 30-year-old client reported to an outpatient clinic for complaints of fatigue and sore throat lasting more than three weeks in spite of frequent rest periods and use of OTC (over-the-counter) cold medications. Physical examination was essentially normal except for the presence of painful white patches in the client's mouth and throat and enlarged cervical lymph nodes. The client's vital signs were a temperature of 100.2° F, heart rate 90 bpm and regular, respirations 16, BP 118/74. Blood samples were obtained for a mononucleosis test and ELISA (enzyme linked immunosorbent assay). It is now one week later and the client must be informed their ELISA test was positive and they have oral candidiasis.

1. What is the significance of the client's positive ELISA test?

   A positive ELISA test means the client has been infected with and produced antibodies to the human immunodeficiency virus. It does not indicate the client has AIDS or will develop AIDS within a specified period of time. It is a screening test that must be validated by further testing.

2. What further testing is essential at this time?

   A western blot test is indicated to validate the positive ELISA test. It is a more sensitive test for HIV antibodies and helps to establish the diagnosis of HIV infection. Since the client has an opportunistic infection (candidiasis), a complete blood count (CBC), CD4 cell count, and lymphocyte count are appropriate at this time.

3. What is the best response to each of the client's questions?

   a. "What is an HIV infection?"

      HIV (human immunodeficiency virus) is a retrovirus transmitted by direct contact with infected blood or body fluids. The virus infects and ultimately destroys T4 helper cells, leaving the person at increased risk for development of infections. HIV may remain inactive for years (8-10 years is the average), or progress to severe immunodeficiency (AIDS).

b. "What is AIDS?"

Acquired immune deficiency syndrome is a progressive loss of immune function and accompanying opportunistic infections due to HIV and loss of CD4 helper cells, which may result in death within 18-24 months following diagnosis.

c. "Are there medications I can take? If so, what are they?"

Yes. Medications are now available that may suppress the HIV infection itself, decrease symptoms, and prolong life. Medications are also available to treat most of the opportunistic infections and malignancies associated with HIV infection. Drug therapies include protease inhibitors, zidovudine (Retrovir, AZT), and other immune modulator drugs. Your health care provider will discuss drug options with you and help you select the best combination of drugs based on your laboratory data and symptoms.

d. "What is oral candidiasis?"

Oral candidiasis is a fungal infection most commonly seen in newborns. It takes advantage of the host's deficient immune system to produce disease. If left untreated, candida can affect your lungs and gastrointestinal tract. You will be treated with oral and topical anti-fungal medications to control this infection.

e. "Am I at risk for other infections? If so, what?"

Yes. You are at increased risk of developing other opportunistic infections, such as Pneumocystis pneumonia, mycobacterium avium pneumonia, tuberculosis, toxoplasmosis, or cytomegalovirus.

f. "Am I going to die?"

This is a difficult question to answer. Most people have a long period of wellness after diagnosis and very good responses have been obtained from use of antiretroviral and anti-infective drugs. There is no known cure for HIV infection or AIDS at this time, but promising research is continuing. Death is usually due to overwhelming opportunistic infections. It is important you maintain a well-balanced diet and continue close follow-up care. Your prognosis (future outlook) will depend on the extent of immune damage you are suffering and your response to medication.

4. Cite the two nursing diagnoses that are of highest priority at this time.

a. Nursing diagnosis # 1

Risk for ineffective individual coping related to changes in lifestyle.

b. Nursing diagnosis # 2

Knowledge deficit regarding disease process, medications, and follow-up care

5. After additional testing, the client is found to have a CD4 T-cell count of 150/mm3 (per cubic millimeter) and an HIV/RNA count of 110,000. What does this mean?

> The findings indicate the client is at high risk for developing AIDS, especially since he is symptomatic (candidiasis).
>
> The CD4 T-cell count measures the extent of immune damage due to HIV infection. Counts >500 cells/mm3 require 6-month evaluations; counts of 200-499 cells/mm3 require 3-month evaluations; counts <200 require even more frequent client evaluations.
>
> HIV/RNA levels measure the amount of HIV virus in the client's serum. Plasma HIV/RNA level <10,000 cells/mL is considered low risk for developing AIDS, levels of 10,000- 99,999 cells/mL indicate a risk of developing AIDS that is twice that when HIV/RNA level <10,000 cells/mL, and levels >100,000 cells/mL indicate high risk for developing AIDS.

6. What should the client be taught about follow up care?

> Close follow-up care is essential since the client has suffered significant damage to their immune system (CD4 cell count below 200/mm3). The client will be treated with various medications that may produce side effects and the client is at significantly increased risk for development of opportunistic infections.

Nursing Management of the Client with Candidiasis Answer Key

Situation: A 35-year-old client is undergoing chemotherapy following a modified radical mastectomy for breast cancer. Her mouth is fiery red with white patches on her tongue and oral mucous membranes. She complains of pain when eating and attempting to brush her teeth. Oral candidiasis is suspected.

1. Why is candidiasis considered an opportunistic infection?

   Candida is a common yeast harbored by most all individuals. It does not, however, produce infection in immune-competent people. When a person's immune system is deficient or suppressed, as occurs with cancer chemotherapy, candida takes advantage of the suppressed state and causes disease; thus, it is labeled an "opportunistic" infection.

2. Which nursing actions will be most effective in addressing the client's oral pain?

   X Encourage the use of a soft-bristled toothbrush

   _____ Add orange juice or grapefruit juice to the client's diet

   _____ Encourage use of an alcohol-based mouth rinse

   X Administer antifungal medications as prescribed

3. Which statements are true about candidiasis? Correct false statements.

   a. Candidiasis is a disease of infants and older adults.
      False. Candidiasis can affect all age groups.

   b. Candidiasis is a primary fungal infection caused by candida albicans.
      False. Candidiasis is a secondary fungal infection most commonly caused by candida albicans.

   c. Candidiasis commonly occurs in persons with a deficient or immature immune system.
      True.

   d. Treatment of candidiasis often involves treatment of an underlying immune problem.
      True.

Nursing Management of the Client with Systemic Lupus Erythematosus (SLE) Answer Key

Situation: A 26-year-old female has been admitted to the acute care facility for re-evaluation and control of her systemic lupus erythematosus. She is receiving NSAIDs and Prednisone (corticosteroid) to control her symptoms.

1. Why is lupus erythematosus considered an autoimmune disease?

   Lupus is considered an autoimmune disease because the body's immune system attacks its own connective tissues, producing inflammation and injury. Q₁

2. Which are common clinical manifestations of lupus erythematosus?

X Reddened facial rash	_____ Fever >102°
_____ Weight gain	**X** Anemia
_____ Peripheral edema	**X** Photosensitivity
_____ Headache	**X** Proteinuria
X Weakness	_____ Cough

3. Which nursing activities are useful in reducing the pain associated with SLE (systemic lupus erythematosus)?

   _____ Performing active range of motion exercises.

   X Placing heat on the affected joints

   X Administering anti-inflammatory agents routinely.

   _____ Administering narcotic pain relievers.

4. Which symptoms will be relieved by use of NSAIDs or corticosteroids?

X Fever	**X** Joint swelling
_____ Fatigue	_____ Weakness
X Joint pain	_____ Anemia

Nursing Management of the Client with Hepatitis Answer Key

Situation: A nurse is caring for two clients. One, an older male, has Hepatitis B. The second client, a young female, has Hepatitis A.

1. Match the type of hepatitis (A or B) with the appropriate description.

    A   The fecal-oral route is the primary route of transmission ✓

    B   Ten percent of clients infected will develop chronic hepatitis

    B   A DNA virus

    A   Contracted from contaminated foods or fluids

    B   The virus is found in semen, vaginal secretions and saliva

    A   Incubation period ranges from 2-7 weeks

    B   Transmitted primarily through blood

2. Match the type of hepatitis (A or B) with its characteristic sign or symptom. Clients may be asymptomatic.

A	Low-grade fever	**A,B**	Abdominal pain
A,B	Fatigue, malaise	**A,B**	Dark, brown urine
A	Nausea, vomiting	**A**	Pruritus
B	Anorexia	**A,B**	Enlarged, tender liver
A,B	Jaundice	**B**	Dyspepsia
A,B	Clay-colored stools	**A**	Mild, flu-like symptoms
A	Headache	**B**	Enlarged posterior cervical lymph nodes

3. Cite the etiology for the nursing diagnoses that apply to both clients.

   a. Risk for altered nutrition: less than body requirements
      Anorexia

   b. Risk for injury: others
      Transmissibility of disease

   c. Risk for activity intolerance
      Fatigue, weakness

   d. Abdominal pain
      Liver inflammation

   e. Anxiety/fear
      Threat to own well-being

Nursing Management of the Client with Cancer Answer Key

Situation: A 49-year-old male has a 32-year history of cigarette smoking. He often eats out with associates and typically eats red meat and potatoes. One of his associates is a 51-year-old female whose mother died of breast cancer. She is 40 pounds over her ideal weight because she likes to snack during the day. She is also a heavy coffee drinker.

1. What risk factors does each of these clients have for development of cancer?

   a. Male:

      Cigarette smoker, diet

   b. Female:

      Obesity, genetic predisposition, caffeine intake

2. Which statements are true about cancer? Correct inaccurate statements.

   a. Cancer involves abnormal cell growth and differentiation.

      True.

   b. Viral agents cause the majority of cancers.

      False. Chemical and physical agents, as well as viruses, cause cancers.

   c. Diet is thought to be a factor that triggers abnormal cell growth.

      True.

   d. Metastasis occurs when cancer directly spreads to distant organs.

      False. Metastasis occurs when cancer spreads directly into adjacent tissues (or indirectly to distant sites) via blood or lymphatics.

   e. Cancer may involve the skin, bone, any organ, or blood.

      True.

   f. Few cancers are curable even when diagnosed early.

      False. Early detection may result in improved prognosis for many types of malignancy.

3. What is the rationale for each nursing intervention?

    a. Monitor for secondary problems.

    Clients with cancer are at increased risk for secondary problems (infection, thrombocytopenia, neutropenia, bleeding, skin breakdown, and weight loss) due to tissue damage from the cancer and from cancer treatments (chemotherapy, radiation, surgery).

    b. Promote adequate food and fluid intake.

    Clients with cancer need additional nutrients and fluids to counteract the effects of cancer growth, chemotherapy, radiation, and surgery.

    c. Educate clients regarding early detection, including CAUTION model.

    Many cancers can be cured when diagnosed early; therefore, it is essential to educate clients about the early warning signs of cancer.

    d. Plan activities to conserve client's energy.

    Clients with cancer are often fatigued from both the cancer and its treatment, therefore to conserve energy are an important part of treatment.

    a. Offer emotional support regarding grieving, loss, and anxiety.

    Clients with cancer must undergo treatments that are often debilitating and painful. They face an uncertain future; therefore, emotional support is essential.

4. What does CAUTION stand for in relation to cancer?

    C: Changes in bowel or bladder habits

    A: A sore that doesn't heal

    U: Unusual bleeding or discharge

    T: Thickening or lump in the breast or elsewhere

    I: Indigestion or difficulty swallowing

    O: Obvious changes in warts or moles

    N: Nagging cough or hoarseness

Nursing Management of the Client with Liver Cancer Answer Key

Situation: A 65-year-old male client is being evaluated for possible primary hepatocellular carcinoma. The client is slightly jaundiced, and he has been experiencing nausea, anorexia, and abdominal pain. His health care provider has also discovered a small abdominal mass in the right upper quadrant. The client is scheduled for a liver biopsy.

1. Which are accurate steps for the nurse to take when preparing a client for a liver biopsy?

    _____ Instruct the client to take nothing by mouth for one to two hours prior to the procedure.

    X Explain the procedure, its purposes and risks.

    X Discuss how important it is for the client to follow instructions during the procedure.

    _____ Administer sedation an hour and a half prior to the procedure.

    X Assist the client into a supine or left lateral position.

2. Which are clinical manifestations of pneumothorax during liver biopsy?

_____ Decreased respiratory rate	**X**	Pleuritic chest pain
X Shoulder pain	_____	Inability to inhale
X Shortness of breath	**X**	Decreased breath sounds

3. Why are pain medications administered with caution to clients with liver cancer?

    Pain medications must be administered with caution to clients with liver disease because they are metabolized in the liver. When liver function is impaired, medications cannot be biotransformed by the liver into inactive metabolites resulting in altered effectiveness or toxicity of the drug and further damage to the liver.

4. What is the etiology of the client's nursing diagnoses?

   a. Risk for impaired skin integrity

      Related to bile deposits in the skin and resultant inflammation and pruritus

   b. Self-care deficit

      Related to fatigue and body wasting, secondary to cancerous process

   c. Altered nutrition: Less than body requirements

      Related to anorexia, nausea, vomiting, and/or chemotherapy

   d. Pain

      Related to liver inflammation and tissue destruction, secondary to cancerous process

Nursing Management of the Client with a Common Cold or Influenza Answer Key

Situation: A 71-year-old woman who lives with her daughter is exposed to a child who has a cold when they visit nearby relatives. The woman has already had pneumonia this winter and she is concerned about becoming ill again.

1. In general, which interventions may help the client to avoid contracting a cold during cold season?

   _____ Gargling with mouthwash   **X** Obtaining adequate rest

   X Increasing her fluid intake   _____ Taking prophylactic aspirin

   X Taking zinc after exposure   **X** Washing her hands frequently

2. If the client develops a cold, which activities may speed her recovery?

   _____ Vitamin supplements   **X** Increased rest

   X Well-balanced diet   _____ Antibiotics

   _____ Restricted fluid intake   _____ Pallor

Nursing Management of the Client with Rheumatoid Arthritis
Answer Key

Situation: A 47-year-old woman visits the outpatient clinic due to exacerbation of her rheumatoid arthritis. She has joint tenderness, symmetrical joint swelling, and subcutaneous nodules.

1. What symptoms, in addition to those being experienced by the client, are common with rheumatoid arthritis?

   - **Fatigue**
   - **Malaise**
   - **Low-grade fever (below 101° F)**
   - **Anorexia**
   - **Localized articular joint stiffness after inactivity (especially in the morning)**
   - **Edema, warmth, and congestion of affected joints**
   - **Tender, painful joints**
   - **Diminished joint function**
   - **Joint deformity**

2. Which laboratory values are likely to be elevated when a client is experiencing exacerbated rheumatoid arthritis?

X Erythrosedimentation rate (ESR)	_____	Red blood cell (RBC) count
X White blood cell (WBC) count	**X**	Antinuclear antibody (ANA) titer
_____ Serum complement	**X**	C-reactive protein (CRP)

3. What is the rationale for applying ice to the client's inflamed joints, rather than heat?

   The application of ice prevents vasodilation and inflammation, which reduces swelling and promotes comfort.

4. What is the desired client outcome for each nursing intervention?

   a. Encouraging active range of motion exercises.

      Client will maintain joint function and experience minimal joint deformity.

   b. Administering salicylates or NSAIDs as prescribed.

      Client will experience reduced joint inflammation and controlled autoimmune process.

   c. Splinting inflamed joints.

      Client will be free of pain or experience reduced pain.

Nursing Management of the Client Requiring Immunizations
Answer Key

Situation: An 18-year-old female who recently graduated from high school is visiting her primary care provider prior to taking a vacation in Mexico. Afterwards, the teenager plans to start a job as a waitress in a fast-food restaurant while attending college. The nurse is preparing to administer appropriate immunizations.

1. Prior to administering immunizations, what questions should the nurse ask the client?

   Have you ever had a local or systemic reaction to a vaccination?

   Are you pregnant?

   Have you been recently moderately or severely ill?

   Have you had a tetanus diphtheria (Td) shot within the last 10 years?

   Have you received the MMR (measles, mumps, rubella) vaccination?

   Have you had chickenpox?

2. What immunizations should this 18-year-old client receive?

   The client has had no prior reactions to vaccinations, is not pregnant or ill, has not had a tetanus shot within the last 10 years, has not received the MMR, and has had chickenpox. The nurse should administer the Td, MMR, hepatitis B, and hepatitis A immunizations.

3. What immunizations should older clients receive?

   Clients who are 50 years or older should receive influenza vaccine every year preferably between October and mid-November. Clients who are 65 years or older should receive the pneumococcal polysaccharide vaccine as a one-time dose. Clients at highest risk of fatal pneumococcal infection should receive a one-time revaccination five years later.

4. What are the signs and symptoms of an anaphylactic reaction to a vaccine, and what is the emergency treatment?

   The Arthus reaction is a severe local inflammatory reaction that develops at the site of injection of an antigen in a client who has been previously sensitized to that antigen. Anaphylactic shock is a life-threatening hypersensitivity reaction that is characterized by severe dyspnea, circulatory collapse, rash, edema, shock, convulsions, and cyanosis. Intervention includes administration of (a) epinephrine, (b) antihistamines, (c) steroids, (d) oxygen, and (e) intravenous fluids given rapidly.

Nursing Management of the Client Undergoing Angiography and Angioplasty Answer Key

Situation: The client arrived to the intensive care unit following a PTCA. He still has a sheath in place is alert and oriented and his only complaint is that he is tired of lying still.

1. The client is asking you if he can sit up or take a couple of steps. What is your answer?

   Specific answers may vary, however the client needs to be instructed to remain on bedrest for 6-8 hours following the procedure; otherwise, the forming clot may get dislodged and bleeding/hematoma will occur. After that time, he may ambulate with assistance and the nurse will continually reassess for hematoma formation or hemorrhaging.

2. You have done your head-to-toe assessment with particular emphasis on the extremity where the sheath is. The client's pulses already weak due to advanced CAD. Every time you come to check them, you are not sure which spot to look at and if the pulses are present at all. What will you assess in that extremity and what interventions can you provide?

   Pulses should be present and equal bilaterally; assess for color, sensation, capillary refill distal to the catheter insertion site. A priority intervention includes marking the spots where you were able to find the pulses (usually dorsalis pedis or posterior tibial) preprocedure. If unable to palpate the pulses, use a Doppler to auscultate them. Otherwise, the client's leg should remain flat and still for the prescribed length of time.

3. In an hour, the client states that he needs to urinate, but cannot do so lying down. What intervention can the nurse provide in this instance?

   Although the client's affected leg must be immobilized and extended, it may help to tilt the whole bed up (reverse Trendelenburg) unless contraindicated. Contraindications include lightheadedness, nausea, pain, or hypoxia. If voiding is unsuccessful and the client is growing increasingly uncomfortable, insert a urinary catheter.

Nursing Management of the Client with Bronchitis Answer Key

Situation: A 32-year-old woman with a 16-year history of cigarette smoking is experiencing her third episode of bronchitis within the past 12 months. She has a productive cough that has persisted between episodes of acute illness, fever, chest discomfort, and fatigue. Her chest x-ray is negative, but her WBC (white blood cell) count is elevated. Based on her data, the medical diagnosis of bronchitis is established. Her health care provider prescribes an albuterol sulfate inhaler and antibiotic therapy.

1. What is the most important information to provide the client about her recurrent episodes of bronchitis?

   The most important information to provide the client is that her cigarette smoking is preventing her from recovery and places her at increased risk for permanent lung injury.

2. Cite three nursing activities to help reduce the client's risk for future episodes of bronchitis.

   Encourage the client to:
   - **Increase her intake of water and other fluids**
   - **Avoid cigarette smoking and other lung irritants**
   - **Obtain immunizations against common viral agents such as influenza and pneumonia.**

3. Differentiate between acute and chronic bronchitis.

   - **Acute bronchitis is an episode of bronchial airway inflammation related to smoke, other irritants, or infection.**
   - **Chronic bronchitis is the presence of a productive cough that lasts approximately three months a year for two consecutive years.**

4. What type of bronchitis is the client experiencing? Provide rationale for your answer.

   Chronic bronchitis. This is her third episode of bronchitis within one year and a productive cough that has persisted between episodes of acute illness.

Nursing Management of the Client
with Pneumonia Answer Key

Situation: An 88-year-old woman underwent a hip pinning four days ago after she fell and fractured her hip. She has a poor appetite and refuses to eat or drink most of the time. While the nurse was attempting to feed the woman two days ago, the woman moved her affected hip and gasped with pain. As she did, she aspirated the milk she was holding in her mouth and began coughing violently. Today the woman is lethargic, has an oral temperature of 101° F, crackling lung sounds on the left, and an elevated heart rate. It is determined the woman has pneumonia.

1. Complete these sentences:

   Pneumonia may be a **primary** disease or **complication** of another disease.

   Pneumonia is a significant cause of **death** among **older** adults.

   Immobility is a significant **contributing** factor for development of **pneumonia**.

   Pneumonia related to a **foreign** substance in the **lung** is known as **aspiration** pneumonia.

2. Prioritize the client's nursing diagnoses, with "1" representing the most important diagnosis.

   3 Altered nutrition: less than body requirements
   1 Ineffective breathing pattern
   4 Anxiety/fear
   2 Pain
   5 Knowledge deficit

3. How does the woman's pneumonia differ from other types of pneumonia?

   The woman's pneumonia is due to a foreign substance within her lungs, which causes an acute inflammatory process. Microorganisms, such as viruses or bacteria, cause other pneumonias. Regardless of cause, the resulting inflammatory process is similar for all types of pneumonia.

4. What assessments does the nurse need to make that directly relate to the client's pneumonia?

_____	Skin integrity	**X**	Temperature
_____	Urine output	_____	Peripheral pulses
X	Heart rate	**X**	Lung sounds
_____	Gag reflex	_____	Pain status

Nursing Management of the
Client with Asthma Answer Key

Situation: A 59-year-old man lives in a cool, dry part of the country. Upon visiting his daughter who lives in a warm, humid part of the country, the man begins to experience chest tightness, wheezing, and a hacking, non-productive cough. The man has a history of asthma and allergy to molds.

---

1. Which are the common risk factors for asthma?

   _____ Colds   **X** Dust

   X Genetics   **X** Smoking

   _____ Mold   _____ Drugs

   X Exercise   _____ Humid air

2. What is the etiology for the client's nursing diagnoses?

   a. Ineffective breathing pattern

      Related to bronchoconstriction and airway inflammation

   b. Anxiety/fear

      Related to inability to breathe

   c. Fatigue

      Related to increased energy required for breathing

3. Prioritize the following nursing interventions for the client experiencing an asthmatic attack, with "1" representing the first intervention to implement.

   3   Offer emotional support

   2   Raise the head of the bed

   1   Establish a patent airway

   4   Assess vital signs

Nursing Management of the Client
with Status Asthmaticus Answer Key

Situation: A 45-year-old female client with status asthmaticus has just been transferred to the ICU (Intensive Care Unit) from the emergency department. The client's husband states his wife has been experiencing episodes of asthma for several days, which have not been relieved by using her metered-dose inhaler. The client is experiencing severe dyspnea and wheezing. In addition, the client is restless and very fearful.

1. Prioritize nursing activities for the client, with "1" representing the activity to implement first.

   4   Administer prescribed medications.

   3   Use calm, reassuring approach.

   1   Maintain patent airway.

   2   Administer oxygen.

   5   Monitor for drug side effects.

2. How does status asthmaticus differ from the usual asthma attack?

   Status asthmaticus is a severe, persistent, and life-threatening attack of asthma, which does not respond to regular treatment. Status asthmaticus may require the use of mechanical ventilation.

3. What is the purpose of increasing intravenous fluid intake in the client suffering status asthmaticus?

   Intravenous fluids help hydrate the client, loosen and liquefy secretions, and facilitate expectoration (which makes breathing easier).

Medical Surgical

4. Which are goals of mechanical ventilation for the client with status asthmaticus?

- Supplemental oxygen is needed for clients with status asthmaticus if the alveolar oxygen tension (PaO_2) falls below 50 mmHg. The client should be monitored closely for signs of respiratory distress, anxiety, and indications of tiring. Endotracheal intubation and mechanical ventilation may be necessary if respiratory deterioration occurs. Severe, prolonged cases that are unresponsive to conventional treatment may be treated medically with paralysis.

- The goal of mechanical ventilation is to optimize the gas exchange by correcting inadequate ventilation and oxygen perfusion. Mechanical ventilation is used to ease the client's work of breathing by supporting inhalation and exhalation efforts. Increased tidal volume and oxygen delivery is provided through various modes of mechanical ventilation.

- Blood gas findings indicating satisfactory gas exchange are PaO_2 >60 mmHg and $PaCO_2$ <50 mmHg, with an optimum pH in the range of 7.35-7.45 range.

5. What is the purpose of administering these drugs to clients with status asthmaticus?

a. Corticosteroids

   Administered to reduce inflammation of the bronchial airways

b. Theophylline

   A bronchodilator, to help relieve bronchoconstriction and dyspnea

Nursing Management of the Client with Chronic Obstructive Pulmonary Disease (COPD) Answer Key

Situation: A 60-year-old male is being treated for COPD (chronic obstructive pulmonary disease). Assessment reveals a thin, frail man with a barrel chest who leans forward to breathe. Breath sounds are decreased bilaterally and the client is tachycardic with a respiratory rate of 36. Low dose oxygen therapy, an aminophylline drip, and bed rest have been prescribed.

1. Place an "S" in front of those nursing diagnoses that are **supported** by the client's data and a "P" in front of those that are **possible**, but unsupported by the client's data.

   S   Ineffective airway clearance   S   Activity intolerance

   P   Anxiety/fear   P   Ineffective individual/family coping

   S   Fatigue   P   Powerlessness

   S   Potential complications of COPD   P   Knowledge deficit

   P   Ineffective individual/family management of therapeutic regimen

   P   Altered nutrition: less than body requirements

   P   Self-care deficit

2. What is the rationale for administering low-dose oxygen to the client?

   A hypoxic state (decreased PO_2) drives respirations in clients with COPD; therefore, administration of high concentrations of oxygen, which elevate PO_2 levels, suppresses breathing.

3. Which criteria will the nurse use to evaluate the effectiveness of the client's oxygen therapy?

   X   Reduced dyspnea   X   Improving respiratory rate

   X   Normal skin color   X   Mental alertness

   ____ Increased fluid intake   ____ Quiet sleep

   X   Pink nail beds   X   Increased appetite

4. Prioritize the following nursing interventions, with "1" representing the most important intervention.

5   Initiate infusion of intravenous antibiotic as prescribed.

1   Check O$_2$ saturation.

2   Auscultate breath sounds.

3   Administer acetaminophen (Tylenol™) for fever as prescribed.

4   Collect and send sputum specimen to laboratory for culture.

5. What is the purpose of the aminophylline drip and what symptoms will it help improve or eliminate?

Aminophylline is a bronchodilator. It relaxes bronchial smooth muscle, causing bronchodilation and increased vital capacity. It will improve or help eliminate the client's dyspnea, rapid respiratory rate, and decreased breath sounds by increasing vital capacity.

Nursing Management of the Client with Hemothorax/Pneumothorax Answer Key

Situation: A 25-year-old man is admitted to the trauma unit following a motorcycle accident in which he suffered rib fractures and a pneumothorax. He has a chest tube in place on the right that is connected to water seal drainage with 20 cm of suction.

1. Match the description with the type of problem it produces. Use "P", "H" or "B" as a response.

P = Pneumothorax	**P**	Air enters the pleural space due to trauma or disease.
H = Hemothorax	**B**	Produces collapse of the lung or portion of the lung.
B = Both	**H**	Trauma allows blood to collect in the pleural cavity.
	P	Causes increased intrathoracic pressure.
	P	Results in decreased vital capacity.
	P	May be spontaneous or traumatic.

2. Of the following, which four assessments are of highest priority for the client with a chest tube in place?

X	Respiratory status	**X**	Oxygen saturations
____	Bowel sounds	____	Urinary output
X	Pain	____	Appetite
X	Fever	____	Anxiety

3. While getting out of bed, the client pulls his chest tube out of his chest wall. What is the first response on the part of the nurse, to this incident?

Immediately cover the insertion site with plastic, Vaseline gauze, or other impermeable dressing to prevent the client from sucking air back into his pleural cavity.

4. Which nursing diagnoses need to be placed on the client's care plan?

   X   Risk for ineffective breathing pattern

   _____   Risk for ineffective airway clearance

   X   Anxiety/fear

   X   Risk for activity intolerance

   _____   Risk for infection

Nursing Management of the Client with Acute Respiratory Distress Syndrome (ARDS) Answer Key

Situation: A 40-year-old male in acute respiratory distress has been admitted to the ICU (Intensive Care Unit) following an automobile accident during which he suffered direct lung trauma. The client has been placed in a prone position and his vital signs and ABG (arterial blood gas) values are being continuously monitored. The client initially received oxygen via a mask with a high flow system, but he is now on a mechanical ventilator using PEEP (positive end-expiratory pressure). The client is extremely anxious and is also frustrated that he cannot speak due to the placement of an endotrachea tube.

1. Which of the client's symptoms indicates his ARDS is progressing?

_____	Hypertension	**X**	Intracostal retraction	_____	Bradycardi
X	Tachypnea	_____	Complaints of nausea	_____	Blurred vision
X	Tachycardia	_____	Warm, dry skin	**X**	Changes in sensorium
X	Pallor	**X**	Cyanosis	_____	Non-productive cough

2. What does PEEP stand for and what does it do?

PEEP stands for positive end-expiratory pressure. The process applies airway pressure during expiration. PEEP keeps the lungs partially expanded and the alveoli open, thereby improving oxygenation.

3. Which is/are the primary purpose(s) for monitoring the client's ABGs (arterial blood gases)?

X   To determine if the client is being adequately oxygenated

_____   To assess the client's fluid balance

_____   To establish what medications are needed

X   To identify the clinical findings associates with hypoxemia

4. List at least three nursing interventions to allay the client's anxiety, fear, and frustration.

Nursing interventions include, but are not limited to:

- Reassuring the client he needs only to touch his call light, and help will be at his side immediately
- Explaining the purpose of procedures and describing any sensations the client may experience
- Supplying the client with paper and pencil so he can communicate his needs
- Administering sedatives PRN (pro re nata = whenever necessary) per order

Nursing Management of the Client with
Acute Respiratory Failure Answer Key

Situation: While caring for an older client with COPD (chronic obstructive pulmonary disease), the nurse notes that he is unusually lethargic, diaphoretic, and difficult to rouse.

1. What is the client's primary risk factor for developing respiratory failure?

    The client's primary risk factor for respiratory failure is his chronic lung disease.

2. Assuming that all need to be performed, prioritize the order of performance of nursing actions for the client, with "1" representing the most important.

    3   Place the client in a high-Fowler's position.

    1   Establish a patent airway.

    5   Change the damp sheets beneath the client

    2   Administer prescribed oxygen

    4   Obtain intravenous access.

3. What are the two highest priority client outcomes for the client experiencing respiratory failure?

    _____ Preventing infection

    X   Correcting underlying cause

    X   Restoring ventilation and oxygenation

    _____ Preventing recurrence

4. List four other signs and symptoms commonly associated with respiratory failure.

    - **Dyspnea**
    - **Headache**
    - **Confusion**

- Rapid shallow respirations
- Hypoxemia
- Hypercarbia
- Respiratory acidosis
- Cyanosis
- Dysrhythmias
- Decreased level of consciousness
- Abnormal lung sounds (pulmonary edema

Critical Thinking Exercise: CHAPTER 71

Nursing Management of the Client with Pulmonary Edema Answer Key

Situation: A 51-year-old man with a history of CHF (congestive heart failure) arrives at the emergency department after a two-day illness, during which time he developed severe dyspnea. He has distended neck veins, audible bilateral crackles, is restless and confused to place and date. The nurse immediately recognizes the client is suffering from pulmonary edema.

1. Which priority nursing diagnoses need to be added to the client's care plan based on the data provided?

X	Ineffective breathing pattern	___	Anxiety/fear
X	Risk for activity intolerance	X	Fatigue
___	Ineffective individual/family coping	___	Altered nutrition: less than body requirements
___	Decreased cardiac output	X	Decreased cerebral perfusion
___	Fluid volume excess	___	Self-care deficit

2. What other clinical manifestations is the client likely to experience?

___	High fever	X	Productive cough
X	Frothy sputum	___	Bradycardia
___	Cheyne Stokes respirations	X	Cyanosis
X	Wheezing	___	Hot, dry skin
X	Ashen gray color	X	Stupor

1. What is the rationale for administering each medication/drug to the client experiencing pulmonary edema?

    a. Oxygen

    To increase oxygen to the heart

    b. Morphine sulfate

    To reduce anxiety and dyspnea

c. Diuretics
    To produce rapid diuresis

d. Digitalis
    To improve cardiac function

e. Dobutamine
    To increase cardiac contractility

Nursing Management of the Client with a Pulmonary Embolism Answer Key

Situation: A 65-year-old woman returned to her room at 2:00 p.m. yesterday following an abdominal hysterectomy. Her vital signs have been stable and her dressings dry and intact. She was up to the side of the bed and ambulated a few feet before returning to bed. A few minutes later, she turned on her call light stating she was having difficulty breathing. The nurse found the client anxious, tachycardic, diaphoretic, gasping for air, and complaining of chest pain.

1. Which diagnostic tests help differentiate between pulmonary embolism and heart attack?

   _____ Oxygen saturation   **X** Ventilation-perfusion scan

   X Electrocardiogram (ECG)   _____ White blood cell (WBC) count

   X Pulmonary angiography   _____ Serum electrolytes

2. What known risk factors does the client have for development of pulmonary embolism?

   _____ Deep vein thrombosis   **X** Surgery

   _____ Hypercoagulability   _____ Prolonged immobility

   X Advanced age   _____ Obesity

3. There is sufficient data to support placing which nursing diagnoses on the client's plan of care?

   X Decreased cardiac output

   _____ Altered nutrition: less than body requirements

   X Fear/anxiety

   _____ Self-care deficit

   _____ Impaired skin integrity

   X Impaired gas exchange

   _____ Ineffective individual/family coping

Situation: A 74-year-old woman who lives independently developed night sweats, loss of appetite, and chronic nonproductive cough. After losing more than ten pounds and undergoing numerous tests, the client was diagnosed with tuberculosis.

1. Which statements are true about tuberculosis? Correct any false statements.

   a. Tuberculosis is a contagious disease that is highly sensitive to current chemotherapies.

      False. Tuberculosis is a contagious disease, but it is becoming resistant to current chemotherapies.

   b. Tuberculosis may affect any organ in the body, but primarily affects the lungs.

      True.

   c. Initial infection with tuberculosis occurs within 6-12 weeks of exposure.

      False. Initial infection with tuberculosis occurs within 2-10 weeks of exposure.

   d. Dormant tuberculosis bacillus can be killed by prolonged chemotherapy.

      False. Dormant tuberculosis bacillus can go undetected and is not affected by chemotherapeutic agents.

   e. Tuberculosis is transmitted via respiratory and gastrointestinal secretions.

      False. Tuberculosis is transmitted via respiratory droplets.

2. Provide an etiology for each of the client's nursing diagnoses:

   a. Noncompliance

      Noncompliance related to lack of knowledge regarding the importance of maintain therapeutic regimen or side effects of drugs.

   b. Activity intilerance

      Activity intolerance related to decreased energy secondary to debilitating disease process or decreased oxygenation secondary to lung disease.

c. Impaired gas exechange

Impaired gas exchange related to tuberculin tubercles within lung and decreased lung tissue.

d. Fatigue

Fatigue related to impaired gas exchange secondary to diseased lung tissue.

e. Fear/anxiety

Fear/anxiety related to chronic disease state, debilitation, or uncertain future.

f. Altered nutrition: less than body requirements

Altered nutrition: less than body requirements related to loss of appetite secondary to chemotherapy or secondary to debilitating disease.

3. The client is placed on Isoniazid (isonicotinic acid hydrazide (INH)) and Rifampin (RIF). What parameters will the nurse use to determine the effectiveness of the drugs?

- Weight gain
- Return of appetite
- Cough will decrease or subside
- Return of energy
- Freedom from side effects of chemotherapy.

Nursing Management of the Client with Atelectasis Answer Key

Situation: A 27-year-old man who underwent abdominal surgery is reluctant to move because of incisional pain. He coughs frequently because he is a cigarette smoker. He complains he cannot take a deep breath because it hurts. The nurse is concerned that he is going to develop atelectasis.

1. Why is it essential that postoperative clients take deep breaths and ambulate as early as possible?

   Coughing and deep breathing, as well as early ambulation, help prevent the development of hypoventilation, and collapse of lung tissue (atelectasis).

2. What are the client's risk factors for atelectasis?

   Smoking, surgery, and surgical pain

3. What are the common clinical manifestations of atelectasis?

_____ Diaphoresis	**X** Dyspnea
X Anxiety	_____ Bradycardia
_____ Hypertension	**X** Tachypnea
X Decreased breath sounds	**X** Fever

4. List at least three nursing actions that can prevent the development of atelectasis?

   - **Administer pain medication and wait 20 minutes. Then coach the client to cough and take deep breaths.**
   - **Obtain an incentive spirometer (IS) and demonstrate its use.**
   - **Stay with the client while he uses the IS and praise him for progress.**
   - **Encourage increased fluid intake to maintain secretions that can be readily expectorated.**
   - **Encourage early ambulation when permitted.**

Nursing Management of the Client with Lung Cancer Answer Key

Situation: A 68-year-old male client who has smoked three packs of cigarettes a day since his teen years is seeing his physician for pulmonary symptoms including dyspnea and a chronic productive cough. The client also states he has pain in his chest, shoulder, and back. The physician suspects the client has lung cancer and is ordering diagnostic tests.

1. What are the warning signals of lung cancer that the nurse may teach the client and family?

    Teach the client and family the warning signals of lung cancer:
    - **Persistent cough**
    - **Any change in respiratory patterns, or dyspnea out of proportion to exertion**
    - **Blood in the sputum, blood-streaked, or frank hemoptysis**
    - **Rust-colored or purulent sputum**
    - **Chest, shoulder, or arm pain**

2. What can the nurse do to help chronic smokers overcome habitual tobacco use for lung cancer prevention?

    Nurses can help chronic smokers quit their habit by:
    - **Emphasizing the health and social benefits of quitting**
    - **Setting realistic goals with the client**
    - **Developing a stop-smoking plan with the client**
    - **Referring the client to self-help stop-smoking programs**

3. How may the nurse educate the client to perform diaphragmatic breathing?

    Diaphragmatic breathing will help the client with lung cancer improve the ease of breathing. The nurse should instruct the client to:
    - **Clear airway with turning, coughing, and deep breathing.**
    - **Assume a comfortable position.**

- Inhale deeply through the nostrils with mouth closed. Try to move the diaphragm down and the abdominal wall outward.
- Pause at the end of the inhalation.
- Exhale passively through pursed lips.
- Use diaphragm and abdominal muscles to push air out. It should take three times longer to exhale than inhale.
- Practice this procedure for 15 minutes, four times a day.

4. Describe the most common surgical procedures that are used to remove tumors of the lung.

a. Wedge resection:
   Removal of small tumors

b. Segmental resection:
   Removal of a segment of lung

c. Lobectomy:
   Removal of a complete lobe

d. Pneumonectomy:
   Removal of an entire lung

5. What outcomes should the client with lung cancer experience following interventions?
- **Breathe without using accessory muscles**
- **Have an oxygen saturation greater than 90%**
- **Feel less anxious about breathing**
- **Have a respiratory rate of 12-20 breaths per minute.**

Nursing Management of the Client with Laryngeal Cancer Answer Key

Situation: A 50-year-old woman, who has been singing in various church and civic choirs for the past 30 years, developed a raspy voice. Since the problem interferes with her ability to sing, she decided to seek medical attention. Visualization of the woman's throat reveals the presence of a small nodule on the client's vocal cord.

1. What questions should the nurse ask the client in order to gain additional data about her hoarseness?

   - **When did you first notice a change in your voice?**
   - **Do you experience pain or burning in your throat when drinking acidic or hot fluids?**
   - **Do you have a cough?**
   - **Do you feel like you have a lump in the back of your throat?**
   - **Do you have difficulty swallowing?**
   - **Do you experience pain that radiates to another area, such as your ear?**
   - **Is your weight stable or have you lost weight?**

2. What additional assessments need to be made?

   The nurse should assess for:
   - **Lumps in the client's neck**
   - **Evidence of breathing difficulties**
   - **Nasal discharge**
   - **Foul breath odor**
   - **Enlarged cervical lymph nodes.**

3. The presence of laryngeal cancer is verified via biopsy and a hemi-laryngectomy is scheduled. What is a hemi-laryngectomy and how does it differ from a total laryngectomy?

   - **Hemi-laryngectomy is a partial laryngectomy performed when the malignancy is less than 1 cm and extends beyond the vocal cord, but is within the subglottic area.**
   - **Total laryngectomy is performed when the malignancy extends beyond the vocal cords and subglottic area.**

4. How can the nurse help the client prepare for the needed surgery?

- **Offer emotional support**
- **Allow the client to talk about her fears**
- **Explain all new procedures and surgical preparations**
- **Offer realistic hope for a positive outcome.**
- **(Other actions are possible.)**

Nursing Management of the Client with a Laryngectomy Answer Key

Situation: The 62-year-old client who was diagnosed with laryngeal cancer earlier has been transferred to the surgical unit from the PACU (post anesthesia care unit) following a total laryngectomy. The client has a tracheostomy, and a nasogastric tube is attached to suction. The nurse suctions the client's tracheostomy tube every two hours, deflates the tracheostomy cuff every eight hours during expiration, and changes the tracheostomy tube daily. Although the nurse is trying to communicate with the client using a magic slate, the client is very apprehensive and frustrated because he cannot speak. The nurse assures him he will be meeting with a speech therapist as soon as he feels stronger.

1. What are some likely etiologies for the client's preoperative nursing diagnoses?

   a. Anxiety:

   Related to fear of surgery, fear regarding outcome of surgery, fear of prognosis or fear of inability to communicate needs.

   b. Knowledge deficit:

   Regarding surgical procedure, postoperative expectations, and methods of communication.

   c. Risk for ineffective individual coping:

   Related to fear regarding inability to speak and temporary inability to communicate needs.

2. Prioritize the client's postoperative nursing diagnoses, with "1" representing the most important diagnosis.

   4   Knowledge deficit

   2   Risk for altered nutrition

   3   Anxiety

   1   Risk for ineffective airway clearance

3. Why is it necessary to deflate the tracheostomy cuff during exhalation?

   The tracheostomy cuff should be deflated during exhalation to prevent the aspiration of secretions that have accumulated above the cuff.

4. Describe the three speech methods available to clients following laryngectomy.

    a. Artificial larynx (electrolarynx):

       A handheld, battery-operated device that is held against the neck. It produces mechanical-sounding speech.

    b. Esophageal speech:

       A technique that involves swallowing air and then holding the air in the upper esophagus while pronouncing words.

    c. Tracheoesophageal puncture (TEP):

       A surgical procedure involving the making of an opening between the tracheostoma and the esophagus. A speech prosthesis is inserted into the puncture site.

Nursing Management of the Client with Emphysema Answer Key

Situation: A 62-year-old retired coal miner is being treated for advanced COPD (chronic obstructive pulmonary disease). He has dyspnea with minor exertion, obvious barrel chest, wheezing, tachypnea, and tachycardia.

1. Which statements are true of emphysema? Correct any false statements.

   a. Emphysema is an acute, rapidly progressive lung disease.
   False. Emphysema is a chronic, slowly progressive lung disease.

   b. Emphysema and bronchitis rarely occur in the same client.
   False. Emphysema and bronchitis are both significant components of COPD.

   c. Prevention is an important component of treatment.
   True.

   d. Restoring maximum respiratory function is a goal of collaborative management.
   True.

   e. Emphysema is characterized by permanent shrinkage of air spaces.
   False. Emphysema is characterized by permanent enlargement of air spaces, destruction of alveolar walls, and reduced capillary perfusion.

2. Based on the client's data, the nurse is correct in placing which nursing diagnoses on the client's care plan?

X	Ineffective breathing pattern	**X**	Anxiety/fear
X	Fatigue	**X**	Potential complications of emphysema
____	Self-care deficit	**X**	Activity intolerance
____	Altered nutrition: less than body requirements		
____	Ineffective individual/family coping		

3. "Ineffective airway clearance" is included as a nursing diagnosis on the client's plan of care. Which nursing activities best address this nursing diagnosis?

_____ Encourage the client to take short, shallow breaths.

X Teach the client to use relaxation techniques.

X Encourage increased fluid intake.

_____ Position the client flat in bed for maximum ventilation.

_____ Administer high dose oxygen therapy.

Nursing Management of the Client
Requiring Oxygen Therapy Answer Key

Situation: An older man is receiving oxygen therapy via a nasal cannula while being treated for exacerbated COPD (chronic obstructive pulmonary disease). The oxygen is prescribed to run at 2 L per minute.

1. How can the nurse prevent the client's skin from breaking down beneath the oxygen tubing?

   Examples: Perform daily assessments to detect changes that indicate skin alteration; place cotton balls or suitable padding beneath the tubing that lies over his ears and rests against his face; clean his nares and reposition the tubing frequently so that it does not rest or rub against the same place continuously; maintain nutritional status to promote healing; humidify delivered oxygen. (Other interventions are possible.)

2. Why is low dose oxygen therapy prescribed for a person with COPD (chronic obstructive pulmonary disease) even though they may be experiencing difficulty breathing?

   Hypoxia drives respirations in the person with COPD. When high doses of oxygen are administered, hypoxia is relieved, thereby eliminating the hypoxic drive for breathing.

3. Prioritize the nurse's activities for the client receiving oxygen, with "1" representing the first activity to be implemented.

   3   Assess for skin alterations beneath oxygen tubing.

   1   Place client in Fowler's position.

   2   Teach client relaxation to enhance breathing.

   4   Encourage client to participate in own care.

Nursing Management of the Client with
Arterial Blood Gas (ABG) Abnormalities Answer Key

Situation: The nurse has just received the ABG (arterial blood gas) analysis report on a client with pneumonia.

1. When assisting with drawing an arterial blood gas, it is important for the nurse to perform which actions?

_____ Administer oxygen

X Assess radial and ulnar arterial circulation.

_____ Maintain direct pressure over arterial puncture site for two minutes after drawing ABG.

X Avoid oxygen contamination of arterial specimen.

_____ Report drawing of specimen to practitioner as soon as possible

2. Which of the following findings are normal/abnormal?

ABGs (arterial blood gases)			Normal	Abnormal
Blood pH	7.38	pH	X	
PaCO$_2$	58	mmHg		X
PaO$_2$	56	mmHg		X
HCO$_3$	18	mEq/L		X
SaO$_2$	96	%	X	

3. Determine the primary type of acid-base imbalance in the arterial blood sample.

Samples					
	1	2	3	4	5
pH	7.50	7.53	7.45	7.28	7.24
PaCO$_2$	29	43	43	54	45
PaO2	91	84	63	88	102
HCO$_3$	25	31	23	26	34

Begin by systemically evaluating the $PaCO_2$ and HCO_3- in relation to the pH.

Sample 1: The primary disturbance is respiratory alkalosis because the pH is >7.45 and the $PaCO_2$ is <35 mmHg.

Sample 2: The primary disturbance is metabolic alkalosis because the pH is >7.45 and the HCO_3- is >26 mEq/L.

Sample 3: The primary disturbance is hypoxemia because the pH is within normal limits and the PaO_2 is <80 mmHg. The $PaCO_2$ and HCO_3- are normal.

Sample 4: The primary disturbance is respiratory acidosis because the pH is <7.35 and the $PaCO_2$ is >45 mmHg.

Sample 5: The primary disturbance is metabolic acidosis because the pH is <7.35 and the HCO_3- is >26 mEq/L.

4. List a possible etiology for the following ABG abnormalities.

Respiratory alkalosis: **Hyperventilation**

Metabolic alkalosis: **Excess intake of an alkaline solution (sodium bicarbonate, improper constitution of total parental nutrition, or overuse of antacids)**

Hypoxemia: **Pneumothorax, status asthmaticus, pneumonia, congestive heart failure with pulmonary edema, embolism, obstruction of the airway, and various other pulmonary disease states affecting the upper and lower airways or parenchyma**

Respiratory acidosis: **Hypoventilation**

Metabolic alkalosis: **Direct bicarbonate loss (renal wasting) or accumulation of lactic acid or ketones (DKA: Diabetic ketoacidosis)**

Nursing Management of the Client
Undergoing a Bronchoscopy Procedure Answer Key

Situation: A young female client, who has a chronic cough and low-grade fever, is about to undergo a diagnostic bronchoscopy. She is unfamiliar with the procedure and is anxious.

1. Complete the sentences regarding teaching of clients undergoing bronchoscopy.

   a. You will be given a mild **sedative** prior to the procedure.

   b. The back of your **throat** will be **anesthetized**.

   c. A long, **flexible scope** will be inserted into your **throat** and **airways**.

   d. The procedure allows your **airways** to be **examined** and **specimens** obtained.

   e. You will **not** feel any **pain** during the procedure.

   f. Your throat may be **sore** immediately **following** the procedure.

   g. You will **not** be allowed to **eat** or **drink** until your <u>gag</u> reflex returns.

2. Why does the client need to be NPO (nothing by mouth) for 6-8 hours preceding the bronchoscopy?

   The client needs to be NPO prior to a bronchoscopy to prevent the client from vomiting and aspirating stomach contents.

3. Which assessments are essential following a bronchoscopy?

   _____ Pupillary reaction   **X** Heart rate   **X** Blood pressure

   X Bowel sounds   _____ Respiratory rate   **X** Skin color

   X Lung sounds   _____ Temperature   _____ Pedal pulses

Nursing Management of the Client with a Tracheostomy Answer Key

---

Situation: A 62-year-old male client who has undergone a total laryngectomy for laryngeal cancer is being cared for on the surgical unit. He has a tracheostomy tube in place. In addition to providing tracheostomy care, the nurse it also trying to help the client communicate his needs to the staff, as he is unable to speak.

---

1. Why is it so important for the client with a tracheostomy to be adequately hydrated?

   The client who does not receive adequate hydration and humidification will have dried, retained tracheobronchial secretions. These secretions can cause an increased resistance to airflow, infection, and altered respiratory gas exchange.

2. By what means can the client with a tracheostomy communicate his needs to the staff?

   To help the client with a tracheostomy communicate:
   - **Provide the client with paper and pencil**
   - **Provide a magic slate**
   - **Prepare a list of needs (urinal, bedpan, pain medication, emesis basin, water), and have the client point to what he needs.**

3. Why must the client with a tracheostomy take laxatives and stool softeners?

   The client with a tracheostomy must take laxative and stool softeners because he cannot perform the Valsalva maneuver, which makes it difficult to have a bowel movement. The glottis and vocal cords have been bypassed by the tracheostomy. To perform the Valsalva maneuver, it is necessary to close the glottis.

4. If accidental extubation occurs, what can the nurse do while waiting for emergency help to arrive?

> If accidental extubation occurs, and the tracheostomy tube has been in place for less than four days, the nurse should immediately summon help. While waiting, the nurse should use an Ambu-bag and mask to ventilate the client. If unable to provide adequate ventilation, the nurse should next try to reinsert the tracheostomy tube. If the tracheostomy tube cannot be reinserted, the nurse should initiate the code for respiratory arrest.

Nursing Management of the Client
with a Thoracentesis Answer Key

Situation: A 73-year-old male client who has been experiencing severe dyspnea is scheduled to undergo a thoracentesis for diagnostic purposes and also to relieve lung compression due to an accumulation of fluid in the pleural space. The client has arthritis and finds it very difficult to remain still during the procedure. To assist the client, the nurse holds the client and encourages him to remain quiet, particularly as the needle is being inserted. The thoracentesis takes approximately 15 minutes to perform. A chest x-ray is performed following the procedure.

---

1. Prioritize the client's nursing diagnoses immediately following the thoracentesis, with "1" representing the most important diagnosis.

   2   Pain

   3   Risk for infection

   1   Risk for ineffective breathing pattern

2. What is the rationale for each of the nurse's actions related to the thoracentesis:

   a.   Positioning the client in an upright position prior to the procedure.

   Positioning the client in an upright position allows the pleural fluid to accumulate in the base of the thorax, where it can be more easily withdrawn.

   b.   Holding the client and helping him to remain absolutely still during the procedure.

   The client must remain absolutely still during thoracentesis because a sudden movement could cause the needle to enter the pleural space and damage the visceral pleura or lung parenchyma. This damage could result in pneumothorax.

   c.   Turning the client to the unaffected side following the procedure.

   Turning the client to the unaffected side for one hour following thoracentesis allows the lung on the affected side to expand.

3. Which are potential complications associated with thoracentesis?

   _____ Acute myocardial infarction   **X**   Shock

   X   Pneumothorax   _____ Pulmonary embolism

   X   Infection   **X**   Bleeding

   _____ Bradycardia   **X**   Subcutaneous emphysema

4. Why did the physician order a chest x-ray following the procedure?

A chest x-ray is ordered following thoracentesis to make certain a pneumothorax has not occurred.

Critical Thinking Exercise: CHAPTER 84

Nursing Management of the Client with a Chest Tube Placement Answer Key

Situation: A 65-year-old-female, who has undergone a pneumonectomy for lung cancer, is receiving care in the ICU (Intensive Care Unit). Chest tubes were inserted in surgery and attached to a disposable Pleur-evac unit. The nurse carefully assesses the client's respiratory function chest tube insertion site, chest drainage, and monitors the closed chest drainage system.

1. Which are primary functions of closed chest drainage following thoracotomy?

_____ To keep the lung collapsed until healing occurs

X To remove air and serosanguineous fluid from the pleural space

X To help re-expand the remaining lung tissue

_____ To prevent hemothorax

X To prevent mediastinal shift

2. Which is the primary sign/symptom of an air leak in a water seal drainage system?

_____ Continuous bubbling in the water seal chamber during inspiration

_____ Intermittent bubbling in the water seal chamber during expiration

X Continuous bubbling in the water seal chamber during inspiration and expiration

_____ Intermittent bubbling in the water seal chamber during inspiration and expiration

3. What should the nurse do if an air leak is suspected in a water seal drainage system?

The nurse should check for a loose catheter, and also thoroughly check the tubing and all the connections. To stop the air leak, the nurse can place sterile petroleum gauze around the insertion site of a loose chest tube, or re-tape loose tubing connections. If these measures do not work, the leak needs to be reported so the entire drainage system can be replaced.

4. Which nursing interventions are appropriate for the client with closed chest drainage?

   X   Place the drainage system two to three feet below the client's chest.

  _____ Place the drainage system on the top of the bed when transporting the client.

  _____ Clamp the chest tube off when ambulating the client.

   X   Record the amount of drainage for each shift.

  _____ Encourage the client to lie quietly whenever possible.

Nursing Management of the Client
with Peptic Ulcers Answer Key

Situation: A 39-year-old man visits his health provider with complaints of burning, epigastric pain occurring about two hours after he eats. He consistently feels bloated and obtains little or no relief from OTC antacids. His past medical history reveals cigarette smoking, stressful job, and chronic use of NSAIDs (Non-steroidal anti-inflammatory drugs) for low back pain.

1. What are the client's risk factors for peptic ulcer disease? Which is the most serious risk factor and why?

> **Stress, smoking, and NSAID use. The client's most serious risk factor is his chronic use of NSAIDs because NSAIDs (Nonsteroidal anti-inflammatory drugs) encourage ulcer formation by inhibiting prostaglandin secretion, a substance that inhibits ulcer formation. NSAIDs (Nonsteroidal anti-inflammatory drugs) are also associated with gastric bleeding, a serious complication of peptic ulcer disease.**

2. Why is smoking contraindicated for clients with peptic ulcer disease?

> **Smoking exacerbates the disease process because it is associated with increased duodenal acidity. Smoking also significantly inhibits ulcer repair.**

3. Which nursing diagnoses are supported by the client's data?

_____ Alteration in nutrition: less than body requirements

X Pain

X Anxiety

_____ Ineffective individual coping

_____ Ineffective individual management of therapeutic regimen

_____ Altered elimination: tarry stools

4. What is the primary reason the practitioner prescribed these medications for the client?

  a. H$_2$-receptor antagonist

   Decrease stomach acid secretion

  b. Antibiotic

   Suppress *Helicobacter pylori* bacteria associated with ulcer formation

  c. Cytoprotective agent

   Protect the stomach lining from acid and NSAIDs (Non-steroidal anti-inflammatory drugs)

Nursing Management of the Client with Gastrectomy Answer Key

Situation: A 44-year-old woman is first day postoperative subtotal gastrectomy for stomach cancer. Her vital signs are stable, and she has been up to the side of the bed one time. She has a nasogastric tube in place, which is connected to low intermittent suction.

1. Which nursing diagnoses are appropriate for the client during this phase of her surgery?

  X   Pain
  _____ Altered nutrition: less than body requirements
  _____ Knowledge deficit regarding home care
  _____ Nausea
  X   Risk for infection
  X   Risk for fluid volume deficit

2. What is the etiology of each of the nursing diagnoses you selected?

   - **Pain related to surgical incision**
   - **Risk for infection related to presence of surgical incision**
   - **Risk for fluid volume deficit related to prescribed nasogastric suction**

3. What is dumping syndrome and how can it be reduced or prevented?

   Dumping syndrome refers to the rapid emptying (dumping) of stomach contents into the small intestine, which frequently occurs following gastric surgery. It is associated with diaphoresis and weakness after eating. It can be reduced or prevented by eating small meals without fluids, and lying down after eating to slow the movement of food through the alimentary canal.

Nursing Management of the Client
with Dumping Syndrome Answer Key

Situation: A 45-year-old client with peptic ulcer disease who has undergone a Billroth II surgical procedure has been discharged home and has developed dumping syndrome. During her first postoperative visit to the clinic, the client tells the nurse practitioner she experiences weakness, diaphoresis, tachycardia, faintness, and abdominal distention 15-30 minutes after every meal. The client also mentions that two or three hours after eating she experiences the symptoms of a hypoglycemic reaction: sweating, mental confusion, anxiety, weakness and tachycardia. The nurse practitioner provides the client with a Teaching Guide, which lists dietary regulations and restrictions for people with dumping syndrome. She also advises the client to lie down following meals.

---

1. What causes the symptoms associated with dumping syndrome?

    Dumping syndrome can result when stomach capacity is decreased (as occurs with the Billroth II procedure). The decreased stomach capacity allows an abnormally large bolus of hypertonic fluid to rapidly enter the intestine. As a result, the intestine pulls fluid from the extracellular space in order to convert the hypertonic fluid to an isotonic fluid. This fluid shift causes a decrease in circulating blood volume, manifested by weakness and faintness.

2. What type of diet is recommended for clients experiencing dumping syndrome? Why?

    Clients with dumping syndrome are placed on high-fat, high-protein, low-carbohydrate diets to promote healing and prevent symptoms associated with high-carbohydrate intake (dizziness, diarrhea, and abdominal distention).

3. Why is it important for clients with dumping syndrome to lie down after a meal?

    Lying down after eating may help to slow the movement of food through the gastrointestinal tract, which decreases symptoms.

4. Why does postprandial hypoglycemia occur 2-3 hours after eating in clients with dumping syndrome?

> Postprandial hypoglycemia occurs 2-3 hours after eating in clients with dumping syndrome because the sudden entry of a bolus of high carbohydrate fluid into the small intestine causes the release of large amounts of insulin into the circulation.

Nursing Management of the Client with Cirrhosis Answer Key

Situation: A 65-year old male has a history of alcohol abuse. He is hospitalized because he began vomiting blood after eating tacos. Assessment data reveal: pallor, jaundice with petechiae and ecchymotic areas on his arms and legs, and a tight, protuberant abdomen. He also has pedal edema and hepatomegaly. His admission diagnosis is bleeding esophageal varices related to cirrhosis. He is receiving IV Aldactone and Lasix.

1. List all of the nursing diagnoses that may apply to this client. Which nursing diagnoses requires immediate attention?

Nursing Diagnosis	Requires Immediate Attention
Fluid volume excess	X
Ineffective breathing pattern	X
Risk for injury	
Risk for infection	
Impaired skin integrity	
Risk for impaired physical mobility	
Risk for activity intolerance	
Fatigue	
Body image disturbances	
Impaired tissue integrity	

Situation: The client is experiencing respiratory distress related to the ascites and the physician performs an abdominal paracentesis, withdrawing 3 L of fluid. The nurse makes the diagnoses of risk for fluid volume deficit.

2. What is the rationale for this diagnosis?

    Because of the rapid removal of fluid, there is a fluid shift into the peritoneal cavity from the intravascular space.

3. What nursing interventions are most appropriate for the client diagnosed with fluid volume deficit after paracentesis?

- Monitor respiratory rate and rhythm.
- Monitor urine output every four hours.
- Check vital signs q one hour x four.
- Obtain daily weights.
- Measure abdominal circumference q shift.

Lab values are drawn. They are:	
Platelet count	50,000/mm3
Serum ammonia	96mcg/dL
RBC	3.8million/mm3
WBC (white blood cell)	5,000/mm3
PT	40seconds
Hgb	10.1g/dL
Hct	30%

4. Based on the client's lab values, what is the priority problem?

Low platelets, low RBC, elevated PT, low hemoglobin and hematocrit—these indicate bleeding.

5. What nursing interventions are most appropriate related to the priority problem noted above?

- Assess for signs of shock.
- Monitor vital signs frequently: q one hour.
- Assess level of consciousness with vitals.
- Observe for signs of increased bruising, petechiae, hematuria, and occult blood.

Nursing Management of the Client with an Abdominal Paracentesis Answer Key

Situation: A 68-year-old male client who has been hospitalized with cirrhosis of the liver is scheduled to have an abdominal paracentesis. The client has been experiencing abdominal discomfort and dyspnea due to the accumulation of a large amount of ascitic fluid in his abdomen.

1. In what order will the nurse perform these activities prior to the abdominal paracentesis, with "1" representing the first activity?

   4   Place the client in a high-Fowler's position

   2   Obtain the client's weight

   3   Measures the client's abdominal girth

   1   Ask the client to void

2. What is the rationale for:

   a. Asking the client to void just prior to the paracentesis?

   It is important for the client to void before a paracentesis to reduce the risk of puncturing the bladder when the physician inserts the needle or trocar.

   b. Positioning the client in an upright or high-Fowler's position?

   A high-Fowler's or upright position allows the intestines to float back toward the posterior of the peritoneal cavity, and thus reduces the risk of intestinal laceration during needle or trocar insertion.

   c. Administering prescribed albumin infusions following the paracentesis?

   Protein is an important constituent of ascitic fluid. When a large amount of ascitic fluid is removed from the client's peritoneal cavity, the physician may order albumin infusions in order to compensate for the protein losses.

3. Which are complications that can occur during or after an abdominal paracentesis?

   X   Shock   _____ Fluid overload

   _____ Hypertension   **X** Infection

   X   Peritonitis   **X** Bleeding

   _____ Bradycardia   **X** Hepatic encephalopathy

Nursing Management of the Client
with Esophageal Varices Answer Key

Situation: A 50-year-old man, with a 22-year history of alcohol abuse, developed a cough a few days ago. Upon arising this morning, he started coughing up blood, which prompted him to go to the emergency department. During the assessment, the client started coughing again, this time coughing up copious amounts of bright red blood.

1. Prioritize nursing actions for the client in regard to his bleeding, with "1" representing the most important action.

   2   Administer oxygen

   4   Assess vital signs

   3   Initiate intravenous access

   1   Establish airway

   5   Prepare client for surgery

2. Which are risk factors for esophageal varices?

   _____ Pancreatitis   **X**   Cirrhosis

   _____ Esophageal cancer   _____ Gallbladder disease

   X   Alcohol abuse   _____ Chronic acetaminophen use

   X   Hepatitis   **X**   Congenital splenic vein abnormality

3. Which are the two most important nursing diagnoses for the client at this time?

   _____ Risk for infection

   _____ Risk for altered nutrition

   X   Risk for fluid volume deficit

   X   Anxiety

   _____ Self-care deficit

Nursing Management of the Client with Cholecystitis/ Cholelithiasis and Pancreatitis Answer Key

Situation: A 40-year-old woman has been experiencing intermittent, vague epigastric discomfort after meals for several months. This evening after eating a hamburger and french fries, the woman developed severe epigastric pain radiating to her back and right shoulder, which prompted her to go to the emergency department. Assessment reveals an obese female who is in obvious pain with tender distended abdomen, tachycardia, and tachypnea. An acute attack of cholecystitis is suspected.

1. What risk factors does the client have for cholecystitis?

   - **Obese**
   - **Female**
   - **Age 40**

2. Why is morphine sulfate contraindicated for clients with gallbladder disease?

   Opiates, such as morphine sulfate, trigger sphincter of Oddi spasms, increasing the pain and nausea associated with gallbladder or hepatic conditions.

3. What are the etiologies for each of the client's nursing diagnoses?
   a. Pain

      Related to acute cholecystitis

   b. Anxiety

      Related to acute cholecystitis

   c. Knowledge Deficit

      Related to lack of experience with disease and/or surgery

Nursing Management of the Client
with Acute Appendicitis Answer Key

Situation: A 19-year-old college student is rushed to a near-by emergency department due to severe abdominal pain. Initial assessment reveals a well-nourished, healthy-appearing youth who is in obvious pain. He has lower right quadrant pain with rebound tenderness, complains of nausea, and a positive Rovsing's' sign. Acute appendicitis is suspected.

1. Which diagnostic studies are commonly used to confirm the presence of acute appendicitis?

   X Ultrasound studies   **X** Physical examination

   _____ CT (computed tomography) Scan   **X** Differential WBC (white blood cell)

   X Abdominal x-rays   _____ Barium enema

2. Why is a preoperative enema contraindicated when appendicitis is suspected?

   Laxatives or enemas could precipitate perforation (rupture) of the appendix.

3. What is the etiology of the client's postoperative nursing diagnoses?

   a. Pain
   Pain related to surgical incision

   b. Risk for infection
   Risk for infection related to surgical incision (portal of entry for microorganisms)

   c. Knowledge deficit
   Knowledge deficit regarding postoperative care, home care

   d. Risk for ineffective airway clearance
   Risk for ineffective airway clearance related to reluctance to cough secondary to postoperative pain

Nursing Management of the Client with Ulcerative Colitis Answer Key

Situation: A 35-year-old woman is hospitalized for an exacerbation of ulcerative colitis following a stressful holiday season spent with relatives. The client is experiencing severe abdominal cramping, distention, and diarrhea, and she has signs of dehydration. The client tells the admitting nurse she has been eating a lot of high-fat holiday foods which she ordinarily avoids: rich gravies, turkey dressing made with sausage, and creamy pies. In addition, she has been drinking bourbon and several glasses of wine during dinner. The client explains she had become very upset when she allowed her mother, who was visiting, to bring up a lot of painful issues from the past, which they normally never discuss unless they are drinking.

1. How does each factor contribute to the symptoms of ulcerative colitis?

   a. Diet:

   Fatty foods that do not digest properly and raw fruits and vegetables can exacerbate ulcerative colitis.

   b. Alcohol:

   Alcohol irritates the damaged colonic mucosa.

   c. Stress:

   Stress and anxiety can trigger episodes of diarrhea by irritating the "fight or flight" response.

2. Which three nursing diagnoses are appropriate for this client?

   _____ Dehydration secondary to ulcerative colitis

   X Acute pain related to exacerbated ulcerative colitis

   X Noncompliance with therapeutic regimen secondary to stress

   _____ Knowledge deficit regarding disease process

   X Risk for electrolyte imbalance related to diarrhea

3. Which nursing interventions will be most helpful to the client's acute exacerbation of ulcerative colitis?

_____ Encourage the client to remain NPO.

X Provide bedrest.

_____ Serve liquid meals for at least a week.

X Provide emotional support.

_____ Encourage client to avoid alcohol intake.

_____ Administer 3000 mL intravenous fluids per day.

_____ Teach client about disease process.

X Administer prescribed analgesics.

Nursing Management of the Client
with Crohn's Disease Answer Key

Situation: A 25-year-old woman with an exacerbation of Crohn's disease is admitted to the emergency department with complaints of diarrhea, intermittent abdominal pain, flatulence, abdominal distention, and severe fatigue. The client's temperature is 102° F. The client states she has felt under stress because she recently lost her job, and has not yet secured new employment. As a result, she is very anxious about her finances.

1. Which signs/symptoms are the best indicators that the client is developing a fluid volume deficit related to diarrhea?

_____ Hypertension

X Thirst

X Bradycardia

X Decreased urinary output

_____ Weight gain

X Dry oral mucous membranes

X Postural hypotension

_____ Anorexia

_____ Headache

2. List at least three dietary modifications that may reduce the client's symptoms.

- **Eat small frequent meals.**
- **Avoid raw fruits and vegetables.**
- **Avoid foods that contain fat.**
- **Drink at least eight glasses of water a day.**

3. Why are these medications commonly prescribed for clients with Crohn's disease?

   a. Corticosteroids:

   To reduce inflammation of bowel tissues, which aids with healing and reduces pain

b. Antidiarrheals:

To prevent fluid and electrolyte losses that occurs from persistent

c. Antispasmodics:

To decrease pain from inflamed, spasmodic bowel

Nursing Management of the Client with Diverticular Disease Answer Key

Situation: A 65-year-old woman is being admitted to the hospital for diagnostic tests and to be evaluated for diverticulitis. The client is experiencing fever, severe abdominal pain, nausea, vomiting and abdominal distention.

1. What diagnostic tests are usually ordered for clients with possible diverticulitis?

   Sigmoidoscopy, ultrasonography, barium enema, and stool sample

2. What interventions do you expect to be performed to relieve this client's severe symptoms?

   The client will have food and fluid restricted, and receive intravenous infusions to provide fluids and nutrients. A nasogastric tube will be inserted to relieve nausea, vomiting and gastric distention.

3. What complications could this client develop as a result of diverticulitis?

   Partial or complete bowel obstruction, perforation of the bowel, peritonitis, fistula formation, hemorrhage

4. If the client has diverticulitis and fails to respond to medical interventions, what surgical procedure will need to be performed?

   Colon resection of the involved portion of the bowel

Nursing Management of the Client with Colorectal Cancer Answer Key

Situation: A 60-year-old married male client has had an abdominal-perineal resection for colorectal cancer. The nurse is preparing him for discharge home.

1. Following abdominal-perineal resection, why is it important to assess the client for signs of postoperative phlebitis and how can it be prevented?

   Clients who undergo abdominal-perineal resection are at increased risk for postoperative phlebitis because they are placed in a high lithotomy position during the surgery. Signs of phlebitis include redness, swelling, and the presence of Homan's sign (calf pain when the foot is passively dorsiflexed). To prevent postoperative phlebitis, the client may receive heparin subcutaneously every 12 hours following surgery, and also wear sequential pressure stockings. The nurse needs to encourage clients to perform leg exercises before and after surgery.

2. Prior to discharge, what instructions does the nurse give to the client and family about colostomy irrigation?

   The nurse must teach the client to perform the following measures for irrigation of the colostomy:

   - **Assemble the irrigation equipment, pouch, and skin care products and place on a convenient surface.**
   - **Remove and discard the old pouch.**
   - **Cleanse the peristomal skin surface thoroughly.**
   - **Apply the irrigating sleeve and close off the distal end or place it into a container or toilet.**
   - **Using one liter of warm tap water, suspend the solution container about 18 inches above the stoma and flush the air from the irrigation tubing.**
   - **Insert the lubricated catheter with a water-soluble product into the stoma opening to 2-4 inches. Never force the catheter.**
   - **Allow the irrigation solution to flow gently into the colon.**
   - **The majority of the stool will pass into the container or toilet; then close off the pouch until the bowel evacuates the material.**

- After the bowel is emptied, remove the sleeve; clean the stoma; and cover with a gauze pad or new pouch.
- Observe skin care protocol prior to application of the new pouch.

3. The client is concerned about the effect of the surgery and colostomy on his sexual relationship with his wife. What actions should be taken to help lessen concerns?

The client needs to understand that only a small number of men become impotent following perineal resection. If impotence develops, a surgeon may refer the client to a urology expert for treatment of impotence. Also, clients may benefit from a referral to a social worker, sex therapist, counselor, or registered nurse with a counseling background. Counseling can also help the client's wife or sexual partner. Even with counseling, it may take several months for the client and his wife to resume a satisfactory sexual relationship.

Situation: It is the second postoperative day for a 62-year-old male who underwent bowel resection colostomy construction as treatment for a bowel obstruction secondary to rectal cancer. His vital signs are stable, he has ambulated about in his room, and his dressing is dry and intact. His stoma is beefy red in appearance and feces and gas are draining into his pouch.

1. What is the etiology of the client's nursing diagnoses?

   a. Risk for body image disturbance

   Risk for body image disturbance related to inability to integrate anatomical changes into self-concept

   b. Risk for altered skin integrity

   Risk for altered skin integrity related to feces in contact with skin and/or appliance adhesive

   c. Risk for ineffective individual coping

   Risk for ineffective individual coping related to change in body image and/or change in bodily function

2. What client behaviors indicate that he is ready to participate in his own care?

   _____ Informing the nurse when the appliance needs to be changed

   X Asking questions about the stoma and its care

   X Looking at the stoma when the appliance is changed

   _____ Stating that he will care for the stoma when he gets home

3. The client is concerned about odor from the pouch. What suggestions can the nurse offer to decrease or eliminate this problem?

   - **Reassure the client that pouches are made of odor-proof plastic.**
   - **Advise the client to maintain seals so leakage does not occur.**

- Rinse the inside of the pouch with tepid water after emptying it.
- Place deodorizing solutions or tablets (which are available) in the pouch.
- Avoid gas-producing foods, such as broccoli or beans.

Situation: A 25-year-old woman who has been diagnosed with gastroesophageal reflux disease (GERD) is meeting with the nurse practitioner to discuss her condition. The client, who is overweight, has been experiencing dyspepsia, belching, bloating after meals, dysphagia, and chest pain.

1. What pathophysiologic problem is causing this client to experience chest pain?

   Chest pain in clients with GERD is caused by spasms of the esophagus, as a result of the reflux of acidic stomach contents and inflammatory response.

2. What instructions should the nurse practitioner provide this client in regard to diet?

   The nurse should instruct the client to eat small frequent meals; chew foods thoroughly; avoid evening snacks, fatty foods, chocolate, alcohol, coffee, and tea; and start a weight loss program. The client should elevate the head of the bed on blocks, not elevate her head with pillows. She should also keep a food diary to see what foods trigger symptoms. If the client smokes, she should seek assistance in quitting.

3. What classifications of medications will help to relieve the symptoms of GERD that result from the reflux of gastrointestinal contents containing acid?

   Antacids, histamine2 receptor antagonists, and proton pump inhibitors

Nursing Management of the Client
with Salmonellosis Answer Key

Situation: An older adult woman is being treated for abdominal cramping, nausea, vomiting and severe, watery diarrhea. Her symptoms began after attending an all day picnic on a hot day at a family reunion. Stool examination confirms the presence of salmonellosis.

---

1. Why are older adults and infants more susceptible to development of salmonellosis than other age groups?

> **Older adults and infants have less efficient immune systems. Infants have not yet obtained immunity to many common organisms. Older adults often have chronic illnesses or take medications that interfere with the functioning of their immune systems. It takes longer for an older adult to react immunologically than younger adults.**

2. Which are the two most important nursing diagnoses for the older adult client with salmonellosis?

_____ Risk for infection

X Risk for fluid volume deficit

_____ Risk for altered nutrition

X Risk for electrolyte imbalance

_____ Risk for altered skin integrity

3. Which collaborative care measures are appropriate for the client with salmonellosis?

X Initiating protective isolation precautions

X Replacing fluids and electrolytes

_____ Encouraging a full liquid diet

_____ Administering anti-diarrheal medication

_____ Administering antimicrobial therapy

Situation: A 75-year-old man with congestive heart failure (CHF) is being admitted to a long-term care facility. The client develops fatigue and dyspnea upon exertion, and consequently tends to severely limit his activities. The client experienced chronic constipation when at home which, at one point, resulted in an impaction that had to be manually removed by a home health nurse. During admission, the client's daughter told the nurse her father had not had a bowel movement in several days, and had been straining at defecation without results.

1. Why is the client at increased risk for these complications related to his chronic constipation?

   a. Fecal impaction:

   Impaction, and subsequent obstruction, occurs from collection of dry, hard feces within the lower colon and rectum.

   b. Hemorrhoids:

   Straining to eliminate hardened stools can cause hemorrhoids.

   c. Exacerbated angina pectoris:

   Straining at defecations can trigger angina pectoris or cardiac arrest due to the Valsalva maneuver. This maneuver, which involves forcibly exhaling with the nose and mouth closed, causes increased intrathoracic pressure, reduced pulse rate, decreased return of blood to the heart, and increased venous pressure.

2. What procedure will the nurse use to determine if the client has a fecal impaction?

   The nurse will put on a glove and insert a lubricated index finger into the client's anus. If the nurse feels a hard mass, an impaction is probably present.

3. What nursing activities will help keep the client free of constipation on a long-term basis?

   ____ Administer daily laxatives

   X Institute a bowel management program

X   Encourage increased fluid intake

_____ Perform a daily DRE (digital rectal exam)

_____ Encourage bedrest

X   Increase daily physical activities

X   Increase dietary fiber

_____ Administer weekly enemas

Nursing Management of the Client with Hypernatremia Answer Key

Situation: A 47-year-old woman has a rapid heart rate, dry oral mucous membranes, poor skin turgor, and fever of 101.3° F orally. Her serum sodium level is 163 mEq/L.

1. Which are risk factors for hypernatremia?

   X Diaphoresis

   _____ Nasogastric suctioning

   _____ Diuretics

   X Diabetes mellitus

   X Cushing's syndrome

   _____ Vomiting

   _____ Diarrhea

   X Burns

2. Which clinical manifestations are most supportive of the presence of hypernatremia?

   _____ Lethargy

   X Dry oral mucous membranes

   X Fever

   _____ Confusion

   _____ Stupor or coma

   X Tachycardia

   _____ Muscle weakness

   X Thirst

3. Prioritize the client's nursing diagnoses, with "1" representing the most important diagnosis.

   2 Impaired skin integrity

   4 Risk for injury

   3 Altered nutrition

   1 Fluid volume deficit

Situation: An 87-year-old man was admitted to the acute care facility for gastroenteritis of two days duration. He is vomiting, has severe, watery diarrhea, and is complaining of abdominal cramping. His serum electrolytes are consistent with hyponatremia related to excessive sodium loss.

1. Why does hyponatremia result from vomiting and diarrhea?

    Gastric secretions are high in sodium, that are lost from the gastrointestinal tract with vomiting, diarrhea or gastric suctioning.

2. Which clinical manifestations support the diagnosis of hyponatremia?

    X Lethargy

      Poor skin turgor

      Hyperreflexia

      Convulsions

      Agitation

    X Headache

3. Which collaborative interventions will help reduce or eliminate the client's hyponatremia?

    X Administer Lactated Ringer's solution.

      Encourage fluid intake.

      Weigh daily.

    X Encourage foods high in sodium.

Nursing Management of the Client
with Hyperkalemia Answer Key

Situation: An elderly client with a medical history of Type 2 NIDDM (non-insulin-dependent diabetes mellitus) complicated by nephropathy, CHF (congestive heart failure), and rheumatoid arthritis comes to the emergency department because of chest palpitations. She describes a feeling of fatigue and nausea without vomiting. The client's medication record is shown in the table below, left. The primary care provider orders an ECG (Electrocardiogram), chest x-ray, CBC (complete blood count), serum electrolytes, BUN (blood urea nitrogen), and creatinine. The electrolyte panel results are shown in the table below.

Medication Record	
Generic Name	**Brand name**
Spironolactone	Aldactone
Digoxin	Lanoxin
Metformin	Glucophage
Magnesium hydroxide	Milk of Magnesia
Calcium carbonate	Tums

Electrolyte Panel		
Na	139	mEq/L
K	5.8	mEq/L
Cl	102	mEq/L
CO_2	28	mEq/L
BUN	25	Mg/100mL
Creatinine	1.3	mg/dL

1. Should the health care provider be concerned about the client's serum potassium level? Why or why not?

> Yes. The client's serum potassium is elevated, placing the client at increased risk for life- threatening dysrhythmias, including ventricular fibrillation (V-fib) or ventricular tachycardia (V-tach). There are several factors contributing to this client's hyperkalemia. This client is taking a potassium-sparing diuretic (Aldactone). However, in light of the client's renal dysfunction related to her diabetes, she is at increased risk for poor potassium excretion and a subsequent elevated serum potassium level. The increased BUN (blood urea nitrogen) and creatinine levels indicate impaired renal function. Additionally, the antacid (Tums) may interact with digoxin (Lanoxin) to increase the potential for dysrhythmia.

2. Which clinical manifestations are associated with hyperkalemia?

> Headache
>
> Thirst
>
> **X** Cardiac dysrhythmias

      Muscular twitching

X   Vomiting

X   Paresthesia

3. Which nursing diagnoses apply to the client with hyperkalemia?

      Risk for fluid volume deficit

X   Risk for injury

X   Activity intolerance

X   Risk for decreased cardiac output

Nursing Management of the Client
with Hypokalemia Answer Key

Situation: A 69-year-old man has a medical history of congestive heart failure (CHF) controlled by digitalis and furosemide drug therapy. Two weeks ago he developed diarrhea, which has persisted in spite of his taking OTC antidiarrheal medications. His heart rate is 86 bpm, respirations 10 bpm, blood pressure 102/56 mmHg, and he is lethargic and confused.

1. Which client data supports the presence of hypokalemia?

2. Prioritize interventions for the client, with "1" representing the most important intervention.
   - **1** Identify and correct underlying cause as prescribed.
   - **5** Encourage intake of foods high in potassium.
   - **3** Administer oral potassium as prescribed.
   - **2** Administer intravenous potassium as prescribed.
   - **4** Assess vital signs.

3. After his diarrhea is controlled, which foods should the client is advised to eat since they are high in potassium?
   -     Beets
   - **X** Cantaloupe
   -     Lettuce
   - **X** Powdered milk
   -     Corn
   - **X** Dried beans
   - **X** Raw mushrooms
   -     Carrots

Nursing Management of the Client
with Acid-Base Imbalance Answer Key

Situation: Acid-base imbalances can be precipitated by a variety of causes in people who are healthy as well as those with illnesses. Interpret each of the ABG (arterial blood gas) findings, and identify common clinical manifestations with acid-base abnormalities.

1. Which ABG (arterial blood gas) findings need to be reported because they are abnormal?

Lab Results		Normal	Abnormal
Blood	7.38 pH	X	
PaCO$_2$	52 mmHg		X
HCO$_3$	30 mEq/L		X
PaO$_2$	62 mmHg		X

2. Match the clinical manifestation with the correct acid-base abnormality. [Hint: A manifestation may appear in more than one type of imbalance.]

Clinical Manifestation	Type of Acid-Base Imbalance			
	Metabolic Acidosis	Metabolic Alkalosis	Respiratory Acidosis	Respiratory Alkalosis
Tetany		X		X
Headache	X		X	
Diaphoresis				X
Coma		X	X	
Convulsions		X		X
Confusion		X		
Kussmaul's respirations	X			
Hyperpnea			X	
Bradycardia	X			
Visual disturbances			X	

3. Which acid-base imbalance should the nurse be prepared to encounter when caring for clients with:

Diagnosis	Type of Acid-Base Imbalance			
	Metabolic Acidosis	Metabolic Alkalosis	Respiratory Acidosis	Respiratory Alkalosis
Fever				X
Cushing's Syndrome		X		
Head injury			X	
Gastric suctioning		X		
Renal failure	X			
Anesthetics			X	
Diabetes mellitus	X			
Vomiting	X			

Nursing Management of the Client with Extracellular Fluid Volume Deficit—Dehydration Answer Key

Situation: A 45-year-old female client, who had prolonged vomiting and diarrhea due to an episode of flu, is being seen in the emergency department. The woman complains of thirst, has cracked dry lips, poor skin turgor, a pulse rate of 110, a temperature of 101° F, and a blood pressure of 80/50. The client's urinary elimination is <30 mL per hour, and her urine is dark and concentrated. When in a supine position, the client's neck veins are flat. The client is seriously dehydrated and the physician orders the administration of 2 L of normal saline IV. Prior to discharge, the nurse talks with the client about methods for replacing her fluids once she goes home.

1. How do the symptoms of dehydration differ between younger clients and elderly clients?

   Unlike younger clients, many elderly clients with dehydration do not experience thirst, nor does their urine become concentrated. Skin turgor and orthostatic blood pressure are also unreliable indicators of dehydration in the elderly.

2. When the client is being treated for dehydration with IV infusions, what can the nurse do to prevent a fluid volume overload?

   When administering IV fluids to clients with dehydration, the nurse should use minigroup IV tubing or an IV pump to reduce the risk of fluid overload. Preventing fluid overload is particularly important in older clients, because many of these individuals have cardiac or renal conditions, making them particularly susceptible to this complication.

3. How can the client continue to replenish her fluid losses once she is discharged home?

   The nurse should advise the client with dehydration to drink eight ounces of water and other fluids at least hourly and to record her intake. The client should also call the physician or nurse if her urine continues to look dark or concentrated, and if she loses more than two pounds in a day. Remind the client that in the future she should seek medical attention for severe vomiting or diarrhea before dehydration develops.

Nursing Management of the Client with Fluid Volume Excess Answer Key

Situation: An older client with CHF (congestive heart failure) is readmitted to the acute care facility with dyspnea, weakness, weight gain, 3+ pitting edema of both lower extremities, and bilateral crackles in the bases of his lungs. The client has a bounding pulse and elevated blood pressure.

1. Which findings, in addition to those exhibited by the client, are supportive of fluid volume excess?

_____ Decreased pulse pressure

X Headache

X Confusion

X Ascites

_____ Postural hypotension

X Decreased hematocrit

2. Prioritize the goals of medical management for clients with fluid volume excess, with "1" representing the most important goal.

4 Preventing complications (pulmonary edema, coma)

2 Early recognition and treatment

1 Identifying persons at risk

3 Eliminating excess fluid volume

3. Which statements are true about fluid volume excess? Correct false statements.

a. Osmosis refers to the flow of particles from an area of high to low concentration.

False. Osmosis refers to the flow of water from an area of high to low concentration.

b. Changes in intracellular fluid volume are often related to changes in potassium balance.

False. Changes in extracellular fluid volume are often related to changes in sodium balance.

c. Fluid volume excess most often occurs from inadequate sodium intake.

False. Fluid volume excess may occur from excessive sodium intake, overhydration, or failure of renal or hormonal regulatory mechanisms.

d. Disease can affect osmolarity and cell permeability to water.

True.

Nursing Management of the Client Requiring Total Parenteral Nutrition (TPN) Answer Key

Situation: A 54-year-old man with pancreatitis is unable to tolerate oral food or fluids due to pain, nausea and vomiting. He is in a severely weakened state, has lost 12 pounds, and has a fever of 101.5o F PO   Following assessment of the client, the practitioner prescribes TPN (total parenteral nutrition) Subsequently, a central line is placed and TPN is initiated, which contains 50% dextrose.

1. What health care condition might a client have that would necessitate the use of TPN?

   - **Weight loss**
   - **Weakness**
   - **Fever**
   - **Nausea**
   - **Vomiting**
   - **Presence of a serious illness**

2. Which nursing diagnoses are appropriate for this client, based on the data given?

   X Fatigue

   X Risk for fluid volume deficit/excess

   _____ Infection

   X Nutrition: less than body requirements

   _____ Impaired skin integrity

3. Which findings support the effectiveness of TPN?

   X Weight gain or stabilization

   _____ Reduced pain

   X Serum sodium of 139 mEq/L

   X Serum glucose of 80 mg/dL

   _____ Urinary output > 30 cc/hour

Nursing Management of the Client with a
Urinary Tract Infection (UTI)—Cystitis Answer Key

Situation: A 23-year-old client visits her health practitioner stating she thinks she has a UTI (urinary tract infection). She has a low-grade fever of 100.6° F PO, and lower abdominal tenderness on palpation.

1. What other symptoms are commonly associated with UTI (urinary tract infection)?

   X Frequency   **X** Polyuria

   X Urgency   **X** Low back pain

   _____ Increased blood pressure   _____ Dizziness

   X Dysuria   _____ Anuria

   X Foul smell   **X** Nocturia

2. Why are women at greater risk for UTI than men?

   Females have a shorter urethra and use a variety of products that may predispose them to infection.

3. What is the most common and important cause of UTI in older adults, and why?

   The use of indwelling urinary catheters for older adults who have decreased resistance to infections related to other chronic illnesses and nutritional and fluid deficit.

Nursing Management of the Client
with Renal Calculi Answer Key

Situation: While working at his desk, a 46-year-old male suddenly develops severe back pain, nausea, and diaphoresis. He is rushed to the emergency department where urinalysis is positive for hematuria. Diagnostic tests indicate the presence of a renal calculus in the lower right ureter.

1. Prioritize nursing activities for the client, with "1" representing the most important activity.

   4   Strain his urine

   3   Take vital signs

   2   Administer prescribed pain medication

   1   Obtain a brief history

2. Which nursing diagnoses are appropriate for the client at this time?

   _____ Infection

   X   Altered urinary elimination

   X   Anxiety/fear

   _____ Knowledge deficit

3. What is extracorporeal lithotripsy and how is the client prepared for the procedure?

   Extracorporeal lithotripsy is a procedure whereby sound waves are passed through water and directed at the client's renal stones. The sound waves fragment the stones, allowing them to be passed out of the ureter into the urinary bladder for elimination.   There is no special preparation for the procedure, although the client must provide written consent. A mild sedative may be administered prior to the procedure.

Nursing Management of the Client with Urinary Incontinence Answer Key

Situation: A 54-year-old woman visits her health provider because she is embarrassed about losing urine when she coughs, laughs, or sneezes.

1. The client is describing what kind of urinary incontinence?

   The client is experiencing stress incontinence.

2. Match the types of incontinence with the correct descriptors. Use the first letter of each type of incontinence as the form of answer.

F = Functional	**O**	Related to obstructed urinary outflow
O = Overflow	**T**	Involuntary, unpredictable loss of urine
R = Reflex	**U**	Related to over-activity of urinary bladder
S = Stress	**T**	Not generally responsive to treatment
T = Total	**R**	Loss of urine due to neurological dysfunction
U = Urge	**U**	Occurs with strong feeling of need to urinate
	R	Results in incomplete emptying of the bladder
	S	Urine loss follows increased intra-abdominal pressure

3. Explain Kegel exercises to the client.

   You will contract the muscles you use for urinating or defecating. Contract your muscles for 10-20 seconds at least four times each day. You may do the exercises at any time during the day. The more exercises you do, the greater benefit you will derive from them.

4. Why are indwelling urinary catheters contraindicated for control of urinary incontinence in older adults?

Indwelling urinary catheters increase older adults' risk for infection and subsequent urosepsis, and should be avoided if possible.

Situation: A 55-year-old female client has been admitted to the medical unit with fever, chills generalized edema, ascites, tenderness of the CVA (costovertebral angle), and flank pain. She also has smoky urine that contains red cell casts and traces of blood. Around 21 days prior to this hospitalization, the client was diagnosed with a beta-hemolytic streptococcal infection of the respiratory system. The client's physician has now confirmed she has developed AGN (acute glomerulonephritis).

1. What are the three "classic" clinical manifestations of AGN?

- **Hematuria**
- **Proteinuria**
- **Hypertension**

2. Explain why beta-hemolytic streptococcal infections of the throat predispose clients to AGN?

The immune response produces antibodies against the offending organism (beta-hemolytic streptococcus). The antibodies attached to the streptococcus bacteria are filtered through the kidneys. However, they become lodged in the glomerulus due to their large size, which causes inflammation within the glomerulus and resultant AGN.

3. What is plasmapheresis and why is it beneficial to clients with AGN?

Plasmapheresis is a procedure that filters the client's blood, ridding it of cellular components, antibodies, immune complexes, and protein-bound toxins. It reduces the number of antibody-antigen complexes that can become lodged in the glomerulus, thus reducing glomerular inflammation and damage.

4. Match the following drugs with the reason they are prescribed for clients with AGN.

b,c Corticosteroids	a. Hypertension
d Diuretics	b. Reduce inflammation
e Antibiotics	c. Inhibit immune response
b,c Immunosuppressants	d. Relieve edema
e Antihypertensives	e. Eradicate strep infection

Nursing Management of the Client with Acute Renal Failure (ARF) Answer Key

Situation: A 39-year-old man was admitted to the critical care unit following an automobile accident in which he suffered multiple injuries, blood loss and hypovolemic shock. He has been diagnosed with ARF (acute renal failure) in spite of aggressive fluid resuscitation.

1. What risk factor(s) does the client have for ARF (acute renal failure)?

   Hypovolemic shock related to blood loss leads to diminished renal perfusion. Decreased blood supply can cause damage to kidneys with subsequent ARF.

2. Match the phases of acute renal failure with their correct descriptors. Use the numbers 1, 2, and 3 as the form of answer.

1 = Phase 1	3	Nocturia
2 = Phase 2	1	Lasts 3-12 months
3 = Phase 3	3	Period of oliguria
	1	Begins when the kidneys start to recover
	1	May last 1-3 weeks
	1	Renal function is fully restored
	3	Lasts 7-14 days
	2	Period of diuresis

3. Which five assessments are essential for the client who is in acute renal failure?

Cardiac enzymes	X	Blood pressure	X	Urine output
Blood glucose	X	Serum creatinine		RBC (red blood cell) count
Serum sodium	X	Lung sounds	X	ABGs (arterial blood gases)

4. Prioritize the client's nursing diagnoses, with "1" representing the most important diagnosis.

3 Risk for Infection

4 Impaired skin integrity

2 Pain

5 Knowledge deficit

1 Fluid volume excess

Nursing Management of the Client with Chronic Renal Failure (CRF) Answer Key

Situation: A 55-year-old woman is admitted to the acute care facility for weight gain, pedal edema, hypertension, and decreased urine output. Her past history reveals chronic use of NSAIDs (Nonsteroidal anti-inflammatory drugs) for low back pain and Type 2 Diabetes Mellitus of twelve years duration. Her family history is positive for coronary artery disease and diabetes mellitus.

1. What risk factors does the client have for CRF?
   - **Diabetes mellitus**
   - **Chronic use of NSAIDs (Nonsteroidal anti-inflammatory drugs)**

2. How does chronic renal failure differ from acute renal failure?
   - **CRF takes months to years to develop. It is progressive and irreversible.**
   - **ARF (Acute renal failure) occurs within hours to days and, if treated promptly, is reversible.**
   - **Both conditions produce the same clinical manifestations.**

3. Match the characteristics with the correct stage of chronic renal failure. Use the Stage number as your response for each answer.

Stage 1: Decreased renal reserve	2	Nocturia
Stage 2: Renal insufficiency	4	Anemia
Stage 3: Renal failure	1	Normal BUN (blood urea nitrogen)
Stage 4: End stage renal failureuremia	4	CHF (congestive heart failure)
	3	Headache
	4	Anuria
	2	Polydipsia
	3	Metabolic acidosis
	1	Normal serum creatinine
	4	Marked azotemia

4. Prioritize nursing activities for the client, with "1" representing the most important activity.

1   Monitor serum potassium levels.

3   Turn every two hours.

4   Offer emotional support to family.

2   Assess lung sounds.

5. Which are the two most important collaborative interventions for the client at this time?

       Providing adequate pain control

X   Preventing complications

X   Correcting electrolyte imbalance

       Teaching the client about dialysis

Nursing Management of the Client Requiring Hemodialysis/Peritoneal Dialysis Answer Key

Situation: A 35-year-old male has received hemodialysis for renal failure or End-Stage Renal Disease (ESRD) for the past seven years due to diabetes mellitus. While awaiting renal transplant, he receives hemodialysis three times each week via an arteriovenous fistula created in his left arm.

1. Which nursing interventions are most important to perform immediately prior to initiating the client's hemodialysis?

    _____ Determine current medications being taken by client.

    X Assess AV fistula for bruit.

    _____ Calculate total urine output for the night.

    _____ Assess dietary intake.

    _____ Obtain blood glucose level.

    X Obtain a current weight.

    _____ Assess hydration status.

    X Draw serum electrolytes.

    X Obtain a current blood pressure reading.

2. Which nursing interventions need to be implemented following the client's hemodialysis procedure?

    X Obtain BUN (blood urea nitrogen) and serum creatinine.

    X Assess for headache and/or confusion.

    _____ Obtain blood glucose level.

    _____ Administer antihypertensive medication for hypertension.

    X Obtain serum electrolytes.

    X Assess access site for indications of bleeding.

3. Provide rationale for the client's nursing diagnoses.

    a. Risk for fluid volume deficit

    Rationale: Fluid is rapidly removed during hemodialysis, increasing the potential for the removal of too much fluid, leaving the client with a fluid deficit.

b. Risk for injury

    Rationale: Hemodialysis involves the use of heparin to prevent blood clotting during the procedure. Heparinization increases the risk for bleeding.

c. Risk for activity intolerance

    Rationale: Fluid overload produces fatigue, which decreases the client's activity tolerance.

d. Risk for ineffective breathing pattern

    Rationale: Fluid overload results in fluid accumulation within tissues and the lungs.

Situation: A 40-year-old male client with failing renal function has undergone a renal transplant and is four days postoperative. He is being treated on the surgical unit. The urinary catheter has been removed, and the client is able to void. The client is still receiving intravenous infusions with electrolyte replacements, but will be started on oral fluids today. Thus far, the client has not had any signs of transplant rejection.

1. Which fluid and electrolyte imbalances is the client at greatest risk for?

  X Hypokalemia   _____ Hypercalcemia

  X Hyponatremia   _____ Hypomagnesemia

  X Fluid overload   **X** Hypovolemia

2. Which are the four priority nursing diagnoses during the early postoperative phase following organ transplantation?

  X Risk for fluid volume deficit

  _____ Risk for constipation

  _____ Body image disturbance

  X Risk for infection

  X Fear and anxiety

  X Altered nutrition: less than body requirements

  _____ Noncompliance with therapeutic regimen

3. Which are clinical manifestations of organ rejection?

  X Malaise   _____ Elevated serum creatinine

  X Bradycardia   **X** Tender kidney

  X Weight gain   _____ Hypotension

  _____ Decreased serum BUN (blood urea nitrogen)   _____ Headache

  X Fever   **X** Oliguria

4. Why is the client undergoing organ transplantation at greater risk for infection than other surgical clients?

Clients undergoing organ transplantation are at greater risk for infection than other surgical clients because they are immunosuppressed to prevent organ rejection.

Situation: An older man with a 30-year history of diabetes mellitus is experiencing excessive protein wasting, edema, and hypertension. Based on the client's clinical manifestations and proteinuria of 3.7 g/day, the client is diagnosed with nephrotic syndrome.

1. Which areas of the client's body will the nurse assess to determine the presence of edema related to nephrotic syndrome?

_____ Posterior neck	**X** Hands	_____ Buttocks
X Sacrum	_____ Elbow	**X** Ankles

2. Which statements are true about the client's condition? Correct false statements.

   a. Nephrotic syndrome is a disease that causes edema and proteinuria.

   False. Nephrotic syndrome is not a disease but a complex of signs and symptoms, which includes edema and proteinuria.

   b. Hypoalbuminemia, hyperlipidemia, and lipuria are consequences of nephrotic syndrome.

   True.

   c. Nephrotic syndrome is a reversible condition when diagnosed and treated early.

   False. Nephrotic syndrome is not a reversible condition. It generally results in renal failure within five years.

   d. Periods of exacerbation and remission are common in clients with nephrotic syndrome.

   True.

   e. Nephrotic syndrome is related to glomerular disease or injury.

   True.

3. Prioritize nursing activities for this client, with "1" representing the most important activity.

3   Encourage bedrest.

1   Limit potassium intake.

4   Teach regarding exacerbating factors.

2   Provide low protein, high carbohydrate diet.

Nursing Management of the Client with Prostate Cancer Answer Key

Situation: A 70-year-old man is scheduled for a radical prostatectomy for prostate cancer. The client has been experiencing back pain, difficulty initiating his urinary stream, and bloody urine. Both his PSA (prostate specific antigen) and PAP (prostatic acid phosphate) were positive.

1. Why are the client's laboratory findings (PSA and PAP) important?

   A positive PSA is associated with prostatic cancer. An elevated PAP is associated with prostatic cancer that has metastasized beyond the capsule to other parts of the body, especially bone. Both are indicative of the presence of prostate cancer.

2. What is the difference between a radical perineal prostatectomy and a TURP (transurethral resection of the prostate)?

   Radical prostatectomy involves removal of the prostate gland and seminal vesicles through a suprapubic, perineal, or retropubic incision. It is indicated for prostate cancer. A transurethral prostatectomy involves inserting instruments through the penis and removing the prostate gland. It is indicated for benign conditions.

3. Which nursing activities will be most effective in reducing the client's anxiety over his diagnosis and impending surgery?

   _____ Explaining the pathophysiology of prostate cancer

   X Establishing a trusting relationship

   X Encouraging the client to verbalize his concerns

   _____ Encouraging the client to not worry unnecessarily

   X Answering the client's questions simply but honestly

   X Including the client in all care planning

Nursing Management of the Client with Benign Prostatic Hypertrophy (BPH) Answer Key

Situation: A 70-year-old male is being admitted to the surgical unit to undergo a TURP (transurethral resection of the prostate). The client has been experiencing dysuria, urgency, and nocturia for over a year.

1. What is the most common surgery for BPH and how is it performed?

TURP (transurethral resection of the prostate) is the most common surgery for BPH. The surgeon inserts an endoscope through the urethra in order to remove a small amount of prostate tissue.

2. Describe the other major surgeries for BPH.

Suprapubic prostatectomy:

Suprapubic prostatectomy involves inserting an endoscope through a lower abdominal incision and then through the bladder to access and assess the prostate.

Retropubic prostatectomy:

Retropubic prostatectomy involves inserting an endoscope through a lower abdominal incision into the prostate capsule without entering the bladder.

Preinial prostatecomy:

Perineal prostatectomy involves removing prostate tissue through an incision between the scrotum and the anus.

3. Why are alpha-blocking agents administered to clients with BPH?

Alpha-blocking agents are given to constrict the prostate, which helps to reduce urethral pressure, increase urine flow, and decrease residual urine.

4. As the prostate enlarges, there is a danger of complete urinary obstruction and retention. What are the precipitating factors that may lead to retention?

- **Infection**
- **Alcoholic and caffeinated beverages**
- **Delayed voiding**
- **Bedrest**
- **Client becoming chilled**
- **Decongestant use or sympathomimetic drugs found in common cold and cough remedies**
- **Some antidepressants**

Nursing Management of the Client with a
Transurethral Resection of the Prostate (TURP) Answer Key

Situation: A 70-year-old client with BPH has been discharged home with an indwelling catheter following a TURP. Prior to discharge, the nurse carefully instructed the client and his wife on the way to care for the catheter and drainage system.

1. Which important points does the nurse need to teach the client and his wife about home catheter care?

    X Wash hands thoroughly prior to caring for the catheter.

    X Use clean technique when caring for the catheter.

    _____ Securely tape the catheter to his penis.

    _____ How to irrigate the catheter

    X How to change the catheter

    X Monitor and record fluid intake and output.

    X Keep the area around the catheter clean.

2. Which instructions should the client be given about his surgery and recovery?

    X He should avoid heavy lifting (> 10 lb or 4.5 kg).

    _____ He can take car trips no further than 500 miles.

    _____ Stair climbing and driving short distances are okay.

    X Sexual activity should be avoided until approved by the physician.

    X Take a daily stool softener.

3. Which two complications is the client most at risk for developing within the first week postoperatively?

    Post- TURP clients are at greatest risk for infection and bleeding within the first week following surgery.

4. What is the rationale for advising the client to increase his intake of fiber and drink 2000-3000 mL of fluid per day?

The client is advised to increase fluid intake and fiber in order to prevent constipation and straining at defecation, which can result in stress on the surgical incision and bleeding.

Nursing Management of the Client with a Radical Prostatectomy Answer Key

Situation: A 65-year-old male client who was diagnosed with a grade C prostate tumor has undergone a radical prostatectomy using a perineal approach. The client is now being prepared for discharge from the hospital. The client is concerned about erectile dysfunction. The client also has some degree of urinary incontinence. If urinary incontinence continues, the client will be evaluated for implantation of an AUS (artificial urinary sphincter).

1. The perineal approach to radical prostatectomy places the client at increased risk for which complications?

X Infection	**X** Impotency	_____ Fecal incontinence
X Urinary incontinence	**X** Erectile dysfunction	**X** Hemorrhage

2. Prioritize nursing activities for this client, with "1" representing the most important activity.

4 Instruct client regarding hormonal therapy.

2 Change dressing when soiled.

3 Provide skin care to prevent breakdown.

1 Administer pain medication as prescribed.

3. Why is the client taught to avoid these activities for the first two months following radical prostatectomy?

a. Valsalva maneuver during bowel movements:

The Valsalva maneuver increases venous pressure, which can result in hematuria.

b. Strenuous activities:

Strenuous activity may cause bleeding.

c. Long motor trips or prolonged sitting:

Prolonged sitting can result in clot formation.

4. What is an AUS (artificial urinary sphincter), and why is it used?

An AUS (artificial urinary sphincter) is a fluid-filled system composed of a silicone rubber cuff that encircles the urethra, and a synthetic pump implanted into the scrotum via an abdominal incision. AUSs are implanted in individuals with refractory urinary incontinence. Complications of an AUS include infection, mechanical failures, and erosion of the urethra.

Nursing Management of the Menopausal Client Receiving Hormone Replacement Therapy (HRT) Answer Key

Situation: A 45-year-old client has been experiencing irregular menstrual periods, hot flashes, and night sweats. After a thorough history and physical, the primary care provider recommends HRT. First, the primary care provider schedules the client for a conference with the nurse practitioner who discusses the advantages and disadvantages of HRT.

1. What are the major advantages of HRT?

   - The major advantage is the reduction of the vasomotor (hot flashes, night sweats) symptoms of menopause.
   - Helps to prevent atrophic vaginitis, osteoporosis, and atherosclerosis

2. What are the major disadvantages of HRT?

   - Can increase the risk of uterine cancer in a woman with an intact uterus who is not also taking progesterone
   - Increases the risk of thrombophlebitis and stroke in women who smoke heavily
   - Women who have had breast or uterine cancer are at greater risk of a recurrence if they take HRT.

3. What are the causes and symptoms of atrophic vaginitis, and how is it treated?

   - Cause: Thinning and dryness of the vaginal walls characterize atrophic vaginitis, which develop due to low estrogen levels.
   - Symptoms: Include vaginal irritation, burning, pruritus, leukorrhea, bleeding, and painful intercourse.
   - Treatment: HRT taken orally. HRT is also administered via a vaginal cream or suppository tablets.

Nursing Management of the Client with a Cystocele and/or Rectocele Answer Key

Situation: A 65-year-old woman diagnosed with serious cystocele and rectocele is being discharged home with an indwelling catheter following an anterior/posterior repair. If the client has difficulty voiding following removal of the catheter, she will need to perform CISC (clean intermittent self-catheterization). For the two years previous to the surgery, the client attempted to control symptoms with the use of a pessary and Kegel exercises.

1. What instructions should the nurse provide the client who is wearing a pessary?

- **Immediately report to their health care provider:**
    - **Any discomfort from pessary**
    - **If pessary falls out**
    - **Any change in color, amount, odor, or consistency of vaginal discharge**
    - **Vaginal itching**
- **Return for follow-up examinations within 3 days following initial insertion of pessary**
- **Schedule reexaminations every 6 weeks thereafter**

2. What instructions should the nurse provide to the client concerning Kegel exercises?

- **Contract the circumvaginal or perirectal muscles**
    - **Starting with 10 repetitions**
    - **Gradually increasing to 35-50 repetitions**
    - **Hold the contraction for 6-10 seconds followed by a 10-second relaxation period**
- **Exercises need to be performed every day for 6-12 weeks.**

3. What measures can the client take to prevent UTI (urinary tract infection) related to the use of an indwelling catheter?

Instruct the client with an indwelling catheter to:
- **Thoroughly wash hands before and after handling catheter or drainage system.**
- **Drink at least 2000 mL of fluid a day.**

- Perform perineal care to remove any crusts or debris from around the catheter itself.
- Take antibiotics and urinary antiseptics as ordered.

4. What instructions should the nurse provide to the client concerning CISC (clean intermittent self-catheterization)?

- Attempt to void prior to the catheterization.
- If unable to void, wash hands thoroughly.
- Assume a comfortable position.
- Separate the labial folds with thumb and midfinger of nondominant hand
- Wash the perineal area from front toward the anus.
- Keep labial folds separated and insert catheter into the urinary meatus.
- Allow urine to flow until flow stops.
- Remove catheter slowly.

Nursing Management of the Client with a Hysterectomy Answer Key

Situation: A 53-year-old woman just returned from the PACU (postanesthesia care unit) after undergoing an abdominal hysterectomy and oophorectomy. Her vital signs are stable and her dressing is dry and intact. She is able to administer her own pain medication by means of a PCA (patient-controlled analgesia) pump.

1. What other essential assessments need to be made by the nurse?

  X   Vaginal drainage   **X**   Abdominal distention

  _____ Pupillary response   **X**   Bowel sounds

  X   Urinary output   _____ Gag reflex

  X   Homan's sign   **X**   Pain status

2. List two positive and two negative effects a hysterectomy can have on a woman's self-image.

    Positive:
   - **Relief related to loss of fertility**
   - **Cure of illness**

    Negative:
   - **Loss of femininity**
   - **Loss of self-worth**
   - **Grief related to loss of fertility**

3. Prioritize nursing activities for the client at this time, with "1" representing the most important activity.

    1   Assess effectiveness of prescribed pain medication.

    3   Provide emotional support to client and family.

    4   Encourage ambulation to the chair or bathroom.

    2   Encourage active leg exercises.

    5   Teach client regarding cessation of menstruation.

Nursing Management of the Client with an Ovarian Cyst Answer Key

Situation: A 25-year old woman is visiting her health care provider because she has missed several menstrual periods. The client has also been experiencing lower abdominal pain and tenderness. Upon examination, the nurse practitioner finds a palpable pelvic mass. Following diagnostic tests, the client is diagnosed with a corpus luteum ovarian cyst.

1. What is the cause of a corpus luteum ovarian cyst?

   The corpus luteum is a small endocrine structure that forms within a ruptured ovarian follicle and secretes estrogen and progesterone. Corpus luteum cysts are caused by increased secretion by the corpus luteum after ovulation.

1. A suspected ovarian cyst must be differentiated from what other female reproductive disorder?

   Perimenopausal or postmenopausal women with a palpable ovarian mass are more likely to have ovarian cancer than an ovarian cyst. The primary symptoms of ovarian cancer are an enlarged abdomen due to ascites or abdominal or pelvic masses.

1. What diagnostic tests are used to differentiate an ovarian cyst from a neoplasm?

   Ultrasound and abdominal radiograph are the primary diagnostic tools used to differentiate ovarian cysts from neoplastic cysts.

Situation: A 62-year-old female client is being evaluated for possible ovarian cancer. She has been experiencing vague gastrointestinal symptoms and urinary urgency for several months. The physician has discovered a small pelvic mass and has ordered a group of diagnostic studies.

1. Why is a PAP (Papanicolaou) test of limited value in diagnosing ovarian cancer?

   A PAP test has limited value as a diagnostic agent because it produces abnormal results in only 20%-30% of women who have a malignancy, and therefore misses the diagnosis in 70%-80% of clients.

2. What is the purpose of exploratory surgery?

   - **Obtain a definitive diagnosis of ovarian cancer**
   - **Establish the precise clinical stage of the cancer**

3. What are the stages of ovarian cancer?

   The four major stages of ovarian cancer are:

   Stage I: Growth is limited to the ovaries.

   Stage II: Growth extends to both ovaries and there may be metastasis to the fallopian tubes and the pelvis; ascites may develop which contains malignant cells.

   Stage III: Malignant tumor involves both ovaries; abdominal implants, not exceeding two cm in diameter, and inguinal nodes may be present.

   Stage IV: Distant metastases may occur. Pleural effusion and parenchymal liver metastases can develop.

4. What is the treatment of choice for clients with ovarian cancer?

The surgery of choice for ovarian cancer is total abdominal hysterectomy with removal of both ovaries and the fallopian tubes (bilateral salpingo-oophorectomy or TAH-BSO), removal of the tumor, and omentectomy (removal of the peritoneal covering). The surgery is followed with chemotherapy for 6-12 months to destroy any remaining cancer cells. TAH-BSO alone may be sufficient to treat younger clients with borderline malignancies.

Nursing Management of the Client with Cervical Cancer Answer Key

Situation: A 33-year-old woman underwent a loop electrosurgical excision procedure (LEEP) for cervical cancer one week ago. Pathology reports confirmed the cancer was preinvasive and due to dysplasia. The client is greatly relieved, but understands she will have to maintain close follow-up care for the next few years.

1. Place a "P" in front of statements that are true for **Preinvasive** cervical carcinoma and an "I" in front of statements that are true for **Invasive** cervical carcinoma.

   P   Abnormal cells within the lower third of cervical epithelium

   I   Involves the basement membrane

   I   Metastasis via the lymphatic system

   P   Abnormal cells contained within full thickness epithelium

   P   Has a 75%-90% cure rate if diagnosed and treated early

   I   Directly spreads to adjacent pelvic structures

2. Prioritize the goals of collaborative care for the client with preinvasive cancer of the cervix, with "1" representing the most important goal.

   3   Prevention of complications

   1   Surgical elimination of the cancer

   4   Prevention of recurrence

   2   Absence of pain

3. Prioritize nursing activities to reduce the client's anxiety while waiting for diagnostic study results or treatment for carcinoma of the cervix, with "1" representing the most important activity.

   2   Encourage the client to verbalize her fears and concerns.
   Verbalizing fears and concerns often reduces them.

4 Assess the client's feelings about having a hysterectomy.
To determine the need for further intervention or different interventions; cannot assess the client's feelings unless the client verbalizes them.

3 Acknowledge the client's feelings.
It is important to acknowledge feelings so the client will continue to share those feelings.

1 Establish a trusting relationshi
Must be established before honest communication and client sharing will occur.

Nursing Management of the Client with Breast Disorders: Breast Cancer and Fibrocystic Breast Disease Answer Key

Situation: A 37-year-old female is scheduled to undergo breast biopsy for a lump she discovered in her left breast four days ago. Her history includes cigarette smoking for seventeen years, use of oral contraceptives, one child who is four years old, and family history of coronary artery disease. She denies breast trauma, alcohol use, or exposure to radiation. She is 20 pounds above desired weight for her height.

1. What are the client's risk factors for breast cancer?

   - **Cigarette smoking**
   - **Pregnancy after the age of 30**
   - **Use of oral contraceptives**
   - **Excessive body weight.**

2. What is the most significant screening conducted for breast cancer? Why?

   - **SBE (breast self-examination). The American Cancer Society recommends women perform a SBE to be performed on a monthly basis. Women are often the first to discover lumps in their breast while tumors are very small, enhancing the opportunity for early treatment and better outcomes.**
   - **Mammogram is a more sensitive, accurate screening test. Abnormalities can be detected much earlier than by BSE. Some practitioners claim palpable lumps are often beyond the early stage. Current guidelines for mammogram screening include:**
     - **Yearly for all women over age 40**
     - **Baseline screen for women between 35-40 years of age**
     - **Prior to age 35 for women with family history of breast cancer, fibrocystic disease, breast implants, or unusual breast findings.**

3. Which statements are true regarding breast cancer? Correct false statements.

   a. Breast cancer is the most common cancer among women age 45-75.

   False. Breast cancer is the most common cancer among women age 25-75.

b. Breast cancer is the leading cause of death in women age 55-65.

False. Breast cancer is the leading cause of death in women age 40-44.

c. Women detect most breast cancers during their annual mammogram.

False. Women detect most breast cancers during their own BSE (breast self- examination).

d. The majority of breast cancers occur in the lower inner quadrant of the breast.

False. The majority of breast cancers occur in the upper, outer quadrant of the breast.

e. An important goal of care is early recognition and treatment of breast cancer.

True.

4. Prioritize nursing activities for the client with breast cancer, with "1" representing the most important activity.

4 Encourage client to lie on affected side to relieve pain.

3 Administer pain medications as prescribed.

2 Maintain surgical asepsis of dressings, incision and drains.

6 Support arm on operative side with sling while ambulating.

5 Encourage early arm exercises to avoid lymphedema.

1 Prepare client for surgery as indicated.

Nursing Management of the Client with a Sexually Transmitted Disease (STD) Answer Key

Situation: A 19-year-old college student comes to the clinic because she has developed a yellowish vaginal discharge and painful urination. The client has a history of pelvic inflammatory disease and infrequent menses.

1. Upon initial assessment, what other information does the nurse need to gather from the client?

- **History of sexual activities and partners**
- **Temperature, pulse, respirations, body weight, and urine sample**
- **History of menstrual cycle**
- **History of vaginal itching**
- **Appearance of genital area**

2. Describe the types of laboratory and physical exams likely to be performed. Give the rationales for the test or exam. (Hint: Answer key lists at least six.)

Test / Exam	Rationale
VDRL	To determine presence of venereal disease
CBC (complete blood count)	To determine infection or anemia
WBC (white blood cell)	To determine infection or anemia
Pelvic exam	To examine vaginal and cervical area
Vaginal culture	To identify organism
Gram stain	To rule out gonorrhea
Urinalysis	To rule out UTI (urinary tract infection) and pregnancy.

After the client's lab tests are reviewed, the physician tells her she has gonorrhea and is pregnant.

3. What are the key points the client needs to know about gonorrhea and pregnancy?

- The gonococci microorganism can ascend to the uterus and fallopian tubes causing pelvic inflammatory disease.

- Gonococcal infections can be spread to the pharynx so it is important to know if she has had oral sex with any of her partners and that while she is infected she should not engage in any sexual activity in order not to spread the disease.

- If untreated, gonorrhea can be passed to a newborn during birth and the newborn can, at the worst, suffer vision problems from the infection.

- A gonococcal infection in her male partner or partners is usually apparent as urethritis and men have urinary symptoms.

- Chlamydia infections often accompany gonococcal infections and also need to be diagnosed and treated.

- Sexual partners also need to be assessed and treated.

Nursing Management of the Client Requiring Preoperative Care
Answer Key

Situation: A 55-year-old-female client is scheduled for an exploratory laparotomy. The client has been experiencing abdominal symptoms for several months. A baseline assessment of all symptoms was conducted. The client has received instructions concerning (a) the procedure, (b) pain control following the surgery, and (c) the importance of coughing, deep-breathing, and leg exercises. The client has also signed an informed consent for the surgery. The nurse has completed the client's physical preparation for the surgery. The client is now being transported to the preanesthesia care unit with her records and the completed preoperative checklist.

1. What are the nurse's responsibilities in regard to obtaining the client's informed consent for the surgery?

> Although it is the surgeon's responsibility to explain the procedure and obtain the informed consent from the client, the nurse needs to (a) ensure that the client has not received a sedative before signing; (b) the client understands the surgeon's explanation of the procedure; and (c) document the signing of the informed consent. Minors, some elderly clients, confused clients, and unconscious clients will require the signature of a legal guardian.

2. What measures can the nurse take to reduce the client's anxiety concerning the surgery?

> Measures the nurse can take to help allay a client's anxiety prior to surgery are: (a) observe and document the client's anxiety level; (b) answer any last-minute questions; (c) address any last-minute concerns; (d) arrange for comforting spiritual or transcultural rituals; and (e) arrange for the family and significant others to accompany the client to the preanesthesia care unit if possible. If the client is still very anxious in spite of these measures, the nurse should notify the surgeon.

3. What important transcultural considerations should the nurse recognize when preparing clients for surgery?

> The nurse needs to recognize that in some cultures (a) the decision to have surgery may be decided by a group of elders rather than the client; (b) shaving body hair violates some cultural beliefs and taboos; and (c) a stoic attitude is maintained toward pain control, and thus clients may refuse adequate postoperative pain medication.

4. What are the major items on the preoperative checklist the nurse must ensure have been carried out?

> Major items on the postoperative checklist include (a) the client identification number; (b) vital signs; (c) blood type; (d) ECG (Electrocardiogram) and chest radiograph records; (e) note that the consent form was signed; (f) note that the history and physical examination were competed; (g) note that consultations were done and laboratory results charted; (h) note that client voided and at what time; (i) note that makeup, dentures, jewelry, hairpins, nail polish, glasses, and prostheses were removed; (j) note whether valuables were given to family; (k) last time client ate or drank; and (l) when preoperative medications were administered.

Nursing Management of the Client Requiring Postanesthesia Care
Answer Key

Situation: A 55-year-old-female was admitted two hours ago to the PACU following an exploratory laparotomy. The nurse has been continually assessing the client for airway patency and adequate ventilation. The nurse has also been monitoring the client's vital signs and dressing every 15 minutes. The client is receiving an intravenous infusion of normal saline, and a PCA pump is set to administer 1 mg of morphine every 6 minutes. The client is now responding to the nurse's voice and moving her extremities. Her Aldrete Score is satisfactory.

1. Prioritize the client's nursing diagnoses while in the PACU, with "1" representing the most important diagnosis.

   3   Risk for fluid volume imbalance

   1   Ineffective breathing pattern

   6   Risk for infection

   2   Pain

   5   Risk for impaired skin integrity

   4   Risk for altered oral mucous membranes

2. What should the nurse do if the client's oxygen saturation levels start to drop?

   If the client's oxygen saturation levels begin to drop, the client needs to be awakened and requested to take several deep breaths.

3. List at least three advantages of PCA (patient-controlled analgesia).

   • **Improved pain relief**

   • **Reduced anxiety**

   • **Increased willingness to turn, cough, and deep breathe**

   • **Reduced sedation**

   • **Reduced narcotic usage**

- Greater sense of control over pain
- Enhanced sense of well-being
- Increased client satisfaction

4. The client is awake, but having difficulty voiding. What measures can the nurse take to help her void?

- Run tap water so client can hear
- pour water over the female client's perineum
- Help the male client to sit or stand if permitted
- Increase amount of pain medication
- Place the client's hand in warn water

5. What is the Aldrete Scoring System, and what is its purpose?

A scale PACUs (postanesthesia care units) are used to determine if a client is ready to be transferred to the surgical unit. The Aldrete system provides criteria that is used to apply numerical score for each of the following: the client's activity, reparation, circulation, consciousness, and skin color. Each of the five items is assessed by a numerical score of 0, 1, or 2. The five scores are then summed together. A total score of 9-10 indicates the client is ready to be discharged from the PACU.

Nursing Management of the Client Requiring Intermediate and Extended Postoperative Care Answer Key

Situation: A 55-year-old-female who has undergone an exploratory laparotomy has been discharged from the PACU and admitted to the surgical unit. The nurse reviewed the client's condition with the PACU staff, performed a baseline assessment and set-up a plan of care for the intermediate and extended postoperative period. The plan of care included preventative measures for complications that may arise during these periods.

1. During the intermediate postoperative period, what signs should alert the nurse to immediately call the surgeon?

   Notify the surgeon at once if client develops (a) changes in vital signs; (b) increased bleeding; (c) fever; (d) dyspnea; (e) tachycardia; (f) decreased or absent bowel sounds; (g) restlessness; (h) reduced urine output; (i) swelling in incisional area; and (j) severe pain unrelieved by analgesia.

2. What is the purpose of incentive spirometry, and what instructions should the nurse provide the client?

   Incentive spirometry is a deep-breathing exercise that encourages the client to take deep breaths by using equipment that provides a visual cue indicating the depth of each breath. The client should (a) assume a comfortable position; (b) put mouth over the mouthpiece of the spirometer and seal lips around it; (c) inhale deeply; and (d) hold breath to let lungs expand. The client needs to perform this procedure 10-15 times, 5-6 times a day, for the first 2 days postoperative.

3. What are the manifestations of pneumonia (a complication of the intermediate period), and how can pneumonia be prevented?

   Pneumonia, which is an inflammatory process in the lungs, may develop within the first 36 hours following surgery. Elderly clients are particularly at risk. Manifestations include increased fever, dyspnea, thick sputum, and altered breath sounds. To prevent pneumonia, the client needs to cough, deep breath, turn, ambulate, and receive sufficient fluids. The client will also benefit from using incentive spirometry.

Bibliography

Ahmad, M., Longworth, D., & Stoller, J. (2002). *Cleaveland clinic intensive review of internal medicine* (3rd ed.). Philadelphia: Lippincott, Williams, & WIlkins.

Al-Ataie, M.B. & Shenoy, V.N. (2005, January). *Ulcerative colitis*. Retrieved May 10, 2005, from http://www.emedicine.com.

American Cancer Society. (2004, August). *Cervical cancer: Treatment options by stage*. Retrieved May 14, 2005, from http://www.cancer.org.

American Cancer Society. (2004, August). *Cervical cancer: How is cervical cancer staged?* Retrieved May 14, 2005, from http://www.cancer.org.

American Medical Directors Association (AMSA). (2002). *Heart failure*. Retrieved April 9, 2005 from http://www.guideline.gov.

Bennett, J.C., Cecil, R., & Goldman, L. (Eds). (2000). *Cecil textbook of medicine* (21st ed.). Philadelphia: W.B. Saunders.

Bickley, L.S. & Szilagyi, P.G. (2002). *Bate's guide to phyisical examination and history taking* (8th ed.). Philadelphia: Lippincott, Williams, & Wilkins.

Bosker, G. (Ed). (2002). *Adult and pediatric emergency medicine: principles, protocols, pathways* (2nd ed.). Portland, OR: American Health Consultants.

Bousquet, J. (chair). (2001). *Management of allergic rhinitis and its impact on asthma: Pocket guide*. World Health Organization.

Bryan, C. (2002). *Infectious diseases in primary care*. Philadelphia: W. B. Saunders.

Bruce, M. & Peck, B. (2005). New rheumatoid arthritis treatments. *The Nurse Practitioner, 30(4)*, 28-39.

Carlton, B.G. (2003). Case in review: Asthma management in the elderly. *CE-Today for Nurse Practitioners, 2(7)*, 23-28.

Celli, B. (2003). Justified optimism for COPD: Progress in disease management. *The Journal of COPD Management, 4(2)*, 10-14.

Centers for Disease Control (CDC). (2005, January). *TB elimination. Document #250010*. Retrieved May 8, 2005, from http://www.cdc.gov.

Centers for Disease Control: Advisory Committee on Immunization Practices. (2004-2005). *Recommended adult immunization schedule, United States, October 2004-September 2005*. Retrieved April 29, 2005 from http://www.cdc.gov.

Chernecky, C., Alichnie, M., Garrett, K., George-Gary, B., Hodges, R., & Terr, C. (2002). *Real-world nursing survival guide: ECGs and the heart*. Philadelphia: W.B. Saunders.

Chutka, D., Edson, R., Habermann, T., Litin, S., McCallum, K., & Rajkumar, S.V. (2002). *Mayo clinic internal medcine board review 2002-2003*. Philadelphia: Lippincott, Williams, & Wilkins.

Dambro, M.R. (2005). *2005 Griffith's 5 minute clinical consult*. (PDA software). Available from http://www.skyscape.com: LWWmobile.

Elliott, N. (2000). *Chest tubes*. Retrieved May 9, 2005, from http;//www.nursewise.com.

European Society of Cardiology. (2001, September). *Guidelines on diagnosis and management of acute pulomary embolism.* Retrieved May 8, 2005, from http://www.guidelines.gov.

Fang, E. (ed.). (199-2003). *Epocrates rx pro* (ver. 6.13). (PDA software). Available from http://www.epocrates.com: epocrates.

Feld, S. (Chair). (2002). The American Association of Clinical Endocrinologists medical guidelines for the management of diabetes mellitus: the AACE system of intensive diabetes self-management - 2002 update. *Endocrine Practice, 8*(Suppl.1), 41-82.

Galvao, M. & Paul, S. (2004). A rational approach to improve clinical outcomes in cardiac failure. *CE-Today for Nurse Practitioners, 3(8),* 17-26.

Gilchrist, K. (2004). Benign prostatic hyperplasia. *The Nurse Practitioner, 29(6),* 30-37.

Holcomb, S.S. (in press). Addison's disease. *Nursing2005.*

Holcomb, S.S. (in press) Cushing's syndrome. *Nursing2005.*

Holcomb, S.S. (2005). Diabetes update: 2005 ACE guidelines. *The Nurse Practitioner, 30(5),* 12-14.

Holcomb, S.S. (2005). Evaluating chronic kidney disease risk. *The Nurse Practitioner, 30(4),* 12-14, 17-18, 23-27.

Holcomb, S.S. (2005). Boning up on osteoporosis. *Nursing Made Incredibly Easy, 3(2),* 6-17.

Holcomb, S.S. (2004, April). *Menopause: What's in, what's out, when hot flashes abound!* (Available from Kansas City Kansas Community College, Continuing Nursing Education, 7250 State Ave., Kansas City, KS 66112)

Holcomb, S.S. (2002). Thyroid diseases: a primer for the critical care nurse. *Dimensions in Critical Care Nursing, 21(4),* 127-133.

Holcomb, S.S. (2002). An update on hepatitis. *Dimensions in Critical Care Nursing, 21(5),* 170-179.

Immunization Action Coalition. (2002). *Guide to contraindications and precautions to commonly used vaccines in adults.* Retrieved April 29, 2005, from http://www.immunize.org.

Immunization Action Coalition (2002). *Medical management of vaccine reactions in adult patients.* Retrieved April 29, 2005, from http://www.immunize.org.

Institute for Clinical Systems Improvement (ICSI). (2004, February). *Hypertension diagnosis and treatment.* Retrieved April 9, 2005, from http://www.guideline.gov.

ICSI. (2004, July). *Management of initial abnormal pap smear.* Retrieved May 14, 2005, from http://www.guideline.gov.

ICSI. (2004, November). *Management of type 2 diabetes mellitus.* Retrieved February 23, 3005, from http://www.guideline.gov.

Jones, C. ((2004). Improving long-term care for patients living with COPD. *CE-Today for Nurse Practitioners, 3(1),* 7-17.

Kazzi, A.A., & Tehranzadeh, E.A. (2004, August). *Glomerulonephritis, acute.* Retrieved May 13, 2005, from http://www.emedicine.com.

Kozier, B., Erb, G., Berman, A., & Burke, K. (2000). *Fundamentals of nursing concepts, process, and practice* (6th ed.). Upper Saddle River, NJ: Prentice Hall Health.

Locke, D. (2005). Establishing a GOLD standard for managing COPD in your practice. *CE-Today for Nurse Practitioners, 4(1),* 17-27.

Lombard, L. (2003, August). *Laryngectomy rehabilitation.* Retrieved May 8, 2005, from http://www.emedicine.com.

Lung, M.C.L. (2003). Asthma management update: Support for early recognition, effective monitoring, and optimal treatment. *CE-Today for Nurse Practitioners, 2(7)*, 15-20.

Moses, S. (2005, March). *Nosocomial pneumonia: Hospital acquired pneumonia*. Retrieved May 7, 2005, from http://www.fpnotebook.com.

National Comprehensive Cancer Network and American Cancer Society. (2004). *Breast cancer treatment*. Retrieved May 14, 2005, from http://www.ncc.org.

National Heart, Lung, and Blood Institute/National Institutes of Health. (2000). *Guidelines for the diagnosis and manaement of asthma, publication no. 98-4051, and the practical guide for the diagnosis and management of asthma, publication no. 97-4053*. PDA version of guidelines available from http://www.NHLBI.NIH.GOV.

National Kidney Foundation. (2000). *NKF K/DOQI clinical practice guidelines for chronic kidney disease: Evaluation, classification, and stratification*. Retrieved February 11, 2004, from http://www.kidney.org.

Neff, M. (2003). ATS, CDC, and IDSA update recommendations on the treatment of tuberculosis. *American Family Physician, 68(9)*, 1854, 1857-8, 1861-2.

Onusko, E. (2003). Diagnosing secondary hypertension. *American Family Physician, 67(1)*, 67-74.

Padda, S. & Ramirez, F. (2002, September). *Dumping syndrome*. Retrieved May 9, 2005, from http://www.emedicine.com.

Rosdahl, C. B., & Kowalski, M.T. (2003). *Textbook of basic nursing* (4th ed.). Philadelphia: Lippincott, Williams, & WIlkins.

Sabatine, M. (2002). *Pocket medicine*. Philadelphia: Lippincott, Williams, & Wilkins.

Salifu, M.O. & Delano, B.G. (2004, December). *Glomerulonephritis, chronic*. Retrieved May 13, 2005, from http://www.emedicine.com.

Saslow, D., Runowics, CD., Solomon, D., Moscicki, AB., Smith, RA., Eyre, HJ., & Cohen, C. (2003, August). *American Cancer Society guideline for the early detection of cervical neoplasia and cancer*. Retrieved May 14, 2005, from http://www.guidelines.gov.

Sinert, R. & Erogul, M. (2004, September). *Transplants, renal*. Retrieved May 14, 2005, from http://www.emedicine.com.

Stoner, G.D. (2005). Hyperosmolar hyperglycemic state. *American Family Physician, 71(9)*, 1723-1730.

Thelan, L., Urden, L., Stacy, K., & Lough. M. (2001). *Critical care nursing: diagnosis and management* (4th ed.). Philadelphia: Elsevier Science Health.

Trachtenbarg, D. (2005). Diabetic ketoacidosis. *American Family Physician, 71(9)*, 1705-1714.

Uphold, C. & Graham, M.V. (2003). *Clinical guidelines in family practice*. Gainesville, FL: Barmarrae Books, Inc.

Wollner, T. (2004). Eradicate *H. pylori* with effective treatment regimens. *The Nurse Practitioner, 29(6)*, 40-44.